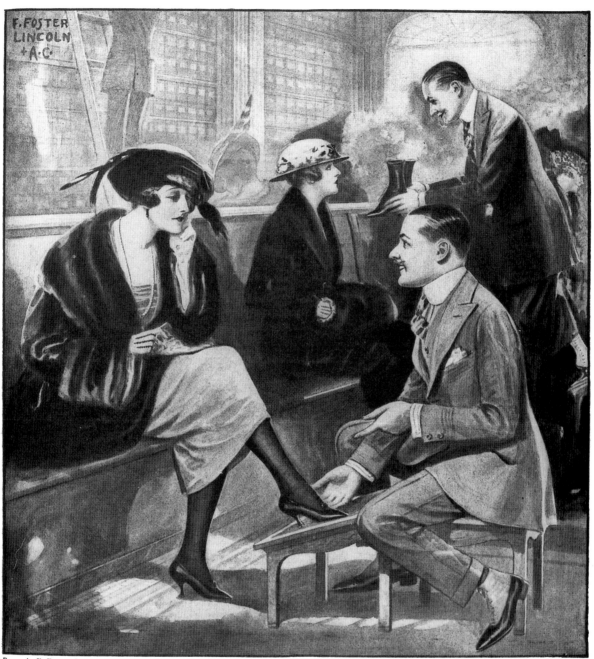

Drawn by F. Foster Lincoln

Shoe Salesman—How does that feel?
Lady Customer—Try a size smaller.   I can bear a lot more pain than that.

From the magazine *Judge*, January 10, 1920, drawn by F. Foster Lincoln.
Smithsonian Institution Photo No. 83-890.

women's shoes

in america, 1795–1930

written and illustrated by **nancy e. rexford**

the kent state university press
kent, ohio, and london

© 2000 by The Kent State University Press, Kent, Ohio 44242
All rights reserved
Library of Congress Catalog Card Number 99-055197
ISBN 0-87338-656-6
Manufactured in China

08 07 06 05 04 03 02 01 00   5 4 3 2 1

Library of Congress Cataloging-in-Publication Data
Rexford, Nancy E., 1947–
    Women's shoes in America, 1795–1930 / written and illustrated by Nancy E. Rexford.
        p.   cm.
    Includes bibliographical references and index.
    ISBN 0-87338-656-6 (cloth: alk. paper) ∞
        1. Shoes—United States—History. 2. Shoes—Collectors and collecting—United States. I. Title.

GT2130.R48 2000
391.4'13'0820973—dc21   99-055197

British Library Cataloging-in-Publication data are available.

For all those who care for the material culture of the past and labor with little recompense to preserve the body of surviving American dress.

Many a man's heart has been kept from wandering
by the bow on his wife's slipper.
—*Demorest's* (1883)

Contents

Acknowledgments

My interest and expertise in costume took root in the world of small, underfunded, and understaffed historical societies that (no matter how sympathetic they were) could not possibly support scholarly work of this scope. Therefore, it is entirely due to financial support from the National Endowment for the Humanities that this volume could be written at all. The National Endowment for the Humanities (NEH) is a federal agency that supports the study of such fields as history, philosophy, literature, and languages, and through its grants it has repeatedly acknowledged costume history to be a worthwhile field of investigation in the humanities. I am grateful that the NEH recognized the validity of work that not only was done outside academia by an independent scholar but that also grew out of familiarity with the evidence of material objects rather than of written documents. It was my good fortune to have as my program officer at NEH David Wise, who for more than a decade consistently encouraged me in my work, and whose very name was a consolation in times of trouble.

I would like to acknowledge the first publisher who took an interest in this book, Holmes & Meier, especially Barbara Lyons, Miriam Holmes, Sheila Friedling, and the late Max J. Holmes. Their work enormously influenced its development, although they were unable to carry the project to completion.

Women's Shoes in America has been a particularly complex publication, and I deeply appreciate the willingness of The Kent State University Press to take it on, especially Julia Morton, the first editor who encouraged the project; Christine Brooks, the designer; and Joanna Hildebrand Craig, the editor who managed to pilot this unwieldy ship into harbor.

During the preparation of this volume, I have benefited from the advice and encouragement of many friends and colleagues, particularly Jean Druesedow, Claudia Kidwell, Edward Maeder, Joan Severa, and the late Otto Thieme. Arthur S. Tarlow of the Alden Shoe Company, Saundra Ros Altman, Jan Armstrong, Dr. Stephen Blomerth, Jeffrey Butterworth, Colleen Callahan, Louise Coffey, Paige Savery, June Swann, and Jonathan Walford have kindly shared information related to shoes. Doris May spent significant time researching the history of Viault-Esté for me in Paris. I also thank the many costume enthusiasts who allowed me to make use of material from their personal collections, including Elizabeth Brown, John Burbidge, Elizabeth Enfield, Heidi Fieldston, Mr. and Mrs. Charles Fisher, Peter Oakley, William Streeter, and Merideth Wright. David Rickman kindly shared his expertise on the art and craft of illustration and on early California costume. Barry Kaplan and the staff of The Finer Image deserve the credit for anything good about the photographs taken by the author. They were unfailingly generous with their advice even when they really didn't have the time, and when I still made mistakes, they fixed them in the lab. I am grateful to Gaza Bowen, Jean Druesedow, Claudia Kidwell, Edward Maeder, Fred Prahl, Nen Rexford, Gillian Skellinger, Charles Turner, Laurel Thatcher Ulrich, Jonathan Walford, Joan Walther, and Merideth Wright, who read and commented on part or all of the manuscript.

As researcher or consultant, I have visited a great many museums and historical societies in the course of my work on American women's dress, and to all of them I am grateful for their generosity in making their collections available. For this volume on shoes, I owe particular thanks to Ken Turino, Sophie Garrett, Laurel Nilsen, and the staff of the Lynn Museum, which opened its collections to me without reservation; to Paula Richter and many other current and past staff members at the Peabody Essex Museum (formerly the Essex Institute), and especially to Anne Farnam, curator and director, whose generous encouragement of my work on shoes extended an entire decade until her untimely death in 1991; to Sandy Rosenbaum and Edward Maeder at the Los Angeles County Museum of Art, who introduced me to the costume of early California; to Jessica Nicoll, Peter Oakley, and Sarah LeCount at Old Sturbridge Village (they suffered lengthy discussions on early nineteenth-century women's work shoes and shared both their collections and their files); to Lynne Bassett and Pamela Toma at Historic Northampton, and before them to Ruth Wilbur, without whose encouragement and guidance I would not be working in the field of costume today; to Colleen Callahan at the Valentine Museum in Richmond; to Joan Walther and the Costume Committee at the Colonial Dames in Boston, and especially to Liz Ballantine, to whose angelic interference I owe a great deal.

I am grateful as well to the following museums that allowed me to study their shoes: in Massachusetts, to the Bedford Historical Society, Danvers Historical Society, Duxbury Rural Historical Society, Haverhill Historical Society, Museum of Fine Arts–Boston, Old Sturbridge Village, the Society for the Preservation of New England Antiquities, Topsfield Historical Society, and Wellesley Historical

Society; in Vermont, to the Aldrich Public Library in Barre, the Ferrar Mansur House in Weston, the Morristown Historical Society, the Old Constitution House in Windsor, the Old Stone House Museum in Brownington, and the Vermont Historical Society in Montpelier; in Pennsylvania, to the Philadelphia Museum of Art and the Tioga County Historical Society in Wellsboro; to the Connecticut Historical Society, the Rhode Island Historical Society, the Natural History Museum of Los Angeles County, the Valentine Museum in Richmond (Virginia), the Kansas City Museum in Kansas City (Missouri), the Oakland (California) Museum, and the Costume Institute at the Metropolitan Museum of New York; and to the staff of the Division of Costume at the Smithsonian Institution, who were willing to share the rich picture files they had developed during the years of preparation for the book *Men and Women: Dressing the Part* and its attendant exhibition on gender and dress.

And finally, I am grateful to my family for doing everything in their power to make it possible for me to write this book: to my father, Don Rexford, for desks, shelves, and all the practical domestic conveniences it was in his power to provide; to my mother, Nen Rexford, for assistance with research and for discovering critical illustrations and quotations, not to speak of a lifetime of intellectual encouragement and support; to my son, Gerritt, who made sure his mother remembered that basketball was just as important as shoes; and most humbly and deeply, to my husband, Charles Turner, whose belief in the value of my work led him, day in and day out, to make the countless sacrifices of time, money, pleasure, and personal convenience that made it possible for me to continue my research and writing.

Fig. 1. Parts of the Shoe

General Areas of the Feet and Footwear:

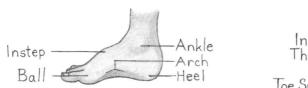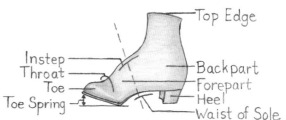

Common Parts and Pieces of Shoes:

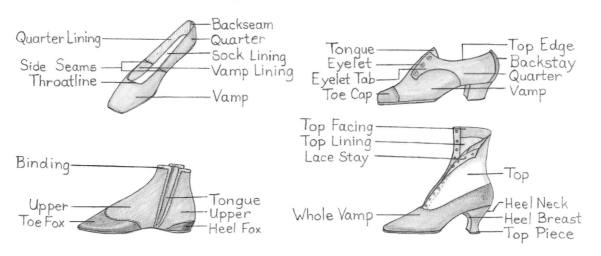

Basic Types of Front-Lacing Footwear:

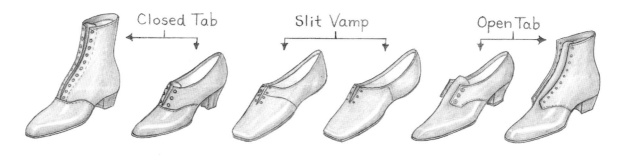

Common Heel Types:

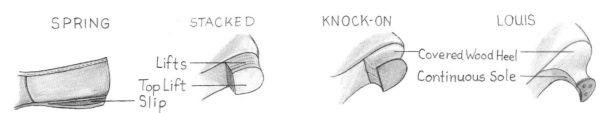

A Note on Terminology

Shoe terminology may confuse the beginner, not merely because many terms refer to variations in detail that are difficult for the novice to distinguish but also because the words have changed over time and are not consistent between Britain and United States. To simplify matters in *Women's Shoes in America*, technical vocabulary is kept to a minimum in the text, and when there is a choice, the term preferred is one that describes the characteristic to which it refers (for example, "side lacing" rather than "Adelaide"). The glossary provides extended definitions of many shoe terms and explains the distinctions between British and American usage.

For the purposes of this book, footwear is broadly divided into shoes, boots, and overshoes. Shoes are defined as encasing only the foot, while boots encase the ankle and sometimes part of the leg. Overshoes are worn over another pair of shoes or boots for warmth or protection from wet and dirt.

In order to produce a more organized discussion, shoes and boots are further divided according to the way they are kept on the foot, whether by front lacing, side lacing, buttons, straps, or elastic. Front-lacing boots and shoes are further divided into open-tab, closed-tab, and slit-vamp styles (see figure 1).

Shoes that have no fastening at all are in this book called slippers (see the glossary for the reasons behind this decision). Slippers are still called slippers even if they have ribbons stitched to the edges to help keep them on, but if the actual shoe upper is cut into straps that fasten with buttons, buckles, or ties, the term "strapped shoe" is used. Boots that have no fastening but simply pull on are called leg boots.

The word "upper" refers to all parts of the shoe above the sole. The word "bottom" includes all parts of the sole and the heel. "Forepart" refers to the front half of the shoe, from the toe to the waist, and "backpart" to the back half, from the waist to the heel.

Introduction

Women's Shoes in America, 1795–1930 is organized into two parts: a narrative history and a detailed reference for dating. "Makers and Marketers," which opens Part I, briefly outlines the development of the shoe industry from the early nineteenth century, when much of the work was done by hand in small shops, through its dramatic mechanization in the 1850s and 1860s, to the complex organization that characterized it in the early twentieth century, before labor unrest, internal competition, and other pressures caused the beginning of its long decline. This chapter also explains how shoes were distributed, how new styles were developed, and why the rapid growth of the shoe industry discouraged regional style variations within the United States. Not until the explosion of novelty shoes in the 1910s and 1920s were Americans able to express subtle local differences in taste through their choice in footwear.

Chapter 2, "Stepping Out or Staying In? Women's Shoes and Female Stereotypes," discusses the relationship between women's footwear and women's roles as reflected in popular periodicals, and explores the nineteenth-century view that gave to men the public world of business, politics, and the mind while giving to women the private world of home, family, and the spirit. This chapter broadens the discussion beyond footwear in order to clarify the social context in which shoes acquired their particular significance. It concentrates chiefly on the middle and upper-middle classes, for whom gender stereotyping was most relevant, and suggests that the strength of such stereotyping, coupled with the fluidity of class structure in the United States, may have encouraged middle-class American women to wear thin and impractical shoes for a wider range of occasions than was common practice among their English cousins.

The last four chapters in Part I describe the variety of shoes available through the period 1795 to 1930, beginning with "A Chronological Overview of Shoe Fashions." The rules of etiquette that applied to footwear are the subject of "The Correct Dress of the Foot," including such troublesome matters as whether one should wear a black slipper or a white satin boot to a ball in the 1860s and what exactly was the proper sphere of tan leather in the 1890s. Chapter 4 also addresses the problematic question of what shoes were worn by rural women and working women who were not attempting to dress at the height of fashion. The last two chapters in Part I, "Shoes Adapted for Sports" and "Shoes Adapted for Protection" deal with the specialized shoes that developed as women's lives broadened to include a greater range of activity.

Precise information about dating shoes is reserved for Part II, chapters 7 through 11. This part is intended as a reference guide for dating shoes and is organized so as to be most functional "in the field." Like a naturalist's field guide, it is arranged according to salient visible characteristics. This arrangement allows the reader to see, for example, all the variations in sole shapes laid out chronologically in columns, so that distinctions can be more easily made between similar styles. The discussion of upper patterns is divided first by whether they are shoes or boots and then by their means of fastening. Thus, if the reader is trying to date a front-lacing boot, it becomes simple to compare all styles of front-lacing boots together because they are all illustrated on adjacent pages. Then the reader can turn to the pages on soles, heels, and materials and decoration for confirmation of the initial identification. The Guide to Part II explains how to use this reference section efficiently.

Readers using this volume as a reference for cataloging surviving footwear may wish to know to what extent it is reliable for Canadian or European footwear. In most cases, the information ought to prove trustworthy in a general way, especially for Canadian shoes, which seem to have shared stylistic characteristics with those from the United States. European footwear, however, is likely to prove more problematic. While French, British, and American shoes do have much in common, style changes are not always synchronized and therefore they cannot all be dated according to precisely the same rules. It is not a simple matter of saying that one country is a year or two behind another, because the features current in one country do not all appear in the same combination in another. Such differences became especially noticeable in the later nineteenth century when the American shoe industry became strong enough to develop styles here at home rather than slavishly copying what was being made in France.

A brief look at figure 2, a photograph of four boots that was included in June Swann's book *Shoes* (a work to which this author and every scholar on the subject must acknowledge a debt), will suggest the kinds of dating problems that are likely to crop up when attempting to use American information to date British or French shoes, or vice versa. The lace-covered satin front-lacing boot with a rather short vamp and very pointed toe that is shown at center left was made and exhibited in Paris in 1889. This French boot looks nothing like the 1888 English

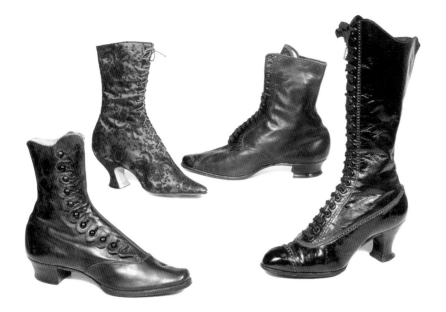

Fig. 2. French, British, and American footwear were not necessarily similar at any one period. *Far left:* Black glacé buttoned boot, probably made by Bailey and Wills of Northampton, England. An arbitration sample, 1888. *Center left:* Front-lacing boot of rust satin covered in black Chantilly lace, made by M. E. Sablonnière, Paris, and shown in the Paris Exposition in 1889. *Center right:* Dark-brown, front-lacing boot with black patent diamond tip made by Cammeyer, New York, June 28, 1893. *Far right:* Black glacé front-lacing boot with patent golosh, National Shoe Stores, London. Christmas, 1917. For the American version of boots in the late 1910s, see plate 10. *Courtesy Northampton Museums and Art Gallery, Northampton, England.*

arbitration example at the far left, even allowing for the great difference in materials, because it was made over a differently shaped last. Nor does the French style have any exact parallel in the United States. The pointed toe was not adopted here until the mid-1890s, and when it was, the vamp was more elongated than this French example. The American boot of 1893 at center right shows what the pointed toe looked like when it did appear in American fashion (the *Shoe Retailer* noted, incidentally, that Americans generally preferred longer vamps than the French, and also pointed out that French lasts did not fit American women's feet[1]). The idea of making a boot in evening materials also ran counter to recent American practice, where boots had not been fashionable for evening wear since the 1870s. Even if Americans did accept a revival of boots for evening, the ostentatiously impractical upper of this French example would have looked particularly odd because it was used on a boot with front lacing. In America in 1889, front lacing was still far less common than button fastening, and when it did appear it was almost exclusively on utilitarian boots.

The tall boot at the far right of figure 2 is an English example dated 1917. Its height and front lacing have contemporary equivalents in American boots, but the English version is made with the short, deep, rounded vamp that had gone out of fashion by 1914 in the United States. Swann reports that this toe style continued in use in England into the early 1920s,[2] but in America the vamp was increasingly long and pointed in the later 1910s. In 1919, the *Shoe Retailer* noted that "there has been much talk of the short vamp shoe, which had its run in this country only a few years ago and which is now so popular in France. To introduce the short vamp, or stage, last would, however, disrupt the whole shoe business as it would minimize the value of present stocks if it should become popular next season."[3] While toe styles were clearly not synchronized in Europe and America, Swann notes that boots went out of use in England in 1922,[4] and they are not commonly advertised in the United States after 1923, so in this respect the two countries are similar. It seems likely that future comparative studies of both shoes and other garments will reveal a similar disalignment of detail that, once charted, may allow us to determine the country of origin for many undocumented garments.

Another area in which English and American practice varies is in terminology. American manufacturers used terms like "foxing" that were not standard in either Britain or Canada. In order to help readers who may be consulting both British and American sources, the lengthy glossary at the end of this volume describes the differences in usage between the two countries. What terminology is necessary for understanding the text is explained through the diagrams included in figure 1, "Parts of the Shoe." Readers interested in the preparation of leather and the technicalities of shoemaking will find basic information about these topics in the appendixes. The appendixes also include a brief history of the role of rubber in the shoe industry and a partial listing of shoe manufacturers drawn from advertisements and shoe labels.

The Evidence

In the study of shoe fashions, the chief primary sources are the surviving shoes themselves and the illustrations and commentaries in fashion magazines, mail-order catalogs, and trade journals. Collections of surviving shoes tend to include large numbers of wedding shoes and other dressy shoes saved in order to remember a special occasion. They also include shoes that were never much worn, perhaps because they did not fit, or because the owner found she had no use for them, or because they went out of style soon after they were bought. None of these is likely to represent the styles commonly worn for ordinary occasions. Most everyday and work shoes were worn out and then discarded, and they are therefore among the rarest of survivals (except at archaeological sites where they have been retrieved from the garbage heaps, usually in poor condition). The usefulness of historical society collections is limited by the prevalence of "wedding whites," although such wedding shoes do provide important documentation within their limited sphere. Art museum collections, on the other hand, lean far too heavily on imported garments and on the dressiest clothing of the wealthiest urban Americans to give anything like a realistic picture of American women's footwear as a whole.

Within the United States, the most important collections to transcend these limitations are in Massachusetts, at the Lynn Museum in Lynn and the Peabody Essex Museum in Salem. While men's shoes tended to be made in the towns south of Boston, such as Brockton (where examples are preserved in the local historical society), the center of the women's shoe industry was north of Boston in Essex County, especially the city of Lynn. The Lynn Museum has an important collection of shoemaking machines and a good library of shoe-related materials as well as a small but interesting collection of shoes. The Peabody Essex

Museum has shoe documents pertaining to Essex County in its research library, and its own large and interesting shoe collection was augmented in 1973 by the gift of the collection formed in the early twentieth century by the United Shoe Machinery Corporation (USMC). The USMC collection includes footwear from around the world, but about half of it (nearly two thousand pairs) consists of American and European footwear, most ranging from the eighteenth century to the 1930s.[5] Particularly important is the large quantity of footwear produced by the American shoe industry from the 1860s through the 1920s. Shoes that are rare elsewhere, such as everyday black serge boots of the 1860s, are here by the dozen. Many of the USMC shoes were never worn, but were preserved by the manufacturers as samples or because they were displayed in the 1876 Centennial Exhibition in Philadelphia, the 1893 World's Columbian Exposition in Chicago, or other international exhibitions. The Bata Shoe Museum in Toronto has a research library, photographic archive, and shoemaking-tool collection in addition to more than seven thousand shoes. Cultures from around the world are represented in the Bata shoe collection, but it is particularly noted for the footwear made by Native Americans and the peoples of the circumpolar region.

Fashion plates can be helpful sources of information only when skirts are short enough to show the shoes, as they often are from 1797 until about 1833, and from 1915 on. Because American magazines were not publishing fashion plates until 1830, we must rely on French and English plates for the first part of the century. "Costume Parisien," the series of costume plates first published in *Le Journal des Dames*, 1797–1839, is a particularly delightful resource because the illustrations are so beautifully drawn.[6]

American women's magazines like *Godey's Lady's Book* began to include separate pictures of shoes from about 1850. At about that same time, American women's magazines also began to feature regular articles on current fashion that included advice about what clothing was appropriate for what occasions. This is particularly helpful in understanding the etiquette governing women's choices in shoes in the latter half of the century. However, it is important to remember that prescriptive writing such as is found in magazines and etiquette books was not a description of what all women actually wore any more than it is today. Most American women did not have the money to buy the variety of clothing needed to follow such advice to the letter. Upper-middle-class women might very well regulate their lives according to the rules of etiquette, but less affluent women could follow them only in a more general way—for example, by dividing their wardrobe into everyday and best dress.

Advertisements become a major element in the documentation of shoe history from the 1890s on, at which time magazines no longer attempted to support themselves by subscription alone. It is important to keep in mind the audience toward which the magazines and the advertisements in them were directed. For example, the figures illustrating new Paris fashions in the *Ladies' Home Journal* in the 1910s and 1920s wear shoes a year or two in advance of the styles the *Journal*'s advertisers were illustrating and (presumably) their middle-class readers were buying. That the more advanced styles were available in America is proven by contemporary advertisements in the *Shoe Retailer.*

Another important resource for the late nineteenth and the twentieth centuries is mail-order catalogs, including not only those from specialized mail-order houses like Sears, Montgomery Ward, and Bellas Hess but also those produced by the larger department stores such as Jordan Marsh, Wanamaker's, and Franklin Simon. Department-store catalogs reflect the tastes of the city clientele they served, while Sears and Montgomery Ward were directed toward middle-class and rural readers and give a better idea of the range of working and practical footwear available in America. With the increase of advertisements in magazines and the development of illustrated mail-order catalogs, our view of everyday footwear becomes a good deal clearer than it is for the earlier nineteenth century.

Because the shoe industry was so important in the United States, it produced a number of specialized publications related to the trade (several of which are available in Boston area libraries). The one consulted for this volume was the *Shoe Retailer,* which was published monthly by the *Shoe and Leather Reporter* beginning in March 1898. In 1901 it combined with *Boots and Shoes Weekly,* an older periodical, taking on the latter's numbering and being published weekly. The set used by the author at the Lynn Museum begins in 1900 and runs through 1928. A description of the *Shoe Retailer* is included in chapter 1. Other industry publications included *Hide and Leather and Shoes* and the *Boot and Shoe Recorder,* whose publishing company produced the *Shoe and Leather Lexicon.* The *Lexicon,* an important glossary of shoe and leather trade terms as used in America, was first published in 1912 and continued to be revised and issued at least into the 1950s.

Among secondary sources, the most important for understanding the chronology of shoe styles is June Swann's *Shoes,* which was published in 1982 as part of Batsford's Costume Accessories Series. Swann was for many years keeper of the enormous shoe collection at Northampton Museum (Northampton was the center of the British shoe industry) and has an unequaled understanding of the history and manufacture of shoes. Other works by Swann and by her predecessor at Northampton, J. H. Thornton, appear in the bibliography. Glimpses of the growing American shoe industry as perceived by men directly involved in it are provided by Richardson (1858), Leno (1885), and Allen (1916). Blanche Hazard's early twentieth-century work on the organization of the industry before 1875 is still required reading today, and more recent American historians have built on her work (see Dawley, Faler, and Melder). For a detailed listing, consult Colazzo's extensive bibliography of materials relating to the foot and shoe.

PART ONE

A History of Women's Footwear in America

CHAPTER ONE

Makers and Marketers

A Brief Look at the
American Shoe Industry

Shoemaking was one of the first great American industries. Even as early as 1768, Lynn, Massachusetts, produced eighty thousand pairs of shoes.[1] By 1795 the city had two hundred master workmen and six hundred journeymen and produced three hundred thousand pairs of women's shoes. While Lynn grew to become for a time the largest shoemaking city not only in the United States but in the world, the industry was also carried on in many other towns in the Boston area. In general, Lynn, Haverhill, and towns to the north of Boston specialized in women's shoes, while the towns to the south such as Brockton, Randolph, and Abington specialized in men's shoes. Towns such as Milford, some miles westward in Worcester County, specialized in brogans.[2]

Marketing Shoes in the Early Nineteenth Century

An important part of the early New England shoe industry was the production of heavy, coarse brogans intended for wear by slaves on the plantations of the West Indies. As early as the year 1771, nearly six thousand pairs of shoes were exported from the American colonies to the West Indies.[3] Casks of American shoes were exchanged for sugar, molasses, coffee, and hides. The sugar was then traded elsewhere, perhaps in Russia for untanned calfskin or in Trieste for opium.[4] The West Indian trade continued into the nineteenth century, but after the invention of the cotton gin in 1791 and the resulting increase in the profitability of both cotton and slavery in the southern United States, southern plantations composed a large and growing market for the products of New England industry. Of course, not all southern slave shoes were made in the North. Some plantation owners kept one slave trained as a shoemaker who was responsible for tanning hides and making shoes for all the hands. An advertisement in the 1845–46 Richmond directory for Hubbard, Gardner and Carlton lists "a very superior article of BROGUES, of their own manufacture, suitable for Plantation and Factory hands," suggesting that at least some of these coarse shoes were made locally. Nevertheless, "Negro shoes," like "Negro cloth," constituted an important part of New England's trade.

Beginning in the late 1790s, wholesale shoe stores in Boston either established branch stores in the South or developed close connections with southern factors in cities such as Richmond, Charleston, Savannah, and New Orleans, and with the keepers of grocery, dry-goods, and hardware stores throughout the South and the expanding West. Blanche Hazard, in her history *The Organization of the Boot and Shoe Industry in Massachusetts before 1875,* mentions one John Houghton who opened a store in Augusta with six hundred dollars worth of goods and who was eventually able to buy russets and brogans for the plantations in lots worth twenty to thirty thousand dollars at a time.[5] Shoes were shipped southward in small trunks covered with leather with the hair on, about the size of latter-day shoe cases (see fig. 16).[6]

At the beginning of the century, these shipments were made through jobbing firms in New York. W. H. Richardson notes that the first ship whose cargo was entirely made up of shoes and boots, the sloop *Delight,* sailed from Boston to New York in 1818, the shoes consigned to the firm of Spofford and Tileston for export. By 1830 this arrangement was no longer found to be profitable, and Boston firms began handling the exports directly, with the result that by 1858, when W. H. Richardson reported these figures, Boston had 218 wholesale and jobbing boot and shoe houses and did $52 million in business a year, while New York had about fifty-five jobbing houses and had sales of $15 million to $16 million a year.[7]

In the earlier nineteenth century, the roles of shoe manufacturer and shoe retailer were not as rigidly specialized as they came to be later on. Hazard offers the example of Quincy Reed of Weymouth, whose father made shoes to order for local consumption and also did some "sale work" on the side; that is, shoes not made for any particular customer. Quincy Reed and his brother sold these extra shoes in Boston, taking the first batches to market in 1809 to sell alongside the chickens on a wheeled cart. Other shoemakers in these early days sent small lots of sale shoes to Boston in saddlebags. Eventually the Reed brothers kept a trunk stored in Boston and sold shoes out of it on market days, $2.00 for the best shoes, $1.25 to $1.50 for those intended for the West India trade.[8] Sometimes a shoemaker, perhaps one with a flair for the marketing side of the business, also bought shoes from other makers to supplement the stock he could produce himself. A small newspaper advertisement of 1812, for example, announced that Benjamin Lovering of Exeter had received a shipment of shoes from a Lynn manufacturer, but also that Lovering himself made boots and shoes in Exeter.[9]

From the very beginning of the nineteenth century, American-made shoes were widely available ready-made, and many women bought even their best shoes off the shelf much as we do today. Tabitha Dana Leach's white kid wedding shoes of 1812[10] have two labels that suggest the degree to which the business was already organized (see fig. 3). The maker's label reads "Shoes, Particularly made for retailing, By Warren Perkins, Reading." In the other shoe, a retailer's label reads: "Warranted Shoes, Made in particular for Josiah Vose's Shoe Store, No. 32, Newbury Street, corner of West Street—Boston." An 1815 wedding shoe worn by a Mrs. Thomas Newcomb is labeled "Chase & Cogswell, Variety Shoe Store, Main Street, Haverhill, Mass."[11]

Alongside these early nineteenth-century American ready-made products, shoes were still being imported from England. Among the English labels found at the turn of the century is that of Jackson, a "Ladies' Shoe Manufacturer" who worked at No. 54 Rathbone Place, Oxford Street, London (see fig. 4).[12] A shoe from the 1790s at the Colonial Dames in Boston is apparently a product of the China trade, since it is stamped in red on the quarter lining "Hon Sing Shoes."[13] Protective tariffs passed in 1816, 1824, and 1842, however, served to discourage foreign imports and encourage the American industry. In 1816 the duty on imported men's boots was set at $1.50 a pair. In 1824 this was extended to men's laced boots and half-boots, and a twenty-five-cent duty was put on leather and prunella shoes and slippers. The tariff on men's footwear was reduced somewhat in 1842, but the duty on women's shoes remained the same.[14]

The duty did not, however, extend to silk slippers, and this perhaps accounts for the fact that it is in silk slippers almost without exception that we find foreign labels in the mid–nineteenth century. By the 1840s the single most common group of labels is from the French exporter Esté, with its later incarnation, Viault-Esté, and its London branch, Thierry and Sons, who, judging from the hundreds of surviving examples, seem to have flooded the American market from about the 1830s through the 1850s with black

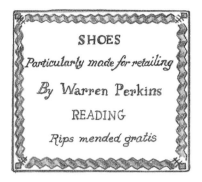

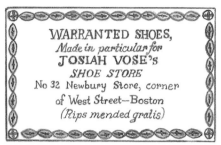

Fig. 3. Both of these labels are found in the 1812 white kid wedding slippers of Tabitha Dana Leach, showing them to be ready-made shoes. Danvers Historical Society catalog #60.7.1.

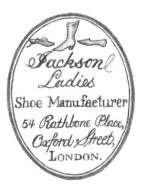

Fig. 4. This label from the English shoemaker Jackson is found in a pair of 1805–15 yellow kid shoes at the Colonial Dames in Boston, #1952.532. See plate 2. Historic Northampton has another pair, dated 1810, with a slightly different label.

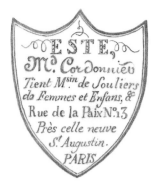
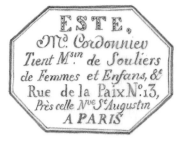
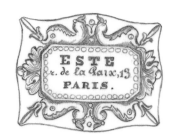

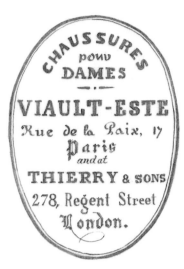
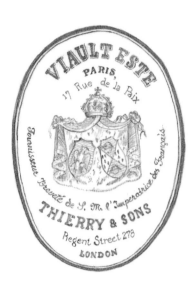
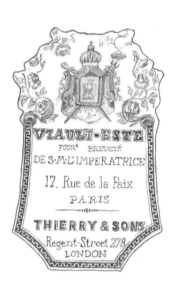

Fig. 5. The labels of the Paris firm Esté (later Viault-Esté) are the most common type surviving in nineteenth-century women's shoes in U.S. collections. The firm was in existence from about 1820 into the 1890s and employed several different labels with variant wordings over the decades. See appendix D for more information about this firm.

Upper left: Shield-shaped Esté label with long address at No. 13, probably the first label in use, ca. 1821–40.

Upper center: Plain octagonal Esté label with long address at No. 13, ca. 1830–45.

Upper right: Octagonal label with scrolled border, ca. 1840–49. Those that still have the phrase "Près celle de N. St. Augustin" are probably earlier than those with merely "Esté, rue de la Paix 13."

An octagonal label may have been made with the old address at No. 13, and the new name Viault-Esté. No example has been noted, but if it exists, it was presumably in use from ca. 1839–49. An octagonal or oval label may also have been made with the new address at No. 17, the new name Viault-Esté, but without

any reference to the Empress or to Thierry. No example has been noted, but if it exists, it was presumably in use from ca. 1849–53.

Lower left: Oval label with No. 17 and reference to Thierry but not to the Empress, ca. 1852–54.

Lower center: Oval label with No. 17, references to both Thierry and the Empress, ca. 1854–60.

Lower right: Label with rosebud border, No. 17, references to Thierry and the Empress, ca. 1860–70.

Current evidence suggests that this label was being used well beyond the fall of the Second Empire in 1870.

A second label is known to have been made with a rosebud border like that at lower right, but the address is No. 20, and the description is "fournisseur de plusieurs cours étrangères." In later examples, the bottom section of the label referring to Thierry has been cut off. It was probably in use ca. 1880–89.

A new label was probably made when the firm moved to Chauveau Lagarde, 18. No such label has been noted, but if it exists, it presumably was in use from 1890 on.

and white satin dress slippers (see fig. 5). One pair made by this exporter after 1853 is also stamped "Made expressly for John D. Rogers, Boston."[15] Other French labels are less common, but there is a pair of purple moiré boots with black leather toe caps in the Natural History Museum of Los Angeles County on whose sole is stamped "Jeanneau Hervé & Cie, Paris, élevès de Renault."[16] These date from about 1850 and come from a Spanish family who lived in the Los Angeles area before the American acquisition of California.

By the mid–nineteenth century, French fashions, including shoes, acquired such authority that American retailers found it expedient to suggest a French connection in their labels. Thus we find an 1835 wedding shoe with the label "J. B. Miller & Co. Ladies' French Shoe Store, 387 Canal St., NY,"[17] and another pair, of 1868, labeled "Henry Tuttle & Co. French and American Shoe Store, 259 & 261 Washington St, Boston, Warranted"[18] (see fig. 6). W. H. Richardson allows us to glimpse the human transactions that provoked such labels in his 1858 *Boot and Shoe Manufacturer's Assistant and Guide.*

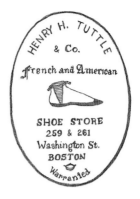

Fig. 6. This label from an 1868 wedding slipper at Historic Northampton (#66.662) reflects the interest in French shoes in the mid–nineteenth century. See fig. 39 for a view of the entire shoe.

> American skill and ingenuity has completely rivalled the most elegant specimens of Parisian handicraft, and the importation of French gaiters, which was once quite extensive, has almost or quite ceased. Most of the so-called French manufacture is the product of American artizans [*sic*]. This "amiable deception" is practiced in order to gratify the whims of those who lack confidence in the skill and taste of American manufacturers. An anecdote illustrative of this prejudice is general in its application. The incident related, occurred in a Broadway establishment, New York.
>
> A lady, after examining the slippers of the tradesman, said, "Mr.——, why do you not import your slippers from Paris?" "Madam," was the reply, "I have already sent out an order, and I expect every day the arrival of an extensive assortment; if you will call in about a week, I think I can furnish you with just the article you desire." The lady left, promising to return, and Mr.—— visited his printer and had a number of "tickets," bearing the name of an imaginary French shoemaker, struck off, and by her next visit he was prepared with a "very extensive assortment." She was fitted with a pair, and after extolling the style, elegance and comfort of her slippers, insulted the tradesman by enquiring "why *he* did not make such shoes."[19]

The same thing was apparently going on in England. Swann says that English and American shoemakers imitated the French style in omitting the back seam,[20] and quotes Henry Mayhew in *London Labour and the London Poor,* who reported that "thousands of ladies' French shoes that never saw France are made at this end of town." It is certainly true that many midcentury shoes have no back seam, and many are also marked *droit* (right) and *gauche* (left) in the sock lining. But in the absence of a French maker's label (perhaps even when it is present!), it is hardly wise to assume that these shoes are French.

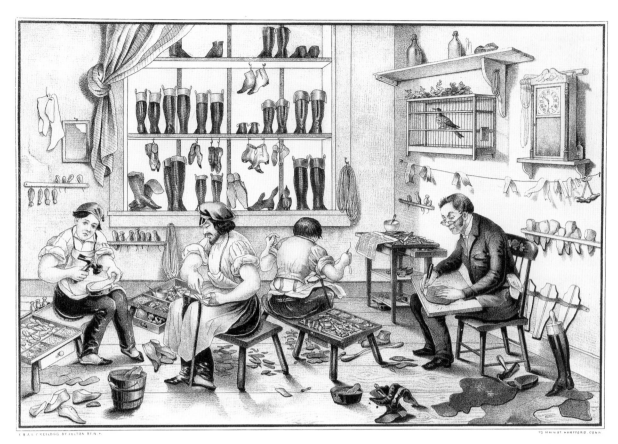

Fig. 7. *The Shoemakers,* ca. 1855 lithograph by E. B. and E. C. Kellogg of Hartford, Connecticut. Although exhibiting a certain degree of artistic license, this view of a "ten-footer" gives some idea of the division of labor that was standard in the early nineteenth century. The worker at left is hammering the sole leather on his lapstone. The soles have been prepared for this condensing process by soaking in the bucket of water near his feet. The bearded man in a visored cap holds a boot in place between his knees with the help of a leather strap called a stirrup. Exactly what he is doing is unclear. He appears to be pricking stitch holes in the sole with a sharp curved awl, but no threads for stitching are visible and the boot has already progressed to the point of having its heel, which is normally put on after the sole is stitched.

There is no doubt, however, that the worker with his back turned is stitching a sole. A shoemaker did not use needles as a seamstress would, but tipped each end of his thread with a boar bristle, working and twisting the feathered end of the bristle into the end of his thread with spit and then waxing the entire length to strengthen and smooth it. The thicker, stiff end of the bristle started the thread through the hole made with the awl. For each stitch, the shoemaker drew first one bristle end of his thread through the hole, and then the other end through the same hole but in the opposite direction. The shoemaker with his back to us is pulling on both ends to tighten the stitch. The thread in his right hand should be wound round the spool-shaped handle of the awl (other similar awls are stored in the rack just below the window) but in fact it appears to be wound around his hand. Normally the shoemaker did indeed wind the other thread round his left hand, which was protected by a hand leather (clearly visible on the bearded worker).

The man in suit and spectacles is cutting a piece of leather, possibly in a spiral to create laces (if he were cutting an upper, he would presumably have used a pattern such as those hanging on the wall by the cracked mirror). Lengths of prepared thread hang on hooks around the room, and lasts are stuck in a rack beneath the clock. Also beneath the clock a pair of hooks used to draw on boots can be seen hanging on the line along with a row of what may be counters (stiffeners placed between the quarters and quarter linings). The floor is littered with leather scraps and tools, including a long bow-shaped instrument called a shoe-peg rasp (underneath the stitcher's bench). This tool was used to reach down inside a shoe or boot and shave off the protruding tops of the wooden pegs used to attach the sole. Each of the three benches has compartments full of these tiny wooden pegs.

The large display window does not ring quite true. Although it is possible that the shoes in the window were sale work or even custom work ready to be picked up, by the 1840s and 1850s most ten-footers were producing shoes for manufacturers who inspected the work and distributed them in larger markets. Real ten-footers were well-lit, but had windows like those in common dwelling-houses. The caged songbird and the newspaper on the table suggest the pleasant working conditions that shoemakers traditionally enjoyed. They may have spent long hours at repetitive work, but their minds were free to range and many accounts speak of the political and intellectual discussions that accompanied their labors. *Courtesy Connecticut Historical Society, negative #801.*

Making Shoes in the Early Nineteenth Century

Although custom shoemaking in which a single shoemaker made the entire shoe persisted well into the nineteenth century in many cities and towns, shoemaking in eastern Massachusetts was already being practiced as a cottage industry in the late eighteenth and early nineteenth centuries. While most of the work was still done by hand (for information about the steps involved in making a shoe, see appendix B), there was considerable division of labor. The leather was provided by a local manufacturer who farmed the work out to teams of shoemakers working in tiny one-room shops called "ten-footers," where they divided up the various steps in lasting and bottoming, etcetera (see fig. 7). The cloth uppers, however, had already been given out to women (often the shoemakers' wives) to stitch and bind at home. Binding shoes was a convenient way for women to earn money without neglecting their household responsibilities, and "'*Hannah binding shoes*' might have been found in almost every home in the shoe towns in eastern Massachusetts" (see fig. 8).[21]

The fact that much of the work making shoes was already being done by women led one anonymous "lady" in 1856 to write a book called *Every Lady Her Own Shoemaker*. She explains in her preface:

> The uppers of thousands of pairs are sent from shoe establishments in cities, to the country to be made. They pay eight cents a pair for those with [leather] tips at the toes only; for toes and heels ten cents, where the [leather] foxing comes half round, and twelve cents where it is all round. This must be stitched twice around, the instep seam stitched on each side, the lining and tongues made and put in, bound around the top and slit, and sixteen eyelets in each shoe; and these gaiters sell from $1.25 to $1.75 the pair. . . .

> Thus the shoemaker's part is confined to cutting out the work and sewing on the soles, for which they receive the profit. To prepare the cloth part takes more time and is quite as fatiguing when the gaiter is foxed—which is generally done

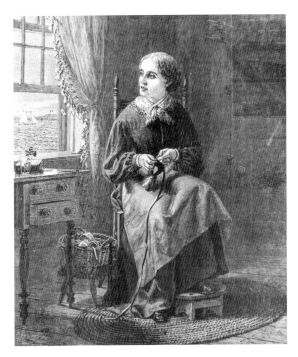

Fig. 8. *Hannah at the Window Binding Shoes* looks out over Marblehead harbor hoping for the return of her sailor husband, lost twenty years before. Her basket of uppers is by her side, and the long galloon, or binding tape, hangs over her knees. Binding shoes was a widespread female occupation in early nineteenth-century New England when it could still be done at home by hand. The poem on which this illustration was based, Lucy Larcom's well-known lyric "Hannah Binding Shoes," was written in 1854, the same year in which the sewing machine began to take over the stitching and binding of uppers, causing this step in the shoemaking process to become centralized in factories. This illustration, based on a painting by W. J. Linton, was engraved and published as the cover of *Every Saturday, An Illustrated Weekly Journal*, September, 23, 1871. *Courtesy Lynn Museum.*

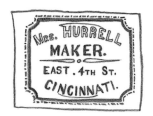

Fig. 9. Mrs. Hurrell's label survives in a pair of plain white kid slippers with rounded square toes, round throatline, and no heel, ca. 1845–55. They are still joined together by a string through the back seams, the device by which mates were kept together during shipping and storage before shoe boxes became standard. Historic Northampton catalog #66.646.

—as to sew on the soles. Why then cannot every lady make her own at a cost of less than half, and thus secure that profit herself.[22]

Swann reports that it was quite fashionable for women in England to make their own shoes from about 1800 to 1820,[23] and thrifty needlewomen may very well have continued to do so. Pamela S. Brown of Plymouth, Vermont, writes in her journal for October 18, 1837, "began a pair of blue shoes for me to wear to the ball," a ball that took place two days later. She does not mention finishing the shoes or taking them to a shoemaker for lasting and bottoming. Earlier that same year she had trimmed moccasins, including a pair for her mother. In November 1837, she "bound a pair of white shoes for myself," and from that month through the end of the diary in March 1838, she mentions eleven occasions on which she bound shoes, many of them after teaching school all day. It is possible that these are all shoes for herself and her family, just part of the endless stream of sewing that occupied so much of her time. But she may also have been binding shoes as a means of earning cash, just as she spun wool, taught school, and knitted stockings. At least one woman had seen the possibilities in not merely making her own shoes but setting up in business. Historic Northampton has a pair of white kid slippers, circa 1845–55, still connected by a coarse string through the back seams, that bear the label of a woman shoemaker, "Mrs. Hurrell, Maker. East 4th St. Cincinnati" (see fig. 9).[24]

The prejudice against American-made shoes that Richardson derides in the story of the lady customer who demanded French shoes probably had a foundation in hard experience. Hazard notes that in the 1830s, shoes were often rather badly made. Makers used flimsy paper stiffeners, poor-quality sewing, and trimmed the uppers so close to the stitching that they ripped out as soon as they were worn. She attributes these problems in part to simple irresponsibility but also to the fact that the manufacturers who put out the work to the binders and makers were not necessarily expert in shoemaking themselves and were not always able to assess the finished work to see if it came up to standard. In addition, new workers entering the field were not as thoroughly taught as the older generation.[25] One wonders if the fact that quality was difficult to control in this decade may be one reason why relatively few shoes clearly datable to the 1830s survive today.

The economic depression that began in 1839, following close on the heels of the financial panic of 1837, forced changes in shoemaking methods. In order to survive in a depressed market, manufacturers had to produce better-quality shoes. On the other hand, with competition for jobs so great, employers had the advantage of being able to choose only the best workers. By 1840, a good worker was no longer one who understood the entire shoemaking process but one who was very skilled in only one aspect of it. Work became increasingly specialized and centralized in the 1840s, and more control was exerted over production methods and standards.[26] For example, from 1848, the patterns used for cutting uppers were made in proportional sizes, and manufacturers required more exactness in matching the lengths and widths of pairs of shoes.[27] Shoe boxes came into general use in the 1830s as a way to protect the finished goods from damage in subsequent handling, and the year 1836 saw the first shoe-box manufacturer to set up production on a large scale in Lynn.[28] At the same time, demand grew for a greater variety of goods. Hazard mentions the special need for ready-made boots among men going to California and settling the West.[29] In the women's market, the development of elastic-sided boots in the late 1840s springs to mind.

The Shoe Industry in the Later Nineteenth Century

From about 1850, practicable machines were invented thick and fast for each stage of shoe manufacture. Among the earliest was a rolling machine that solidified and condensed sole leather to the proper texture, a job that had previously been done by laboriously hammering it on a lapstone. Other early machines included a stripper to cut up sides of sole leather into strips, a splitting machine to split skins or hides into two or more thin sheets, and machines that cut and drove in the wooden pegs used to attach sole and upper in utilitarian footwear. By the mid-1850s a sewing machine had been specially adapted for use in sewing uppers. A "dry thread" sewing machine using a lockstitch (the two-thread stitch normal in today's home sewing machines) was used for fabrics and light leathers, while a "wax thread" chain-stitch sewing machine was used from 1857 on heavier leathers.

This burst of invention in the middle of the century led to centralizing the work in factories where the machines could be housed and where a water- or steam-power supply was available to run them. David Johnson noted in his recollections of Lynn that "the Revolution in the shoe business occurred during the ten years ending [in] 1865. From 1855, or a little later, the workmen began to leave the 'little shop' to work in the factories of the manufacturers; and in a few years vacant shops were seen all over the city, until most of them were transformed into hen houses or coal pens, or were moved and joined to some house to make a snug little kitchen."[30] Although an advertisement in the *Lynn Directory and Almanac* for 1854 recommends "Wheeler & Wilson's Improved Sewing Machines" as "peculiarly desirable to private families who do Gaiter stitching," the sewing machine spelled the end of shoe binding as a job that could be done at home, fitted in around the cooking, cleaning, and child care. In that same year, an adaptation of the sewing machine called a binder was invented that was specifically arranged to carry the galloon.[31] The days of "Hannah Binding Shoes" came to an end just as Lucy Larcom's famous poem was being written, and Hannah now had to leave home for a factory if she was to find work in the shoe industry (see fig. 10).

The advent of the sewing machine made stitching uppers a swift business, but stitching the upper to the sole was still a slow hand operation. The pegging process, however, was mechanized by 1860. Saguto quotes Bishop's 1868 *History of American Manufacture*, which reports that by 1860 "the pegging machine has been so perfected as to cut the pegs from a strip of wood, punch the holes, and drive the pegs at a single operation. A machine will peg a ladies' shoe in seven seconds after the work is placed in the machine. It will average one thousand pairs of such shoes a day, and from four hundred to five hundred pairs of shoes

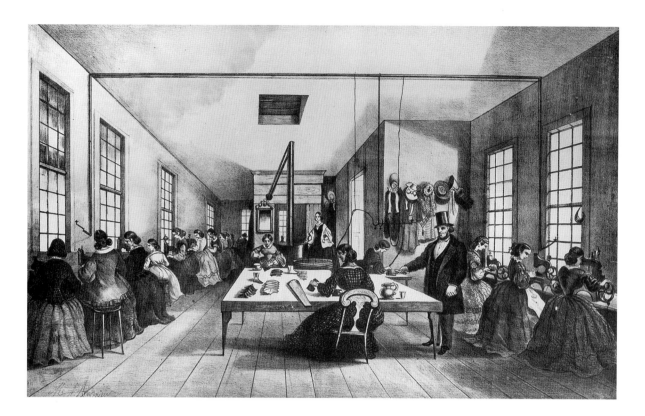

Fig. 10. *Pray's Stitching Shop*, showing women at work stitching uppers by machine about 1860. This work had formerly been done by hand and at home, but once manufacturers acquired sewing machines, this part of the shoemaking process became centralized in factories. Catalog #2170. *Courtesy Lynn Museum.*

with double rows of pegs in the same time." By 1860, we are told, seven-eighths of the shoes made in America were pegged.[32]

Pegged shoes may have been speedy to make, but they were rather stiff and inflexible, and the best-quality shoes still required hand-sewing to attach sole to upper. But a new era commenced in 1860 when the McKay sole-sewing machine was patented. This machine stitched the sole to the upper, allowing the bottoming process to catch up with the speedy production of uppers already possible with the sewing machine. The licensing stamp attached to early shoes made with this machine ("pat Aug. 14, 1860") can still be seen on boots at the Peabody Essex Museum.[33] The machine's value was tested when it was used to make military footwear during the Civil War, and by the late 1860s it was widely adopted. Shoe manufacturer William Rice believed that "no other machine has caused so great a revolution in the business as the McKay sewing machine," and claimed that by 1895 there were four thousand machines in use producing 120 million pairs of shoes annually.[34]

Even by 1858, the point at which W. H. Richardson looked back on it, the growth of the industry was stunning.

The trade has increased to an almost wonderful extent. It now forms one-third of the whole manufacturing power of the country; New England and Pennsylvania retaining two-thirds. . . . The domestic and foreign boot and shoe trade of the state of Massachusetts alone, amounts to between fifty-five to sixty millions annually. The shipments from Boston to San Francisco for 1856 were $2,100,000. The manufacture of boots and shoes is the largest domestic trade in the States, and there is no country or nation that can successfully compete with us, either as regards prices or quality.[35]

The Civil War (1861–65), with its shortages of labor and expanded need for boots, encouraged the transition toward centralizing and mechanizing the shoe industry. After the war, the pace of invention quickened even more, with Americans still the leading innovators. In the 1870s came a heeling machine, edge trimmer, standard screw machine (which used metal screws rather than wooden pegs as a rigid vertical fastener to attach soles to uppers), and most important, the Goodyear welt machines (1877), which could produce welted shoes (welting is the means of attaching sole to upper used in better shoes). One of the last processes to be mechanized was lasting, the process of stretching the upper around the wooden last. It required a great deal of skill and experience to know how tightly to stretch the leather. But even this problem was solved in 1883 by Jan Matzeliger, a black immigrant from Dutch Guiana. It is clearly with a great sense of satisfaction that Mr. Rice, having reviewed the progress of machine shoemaking to date, remarked that "although on going through a modern shoe factory one would think perfection had been reached, no season passes without the introduction of some new machine which works a revolution in its particular sphere."[36]

In spite of the increasing sophistication in both the manufacture and distribution of shoes, the traveling shoemaker existed into at least the 1870s in very remote areas. Nettie Spencer, who was interviewed as part of the Federal Writers' Project in 1938, remembered that in rural Oregon during her childhood, "all of our shoes were made by a man who came around every so often and took our foot measurements with broomstraws, which he broke off and tagged for the foot length of each member of the family. The width

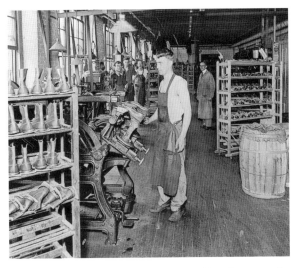

Fig. 11. The "making room" of the Burdett Shoe Company of Lynn in 1919, showing the Sole Leveler machine and racks of partly made shoes. The American shoe industry was at the height of its prosperity in the early twentieth century. Catalog #14.780 pb4.3. *Courtesy Lynn Museum.*

didn't make any difference and you could wear either shoe on either foot—for a long time, too, for the shoes wore well."[37] By this date, ready-made shoes would have been available from coast to coast, but in sparsely settled areas, the traveling shoemaker must have found his last market among families who lived out of reach of the nearest general store.

As the American shoe industry grew in the latter half of the nineteenth century, fewer shoes were imported. Certainly after about 1865 foreign labels in surviving shoes are relatively rare. Those that do turn up are comparable to dresses from Worth and Pingat, brought back as special purchases from Paris rather than imported in bulk for retail sale in the States as had been the case in the mid–nineteenth century. In this class is an embroidered shoe made in Paris by Perchellet in the late 1870s (see fig. 427).[38] By the 1880s American manufacturers were not merely supplying the home market but exporting vast quantities of shoes abroad, and by 1900 the United States surpassed France, Germany, and Switzerland, its shoe exports being valued at $4.25 million. The foreign market expanded beyond the West Indies and other agricultural areas to include even England, which had its own highly developed shoe industry centered in Northampton, and United States products competed directly with British goods for markets in the British colonies. The *Shoe Retailer* reported that in 1900 Australia was America's largest foreign customer, followed by the British Isles and Canada.[39] To this day, the influx of cheap low-quality American shoes in the 1880s and 1890s is remembered with resentment in Northampton as "the American invasion."[40]

Some of the best work of this period, however, survives in the form of exhibition shoes displayed at fairs like the 1876 Centennial Exhibition in Philadelphia and the 1893 World's Columbian Exposition in Chicago. The Los Angeles County Museum of Art has a boot that is hand-sewn with sixty-four stitches per inch, the highest number so far observed anywhere.[41] It was made by Laird, Schober, and Mitchell of Philadelphia, possibly for the Centennial Exhibition. This was by no means the normal standard of work, but it does suggest that the best American workmen were capable of very high levels of craftsmanship. In several cases, exhibition shoes were proudly preserved by the manufacturer until the shoe industry declined and such company collections were dispersed. One of the greatest of these collections was that formed by the United Shoe Machinery Corporation (USMC). USMC did not make shoes but leased shoemaking machines, and therefore had business connections with all the major shoe manufacturers. The USMC collection is now preserved in the Peabody Essex Museum in Salem, Massachusetts. In this collection one finds exhibition shoes from such companies as Hazen B. Goodrich of Haverhill and Selz-Schwab of Chicago, as well as numerous non-exhibition shoes whose manufacturers' names were preserved by the shoe industry collectors.

The Shoe Industry in the Early Twentieth Century

Trade periodicals provide vast quantities of detailed information about shoe styles and the shoe industry at the height of its prosperity in the late nineteenth and early twentieth century. The following information about the industry between

1900 and 1930 is gleaned from a sampling of material from the *Shoe Retailer*, 1900–28, available at the Lynn Museum. The *Shoe Retailer* began publication in March 1898, at first monthly and then weekly (see fig. 12). Each issue contains at least thirty and sometimes well over a hundred pages. Because it came out so frequently and contains so much material, it constitutes a sensitive reflection of fluctuations in the industry. Its readers were, as its name suggests, the people who owned or ran retail shoe stores, and it provided them with a number of important services, including advice on marketing and window-dressing. Each issue is full of advertisements placed by the manufacturers illustrating their in-stock styles. In the spring and fall, it dedicated a group of issues to the styles being planned for the following season, usually one for women's shoes, one for men's, and sometimes one for children's shoes. The information is often divided by manufacturing center, so that new styles coming out of Rochester, New York, or Haverhill, Massachusetts, may each have their own descriptive article. The publishers tended to reflect the manufacturer's point of view. For example, in 1909, the *Shoe Retailer* explained to retailers at length why the price of shoes could not possibly go down in spite of the repeal of the tariff on hides. But it also funneled information back from the retailers to the manufacturers, chiefly about what was selling in various parts of the country, the reports being written by the retailers themselves. All this material deserves a much more thorough analysis than has been possible within this book, but the following is offered as an encouragement to others interested in researching the history of shoes in America.

By the early twentieth century, there was a good deal of specialization within the shoe industry, with certain elements of shoemaking developing their own industries. The leather manufacturers, of course, formed one large class, with companies often specializing in particular leather types, such as kid, calf, or oak-tanned sole leather (see fig. 13). Then there were the makers of a myriad of shoe findings, including elastic goring, shoe buttons, buckles, and ornaments, shoelaces, boxes, labels to keep mates together with the appropriate box, shoe polish, and rubber

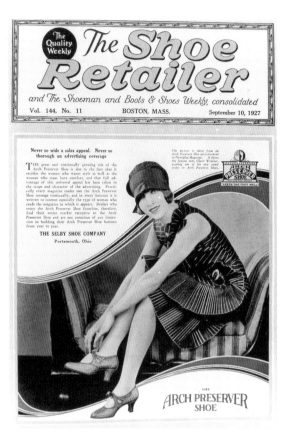

Fig. 12. Cover of the *Shoe Retailer* for September 10, 1927. This trade periodical is an important source of information about shoe fashions and the American shoe industry. *Courtesy Lynn Museum.*

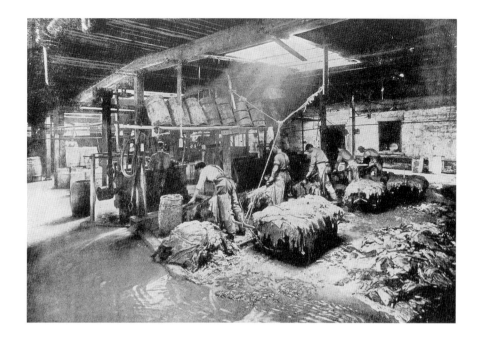

Fig. 13. This "picture of one small corner of our beam house at Lowell, where we remove the hair in making the famous Enamel Box Calf" is from an advertisement placed by the American Hide and Leather Company in the *Shoe Retailer,* April 3, 1901, p. 11. *Courtesy Lynn Museum.*

heels. In so thoroughly mechanized an industry, the production of shoemaking machinery was a whole separate business. The best known of these companies was the United Shoe Machinery Corporation of Beverly, Massachusetts, which built and leased machinery to the shoe manufacturers.

Lasts were made by specialized companies, not by the shoe manufacturers themselves. New lasts were often given names (the Arena last, Stage last, and Modified Stage last are often mentioned). The characteristics of these lasts were universally understood and they were bought and used by more than one company. There were also specialized pattern-making companies that produced the metal or cardboard cutting patterns in graduated sizes from which the various pieces of the uppers were cut. The *Shoe and Leather Lexicon* of 1916 explains that "the proper grading of these patterns in size, so as to bring certain features of the pattern at the right point on the last is a trade in itself, and the producing of a new sample involves cooperation and collaboration between the last-maker and the pattern-maker. That is, a last of a certain form being provided and a certain style of shoe being decided upon, it is then the duty of the pattern-maker to so proportion the parts of the upper that when stitched and lasted it will throw a shoe of the desired characteristics."[42]

Then of course there were the manufacturers themselves. The highest grades of women's shoes, according to the *Shoe Retailer,* were made in New York City, Brooklyn, and Philadelphia, while Lynn and the surrounding towns north of Boston made middle-grade women's shoes. Haverhill was famous for its production of slippers. The cities lying south of Boston, especially Brockton, made men's shoes (and occasionally women's shoes when "mannish" styles were in fashion). Along with the New England manufacturers, New York State (notably Rochester and Endicott-Johnson near Binghamton), Cincinnati, Chicago, Milwaukee, and St. Louis were listed as makers of medium-priced lines in 1921. Ten years earlier, in 1911, Cincinnati was congratulating itself on having caught up with the eastern manufacturers in terms of quality. St. Louis specialized in women's shoes and is often mentioned in connection with "novelty shoes." See appendix D for a partial list of shoe manufacturers.

Traveling salesmen had been part of the shoe marketing system in the early nineteenth century. Hazard mentions a James Littlefield who traveled through the South in 1816–17, selling shoes in exchange for flour, which he sold at high profits in the North, where a bad wheat harvest had raised prices.[43] But Littlefield seems to have been in business for himself rather than representing a company as modern salesmen do. A publication by the Sterling Last Company, which includes a "Chronological Record of Shoemaking in America," gives the date of 1852 for "the first shoe traveler, Joel C. Page, who worked for the wholesale house of James A. Estabrook, Boston. His first sale was to a store in Montpelier, Vt."[44] Certainly by the beginning of the twentieth century, the practice of using traveling salesmen to reach the retailers was well established. In 1909, the P. J. Harney Shoe Company of Lynn had "sixteen salesmen . . . out showing our samples in every state in the Union"[45] (see fig. 14). Most manufacturers also produced catalogs that were sent to shoe retailers on request, and samples were also sent directly. The *Shoe Retailer* mentions jobbing or wholesale houses only occasionally, as if such firms were no longer particularly important. This may be because the manufacturers who supplied most of the advertising revenue to the *Shoe Retailer* found it more profitable when retailers bought directly from them through their own salesmen, and that therefore they chose to play down references to the wholesale-house alternative.

There was, however, an important class of firms who tried to bring all levels of manufacturing and sales under one company umbrella. Endicott-Johnson, situated near Binghamton, New York, for example, was

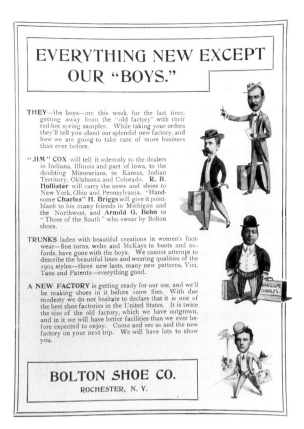

Fig. 14. At the beginning of the twentieth century, shoe salesmen sent out by the manufacturers were an important part of the marketing structure and they are often mentioned by name in the *Shoe Retailer*. Advertisement from the *Shoe Retailer*, September 16, 1903, p.87. *Courtesy Lynn Museum.*

referred to in 1923 as the largest tanner and shoe manufacturer in the world. It had enough business to require its own jobbing warehouses (one is mentioned as being built in St. Louis, from which it sent salesmen out into its southern and southwestern territories), and it also had its own chain of retail outlets. Others used a combination of distribution techniques, including their own stores, mail-order services, and general retailers. Some shoe manufacturers created national brand names like Red Cross Shoes (made by Krohn Fechheimer of Cincinnati) and Arch Preserver Shoes (made by Selby). While most shoe manufacturers advertised their wares to the retail dealers, these companies advertised directly to the consumer and their ads are quite common in women's magazines from about 1890.

The *Shoe Retailer* provides a good deal of information about how new styles were developed and introduced. Through their salesmen, manufacturers kept tabs on what kinds of shoes were selling in what cities, and no doubt also took note of the retailers' reports as published in the *Shoe Retailer*. Occasionally they worked directly with a major retailer to create a new style for which the retailer believed he had a market. The story of how the "Bulgarian sandal" was developed by the Chicago retailer O'Connor and Goldberg and a Lynn manufacturer, for example, is told in the September 20, 1913, issue of the *Shoe Retailer*. Retailers seem to have increased their role in new style development in the 1920s, but otherwise the general practice was to continue making styles that were selling well at the end of the previous season, to drop styles that appeared to be declining, and to introduce a sprinkling of new variations as a means of testing the market for new trends. While manufacturers clearly kept an eye on Paris shoe fashions, one gets the distinct impression that French taste and American taste were by no means synonymous. In the late 1910s and early 1920s, American shoes had long pointed toes while the French shoes had shorter vamps and square toes. The great question in 1919 was whether or not French-style lasts would be introduced. When they did come in a couple of years later, they were altered, because it was felt that "American women do not like stubby foreparts, so that French lasts Americanized are fairly pointed at the end."[46]

In the early twentieth century, there were two main seasons for introducing new shoes: spring (in time for the Easter trade) and fall. As soon as the spring season was sufficiently advanced to know which styles were selling well, manufacturers sat down with their salesmen and began discussing the best prospects for the next year. By July they were experimenting with new patterns and lasts, and the new models were published in the *Shoe Retailer* in September. That same month, the salesmen took samples of the new styles out to the retailers. These sample suitcases usually contained far more styles than the manufacturer really wanted to produce, but manufacturers were induced by the pressure of competition to offer these extra models, as the *Shoe Retailer* explained in 1913: "Of a thousand styles no sane dealer will buy more than a dozen. No shoe store wants a big variety of patterns, nor a too extreme range of lasts. There are lots of shoes in the samples that the manufacturers don't want to sell, and when asked why he

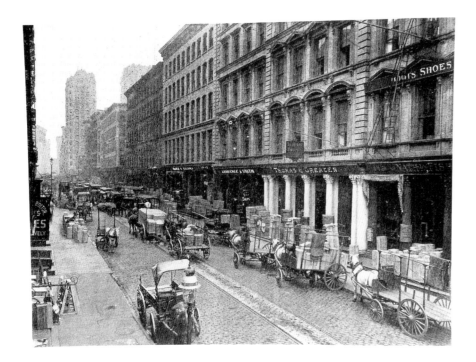

Fig. 15. "Duane Street, noon, looking toward Broadway," from the *Shoe Retailer,* September 16, 1903, p. 108. Duane Street was the center of New York City's shoe trade. The boxes piled on the wagons along the street are filled with shoes. *Courtesy Lynn Museum.*

puts them in, he will give one of the two following replies: 'To show that I can make fancy shoes if necessary,' or, 'I must show them because others have them; dealers would ask my salesmen where they were, and we must have them, of course.'"[47] One manufacturer in 1909 showed nearly one hundred styles in his sample case even while believing that "a great variety of styles . . . are not advisable for next season."[48] The salesman's suitcase contained two broad categories of shoes: staples and novelty shoes. Staples included such styles as basic oxford walking shoes that did not change radically from year to year and could be settled well in advance of the new season. Novelties included shoes made of nonstandard leathers or colors, or those made with fancy-cut uppers or fancy ornamentation. These were designed in response to shorter fluctuations in the market and could appear at any time during the year. Occasionally what began as a novelty ended as a staple of the trade.

What concerned manufacturers in the 1910s was the tendency for novelties to form an increasingly important part of the shoe business. Even in the smaller towns, novelty shoes began to supplant the staple boots and oxfords that had previously formed the backbone of the trade. This had its pros and cons. On one hand, there was less risk when buyers were interested chiefly in staple styles that changed little from season to season. Manufacturers enjoyed the advantages of scale when they could make up large quantities of shoes in only a few basic easy-to-sell styles. It was more expensive and more risky to produce a great variety of styles, all of which required the initial outlay in design, lasts, and patterns, but only a few of which would sell to any large extent. On the other hand, since

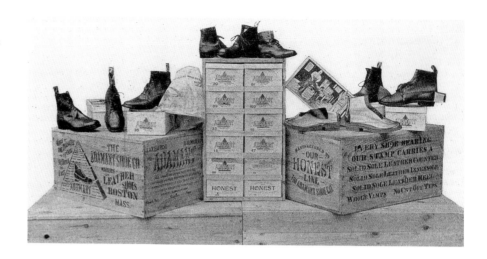

Fig. 16. Shoes and their packing boxes, from the *Shoe Retailer*, September 16, 1903, p. 119. The wooden crate at left is marked "Like the Builders of Old, We Build to Last. The Adamant Shoe Co. Makers of Leather Shoes, Boston Mass. Kangaroo Balmoral." The trademark illustration is a shoe within a pyramid. The right-hand packing case is marked "Manufactured by The Adamant Shoe Co., Our Honest Line. Every shoe bearing our stamp carries a solid sole leather counter, solid sole leather innersole, solid sole leather heel, whole vamps, no cut off tips." The boot sitting directly on the right-hand wooden case has been cut in half, showing the white lining and the layers of the sole (the left half has been folded down slightly to show the photograph on the wall behind it). *Courtesy Lynn Museum.*

novelty shoes went in and out of fashion faster, there was an inducement for women to buy shoes more often, resulting in more business and greater turnover. This tension resulted in apparently conflicting remarks from the *Shoe Retailer* in 1911. "Retailers should not lose sight of the fact that it is not novelties that sell best, and that good strong lines in oxford ties, in lace and button patterns, with fabric tops, will be the strong feature for the conservative trade."[49] In the same issue we are told that "the 'millinery' [i.e., novelty] side of the shoe business shows up more on spring and summer goods than for fall and winter, and with the making of novelties manufacturers should very materially improve the price situation. With the business getting more on the 'millinery' basis there naturally should be more profit in trade."[50] This use of the word "millinery" to refer to novelty shoes, or shoes that are more than commonly ornamented, harkens back to the eighteenth-century milliner, who specialized in trimming not only hats but dresses and other articles of clothing as well.

As novelty shoes became more important, manufacturers became unwilling to publish their designs a full six months before they reached the shelves. As early as 1909, the *Shoe Retailer* was noticing that "manufacturers of some lines are not going to 'give away' exclusive spring ideas at this time. 'Tis too early. There is yet time to show that the so-called 'style experts' are out of tune. It was ever thus. Last year a prominent Lynn manufacturing house was late in introducing a special tie. But the fact of its coming late saved it from being hocked about and copied in the cheap lines."[51]

Not only was it a disadvantage to publish new styles far in advance, it was also risky to make up the shoes without having orders in hand, because the market for novelty shoes was so volatile. All these factors contributed to the breakdown of the two-season system in the early 1920s. In September 1921, when the *Shoe Retailer* was attempting to report on new spring styles in St. Louis, the periodical could only say that "the real spring line has not been laid out in St. Louis yet, except insofar as it embraces strictly staple numbers in medium priced goods, and these do not vary much from the usual patterns. Makers of novelty shoes do not expect to assemble their spring season sample lines before the middle of November. Many seem to feel that the real spring sellers will hardly be materialized in the trade for several months, presumably after the NSRA [National Shoe Retailers Association] convention in January."[52] By 1923, the *Shoe Retailer* reported that Rochester manufacturers recognized "six well defined seasons, which explains in part why so many merchants will not place their orders more than 60 days ahead."[53] These six seasons were listed as January to Easter, Easter through June, July and August, late summer/early fall (September/October), and late fall/early winter (November/December).

Besides the fragmentation of the year into six style seasons, there was also a fast-growing tendency to produce an enormous number of different styles at any one time, and also to produce shoes that were extremely elaborate in cut. With shoes going in and out of style so quickly and no strong seasonal etiquette to govern the suitability of certain patterns or materials, it became very difficult to project what would sell two or three months in the future, and the risks involved in making and selling shoes became steadily more intimidating through the 1920s. An article printed in the *Shoe Retailer* early in 1928 describes with dismay the frantic pursuit of novelty in the shoe trade.

> Too much emphasis cannot be laid on the gravity of this indictment against the over-styling that is abundantly manifest in the trade. We are in deep, whirling rapids and the canoe is frail. . . . [The retailer faces a serious problem when there is so great a] profusion of entries in the race for orders. A retailer is not likely to pick just a few. He is afraid that his competition will adopt what he has neglected and beat him to the punch, and the final result will more likely be a long, thinly spread stock that will not provide adequate sizes and widths with which to do business. The manufacturer is not at fault. Some retailers, and too many of them, want to be style leaders and they search outside of their legitimate field for fabrics and leathers that are distinctive, and primarily suited only for the luxury trade. They turn these ideas over to a manufacturer, insist on his submitting shoes to them of these materials; and it is not long before other manufacturers learn of the new things and for fear they may be out-stripped by their competitors, they rush to secure these samples for their trade.
>
> Right now, the sample rooms of manufacturers are more colorful than a summer garden. The displays are fascinating but behind the multitude of magnificent materials is the menace of red ink that represents losses.[54]

In 1923, one contemporary shoe man connected this "overstyling" with the overcapacity of American shoe factories and would have solved the problem by somehow enlarging the market.

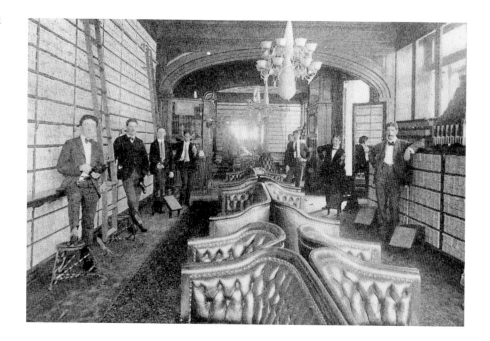

Unquestionably the biggest issue in the minds of women's shoe manufacturers today is the style question. I think most of us regard it as a disease, whereas as a matter of fact it is only a symptom. A real disease is the necessity for getting more business.

It has been variously estimated that the shoe factories in this country can produce from 50 per cent to 250 per cent more shoes than are consumed. As long as that condition exists to the extent that it does exist, the style issue is going to be over-played. . . . Figures which I think are reliable show that the consumption of shoes per capita in this country is about three pairs a year, and figures show that the consumption 30 years ago was three pairs per year. . . .

I believe that this great industry, if it can fully appreciate that the per capita consumption of shoes has not increased in 30 years, will be willing sooner or later to take up that subject and make plans to increase the per capita consumption of shoes.[55]

John Slater, president of the National Shoe Retailers Association, blamed the retailers, saying that the reason the consumption of shoes had remained flat was that "instead of using the additional styles to increase his business, as merchants do who sell other kinds of apparel, the shoe merchant has merely substituted some different style for the one that was sold before and allowed his customer to believe that this was the shoe she ought to wear on practically every occasion. 'Satin slippers,' said Mr. Slater, 'have been sold for street wear, when they were originally and properly intended only for dress footwear, thus cheating the merchant out of the second pair of shoes he ought to have sold. . . . Much of the trouble arising out of our multiplicity of styles arises from the fact that we have not taught our customers to buy shoes for the occasion."[56]

It seems just as likely, however, that Americans wore for general purposes shoes suitable only for a specific occasion because they could not afford separate shoes for every situation. In the same year in which Slater castigated retailers for their failure to increase consumption, other shoe men reporting on the state of the industry congratulated themselves on having been able to reduce wages to their workers.[57] In a laissez-faire economy that generated much wealth for a few but little purchasing power for the masses, many Americans in the 1920s did not have the money to buy more shoes, no matter how attractively they were advertised.

These alterations in the trade were only part of a larger complex of changes that together led to the decline of the shoe industry in America. The price of leather seems to have steadily increased in the first decades of the 1900s, owing to increased demand and reduced supply (the leather supply is tied to the demand for meat). According to the *Shoe Retailer* (in this case operating almost certainly as spokesman for the manufacturers), these costs were not at first passed on to the consumer, so that by the time the tariff on imported hides was repealed in 1909, it was possible only to hold prices steady, not to decrease them. This seems to have caused a great deal of irritation and misunderstanding between makers and retailers in that year.[58] By 1919, after the close of World War I, the price of leather had risen until it was more profitable to sell stockpiled leather on the open market than to make it into shoes.[59] The resulting high cost of boots was one very important reason they went out of fashion when they did. At the same time, workers were agitating for shorter hours and higher wages, and the strikes in both the shoe and leather industries at first slowed down production and then resulted in higher prices. Thus the signs of distress were evident in the shoe industry as early as the 1920s, and the stock-market crash of 1929 and the depression of the 1930s precipitated the closing of many shoe factories. Even more devastating, however, was the growing tide of imported shoes that inundated the United States in the late 1960s from countries with far lower labor costs. American manufacturers simply could not compete, and the glory days of the American shoe industry were gone forever.

Regional Variations in Shoe Fashions

The shoe industry developed early in American history, and the division of labor within the small shops made the mass production of ready-made shoes a reality long before machines became important in production. Thus as the country expanded westward in the nineteenth century, the shoe industry was already sufficiently mature to send shoes and boots along with the pioneers. When so much of a country's footwear was being made in only two or three manufacturing centers, as was the case in the United States, it is hardly surprising that there should not be very great differences in footwear owing merely to region or geography.

The excavation of the steamboat *Bertrand*, which ran aground in the Missouri River just north of Omaha in April 1865, suggests the range of ready-made footwear, clothing, and other goods that was being sent to the most distant reaches of the United States at midcentury. The *Bertrand* carried some seven hundred pairs of boots and shoes for men, women, and children to merchants in Hell Gate and

Virginia City, Montana. Surviving case labels show that they came from manufacturers in Weymouth, Holliston, Coburn, Randolph, and Boston, Massachusetts, and from a wholesale distributor in St. Louis. The women's footwear included serge Congress and front-lacing boots with leather foxing and stacked heels, essentially identical to those illustrated in figure 64.[60] These shoes were no different from those being worn on the street by middle-class women along the eastern seaboard.

The one place I have found shoes surviving that may clearly reflect a local taste is at the Natural History Museum of Los Angeles County (others probably survive in collections with ties to the Caribbean and the southwestern United States). These dark blue, brown, black, and white satin slippers seem to have been the product of Spanish/Mexican culture in southern California before the American presence became important, although they look very much like those preserved on the East Coast from the period 1825 to 1835. They are hand-sewn, and the silk uppers and linen linings are typically early nineteenth century. The thin heelless soles, oval toes, very narrow waists, and square throatlines all suggest a date in the 1820s or 1830s. They are different, however, in having circular stamps on the sole that appear to have been burnished with some sort of metallic finish so that they look like nail heads. Circular stamps without the metallic finish are not unusual in early nineteenth-century shoes. They were often used around 1830 to close the small holes made in the leather when the sole was tacked to the last. But in the California shoes, the metal-finished stamps are used in addition to conventional circular stamps. Some of the California shoes also have distinctive fish-, bird-, or chain-shaped marks stamped in the sole. A similar pair of shoes, preserved at the Society for the Preservation of New England Antiquities where one would not expect to find them, turns out to come from a family with close ties to the Spanish culture of the Caribbean. Made of brown satin with oval toe, very narrow waist, and elaborate sole stamping (though not with metallic finish), these shoes were worn by the American wife or daughter of Leon de Chappotin, who fled San Domingo (Haiti) during the uprisings of the early 1790s.[61] But the most unaccountable pair of Spanish-style slippers is a pair at the Natural History Museum of Los Angeles County. Hand-sewn in what appear to be early nineteenth-century materials like the other shoes in this group (see fig. 18), they are stamped on the sole with the trade name "Ramirez" in a slanted cursive style that stylistically belongs to the early twentieth century.[62] It is not immediately obvious how to account for the conjunction of early nineteenth-century style and materials and the early twentieth-century maker's label.

Satin shoes were mentioned by contemporary observers as a typical part of women's dress in early nineteenth-century Cuba, Mexico, and California. They were particularly associated with the Mexican national dress known as the China Poblana style, a style also worn in southern California when it was part of the Mexican Republic (1823–46). The main components of this costume were a chemise with embroidered, drawn-work, or lace decoration worn to show, a full skirt whose upper six or eight inches were made of a contrasting color, a shawl known as a rebozo, and satin shoes worn without stockings.

Frances Calderón de la Barca, a Scotswoman who lived in Mexico in 1840 and 1841 as wife of the Spanish ambassador, repeatedly mentions satin shoes in her lively descriptions of Cuban and Mexican dress. Walking from church to church during the Holy Thursday celebration in Mexico City in 1840, she saw wealthy ladies in velvet and satin dresses, wearing diamonds and pearls, and white or colored satin shoes. "The petticoats are rather short, but it would be hard to hide such small feet, and such still smaller shoes."[63] She had been impressed from the first by Mexican women's feet, which "naturally small, are squeezed nearly double, Chinese fashion, into little ill-made shoes still smaller —so that they look in front like little horses' hoofs. Of course they can neither dance nor walk."[64] She herself donned satin shoes for Holy Thursday, and admitted that "the fatigue was terrible, walking for so many hours on that bad pavement with thin satin shoes, so that at length our feet seemed to move mechanically—and we dropped on our knees before each altar like machines touched by a spring, and rose with no small effort."[65] Satin shoes were not, however, limited to the wealthy. On her Holy Thursday pilgrimage, she also noticed "women of the shopkeeper class, or it may be lower, in their smart white embroidered gowns, with their white satin shoes, and neat feet and ankles . . . the peasants and countrywomen, with their short petticoats of two colours, generally scarlet and yellow . . . , thin satin shoes and lace trimmed chemises . . . and above all, here and there a flashing Poblana, with a dress of real value and much taste . . . a bold coquettish eye, and a beautiful little brown foot shown off by the white satin shoe."[66] Even very poor women whose petticoats were in rags wore "dirty white satin shoes, rather shorter than their small brown feet."[67]

Foreign visitors found these satin shoes bizarre not because their style was unfamiliar, but because by the 1820s, European etiquette limited satin shoes to evening wear, and white satin shoes were even more strictly confined to weddings and other very formal occasions. In Spanish America, however, satin shoes were a normal part of everyday public dress, and might be worn even when horseback riding. The

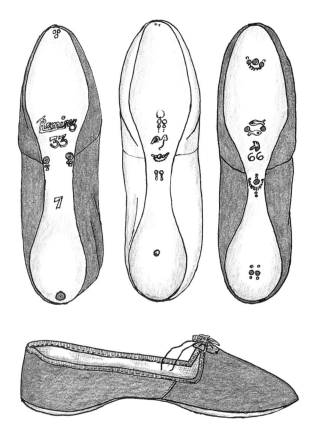

Fig. 18. Hand-sewn satin slippers from the Museum of Natural History, Los Angeles County, having unusual marks stamped on the sole. These may have been worn as part of the traditional China Poblana costume that developed in Mexico and southern California in the early nineteenth century, but it is possible that at least some are early twentieth-century reproductions worn with traditional dress on festival occasions. *Left and below:* Dark-blue satin slipper. The cursive-style marking "Ramirez" suggests a date ca. 1890–1915, even though the materials and making are very similar to early nineteenth-century examples. Catalog #A.3580-1300. *Center:* White satin slipper with bird, chain, and circle stamps, ca. 1820–45. Catalog #A.3580-1322. *Right:* Dark-blue satin slipper with chain and fish stamps and circular stamps that have a burnished metallic finish imitating nail heads, ca. 1820–45. Catalog #A.3580-197.

Spanish population in California in the early nineteenth century was not very large, and after the discovery of gold in 1849, their distinctive dress was overwhelmed by the massive immigration of Americans. The memory of it was preserved in families of Spanish descent (the del Valle and Coronel families eventually gave their clothing to the museum in Los Angeles), but already by the late nineteenth century, people interested in their distinctive costume history had to resort to reproductions for some garments when they put on traditional dress. Among the Coronel clothing, for example, is a man's coat clearly dating from the 1870s or later to which has been applied decorative loops of white braid in the style worn before 1850. It may be that the puzzling "Ramirez" shoes were made to wear for some festival occasion in the late nineteenth or early twentieth century by a Spanish shoemaker old enough to remember how shoes had been made before 1850. Whatever the explanation, it is hard to escape the implication that the Ramirez shoes represent the survival of a much earlier hand shoemaking tradition.

The significant point, though, is not that Spanish California was geographically distant or isolated, but that it enjoyed a different cultural heritage. The Spanish in California were not the only culturally distinct group that wore distinctive shoes. The best known, of course, were the American Indians, whose moccasins were incorporated into white American dress from an early period. There is also evidence that newly arrived immigrants continued to wear the footwear of their native lands, at least for a short time after their arrival in the United States. In 1903, the *Shoe Retailer* prepared a short article on the sidewalk shoe trade carried on in New York City on the Lower East Side, and described how the large population of newly arrived immigrants provided a market for the clothing styles they had worn in their own countries, at least until they were assimilated into the cultural mainstream.

New York has swallowed and is trying to digest a good share of the population of the several nations of the earth and during this process of assimilation trade customs as well as other phases of existence partake of the exotic.

For instance, nobody ever sees wooden shoes, but, as a matter of fact, thousands of pairs are made and sold each year within the confines of the greater city. The embroidered foot covering of the Celestials [the Chinese], the red Russia leather of the Slavs, the sturdy 'brogues' of the newly-arrived son of Erin and the all-too-dainty confections of the Parisian are in evidence in certain quarters, but not for long. The Americanizing usually starts at the foot, and except with those who are too old to heed the changes of the times, the familiar homemade footwear soon succeeds the more picturesque fashions of the old world.

As ever keen to note the pulse of popular demand, the East Side Hebrew devotes his energies toward the proper outfitting of newcomers. He knows what they will want, puts a price on his wares that his trade can pay, and goes after his customers where he can find them, on the street.

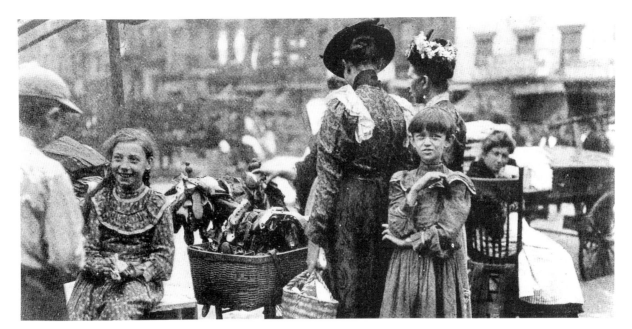

We cannot conceive of anything that a rationally-minded individual wants
that is not displayed by the sidewalk merchants of the East Side. We will not
attempt to describe the multitudinous enterprises that flourish in this densely
populated area, but we assure our readers that shoes are not forgotten. Shoes
for the baby, the bruiser and the belle—nothing is lacking.

Our artist has secured us some typical views of this great but seldom-
mentioned retail district [see fig. 19], and it is but fair to state that in courtesy,
progressiveness and attention to details the sidewalk merchant has little to
learn from his uptown confrere.[68]

As the article points out, the impulse, at least among younger immigrants, was
generally to become as American in appearance as possible, in order to fit in and
get ahead. So while cultural difference did give rise to some variation in footwear,
these variations tended to be short-lived, and were soon swallowed up in the
mainstream of American shoe fashions.

One gets the impression that truly regional variations in taste only became
possible after 1900 and that these developed as a result of the increasing number
of novelty styles being offered by the shoe industry. Before that, within any one
class of footwear, only a few style variations were available. In the 1880s and early
1890s, for example, the same basic dress slipper was offered in black, white, and
bronze kid and in satin in a variety of common evening colors. The buyer could
choose an alternate version with a strap and a bow on it. By contrast, in the 1920s,
dressy shoes were made in hundreds of styles, varying in material, color, cut, and
decoration. Given the newly expanded range of choice, it makes sense that regional variations in taste might for the first time begin to reveal themselves.

Fig. 20. Charts like this one (October 15, 1927, p. 50) detailing "Best Selling Styles" in various cities around the country were published in the *Shoe Retailer* by the late 1920s, reflecting an increasing awareness of regional differences in taste. *Courtesy Lynn Museum.*

Best Selling Styles

Women's Styles

CITIES	PATTERNS	COLORS	LEATHERS AND MATERIALS	LASTS	HEELS
NEW YORK	Oxfords, broad and narrow one-straps, step-ins and opera.	Black and brown.	Suede, patent, reptile leathers, black satin, kid velvet.	Refined toe.	14 and 15/8 Cuban; 17 to 19/8 Spanish and spike.
BOSTON	One strap patterns, oxfords, step-ins and pumps.	Brown shades, including marron, and black.	Suede, patent, kid, lizard, alligator, calfskins and fabrics.	Medium toes.	Cuban averaging 14/8; moderately high French heel.
CHICAGO	Pumps, one-straps, oxfords.	Black, brown, blue.	Suede, patent, kid, reptile.	Medium short vamp.	19/8 and 17/8.
PHILADELPHIA	One-straps, twin-straps and ties.	Black, brown, golden brown and tan.	Patent colt, satin, kid and calf.	Medium toes.	14/8-16/8.
WASHINGTON, D. C.	Oxfords, pumps.	Black, brown and pastel shades of velvets.	Suedes, velvet, reptiles and kid.	Round and medium toes.	15/8-17/8 and 19/8.
ATLANTA	Pumps and straps.	Tan and black.	Suede, kid and patent leather.	Medium toes.	———
NEW ORLEANS	One-straps.	Gray, orchid, black and brown.	Patent leather and kid.	Medium toes.	14/8 and 18/8.
CLEVLAND	Straps, pumps and ties.	Black and brown.	Patents, suedes, calf, kid and satin.	Medium toes.	14/8-16/8.
MINNEAUOLIS and ST. PAUL	Tongue and opera pump, one-strap, high riding three-eyelet ties.	Black and brown.	Patents, kid, satins and suedes.	Vamps slightly longer, toes more shapely.	Spanish and Cuban.
ST. LOUIS	Pumps, one-straps, oxfords and step-ins.	Black and Tan.	Patent, suede, kid, calf and reptile.	Narrow toes.	16/8.
OMAHA	Opera pumps and ties.	Black.	Patent, satin and suede.	Short vamps.	Spike heels.
SAN FRANCISCO	Pumps, straps, step-ins and oxfords.	Black, brown, tan and blue.	Patent, suede, kid and satins.	Medium toes.	12/8-14/8 covered Cuban; 17/8-22/8 Spanish.
LOS ANGELES	Straps, pumps, closed-up tie effects (3 and 4 eyelets).	Black, brown and midnight blue.	Patents and kids.	Medium and round toes.	14½ to 16/8 and 19 to 20/8.

It is in the 1920s that the *Shoe Retailer* began to include reports from retailers around the country about what was selling in their cities. By the late 1920s, this information was being recorded both as verbatim reports from the retailers and also in charts that listed the most popular heel heights, lasts, materials, and patterns for a number of major cities (see fig. 20). This material may eventually prove valuable to researchers attempting to define regional variation in taste within the United States, but differences in reporting terms make quick comparison difficult. The reports may reflect not just the taste of a particular city as a whole, as they purport to, but the specific clientele of the store doing the reporting—does it cater to the upscale or to the middle class? An initial review suggests that a statistical study of this information will be required to discover whether the differences are significant or not, and if they are, whether they correlate more clearly to the size of the town or to the geographic region.

Although the minute detail of the individual reports may be ambiguous, it is clear that the editors of the *Shoe Retailer* were convinced that regional differences in taste were a real force to be reckoned with, and their comments on the subject became a good deal more common after 1910. As we generally do today, they saw the country as consisting of East Coast, West Coast, Midwest, and South. Sometimes regional differences were primarily a practical matter of climate. Suedes were less worn in the South because they were perceived as a cold-weather shoe. Boots hung on longer in the cold reaches of the North than they did elsewhere in the country. The *Shoe Retailer* points out that welted oxfords were likely to sell well in cities that didn't have very good sidewalks or racks of taxis. But in the next breath they note that even small towns were paying more and more attention to style rather than just to utility.

But even after all these practical differences are set aside, some of the regional differences seem to arise purely from differences in taste and temperament. It comes as no surprise to hear that "what will 'go' in a large city will, many times, not be a good seller in the medium sized city or large town. Fads go in New York which have no standing elsewhere in the shoe business."[69] In 1911, a Lynn manufacturer noted that "full round toes are to be the predominating feature in lasts, especially for the Western trade. New York and vicinity still want medium narrow toes and do not seem to care for the high nob effects."[70] Two years later, the same distinction was still being noticed among the samples for 1914.

> The samples show all lengths of vamps, from the extreme 4-inch vamp and very narrow toe for the large city trade to the short vamp and modified high toe for the middle western trade. . . . Even for the country where they "swear by" the comfortable roomy toe and the abbreviated forepart, the new samples show slightly longer vamps and less wood on the toe of the last.
>
> These styles are really much prettier than the exaggerated styles so long in favor, and in the minds of the western salesmen should be adopted as a forerunner to the long vamp styles, which will unquestionably be in general demand before long.[71]

In 1919, when long, pointed toes had been in style for two or three years, there was talk in New York of reviving a short-vamped style called the "stage last" that was already being worn in California. Whether the West Coast was truly ahead of the styles, or whether it had never entirely abandoned the short-vamped styles of the early 1910s is unclear. "This type of last has had quite a vogue on the Pacific Coast, and the talk of reviving it as a style proposition in the East, and more especially New York, results from inquiries for this style shoe by women now in this country who spent one or more years in France during the war, where the stage last always is the fashion."[72] A modified version of the stage last did become standard beginning in 1921.

A 1924 article on shoes in the *Ladies' Home Journal* supports the idea that regionalism in taste (as opposed to merely climatic needs) was a relatively new phenomenon. "The buyer for a chain of very smart shoe stores was nearly distracted. 'That old saying about death and taxes being the only sure thing might have been originated by a boot and shoe man,' he said. 'Women certainly have us guessing. What goes in the East isn't popular in the Middle West. Out on the Coast they are apt to want an entirely different type of slipper. The result is, instead of ordering a half dozen styles and calling it a day, I have to select several dozen,' and he gave a groan of complete exhaustion."[73] Unfortunately the article does not go on to explain what the differences in taste actually were. Such subtleties, if they can ever be revealed, await the next generation of costume scholars.

CHAPTER TWO

Stepping Out or Staying In?

*Women's Shoes
and Female Stereotypes*

Preserved at the Peabody Essex Museum in Salem, Massachusetts, is a small box, only six inches by ten, and three inches deep, covered with white satin and mounted with a hinged glass lid. The only foil to its simplicity is the scrolled gold hook that serves as a latch. Beneath the fastening, stamped in gold, are the initials "C. F. W." and a date, "Sept. 1, 1858." The inside is divided into two compartments, also lined with white satin, and laid in these, like Snow White in her glass coffin, are a pair of dainty white satin shoes with rosettes of papery silk, worn but once. Their thin satin uppers are lined with linen and only barely stiffened round the back, and a long narrow flimsy ribbon is attached to each side, meant to cross and tie round the wearer's slender ankle. The soles, no thicker than thin cardboard, are only two inches wide at the widest point and there are no heels at all. This frail footwear belonged to Caroline Frances Fitz of Ipswich, Massachusetts, and was worn at her marriage to Joseph Wheeler Woods in 1858.[1]

Looking at these little slippers, one is led to imagine that the bride who thus enshrined them must have been a delicate, angelic little creature of exactly the kind praised by contemporary fiction and journalism. We see her in these tiny satin shoes, stepping into a new identity, trying to be like the young wives in countless magazine stories, gliding quietly about the house making all things neat and orderly in preparation for her husband's return, knowing that home ought to be a refuge for a man weary of wrestling with a wicked world. If she read those stories, she would know that in that refuge, her husband would expect to find a prettily dressed, daintily shod figure with a loving heart, a submissive mind, a sympathetic ear, and a well-cooked dinner. He would expect to be able to bring home his friends knowing that the hospitality she offered would be neither embarrassing by its frugality nor sumptuous beyond his means. If she read those stories, she would know how her trusting dependency on his judgment could make her husband feel strong and protective. She would know better than to oppose his will, but she would make him the object of her constant prayers, trusting that he would have little temptation to stray beyond her influence when he found such orderly peace and comfort at home. If she read those stories, we also know how to imagine her a few short years later, now become a mother, her neatly slippered foot in its snowy stocking peeping out from under her skirts to rock a new baby's cradle. Close in her arms she draws a little boy with dirty, tear-streaked face, whose mischief she is gently correcting and whose soul catches in his mother's sweetness its first glimpse of heaven.

A cliché? Of course it is, but it was one pervasive enough in early nineteenth-century America to influence the kind of shoes women were wearing then and for a long time thereafter. Unless we understand the ideal of women as "angels in the house," we will wonder why women didn't (and often still don't) wear solid, practical shoes as men do. Without this perspective, we will remain perplexed to discover that in a collection of early-nineteenth-century women's shoes, almost none are any more substantial than the hallowed white satin wedding shoes. If not actually made of satin, they are very probably silk taffeta or wool serge, or at best thin morocco leather, and like the wedding shoes, they have paper-thin soles. Many appear rather small and quite implausibly narrow. Of course it is true that today's collections represent almost entirely the dressiest shoes. But even the boots are not very stout by modern standards. They, too, are made of cloth, with a mere scrap of morocco or patent leather at the heel and toe to defend against wear. It is hard to believe that such shoes were worn even indoors, considering how cold and drafty old houses must have been when heated only by inefficient fireplaces. Surely no one could have walked—let alone worked—in them outdoors.

But contemporary accounts suggest that American women did indeed wear their thin little shoes and boots for everything but work so heavy it was beneath the reach of fashion. The English writer Frances Trollope, who lived and traveled in the United States from 1828 to 1831, remarked of American women, "They never wear muffs or boots, and appear extremely shocked at the sight of comfortable walking shoes and cotton stockings, even when they have to step to their sleighs over ice and snow. They walk in the middle of winter with their poor little toes pinched into a miniature slipper, incapable of excluding as much moisture as might bedew a primrose"[2] (see fig. 21).

English women also wore delicate shoes indoors during this period, but if Trollope is to be believed, they had enough sense to put on more substantial footwear when they went out. American women of fashion for some reason didn't. "The Cheap Dress," a story published in *Godey's* in 1845, even suggests that substantial shoes were not commonly available to women in the United States. The narrator,

Mrs. Allanby, has foolishly made a dress of cheap fabric. It has shrunk and faded at the first wash, so she decides to use it up as a gardening outfit.

> The completion of my equipment was to be the ugliest, clumsiest, stoutest pair of boots ever intended for a lady's feet—boots that had been expressly imported for me from some provincial place in Great Britain by an English friend, on the hypothesis that the slight, pretty articles manufactured for our use on this side of the ocean, were the cause of a national tendency to consumption. Hitherto I had rebelled against wearing them, but now that I had concluded upon setting up a distinct suit of habiliments for a particular purpose, I rejoiced in the possession of them.
>
> The first warm, bright day suitable for my out-door employments, came on, and I incased myself in my cheap dress, which did not quite join company with the tops of my English boots.

Inevitably, while she is out working in the garden, an old family friend named Mrs. Sanderly comes to call. Mrs. Allanby runs in to bid her welcome only to find that Mrs. Sanderly has brought with her an extremely elegant and refined young man.

> I cannot tell how I received the bow of the elegant Mr. Howard—I take it for granted that he made one. . . . All I saw was a pair of daintily-shaped boots, smooth and shining as polished jet, and the thought struck me of my English foot-garniture. Never was a belle more enraptured with an imported bonnet or mantilla than I was mortified at my imported shoes. If I had another gown, one of usual length, they would have been hidden from view, but at one time I had on *that* dress and *those* shoes. . . .
>
> [After Mr. Howard had left with Mr. Allanby], I exclaimed to Mrs. Sanderly—"Was there ever any thing so provoking? To think of my running into the room before such a stranger as Mr. Howard in such a dress! In my eagerness to receive you, my dear Mrs. Sanderly—"

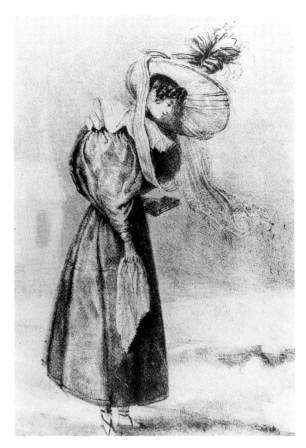

Fig. 21. *Walking in the Snow*, one of the twenty-four original illustrations for Frances Trollope's *Domestic Manners of the Americans* (1832) drawn by Mrs. Trollope's protégé Auguste Hervieu, shows one of those American ladies "who never wear muffs or boots, and appear extremely shocked at the sight of comfortable walking shoes and cotton stockings, even when they have to step to their sleighs over ice and snow. They walk in the middle of winter with their poor little toes pinched into a miniature slipper, incapable of excluding as much moisture as might bedew a primrose."

"But you had already appeared in the presence of your husband in that dress?" interposed the old lady with portentous gravity.

I understood it, yet I returned the very answer I should have avoided. "Oh, yes; but one does not mind one's husband."

"I beg pardon, my dear; you have taken an erroneous view of a very important subject. No woman should present herself before her husband in a dishabille which would cause her to blush if seen in it by any other man. The continuance of affection depends upon a strict attention to what may be trifles in themselves—"[3]

That is the beginning of a long lecture, the details of which we are spared, but that leaves the young wife thoroughly irritated. But the tone of the story leaves us in no doubt that it is Mrs. Sanderly and not the narrator who represents the voice of wisdom in this matter.

Why on earth should a wife's wearing an old dress and thick boots for gardening put her husband's affection in jeopardy? To answer this, one must understand how very thoroughly the early nineteenth century sought to differentiate the spheres of men and women. Sarah Josepha Hale, editor of *Godey's Lady's Book*, included in her editorial column in 1844 a passage from L. Aimé-Martin's *The Education of Mothers*, a French work that had recently been translated and published in Philadelphia. For Mrs. Hale, the attraction of this work was its call for women's education, which was one of her own lifelong concerns. But the passages she chose to quote also reflect another important early nineteenth-century idea, that women were coarsened and degraded by heavy outdoor labor.

"The great misfortune of our villages," says this benevolent author [L. Aimé-Martin in *The Education of Mothers*, describing France], "is the degradation of the women through the labours which belong to men. You see the women bowed to the earth, as labourers, or laden with enormous weights, like beasts of burden. There are districts in France, where they are harnessed to carts with the ox and ass. From that time their skin becomes shrivelled, their complexions like coal, their features coarse and homely, and they fall into a premature decrepitude more hideous than old age. . . . Everywhere is the degradation of the woman a sure proof of the brutishness of the man, and everywhere is the brutishness of the man a necessary consequence and reaction from the degradation of the woman."

These are shocking pictures [comments Mrs. Hale], yet sad as they are, the good Aimé-Martin sees a star or two which may rise and shed lustre on the darkness. He says—

"Two modes of amelioration offer themselves—the first is to . . . [teach young girls] how to direct the interior economy of a house. . . . The second method, a necessary sequel of the first, consists in restoring to the women of the village the natural occupations of their sex, and freeing them from the drudgery of out-door labour."

He says truly—"Never will instruction take deep root and spread in the rural districts, if it does not reach the children through their mothers, and the men through their wives. The public teacher is but a dry instrument that teaches the alphabet; the mother of the family is a moral power, which fertilizes the mind, while at the same time it opens the heart to love and the soul to charity."

No wonder that this philanthropist . . . should exclaim, while dwelling on the blessings which education, freedom and the elevated position of woman had wrought in our United States—

". . . America is the star which brightens the darkness of Europe; and the education of women the light which promises civilization to mankind."[4]

Readers conditioned by the women's movement that blossomed in the late 1960s and 1970s may see beneath rhetoric like this an attempt to shackle women to a domestic role no less restrictive than farm drudgery, to cramp her intellect and confine her achievements to housekeeping or the more trifling arts. Nevertheless, it is important to understand that in the early nineteenth century, the enthronement of woman within the home was generally perceived as an *advance* in civilization and as a sign of the increased respect in which women were held. One need only consider the position of women a century or two earlier to see what gains they had made. In the words of historian Nancy Woloch, the role of seventeenth-century woman was "defined only by deficiencies and limitations; she had no innate assets to distinguish her from a man. On the contrary, God and nature had made her weaker, in wit, will, and physical capacity. First in transgression and tainted by original sin, 'the woman is a weak creature not endued with like strength and constancy of mind,' as English parsons told their congregations. Inferior in brain and morally suspect, she depended on man to protect her interests, ensure her submission, and see that she did as little damage as possible."[5] During the eighteenth century, family structure became less rigidly patriarchal and women began to gain the respect within the home that was an essential first step on the long road to equal rights, a trend that continued in the nineteenth century. The special status women had achieved within the family was one of the American peculiarities observed by Fredrika Bremer, the Swedish novelist who traveled in America from 1849 to 1851. She reported in a letter to Carolina Amalia, Queen Dowager of Denmark,

Probably that which most distinguishes the home of the New World from that of the Old is the dominant sway which is assigned in it to woman. The rule of the American man is to allow his wife to establish the laws of home. He bows himself willingly to her sceptre, partly from affection, partly from the conviction that it is best and most just that it should be so, and from chivalric politeness to the sex; for the American believes that a something divine, a something of a higher and more refined nature, abides in woman. He loves to listen to it and to yield to it in all the questions of the inner life."[6]

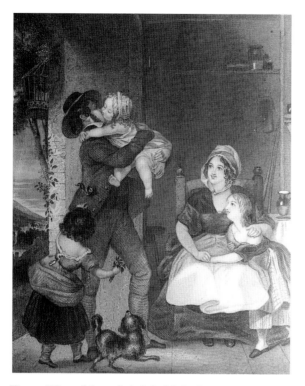

Fig. 22. "Home," from *Godey's Lady's Book,* December 1841. Even in rural America, woman's work revolved around the house and garden. When father came home, he was supposed to find a little paradise, orderly, attractive, and full of sunny, welcoming faces. But creating such a household could be overwhelming for a woman who had no help. In the 1880s, Gene Stratton-Porter wrote to her fiancé, "I sincerely believe that nine girls out of every ten, who earnestly strive to make such a home, half kill themselves at it; . . . to have [a girl] cook, wash, bake, iron, scrub, make beds, sweep, and dust—and she must be bright—oh, yes, always bright and cheerful—is enough to make a scold out of her." (Quoted in the Afterword by Joan Aiken to Stratton-Porter's *A Girl of the Limberlost,* p. 377). *Courtesy Heidi Fieldston.*

The ideology underlying this apparent deference to women is explained by journalist Park Benjamin in an 1844 *Godey's* article called "The True Rights of Woman," though it is only fair to mention that Benjamin's somewhat defensive tone arises from the fact that these ideas were being questioned in the 1840s. The antislavery movement provoked wide discussion of human rights, and some Americans began to ask why property rights and suffrage should be denied on the basis of sex any more than on the basis of color. It was the emergence of a vocal opposition to the subordination of women that provoked Benjamin's definition of woman's sphere.

> On that principle, well known to political economists and called the division of labour, man discharges a certain set of duties and woman another set. The man, for example, transacts out-of-door and the woman in-door affairs. . . . There must be a division of labour; and that which exists is unquestionably the best that could possibly be contrived. . . .
>
> Where, I may be asked, where is the proper sphere of woman? . . . Where is the seat of her dominion? My answer is—HOME!—home, which has been eloquently called "the highest, holiest place in which human agency can act."[7]

The dichotomy between the public male world and the private female world resulted from—or at least was justified by—the nineteenth-century belief that God gave men and women different innate abilities. It was therefore only right that they should operate in different spheres. Men had a virtual monopoly on gifts of the intellect and thus were preeminent in the arts and sciences. But the heart, the seat of emotional life, was underdeveloped in the male. Being kind and loving did not come naturally, and the "baser passions" were a constant temptation. The baser passions included drinking, smoking, gambling, and sex, all of which were encouraged by membership in men's clubs (for the well-to-do) and by visits to local bars (for the poor). Balancing this view of maleness was an image of women that considered them rich in emotion but correspondingly weak in intellect. At its best, a woman's emotional faculty bloomed as a refinement of moral sensibilities and strong religious sentiment. Men, by virtue of their superior intellect and judgment, had ultimate authority within the family and represented the family in the outside world, taking responsibility for the public welfare through the vote and public office. Women had responsibility for running the household and setting the moral tone within the family. Park Benjamin described this difference in innate abilities in his 1844 article:

> A great deal has been said, in these modern days, of the intellectual powers of woman, and an equality with man has, in this regard, been claimed for her. The education of the head has been determined to be of more importance than the education of the heart. I am old-fashioned enough to pronounce this all wrong. The head is educated for time, the heart for eternity. . . . In my eyes, [women] surely are angels on earth. These angelic qualities, however, are emanations from the heart. . . . The most truly sensible women do not contend for a mental equality. . . . I do, unhesitatingly, . . . assert that nothing is more susceptible of demonstration than that women are and always have been intellectually inferior to men. The exceptions confirm the fact. It can be said, with equal truth, that in all qualities of the heart—in all the virtues, it may be,—men are inferior to women.

Benjamin then goes on to describe in rather poetic language how this superior virtue is meant to function in the scheme of life.

> While I oppose the active participation of women in the stern business of life, I would not have them remain passive and indifferent spectators. Far from it;—they have an immense influence, which they ought to exert, and which they can exert in all matters of importance. This influence is greater than it would be, were it openly used. This influence is like that of the moon upon the waters of the sea;—it controls the great tides of public sentiment, and causes them to ebb and flow with majestic regularity. . . . Exert, I pray you, my fair readers, an influence, calm, steady and enduring; . . . pursue, with dauntless resolution and quiet fortitude, that direct and elevated course which the wisdom of past ages has indicated as peculiarly your own, and in which a happiness is found far superior to that bestowed by noisy distinction or evanescent power. . . .
>
> As the peculiar office of man is to govern and defend society, that of women is to spread virtue, affection and gentleness, through it. She has a direct interest in softening and humanizing the other sex. . . . Sister, mother, wife,—dear and hallowed names!—may your lustre never be tarnished, your sanctity never be profaned! May you never cease to be spells to cast out the evil passions of men, and to invoke the pure and tender affections! May you grow forever

in fragrance and freshness on the dreary way of life, causing the desert places to be glad, and the wilderness to blossom as the rose![8]

Exactly how a woman was to exert this mighty influence is not immediately obvious since she was also being exhorted never to oppose her husband's will. Even Park Benjamin's language suggests something magical about it. But note that he describes women not as actively *casting* spells, but as *being* spells, as if he is inclined to find women bewitching, but is unwilling to grant them the dread autonomy of witches. How does a woman go about being a spell? It is clear that for the mid–nineteenth century, the magic of womanhood lay primarily in the attractiveness of her appearance and then in the sweetness of her manner. Lured by a woman's appearance, the man is drawn within her sphere like a bee to a brightly colored flower. Once induced to come near, his continued attention is ensured by the charm of her manners, and through his continuing contact, he is in position to observe the integrity of her principles, the rectitude of her behavior, and the unvarying gentleness of her disposition. Thus, drinking in the sweet nectar of virtue in beautiful dress, he desires to spend more and more time in her company, where he learns to think seriously of serious matters and becomes content to live within the safety of the domestic circle.

Since her appearance was the chief weapon by which a woman forged and maintained her power for good, it was imperative that she care for it and keep it bright. It was for this reason that women were advised to wear pretty, becoming clothes made in the prevailing style. When Mrs. Allanby put on her faded, ill-fitting dress and clomping boots, she effectively disarmed herself and severed one of the silken threads by which a woman attached her husband and family to herself. It was always a mistake to think it sufficient to dress well in public while neglecting one's appearance in the privacy of the home. *Demorest's* was still warning its middle-class readers in 1883 that "the *chaussure* is another item of the home dress, which should never be neglected, for it is certain never to escape observation. A shrewd writer says, 'Many a man's heart has been kept from wandering by the bow on his wife's slipper.' Daintily dressed feet are always admired, so we would advise all young wives, and older ones, too, for the matter of that, to look well to the ways of their feet and dress them in pretty hose and neat slippers."[9]

While the American woman was, like Mrs. Allanby, subject to steady pressure to dress attractively, she was also warned not to pay too much attention to the world of fashion. She had a very fine line to tread in matters of dress. Interest in fashion was legitimate when it served to increase a woman's attractiveness (and as a result, her influence) within the family. But when she followed fashionable styles and manners in order to win personal recognition among the social elite, a woman risked ruining her family by her neglect and at last becoming the "heartless woman of fashion" who spread disaster across many a popular story. A good wife was expected to stay at home, and, in the words of the ever-eloquent Park Benjamin, "much to be deplored is any circumstance which draws a woman from this sacred sphere;—I care not whether it be fashion or fanaticism, pleasure or politics."[10] Fanaticism (in the form of religious revivals) and politics (in the form of abolitionism and women's rights) may have lured a handful of women from the home, but contemporary magazines are full of didactic stories about women who were tempted to neglect their families by the world of fashion and pleasure. In the iconography of magazine fiction, men's clubs and bars with their smoking, drinking, and gambling had their feminine counterpart in the worldliness of high society with its expensive clothing, furnishings, and parties. In one plot line typical of these stories, which were clearly intended to edify middle-class readers, the heroine discovers the hollowness of fashion and society just in time to save her husband, who, left unattended, has been turning to drink but can still be redeemed by a love content to find its duty in creating an attractive home.

Just as clothing that was too costly and fashionable betrayed a cold or straying heart, ill-fitting and unattractive clothing exposed the wearer as too lazy, thoughtless, or disorganized to create an attractive and orderly home, and proved that she was not properly managing her moral and domestic responsibilities. Mrs. Allanby's choice of clothing was doubly unfortunate in that it not only jeopardized her husband's affection for her but it also implied a serious defect in her character. In the nineteenth-century view, as expressed by Sarah Josepha Hale, dress was "something more than necessity of climate, something better than condition of comfort, something higher than elegance of civilization. It is the index of conscience; the evidence of our emotional nature; it reveals, more clearly than speech expresses, the inner life of heart and soul in a people, and the tendencies of individual character."[11]

Because a woman's appearance was felt to be the key to her moral disposition, even garments that were rarely seen played an important symbolic role in the game. Underclothing must always be clean and well-mended, because dirty, ragged underwear beneath an elegant dress suggested that the wearer cared more about outward show than inward perfection of character. Shoes lent themselves naturally to this kind of symbolism, being a part of the costume that was in

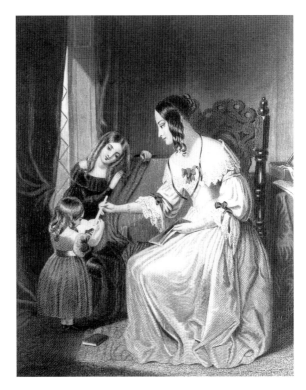

Fig. 23. "Maternal Instruction," from *Godey's Lady's Book*, March 1845. A mother's role in instructing her children and overseeing their moral development became an important reason for encouraging women's education in the early nineteenth century. By the mid–nineteenth century, "maternal instruction" was just one element of the larger sphere routinely referred to as "woman's influence." An attractive appearance played a large part in wielding this influence successfully. *Courtesy Heidi Fieldston.*

the common course of things very easily soiled, and though not immediately visible, being likely to be seen eventually. It was a temptation to let one's shoes get shoddy when they were usually hidden beneath a long skirt, and therefore it was a sign of a well-regulated character to wear shoes that were always whole, clean, polished, and neatly fitted. Neat, pretty shoes appear in nearly every description of the ideal woman well into the twentieth century.

Shoes carried additional meaning in the mid–nineteenth century, however, because they could be used to diminish the apparent size of the foot. Small feet, along with small hands, were one of the traditional attributes of a gentlewoman, evidence that she did not stand all day doing laundry or working in a mill or at any other heavy labor, but that she had a husband or father to provide for her. Just as the word "lady" came to mean not merely a woman of rank but a woman of refined character, small hands and feet often became the "outward and visible sign" used by popular authors to reveal the heroine's "inward and spiritual grace," showing that she was a lady by nature if not by birth.

In order to have little feet, many women apparently wore their shoes as tight as they could manage to squeeze into, a practice that seems to have been associated with French rather than English style. Charles Dickens noticed that "the pinching of thin shoes" was part of a fashionable American lady's appearance during his visit here in 1842,[12] and in 1850, *Godey's* graphically described the discomforts of life in a fashionable watering place, where you were expected to wear a dinner dress "as uncomfortable as stiff laces and tight corsages can make it and steam over the soup, or faint in the odor of the roasts, with your hair in Jenny Lind bandeaux, and your feet in excruciating French slippers."[13]

Flimsy shoes or gaiter boots worn painfully short and tight were a very real discouragement to physical activity, and as a result they tended to foster both dependence and domesticity. Even if a woman disregarded the pressures of fashion and wore shoes that fit, fabric boots and shoes with thin soles and no heels were not comfortable for real walking, especially on the irregular cobbles and paving stones of urban streets. Writing of her childhood in Boston in the 1820s, Mary Livermore recalled being "foot-sore with my tramp, in slippers, over the cobble-stones, for the crowd had forced me off the sidewalk" during an Independence Day celebration that called for her best clothes.[14]

No one describes the difference between men's and women's shoes better than George Sand, the French novelist, who in 1831 began dressing as a man in order to save money and still be able to attend the theater in Paris (women were not allowed in the pit, which was all Sand could afford). Sand got the idea from her mother, who had done the same thing as a young married woman because her dressing as a boy halved the household's bills.

On the Paris pavement I was like a boat on ice. My delicate shoes cracked open in two days, my pattens sent me spilling, and I always forgot to lift my dress. I was muddy, tired and runny-nosed, and I watched my shoes and my clothes—not to forget my little velvet hats, which the drainpipes watered—go to rack and ruin with alarming rapidity. . . . So I had a "sentry-box coat" [long, square, roomy, and figure-concealing] cut for me out of a heavy drab stuff, with matching trousers and waistcoat. With a gray hat and wide woolen tie, I was a perfect little first-year student. I can't convey how much my boots delighted me: I'd have gladly slept in them, as my brother did when he was a lad and had just got his first pair. With those steel-tipped heels I was solid on the sidewalk at last. I dashed back and forth across Paris and felt I was going around the world. My clothes were weatherproof too. I was out and about in all weather.[15]

Sand was not alone in her appreciation of boots. A writer for *Harper's New Monthly Magazine* in 1856 equated boots with the very possibility of male exertion and achievement, unconsciously consigning the bootless female half of humankind to insignificance.

> Do you remember, reader, the first pair of *boots* that ever encased your boyish legs? Is there any acquisition of after-life that *quite* comes up to it? . . .
>
> After all, *men* are not of much account without boots. Boots are self-reliant—they stand alone. What a wretched creature, slip-shod and discordant, is a human being without boots! In that forlorn condition he can undertake nothing. All enterprise is impossible. He is without motion—a thing fit only to have his toes trodden on. But if the thought flashes through his brain that he must be up and doing, what are the first words that rush to his lips?
>
> *"My boots!!"*
>
> Nothing else could express the fixedness of his new-born purpose. Suppose he called for his horse, or his arms, what sort of figure, having them *only*, would he cut *without his boots?* He could not ride a rod, nor hold his ground against a foe for a single inch. But give him time enough to draw on his boots, and a new man starts at once into existence, ready for any thing!
>
> You have only to say that an effort is *'bootless,'* and the folly of attempting any thing without boots becomes at once apparent. [16]

Gaiters, the feminine version of boots worn between 1830 and 1860, were made of fabric, with only little bits of thin leather added at the toe and heel. They were little better than slippers outdoors, and neither afforded much resistance to the wet. *Every Lady Her Own Shoemaker* warned readers in 1856 that "cloth gaiters should not be worn on the damp ground without India-rubbers, as the mud will soil the cloth, and if wet many times, the leather cracks, and the lower part will wear off much sooner than the upper part, and do much less service."[17] Even on a dry road, should it be unpaved, cloth shoes were not very serviceable. *Godey's,* in a September 1849 article called "Dress in Rural Districts," observed "from sad experience, that gaiters and slippers are of no use at all on unpaved roads. The dust penetrates the prunella, and defaces the patent leather in one instance, and sifts through the stocking, to the detriment of that important article of dress, and

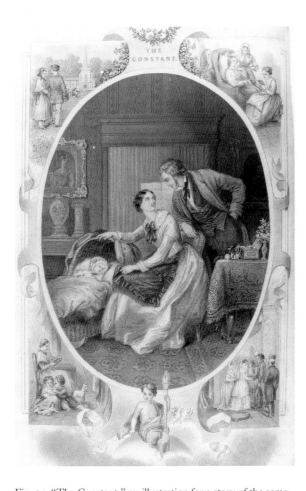

Fig. 24. "The Constant," an illustration for a story of the same name in *Godey's Lady's Book*, January 1851. Although the young husband persists in his bachelor habit of visiting his club every evening, his wife never complains. Only after overhearing an outspoken friend discussing the situation does it occur to the husband to resign from his club and spend more time at home, but the narrator considers the operative influence to be the passive and uncomplaining endurance of the wife. *Courtesy Heidi Fieldston.*

the cleanliness of person so necessary to one's self-respect." The recommended alternative was to wear morocco or kid "buskins," by which was meant shoes cut high enough to require tying. But in spite of the disadvantages, many women preferred cloth gaiter boots, because "gaiters give the foot a much smaller and more genteel appearance than a kid walking-shoe; they are easier to the foot, and if the wind blows one's skirts away from the feet, one's ankles are not so much exposed."[18]

The thin heelless soles, the permeable uppers, and the tight fit of women's fashionable shoes all conspired to keep American women indoors, and to wear them was to signal one's acceptance of the social economy by which men ruled outdoors and women (by grace of their husbands) ruled indoors. There was real risk in doing otherwise because by the terms of the deal, as Park Benjamin makes clear, women were honored only insofar as they kept to their own sphere. Women who stepped outside it and tried to live a man's life gave up their claim to male protection.

One deplorable consequence which would inevitably attend the exercise by women of political and other rights, now wholly delegated to men, would be the withdrawal from the former of that peculiar deference, tenderness and courtesy, which in all modern civilized communities,—particularly in the most refined and cultivated portion of those communities,—is universally paid to their gentleness, their delicacy, and their unostentatious worth. Let women be made ostensibly powerful; let a sense of competition be introduced; let a man be made to feel that he must stand on the defensive, and the spirit of chivalry will speedily cease—and forever extinct will be that lofty sentiment to which women can now appeal with confidence. The insecurity of weakness and the advantage of power cannot both be enjoyed.[19]

Frances Trollope (the English traveler mentioned above who commented on American women's thin shoes) experienced exactly this withdrawal of support because she did not pay sufficient attention to her clothing. One of Mrs. Trollope's projects when she lived in Cincinnati in 1828–29 was to open a sort of department store called the Bazaar. This attempt to enter the man's world of public enterprise failed utterly, we are told by her acquaintance Timothy Flint in a review of Trollope's *Domestic Manners of the Americans*, because she did not heed the business advice of American friends. He was probably right about the causes of her failure. But what is interesting is that he immediately points out that "this was not the sorest evil." The sorest evil was apparently that she was shut out of the best Cincinnati society because she did not dress well. "The ladies of the interior overdo the ladies of the Atlantic cities in dress, as imitators generally overreach their model in show and gaudiness. In such a town as Cincinnati, persons are measured by their exterior. It was to no purpose to urge that she was endowed, amusing and a blue stocking dyed in the wool. None would welcome her or receive her; save in four respectable families, and they were not families that gave parties, she was never admitted."[20] The implication is that this failure to win a place in Cincinnati society was one of the most important reasons her Bazaar failed. The point is important enough for Flint to make twice in the same article. "Had she come with numerous letters [of introduction, which she had it in her power to obtain], and been an elegant figure dressed in the most approved fashion, there is no doubt, that she would have made her way in every circle. As it was, had she made her debut in Boston, where the ladies are somewhat more in the habit of judging beyond the exterior, we dare presume she would have been a rare lioness, and a first rate show."[21]

What was so offensive about Mrs. Trollope's appearance? Flint describes her as

a short, plump figure, with a ruddy, round, Saxon face of bright complexion, forty-five, though not showing older than thirty-seven, of appearance singularly unladylike, a misfortune heightened by her want of taste and female intelligence in regard to dress, or her holding herself utterly above such considerations, though at times she was as much finer and more expensively dressed than other ladies, as she was ordinarily inferior to them in her costume. Robust and masculine in her habits, she had no fear of the elements, recklessly exposing herself in long walks to the fierce meridian sun or the pouring shower, owing a severe fever, no doubt, to those circumstances.[22]

One Cincinnati lady reported seeing Mrs. Trollope "in a green calash, and long plaid cloak draggling at her heels . . . walking with those colossean strides unattainable by any but English women,"[23] strides presumably made possible by the "comfortable walking shoes and cotton stockings" that Mrs. Trollope said American women were so "extremely shocked at the sight of." By such false steps Mrs. Trollope lost both her entrée into Cincinnati society and her success in the world of commerce.

For a woman to wear thick shoes or clumsy boots was personally foolhardy, because she risked, like Mrs. Allanby of "The Cheap Dress," losing her hold on her husband's affections. Such behavior could also be seen, as in Mrs. Trollope's

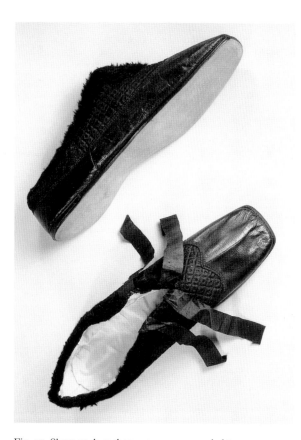

Fig. 25. Shoes such as these were recommended to wear outdoors for dressy occasions in cold weather, rather than the thin-soled prunella or kid slippers stylish American ladies seem to have preferred. While the fact that they survive proves that such shoes were known in America, it must be admitted that these show no sign of ever having been worn. They are made of a black silk woven to imitate quilting, edged with black plush, foxed with black kid, and lined with wadded white silk. The soles are welted and relatively thick. They tie with two pairs of thin black silk ribbons and date ca. 1845–55. A very similar pair, cut slightly higher, is illustrated in *Godey's,* February 1855, and is recommended as being "pre-eminently serviceable," having the advantage of "being adapted to the wear and tear of everyday use." Compare the quilted indoor shoes in fig. 49. *Courtesy friends of the author.*

case, as a challenge to the social order, less dramatic perhaps than the challenge posed by bloomers in 1851, but still potent. How could any woman expect to call up a man's protective instincts if she was clomping around in thick English boots, acting for all the world as if she could get along quite well without him? Even a servant or working girl needed to think twice before sending that message. Generally unequipped by custom or education to make her own way, a woman needed to show that she made no serious claim to the outdoor male world of public endeavor, that she admitted her need for protection, and that she accepted that men should speak for her in that world. American women did this by squeezing into their satin shoes and staying indoors.

All this raises the question why American women in particular should have felt obliged to wear thin slippers at all times and seasons when English women apparently felt free to match their shoes to their circumstances? Even twenty years after Mrs. Trollope's sad experience, American etiquette books remarked on this divergence between English and American practice. "The delicately bred fine lady in [England] puts on cotton stockings and thick shoes to walk out for exercise, and would think it very unlady-like not to be so provided; and on more dressy occasions, when she wears silk hose, she would on no account go out in cold weather without warm shoes, either kid lined with fur, or quilted silk shoes foxed with leather [see fig. 25]. To walk out, as our young ladies do, in cold and wet weather, with thin-soled prunella or kid shoes, would seem to them very vulgar; as betraying a want of suitableness, only to be accounted for by supposing the individual to be unable to provide herself with better."[24] The delicately shod "angel in the house" was not a purely American phenomenon. Her spirit was abroad in England as well. Why was departing from that role so much more difficult here in America, precisely where one would expect a republican philosophy and the practical needs of a frontier country to lead women to embrace clothing suitable for their circumstances?

One plausible hypothesis is that the fluid class structure in American society increased the pressure on women to be dependent and ladylike. In England, supposing a duchess chose to cultivate her own garden, she could wear what she pleased and there would still be no doubt about her rank. She might be an eccentric duchess, but a duchess she was still. The housemaid might dress like a duchess but would only be laughed at for her pains. But in a democracy where hereditary rank did not exist, everybody was theoretically "as good as" anybody else. This was a principle that early-nineteenth-century Americans loudly insisted upon (ignoring the obvious inconsistency of slavery), and pride made them very sensitive to any suggestion that they might be inferior. Contemporary accounts often mention girls who would come and "help" with the housework only as long as they took their meals with the family and were never referred to as servants. Americans did not willingly accept visible symbols that would tie them to an inferior class, nor was there any inducement to do so when classes were indistinct and it was possible to rise. In an era of westward expansion and of urban growth, both individuals and families often moved to areas where their backgrounds were not known. Their position in a new city or county depended on their economic condition coupled with their behavior, manners, and personal appearance. Where each person's rank was neither firmly fixed nor widely known, dress and deportment were the most immediate ways of distinguishing anyone's social class. Thus there was every reason to dress above one's condition, and Mrs. Trollope reports that American women spent proportionally more money on clothes than did their English cousins.[25] When society rewarded women who managed to dress like ladies, and being ladylike meant cultivating an aura of physical delicacy and restricting oneself to indoor pursuits, then thin indoor footwear was bound to be widely worn while heavy shoes would be shunned even when it made sense to wear them.

Public opinion was not entirely unanimous in thinking that women belonged indoors in the early nineteenth century. Even a sympathetic observer like Fredrika Bremer, who described in approving tones the elevation of American women within the family, noted the way in which the idolization of the indoor woman could be taken to an unhealthy extreme. While staying in St. Louis in 1850, Miss Bremer paid a morning visit to a newly married couple who were living in the same hotel. Her reaction to this experience portends an important new development in the evolution of cultural stereotypes regarding women, one that was signaled by a growing concern with the deleterious effects that the confinement of women indoors had on their health and the consequent demand for fresh air and outdoor exercise as a regular part of a woman's daily routine.

It was in the forenoon; but the room in which the bride sat was darkened, and was only faintly lighted up by the blaze of the fire. The bride was tall and delicately formed, but too thin, yet for all that lovely and with a blooming complexion. She was quite young, and struck me like a rare hothouse plant, scarcely able to endure the free winds of the open air. Her long, taper fingers played with a number of little valuables fastened to a gold chain, which, hanging around her neck, reached to her waist. Her dress was costly and tasteful. She looked, however, more like an article of luxury than a young woman meant to be the mother of a family. The faint light of the room, the warmth of the fire, the soft, perfumed atmosphere—everything, in short, around this young bride, seemed to speak of effeminacy. . . .

When I left that perfumed apartment with its hothouse atmosphere and its half daylight, in which was carefully tended a beautiful human flower, I was met by a heaven as blue as that of spring, and by a fresh, vernal air, by sunshine and the song of birds among the whispering trees. The contrast was delightful. Ah, I said to myself, this is a different life! After all, it is not good; no, it is not good, it has not the freshness of Nature, that life which so many ladies lead in this country; that life of twilight in comfortable rooms, rocking themselves by the fireside from one year's end to another; that life of effeminate warmth and inactivity, by which means they exclude themselves from the fresh air, from fresh invigorating life! And the physical weakness of the ladies of this country must, in great measure, be ascribed to their effeminate education. It is a sort of harem-life, although with this difference that they, unlike the Oriental women, are here in the Western country regarded as sultanesses and the men as their subjects. It has, nevertheless, the tendency to circumscribe their development and to divert them from their highest and noblest purpose. The harems of the West, no less than those of the East, degrade the life and the consciousness of woman.[26]

It is only fair to explain that calls made upon a new bride were among the most formal and ceremonious. Etiquette books countenanced the practice of drawing the shades, lighting the gas, and receiving guests in evening dress for both bridal calls and New Year's calls. Fredrika Bremer had been in the United States more than a year when she wrote this letter and presumably was already familiar with this custom. Nevertheless, the vivid contrast between the hothouse bride and the clean, bracing, outdoor air illuminated for Bremer the price a woman paid for her sovereignty indoors.

The importance of fresh air and physical exercise was at least partially understood even in the early nineteenth century. In Jane Austen's *Mansfield Park* (1814), the heroine Fannie Price (in whom sweetness, passivity, and moral strength combine with physical delicacy in a way that would become a Victorian truism) depends on riding daily to preserve her health. "If Fanny would be more regular in her exercise, she would not be knocked up so soon. She has not been out on horseback now this long while, and I am persuaded, that when she does not ride, she ought to walk."[27] Keeping saddle horses was no small expense, and riding was beyond the means of many women. For most of the nineteenth century, walking was the primary outdoor exercise available, but the tight and thin-soled cloth shoes American ladies wore were hardly an encouragement to engage in it.

This situation began very gradually to change in the mid–nineteenth century. The cause of physical exercise had been championed as early as the 1830s by some of the more progressive girls' schools, such as the Gothic Seminary in

Northampton, Massachusetts, and it became an important part of the program in the women's colleges that were founded in the 1860s, 1870s, and 1880s. Advanced education was thought by many in the mid–nineteenth century to be dangerous to female health because the mental effort it required drew blood away from the reproductive organs, resulting in physical weakness even to the point of infertility and mental breakdown to the point of insanity. Women's colleges had a strong interest in protecting their students' health if their grand experiment in higher learning was to prove a success. Therefore physical exercise was required from the beginning. At Mount Holyoke in the late 1830s, girls were required to walk one mile (or forty-five minutes) a day. In addition to the exercise provided by the required domestic work and running up and down stairs, they also interrupted their studies for a half hour of calisthenics each evening. By the 1860s, girls at school were wearing special loose-fitting, short-skirted dresses over bloomers for their gymnastic exercises and were being warned that "corsets and high-heeled boots are out of place in the gymnasium."[28]

The calisthenics of the 1830s, 1840s, and 1850s were followed by a series of sports fads: in the 1860s by croquet, in the mid-1870s by lawn tennis, in the 1880s by walking and hiking, and in the 1890s by bicycling and golf. Bathing had been practiced in America as a health cure from the eighteenth century. In the mid–nineteenth century it was transformed into a pastime, and some women even began to learn to swim (as opposed to bobbing about in wet clothing).

The clothing worn for sports was not necessarily practical. It depended whether a woman participated in games for the social opportunities they furnished or for the sake of the sport itself. Women played tennis in high-heeled shoes and tied-back skirts with trains when such fashions were considered attractive and being attractive was the point of the game. But should a woman be interested in the physical exercise for its own sake, she wore slightly shorter, less complex skirts, roomier bodices, and low-heeled shoes. "French heeled shoes are incompatible with good tennis playing."[29] These compromises were not enough to make any game easy to play, but this mattered less when a woman's success in sports was not a matter of congratulation. An 1890 pamphlet about the new game of lawn tennis remarked that,

In the opinion of some . . . critics, the woman who is unfortunate enough to defeat all others 'plays just like a man,' 'is too ungraceful for anything,' etc. But we of the other sex and, to their credit, the majority of her own, admire the woman who, for the time being, is unconscious of her personal appearance and bravely struggles against the awful handicap imposed upon her, viz., much dress and little strength. The physical superiority of the English women to those of most other nations is well known to be due to the greater amount of exercise which they take; and the English girl plays Lawn Tennis much better than the American simply because she is physically her superior, and can more easily handle a racket of adequate weight.[30]

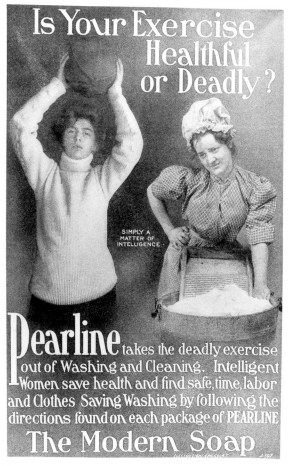

Is Your Exercise Healthful or Deadly?

SIMPLY A MATTER OF INTELLIGENCE

Pearline takes the deadly exercise out of Washing and Cleaning. Intelligent Women save health and find safe, time, labor and Clothes Saving Washing by following the directions found on each package of PEARLINE

The Modern Soap

Fig. 26. Like the story "Rev. Abiel—Convert," this advertisement for Pearline laundry soap from the *Ladies' Home Journal*, March 1903, distinguishes between the strain and fatigue caused by indoor housework and the strength and buoyancy fostered by outdoor sports. *Courtesy John Burbidge.*

By the 1890s, when the craze for bicycling swept the country, the connection between women's health and outdoor exercise was being widely promulgated. One propagandistic story, published in *The Household* in 1896, was clearly written to defend the new sport against the claim that doing housework provided sufficient exercise to make riding on unladylike bicycles entirely unnecessary. The main character, Rev. Abiel Stone, refuses to allow his daughter Clara to have a "wheel" on the grounds that it is immodest and unwomanly, yet he frets at her poor health.

He could not see why she was always tired, with the little she had to do. A girl could certainly keep house for three people, and the duties connected with the parish were slight, so he thought; at any rate it was woman's work, and the Rev. Abiel believed in woman's having her place and keeping it.

[Compared with his pale and stooping daughter, the minister is impressed by the vigor of his two young neighbors, whom he sees going about their household work next door. He considers them] "as pretty and modest girls as can be found; they are satisfied with their own sphere, and are not ashamed to do housework. As for your theory about women, Malcolm [he is speaking to his son, a doctor], that is entirely disproved, for two healthier, brighter girls I never saw. And they have some muscular strength as well. 'Twould be well if Clara patterned after them." . . .

"Oh yes," returned his son, carelessly, "the girls are both members of our tennis club, and fine players, too; Miss Stacey is practicing for the boating race in June, and they are two of the finest bicyclists in town.

"I believe they do their own work, but there are only three of them, their mother is a widow, and three women make light work. In fact, father, that muscle that you admire so much was acquired by outdoor exercise, cycling, rowing and tennis." And the young man, having taken deliberate delight in toppling over his father's idols, withdrew.[31]

Secretly, Malcolm buys his sister a bicycle and teaches her to ride, and before long Clara gains noticeably in color and vigor. The secret is exposed by a neighbor who announces, "I'm glad to see that you have bought Clara a wheel, it will build her up better than anything else; my wife declared she was going into consumption. It's a good thing, pastor, I'm of the opinion that we keep our girls too much in the house." At first Rev. Stone is furious, but he is convinced of the bicycle's virtue when his neighbor Miss Stacey rides off like the wind to retrieve a forgotten sermon just before church, and by the end of the story he is even enjoying the healthful benefits of bicycle-riding himself. And although the reader suspects that Malcolm and Miss Stacey will make a match, the author, intent on his main message, refuses to confirm it.

During the second half of the century an important new ideal of womanhood was evolving, and Rev. Stone's athletic young neighbor Miss Stacey is a good example of it. While not necessarily "strong-minded" or anxious to escape the duties of home, this new American breed of woman, christened the "Gibson Girl" after the illustrations of Charles Dana Gibson in the 1890s, is healthy, strong, active, even muscular. She is competent, self-confident, and able to think and act for herself. Instead of fainting or having hysterics when faced with an emergency, she swings onto her wheel and races for the doctor. The growing fashion for physical culture was one of the most important elements in this metamorphosis. Participating in outdoor sports also gave women new opportunities for enjoying companionship with men, and a whole class of leisure activities that had previously lain within a solely masculine sphere now became common ground. In 1884, one commentator in *Godey's* noted,

> There was a time which most of us remember, when feminine accomplishments had a range wholly different from what they have now. The whole charm of fashionable womanhood once lay in that sweet assiduous languor which suggests a flower-like frailty and a disposition too delicately refined to bear the bustle of life on the ordinary plane. But—other times, other manners! In this enlightened era of society, the Amazon type is much more admired than the statuesque loveliness of a drowsy Cleopatra; Di Vernon takes precedence in popular favor over a whole train of Lydia Languishes. In a word, this is an athletic era, and it is the fashion in elegant society to affect all the rousing, rollicking sports which were once the censured pastime of a hoyden.[32]

The sister of the physically vigorous Gibson Girl in the later nineteenth century was the intellectually vigorous "new woman," often college-educated, often single, often active in social causes. The new woman took the old feminine ideal, disproved the part about female intellectual inferiority by going to college, and then played the card of female moral superiority for all it was worth. Women's sphere may have been the home, but these women argued confidently that home did not stop at the front gate. The holiness of the domestic sphere was contaminated by such "outside" abuses as drunkenness, prostitution, and adulterated

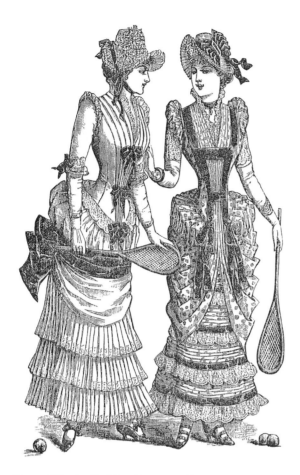

Fig. 27. "Hoydens" of the 1880s were still not very well equipped for strenuous sports. *Godey's Lady's Book*, July 1884.

food products, and the new woman claimed that it lay within her sphere to carry on a public crusade against them. By combining in a wide variety of women's associations, from the Women's Christian Temperance Union to the local literary club, women learned how to work together to create change both within their personal lives and outside the home. Thus the domestic sphere within which women had been granted increased power and authority in the early nineteenth century became the platform from which women made their entrée into the public world of men by century's end.

In tandem with the growing recognition that fresh air and exercise improved women's health and appearance and that women had legitimate business outside the house, public opinion also began to be more tolerant of sensible, thick-soled walking shoes. As early as October 1854, *Godey's Lady's Book* illustrated a cloth boot that it described as being "adapted for rougher weather and for the cold ground, the soles being stouter." The editor then observed, "We need not remark upon the wisdom of selecting this, as prudent ladies (and we trust that our habitual readers are all so) will not require admonition upon this subject. Alas! how many that were among the most prized and lovely have, by thoughtlessness or vanity, sunk into a premature grave from that apparently trifling cause, a thin-soled shoe!"

Having offered this requiem for all those American ladies Mrs. Trollope saw walking through the snow in their satin slippers, *Godey's* in the succeeding years provided growing evidence that a new era was in the making. In February 1860, the fashion editor from *Godey's* announced after having visited Genin's Bazaar, one of the new department stores in New York City: "From Mr. Bowden of the shoe department, we learn that thick walking boots for ladies are universal this winter, and no one will be required by elegance or fashion to shiver along in thin soles. We have examined three or four styles of buttoned boots, and congress [elastic-sided] boots with heels and soles a half inch thick, lined with cloth, Canton flannel, or flannel, and costing $4.50 to $6.50." Elsewhere in the same issue we are also told that "the soles are sensibly thick, the toes and heels compare favorably with a gentleman's boots in that respect." Although the appearance of thick soles sounds here like the sudden whim of some arbitrary fashion deity, the real implication is that there was a growing market within the fashionable world for more sensible footwear.

The idea that men's boots or shoes were a desirable model for women's footwear is a recurring theme in the second half of the nineteenth and early twentieth centuries and the comparison with men's footwear is found in every decade from the 1860s on. The characteristics considered masculine include a broad last that didn't cramp the foot, a thick projecting sole, and a sensible low heel. In 1874, we read that "ladies' walking boots are made with thick projecting soles, like those worn by the gentlemen, and with low, broad heels. The high French heel is entirely out of fashion."[33] The comparisons made with traditional feminine footwear suggest that many women's shoes had been torture to wear. New practical walking boots were praised in 1885 because they had roomy toes and "the sole of the foot is broad enough to allow of promenading without having to stop every few moments to give a rest to the pinched and rebellious foot."[34] "The walking mania promises to be again a feature of the season [in 1883], and ladies who have tried easy shoes, with medium width soles and toes, are in no mood to return again to bondage. Heels are wider and lower . . . and very pretty and stylish shoes are to be found which fulfill all of the conditions of good sense and health."[35]

By 1899, the masculinization of women's walking footwear had become very pronounced. "Shoes made on a man's last, laced in front, with broad, projecting sole, and round, boxed toes, with low, flat heels, are worn exclusively for the street, both in tan and black."[36] "A thin shoe on the street is bad form, as is the narrow pointed toe formerly worn. The shoes must be as roomy as the gloves to allow for moving the toes, and doing their work in making a light, easy carriage. They are made in black, dark red, and tan calfskin, many of them having an inner lining of calf the same as in men's boots."[37] The interest in masculine footwear continued strongly until about 1920. "Speaking of mannish shoes [in 1911], *The Shoe Retailer* has observed one line of mannish button 'half-boots,' which have a strong masculine look in lasts, patterns, whole quarters, calf upper stock, large buttons and heavy perforations. They will evidently fill a large city demand for this kind of footwear, and they have much to recommend them on account of their sturdy and stylish qualities. Women do not appear to be any longer desirous of putting their feet in prison and the masculine idea rather tends to comfort and service."[38] Shoes such as these were made in the factories in Brockton and other towns south of Boston that had always specialized in the making of men's shoes.

Despite the winds of change that had begun to approve sturdier and more athletic types of female beauty, and more intellectual and public-spirited types of female character, the older ideal of the marriage-oriented ladylike woman also persisted. In its July 1904 issue, *McCall's* included a short essay on "Fashions and Manners" that idealized the women of the early nineteenth century and connected their decline to the rise of practical footwear.

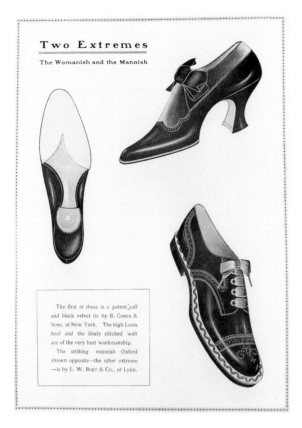

Two Extremes

The Womanish and the Mannish

The first of these is a patent calf and black velvet tie by B. COHEN & SONS, of New York. The high Louis heel and the finely stitched welt are of the very best workmanship.

The striking mannish Oxford shown opposite—the other extreme—is by E. W. BURT & CO., of Lynn.

Fig. 28. "Two extremes, the womanish and the mannish," from the *Shoe Retailer*, May 22, 1901, p. 28. The shoe above is for dressy wear and incorporates feminine qualities such as a high Louis heel, thin sole, and narrow toe. The lower shoe is a woman's walking shoe incorporating masculine qualities, including a low heel, thick extension sole, broad toe, and extensive perforation. The disparity between the two styles reflects the diversity in female roles and ideals at the turn of the century. *Courtesy Lynn Museum.*

This season sees a revival in a prettily modified form, of the dainty and quaint fashions of 1830. They are adapted to modern requirements and tastes but retain their dignity and quaint gentle womanly look, and are therefore becoming to nearly every one and admired by all. . . .

What an excellent thing it would be if, with the revival of 1830 fashions, there should be a revival of 1830 manners, the manners that made our grandmothers, whether they lived in a palace or a cabin, dames of high degree. For in those days rudeness of manners such as one so often finds now, was quite unknown. It seemed to come in together with heavy boots, but in the day when women wore only thin shoes or thinner slippers, their steps and their voices were lighter, less hurried, less boisterous. And yet there were merry times among young people we are told, and far more marriages in proportion to the population than there are now. The stately manners were not only practised in public but in the home as well, and the behavior of children to parents, of husbands and wives to each other and of brothers and sisters was kept to a strict line of politeness. Those were the days of placid faced women and rosy girls, for good manners generally help to make all things go smoothly, and wrinkles will not come nor red cheeks go where there is harmony. Then let us try to regain the manners with the fashions of 1830![39]

In 1913, a writer calling himself "Bob, the Gibson Man" wrote an article for *Ladies' World* called "My Ideal Sweetheart" in which the early twentieth-century incarnation of sweet wifeliness is vividly described.[40] When asked what his ideal girl looks like, the Gibson Man answers that the particular style does not matter, but she should wear no makeup beyond powdering her nose and she must walk and dress modestly. On the subject of dress, he begins by saying, "First, she must be daintily shod. A run-down heel, or a cracked or ugly shoe will ruin the prettiest dress effects that were ever planned."

The only "accomplishment" he really cares about is that she have an "old-fashioned knowledge of housework. This is where nearly all the girls I have known have failed utterly." But his ideal sweetheart knows all about cooking, and "with her needle she is almost magically clever." He doesn't care whether she can sing or paint as long as she doesn't try unless she is very good at it (presumably a mediocre performance would embarrass him). In exchange, he offers a pleasant home, sufficient income, the pledge to remember romantic anniversaries and always to treat her as a sweetheart.

The Gibson Man permits his ideal sweetheart a few faults, especially those that reflect well on himself. "Perhaps she is vain of her personal appearance, and I cannot blame her for it. . . . I know that because she loves me she will wish to appear attractive to my eyes. Wherefore I shall take a pride in her adornment and regard it as a tribute to myself. I can imagine her as being unduly extravagant in some details of her dress. . . . I only ask that none of her expenditures shall be on a scale beyond our means. I can imagine her, too, as having that feminine weakness of always setting an especially elaborate table for guests." It is ironic that a woman is now belittled for what had formerly been a virtue—that her table should reflect well on her husband as a provider.

This statement of the ideal relationship between men and women in 1913 differs little except in tone from the one laid out by writers seventy years before. If anything, the ideal wife has lost ground and is a more trivial person than her grandmother. She is not even granted that moral authority that had been a woman's special contribution to marriage in the 1840s. The ideal sweetheart is permitted a few superstitions "such as lucky days, lucky numbers and lucky stars," as if she is not fully rational, but she is not expected to have any central core of religious and moral rectitude, perhaps because religious sentiment was losing credibility in an increasingly scientific age. It is as if that particular brand of goodness had been siphoned off into the world of the single, college-educated, professional woman, who expressed her inborn yearning for service not within the family but as a settlement worker, librarian, teacher, or nurse. Stripped of these qualities, the ideal wife is prized chiefly as an efficient domestic servant and consumer who in the husband's absence cares for the kitchen and the collar box, and in his presence functions as a prettily dressed sexual toy, building her husband's ego by letting him feel how superior he is to her charming childishness.

Thus the relatively unified ideal of womanhood promulgated in the early 1800s splintered by the 1880s and 1890s into three major types: the athletic comrade to a crowd of admiring young men, who became known as the Gibson Girl; the college-educated, serious-minded career woman, who found her companions among other like-minded women; and the ideal sweetheart and housewife. Stories and articles in women's periodicals in the early twentieth century strongly suggest a need to confine women's advancement within tolerable limits. Perhaps it was just as well that women were better educated and got more exercise, but to allow women the same prerogatives as men raised deep fears.[41] As scientific thinking became increasingly esteemed, it is not surprising that the theory of evolution and other scientific concepts were used to reinforce the boundaries around women's roles. In a 1912 *Ladies' Home Journal* article, "Are Athletics Making Girls Masculine?" Dr. Dudley Sargent goes so far as to imply that to allow women to participate fully in typically masculine public and competitive pursuits was to return to a more animal-like condition.

> In the early history of mankind men and women led more nearly the same life, and were therefore more nearly alike physically and mentally than in the subsequent centuries of civilization. This divergence of the sexes is a marked characteristic among highly civilized races. Co-education and participation in occupations and recreations of certain kinds may have a tendency to make the ideals and habits of women approximate those of men in these highly civilized races. But such approximation would not belong to the progressive stages of the evolution of mankind. . . . These biological theories, although usually considered in connection with the evils of co-education, are equally applicable to the consideration of the evils which have followed the entrance of women into commercial life, and must follow them into competitive athletics which are regulated according to men's rules and standards.[42]

The scientific references may be new, but the essential idea, that limiting women to the domestic sphere is a characteristic of higher civilizations, is in fact identical to the views expressed by Aimé-Martin and quoted by Sarah Josepha Hale in *Godey's* in 1844.

Shoes of the late nineteenth and early twentieth centuries reflect the period's ambivalence about women's proper sphere. Although sensible walking boots or shoes were available from the 1860s on and were sometimes even fashionable, the traditionally feminine factors in footwear (tight fit, thin sole, high heel, and narrow toe) continued without much abatement among the dressier kinds of shoes. The frequency with which the habit of wearing tight shoes comes under attack from the 1870s on suggests that it was still extremely widespread even though it was increasingly hard to justify. In 1881, *Godey's* sputtered, "Why it should be desirable to have a small, weak foot any more than a small and weak brain, is not easy to conceive. For the purpose of having such small feet, not a few wear boots one or two sizes too small and about two-thirds of the width of the foot as it would be at the ball if allowed to spread as it does when standing without the confinement of the boot."[43]

The predilection for tight shoes and boots in the later nineteenth century relates to the demand for a "perfect fit" as one of the critical distinctions of a well-dressed lady. In an age when the dress was expected to conform to the corseted torso with perfect smoothness, a "perfect" fit easily degenerated into one that was merely tight. "Be always careful when making up the various parts of your wardrobe, that each article fits you accurately," wrote one etiquette book in 1876. "A stocking which is too large, will make the boot uncomfortably tight, and too small will compress the foot, making the shoe loose and untidy. . . . A shabby or ill fitting boot or glove will ruin the most elaborate walking dress, while one of much plainer make and coarser fabric will be becoming and lady-like if all the details are accurately fitted, clean, and well put on."[44]

The arguments against tight shoes were made on grounds of both health and beauty, and may owe something to the aesthetic movement of the early 1880s. *Demorest's* remarked in 1883 that "small feet are not as fashionable as they were. The aesthetic craze has even extended to the toes, and a diversion in favor of shapely feet has set in. The current is rather weak as yet, but 'faint lilies' in the agonies of tight boots would never do."[45] The inartistic effects tight boots could produce are graphically described in an etiquette book of the period:

> If a modern artist succeeds in painting a perfect foot, it must be looked upon as the result of inspiration, for surely he can find no models among the shoe-tortured, pinched and deformed feet of the men and women of the present day. The writer of this book not long since had an opportunity to examine the feet of a modern fashionable lady—feet which, encased in their dainty gaiters, were as long and narrow and as handsomely shaped as the most fastidious taste could require. But what a sight the bare foot presented! In its hideous deformity there was scarcely a trace of its original natural shape. The forward portion of the foot was squeezed and narrowed, the toes were pressed together and moulded into the shape of the narrow shoe. The ends of the toes, with the nails, were turned down. . . . [The outline of the big toe] formed one side of a triangle, of which the little toe and the ends of the intermediate toes were the second side. . . . In addition to this, the toes and the ball of the big toe were covered with corns and calluses. This deformity and disease, existing, no doubt, in many a foot, we are called upon to regard as beauty when hidden in its encasing shoe![46]

Another argument leveled by *Demorest's* in 1883 against the fashion for small feet and tight shoes was the toll it took on family harmony: "Nothing so utterly destroys amiability and good temper as ill-fitting or too tight shoes. Many a child has been punished for viciousness when its shoes should have been taken off and destroyed. How many domestic infelicities are traceable to tight shoes and boots, proper consideration for the sanctity of the home circle forbids us to inquire. At all events let us hope for more sunshine as the feet expand."[47]

But women's magazines spoke with forked tongues. The fashion-plate figures with their ridiculously tiny feet outweighed thousands of mere words inveighing against tight shoes. And even the verbal message was ambiguous. In a single breath one writer managed to acknowledge in 1873 the foolishness of tight shoes and yet to describe the beautiful foot as a small one: "The prettiest foot is dearly paid for by the pain a tight boot entails."[48] But as we all know, the price paid, whether in money or pain, never made anything less fashionable.

Unable in good conscience to approve the habit of buying shoes too small for the feet, magazine writers still pandered to fashion by pointing out styles that would make the feet appear smaller. An 1879 article on shoes in *Demorest's* begins by stating dutifully but without conviction that "a foot to be beautiful need not be very small," but quickly betrays the continuing obsession by pointing out that buttoned boots were universally favored because "a large foot has the size broken and interrupted, so to speak, by the line of the buttons, and a small foot appears still smaller so encased."[49] Black shoes were recommended from at least the 1850s right through the 1920s because they made the foot appear smaller. In 1862, *Godey's* felt that "for evening dress . . . black satin slippers are the most suitable and becoming, as they reduce the apparent size of the foot."[50] A contributor to *Ladies' Home Journal* in 1892 could "not recommend a white shoe, for even the foot of a Cinderella looks large and ill-shaped in it."[51] Four years later, the same journal remarked that "a colored shoe makes the foot appear two sizes larger—a fact that makes many hesitate in buying either tan or white ties."[52]

Considering this continuing fixation, it is not surprising that the association of small feet with a ladylike and refined character persisted into the later nineteenth century and beyond. American fiction is full of girls who did not have the advantages of wealth (at least at the beginning of the story) but whose country upbringing gives them kinder hearts and more delicate sensibilities than the beautiful society girls with whom they are regularly contrasted. These late-nineteenth-century heroines may be taller than their predecessors; they may be independent and firm-principled, and committed to education and self-improvement; they may be robust in health and enjoy outdoor activities. But they cannot have big feet. Elnora Comstock, heroine of Gene Stratton-Porter's 1909 *Girl of the Limberlost,* is just such a girl. Although raised on an impoverished farm beside the Limberlost (a great swamp in Indiana), she is a true lady in all the ways that count. As the story opens, Elnora goes to high school for the first time in her country clothes and heavy high shoes and is mortified by the sniggers of the other girls and dismayed at the cost of books and tuition. "She should have remembered how her clothing would look, before she wore it in public places. Now she knew, and her dreams were over. She must go home to feed chickens, calves, and pigs, wear calico and coarse shoes, and pass a library with averted head all her life. She sobbed again."[53] Luckily, Elnora is befriended by her elderly neighbors, Wesley and Margaret Sinton, who buy her the new dresses and shoes she needs both to fit comfortably in her new environment and, the author makes clear, to reflect the delicacy of the inward woman:

> Wesley opened a box and displayed a pair of thick soled, beautifully shaped brown walking shoes of low cut. Margaret cried out with pleasure.
> "But do you suppose they are the right size, Wesley? What did you get?"
> "I just said for a girl of sixteen with a slender foot." . . .
> Wesley picked up one and slowly turned it in his big hands. He glanced at his foot and back to the shoe.
> "It's a little bit of a thing, Margaret," he said softly. "Like as not I'll have to take it back. It don't look as if it could fit."
> "It don't look like it dared do anything else," said Margaret. "That's a happy little shoe to get the chance to carry as fine a girl as Elnora to high school."[54]

When Elnora tries them on, it is no surprise (to this reader at least) that she finds them "just a trifle large." Elnora may have been a modern girl in her love of the outdoors and her quest for education, but she was a daughter of the 1840s when it came to her feet.

For women who procured their small feet by wearing tight shoes, the discomfort was only increased by lasts that had no relationship to the natural shape of the feet. In one of the worst periods, the mid-1890s, vamps were drawn out in long "needle points." When this went out of fashion, toes became oval but still so shallow there was insufficient room for the foot. In 1904 *The Woman's Magazine* remarked caustically, "All dress hats must be large. All dress shoes must be small—they are made to fit fashionable lasts, not feet."[55]

One stratagem for making the feet look smaller was to wear even on the street a turned shoe, which owing to the exigencies of its construction has a single, thin, flexible sole that does not add bulk to the foot. Sears included "A Word to the Ladies" in the beginning of the shoe section in its 1897 catalog, which read "Ladies often complain that the soles of their shoes do not wear well. This is undoubtedly because they wear a light hand-turned shoe, when they really should have a Goodyear Welt or a McKay sewed shoe. The hand-turned shoe has a very thin sole and is designed principally for indoor and dress wear. The McKay sewed shoe has a heavier sole, and consequently will wear longer." Men were told in blunter terms, "A good many men buy a fine calf or kangaroo shoe and expect it to give the same service as a plow shoe. A fine shoe is not intended for heavy wear any more than a top carriage is intended to carry a load of wheat. . . . Don't wear a thin shoe for street or rough wear."

American women did not take the advice. The *Shoe Retailer* is full of remarks about the strong predilection for turned shoes that became particularly noticeable after 1910. It noted in 1913 that "turn footwear is expected to exceed all past records for popularity, notwithstanding that this style of shoes does not give as good nor as satisfactory wear as a light welt, but the demand seems to be for extremely light

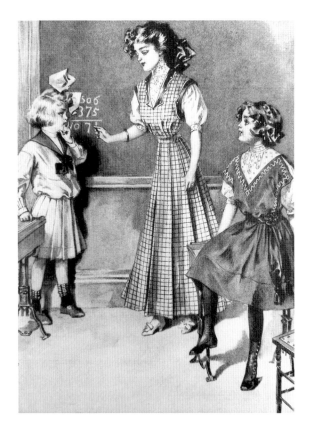

Fig. 29. Elnora Comstock, heroine of *A Girl of the Limberlost*, longed to be dressed like the miniature-footed schoolgirl in this fashion plate from the *Delineator*, September 1908, p. 359. *Courtesy John Burbidge.*

shoes, which women say they have found in shoes made by the turn method."[56] This desire for light, feminine, indoor shoes in the 1910s may possibly be reflecting the contemporary desire to reunite women with the indoor domestic life. But the demand for turned shoes in the teens also clearly relates to the shortening skirt. Once the entire foot was visible all the time, rather than merely peeping in and out, the contrast between large-footed reality and pygmy-footed fashion plate must have come as something of a shock. No wonder turned shoes were popular.

Considering the strength of the cultural preference for small feet, it is interesting to consider why substantial footwear was able to gain even what ground it did. The broadening arena in which women lived their lives has already been mentioned. But it may be equally significant that substantial footwear began to be tolerated only when heels came into widespread use, about 1860. The shift toward shoes in somewhat larger sizes with box toes around 1900 also occurred in conjunction with an increase in the height of the heel. The connection between the two events lies in the fact that heels tend to reduce the apparent size of the foot, thus canceling out the increase in size brought about by wearing stiffer, larger shoes. A *Ladies' Home Journal* article of 1908 suggests that this was one of the most important reasons for wearing heeled shoes. "All women like pretty feet. To enhance the attractiveness of this important point they wear high heels for three reasons. The first is that the coveted highly-arched instep is secured; the second is that the height is increased, and the third is that the foot is actually shortened in its new unnatural position by at least half an inch, measured from toe to heel. This shortening is augmented by placing the shoe heel far forward under the shoe, thus decreasing the apparent length of the foot by from one to two inches."[57]

When heels first returned to general use in the 1850s, theorists had their doubts, chiefly about the aesthetic effect. "Heeled boots are not entirely to be objected to; but care should be taken that the heel be not high, for, if so, it entirely destroys the grace of the body by throwing it out of its perpendicular; and a lady, instead of becoming like a graceful pillar, resembles rather a leaning tower, and that most awkwardly so."[58]

The relationship between heeled shoes and posture was complicated by wearing stiff corsets. The specific effect depended on the cut of the corset and how tightly it was laced. An inflexible corset that limited the natural compensatory tilt of the pelvis would force the wearer to bend her knees slightly in order to keep her balance, as Claudia Kidwell and Gretchen Schneider recognized in their work on eighteenth-century posture and movement.[59] With knees locked, the wearer of a tightly laced corset and high heels tended to tilt forward, a posture that was the butt of satirists when higher heels came into fashion in the later 1860s (see fig. 30). Later nineteenth-century corsets seem to allow enough pelvic tilt and protruding stomach so that wearing low heels would not be particularly difficult. After 1900, however, the new straight-fronted corset must have made it a good deal harder to keep one's balance. The new cut exaggerated the pelvic tilt, but at the same time it suppressed the protruding stomach and created an exaggerated forward pitch of the upper body. The higher heels now fashionable encouraged this forward pitch, and to lead with the bust became a hallmark of the stylish woman's posture. In its day, the straight-fronted corset was considered a healthful development because it did not push in against the abdomen at the waist, but it must in fact have been very hard on the back, and perhaps was the real culprit responsible for the list of ills described in a 1908 article castigating high heels:

> The first and immediate result of wearing high heels is a general bodily discomfort. One tires more easily, is more irritable, and symptoms of nervous breakdown arise . . . the upper part of the body is thrown forward [and] in this position it is impossible to keep the shoulders thrown back. They fall forward and the chest sinks in. Full or normal breathing is impossible, and . . . as a result . . . every organ of the body suffers. . . . Sooner or later [these changes] transform the girl of spirit into a listless person; the rosy cheeks to pale ones; the erect figure to stooped shoulders; the healthy, hearty, robust person to a semi-invalid or a total one.[60]

This is not the impartial voice of reason speaking but the partisan spirit that glorified the virtues of the athletic girl and connected heels with all the negative aspects of the traditional indoor woman: poor health, weakness, and irritability. Doctors today would probably not concur with so extreme an assessment. However, while heels alone are unlikely to cause complete invalidism, it is true that habitually wearing high heels causes measurable anatomical changes. Calf muscles may shorten to such a degree that not only does it become uncomfortable to wear flat shoes, but knee or foot problems may also result. In addition, a woman wearing heels increases the sway of her back to maintain her balance, making her abdomen and buttocks protrude. The medical term for this is *hyperlordosis*. It can aggravate lower back problems and is the reason doctors today recommend against choosing high heels for common wear.

As long as skirts were long, the heel served chiefly to shorten the foot and alter the posture as described

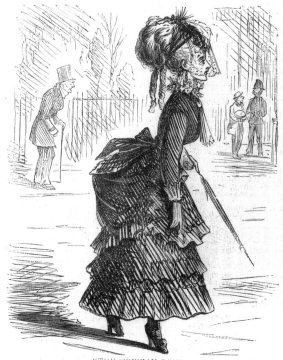

"THE GRECIAN BEND."
Does not Tight-Lacing and High Heels give a Charming Grace and Dignity to the Female Figure?

Fig. 30. "The Grecian Bend," from *Harper's Bazar*, November 6, 1869. The interaction of corset, bustle, and high heels produced a new fashion in posture in the late 1860s. *Smithsonian Institution Photo No. 82-3808.*

above. But once hemlines were shortened sufficiently to reveal the calf as well as the ankle, heels were also valued because they made the leg seem longer, an aesthetic advantage when the body line was broken not only at the waist but also at the bottom of the skirt. In addition to lengthening the leg, high heels cause the shortened calf muscles to distinctly bunch out. This conspicuous musculature of the calf makes the ankle below look longer and more slender by contrast. This was described as early as 1928 in the advertisements of the Julian and Kokenge Company of Cincinnati, makers of Foot Saver Shoes. "Foot Saver Shoes mean slender ankles. . . . Every Foot Saver design is executed in lines of slenderness for the foot—lines that lure the eye to the incurving contours of the ankle, and carry it to the outcurving contours of the calf!"[61] The same effect was described with equal approval as recently as 1989 in a *New York Times Magazine* article by Linda Wells entitled "Ups and Downs." Wells recounts how beauty pageant contestants, no longer permitted to wear high heels with swimsuits, chose to go barefoot instead, "padding down the runway on tiptoes to give their legs a long, tight look," and succinctly explains that "high heels do more to flatter the legs than flats do, mostly because they make the legs look fit and shapely." The *Times* article suggests that the distinct calf muscle is particularly attractive to us today because it suggests a physically fit body. The inconsistency between high heels and healthful physical exercise does not seem to bother anyone.[62]

The "lean and leggy" look has been a mainstay of the fashionable silhouette ever since legs came into view seventy-five years ago. Since the 1920s unnaturally long legs have been routinely incorporated into fashion illustration, where sartorial ideals are blissfully unhampered by the common realities of the female body. And now that photography plays so large a role in fashion advertising, no girl has a chance at serious modeling unless she looks as if she has been stretched on Procrustes' bed. Overpowered by these unrealistic images (one recent ad proclaimed "Legs Can Never Be Too Long or Too Sexy"), the ordinary quantity of leg revealed below the skirt now appears distastefully short and dumpy, especially in the unfortunate woman who is relatively long-waisted and short-legged. High heels help correct this artificial defect and make long legs look more fashionable still.

The kinship between footwear and gender roles is an ongoing theme, and the pattern established in the early twentieth century continues today. On the one hand, women are increasingly accepted as athletic beings, and the interest in physical fitness has encouraged the acceptance of more muscular types of beauty with larger feet. These larger feet appear on almost all occasions in athletic shoes that by the traditional standards of feminine footwear are rather bulky and clumsy. In this category of footwear, men and women may choose from essentially identical shoes. But the farther one moves away from purely practical footwear, the more likely it is that functional differences will be introduced to differentiate male and female footwear, until at the dressiest extreme, women's shoes are distinguished by all the traditional feminine characteristics, thin soles, thin uppers, narrow toes, and very high, slender heels. Although more conservative styles are

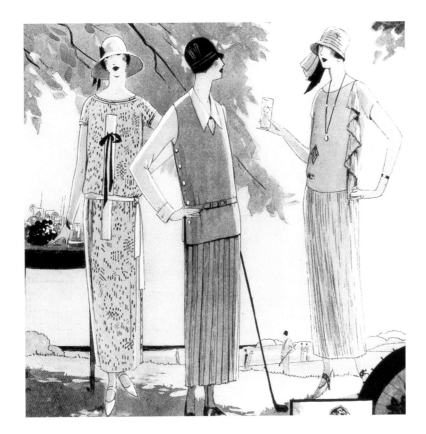

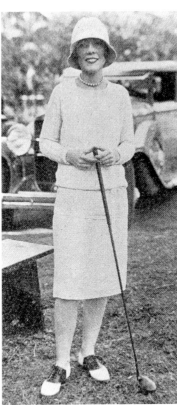

Fig. 31. Most people have a height of seven to eight times the length of their heads. The chic slenderness of the golfer in the *Vogue* illustration is achieved by making her an unlikely nine and a half heads tall. The Philadelphia society woman playing golf at Palm Beach in 1928, no matter how well-dressed she is, cannot compete in elegance with such elongated images. *Left: Vogue,* July 15, 1923, p. 65. *Courtesy Colonial Dames, Boston. Right: Shoe Retailer,* January 28, 1928, p. 31. *Courtesy Lynn Museum.*

usually available for women who aim at a professional look, extremely high thin heels and pointed toes continue to recur often in the fashion cycle, and whenever heels become high enough to make it more difficult to run or walk, they function as powerful symbols of feminine helplessness and sexual opportunity. This has perhaps always been true. An eighteenth-century rhyme runs "Mount on French heels when you go to a ball, 'Tis the fashion to totter and show you can fall."[63]

While high heels may be considered sexy (and taken to the extreme, they are a symbol of female bondage and the object of fetishism), it does not follow that flat shoes signify female independence and equality. Moderate heels that allow easy walking may in fact suggest that a woman wishes to even the field on which she deals with men. And now that heels have been standard formal wear for women for well over a hundred years, a moderately heeled shoe strikes most people today as a necessary part of the image a professional woman needs to project.

In this sense the low-heeled pump functions today much like a moderately laced corset did in the 1880s. Neither one actually increases a woman's capacity for movement or action. Neither one is functional in any practical, physical sense, but both are powerfully functional on the symbolic level. The 1880s woman in her corset and the 1990s businesswoman in her heeled shoes indicates her willingness to bear a certain amount of discomfort in order to create an appearance that will reflect well on her company and on herself. Both high heels and corsets (like the tightly buttoned collar and tie for men) are signs that the wearer is a self-disciplined, well-regulated, mature adult prepared to act in the public world and to accept the rules of that public world even when they conflict with personal comfort.

While the greatest gender differentiation occurs in dressier shoes, significant if subtle differences also appear in footwear worn for everyday. The distinctions in athletic shoes are particularly interesting, because it is here that men's and women's worlds and roles overlap. Apparently, we are so ambivalent about merging gender roles that we feel that it is essential to identify gender at least on the symbolic if not on the functional level. Thus men's athletic shoes sold in the author's neighborhood in 1990 were trimmed with primary colors, usually red and blue, or fluorescent lime green, while the trim on women's athletic shoes was rigidly restricted to the pink/purple range, with the addition of turquoise/aqua. The identical color stereotyping was even more pervasive in children's clothes, presumably because children's bodies do not by themselves always make gender obvious.

An even more thought-provoking example of gender distinction that also appeared in 1990 was an advertisement for Keds's "track shoes."[64] The ad shows an attractive young couple in informal clothing walking arm in arm along a railroad track. The picture speaks strongly of a companionate and egalitarian relationship between the sexes. The man and woman appear to be wearing identical white canvas "sneakers," but in fact the man's version has a padded collar that relates it to the athletic shoe. The woman's version has no padded collar, implying that she is not likely to be as active and would prefer not to have bulk added to her feet. The names of these new Keds shoes are given in fine print at the bottom of the ad, and one glance proves that two centuries of tradition are living still. Although the photograph shows them in a moment of shared experience, the man in this ad, like his grandfathers before him, is striding forth to conquer the world in shoes called "mainsails," while the woman, wearing "anchors," still provides a haven of peace at home.

CHAPTER THREE

A Chronological Overview
of Shoe Fashions

The earlier part of the nineteenth century, up to 1868, can be divided into two very broad periods as far as dress fashions are concerned, with the year 1828 as a convenient dividing date. Before 1828, dresses were more or less high-waisted and had relatively scanty skirts, generally made of gored panels so that they could be set into the waistband without any pleating or gathering in front or on the sides (see figs. 32, 37). From 1828 into the 1860s, nearly all skirts were made entirely of straight, ungored panels that were then pleated into the waistband. This established the new silhouette that was to lead to the hoop skirts of midcentury (see fig. 57). Waistlines returned to a natural level at about the same time, and from then until the mid-1860s fashion focused chiefly on variations in the sleeve.

In the first part of the century, skirts were often short enough to expose the foot, and even when they were long, they were scanty enough that the shoe was normally visible. Therefore, early nineteenth-century shoes tend to be rather colorful and are often attractively trimmed (see fig. 58). But in 1834, the hem dropped to within an inch or two of the floor, and from that time, since skirts were full and held away from the body by the petticoats, the feet were far less often seen (see figs. 38, 53). Naturally, less attention was given to the color and trimming of shoes.

The cycle of very full skirts that concealed the feet came to an end in the late 1860s with the advent of the short walking skirt (once again made with gored panels), the bustle, and the draped overskirt (see fig. 30). The shorter walking skirt immediately resulted in more elaborate and more colorful shoes and higher

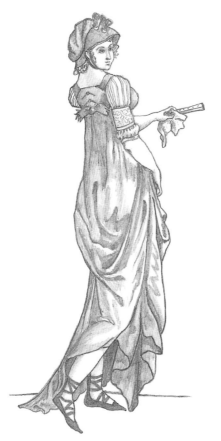

Fig. 32. The ribbons of "sandal slippers" of the 1790s and early 1800s are often shown crossed and tied in rather complex arrangements such as this one from *Le Journal des Dames* series "Costume Parisien," 1800/1801.

boots. Shoes never again suffered quite so great an eclipse as they had from 1835 to 1860. Although skirts were elaborate and sometimes trained, they fell straight enough in front to reveal the shoe in the course of ordinary movement. In the 1870s and 1880s, drapery characterized the skirt while the silhouette fluctuated from bustle to slim verticality, back to bustle, and back to verticality once again. From 1890 to about 1908, the undraped gored skirt held sway while sleeves varied wildly above, from tight in 1890, to full and stiff in 1895, back to tight in 1900, to full and soft in 1905, back to tight in 1910.

But these changes, although conspicuous, were not as important as those happening beneath the surface. At the beginning of the nineteenth century, women's dresses had been soft, light, minimally lined, and easily adjustable. But almost every new decade saw some increase in stiffness, tightness, weight, lining, boning, or complexity of cut until, by the mid-1890s, women's formal clothing, especially in the winter, had become extremely stiff and structured (see fig. 33). Not only did women wear fully boned corsets quite as oppressive as those of the eighteenth century, but the bodice itself was stiffened with as many as sixteen bones. The winter skirt was lined with substantial cotton and often had a layer of horsehair for twelve inches above the hem while the hem itself was further stiffened with a band of thick velvet.

The turn of the new century signaled the swing of the pendulum away from such heavy, stiff, and constricting clothing, and what had taken a century to build up was demolished in a mere fifteen years. From about 1900, new dress fabrics were chosen that were soft and conducive to draping (see fig. 67). The stiff skirt lining was abolished, and the dress was cut loose from its linings both in the bodice and skirt so that the eye began to be accustomed to a look where the clothes did not appear to be pasted to the corseted body. By 1915, the foundation for the entire dress consisted of a broad grosgrain belt suspended on a net underbodice, and a corset was no longer absolutely necessary to a fashionable appearance, although most women still wore one. Skirts cleared the ankle and were neither inconveniently tight nor excessively full, while softly draped bodices were troublesome only by their complex fastenings (see fig. 34).

About 1900, at the same time that women's clothes began to be lighter and less constricting, their shoes became larger, more substantial, and more mannish in style, as if the entire costume had rotated toward something more fitted for action. But the advent of shorter skirts cut this experiment short in the 1910s. The short skirt called attention to the feet, increasing pressure to wear attractive footwear. "Attractive" still meant "small," and shoe manufacturers were quick to recognize the demand for light, turned pumps that minimized the size of the foot. Since footwear was so conspicuous by the 1920s, a market was created for a bewildering variety of novelty styles. The shortened skirt also looked best on a long-legged body type, and this aesthetic need for an elongated lower leg ensured that the high heel became a staple of women's dressy footwear from the 1920s to the present (see fig. 12).

This chapter sketches out in chronological order the stylistic changes in American women's footwear between 1795 and 1930, while the first twelve of the color plates provide a concise pictorial overview of the same subject. The black-and-white figures in Part I illustrate a number of important shoe types not included in the color plates. For more complete and detailed information, or to date a particular pair of shoes, the reader should consult Part II, beginning with its introductory guide, "Procedures and Considerations in Dating Shoes." Part II is organized by shoe type and contains over four hundred figures illustrating most of the common variations found in women's footwear.

Changing Shoe Styles before 1860

In 1856, the "lady" who wrote *Every Lady Her Own Shoemaker* could state with some truth that "one advantage in making [one's own] shoes is, that the fashions do not change. A last, if once purchased, will answer a lifetime."[1] At the time she was writing, neither boots nor shoes had changed significantly for

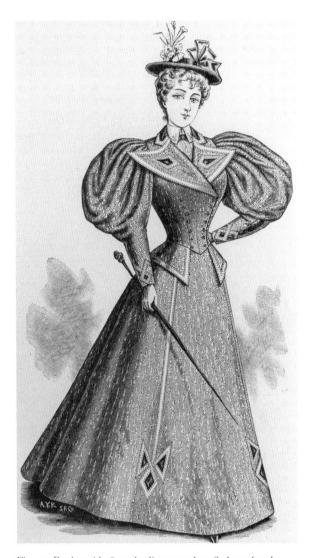

Fig. 33. By the mid-1890s, bodices were heavily boned and skirts heavily lined, producing an extremely stiff appearance. At the same time shoes and boots were made with shallow pointed toes so that the entire costume must have been very uncomfortable to wear. From the *Ladies' Standard Magazine,* April 1896. *Courtesy Heidi Fieldston.*

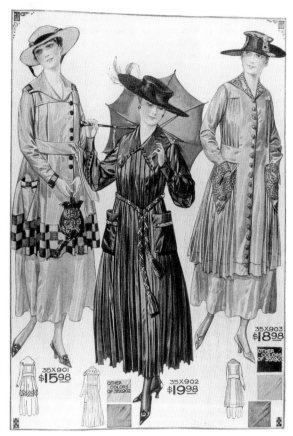

Fig. 34. In the first two decades of the twentieth century, women's clothing became gradually softer in line and looser in cut, until, by 1917, corsets were not really required to create the fashionable line (although most women still wore them), and the body could move with ease even in a fashionable dress. As hemlines rose in the late teens, boots reached a standard height of nine inches above the sole. From *Spring and Summer Fashions 1917*, Bellas Hess and Company, Catalog No. 77, p. 25. *Courtesy Heidi Fieldston.*

about twenty-five years, and shoes not all that much for another twenty-five before that. From her perspective, it must indeed have seemed as if shoe fashions never changed. In spite of the overall similarity, however, the historian can distinguish some variation in style during the first half of the nineteenth century.

1795–1830 (Plates 1–4)

Heels and Toes: As the century opened, women's shoes were changing from the high-heeled buckled style worn for most of the eighteenth century to a flat slipper (see plate 1). The commonest heel type was a wedged Louis known as an Italian heel, and in the twenty years before 1810 it decreased from about two inches in height to next to nothing. The arbiters of fashion, mad for all things classical, had noticed that sandals, not high heels, were worn in ancient Greece and Rome, and therefore flat, low-cut shoes with conspicuous lacings became the fashion. While, technically, shoes continued to be made with some sort of heel—often a single thickness of leather inserted above the sole—in appearance some women's shoes were made flat as early as the mid-1790s, and most were flat from about 1810. A low, stacked heel returned briefly in the 1820s only to retreat again about 1830. The toes were very pointed at the end of the eighteenth century, but from about 1805, a round or oval shape dominated until the late 1820s, when a narrow square toe also appeared.

Slippers: The type of shoe most worn at the beginning of the nineteenth century was the slipper, a thin-soled, low-cut shoe without fastenings, except in some cases a pair of ribbons added to tie round the ankle. In the 1790s and early 1800s, slippers were very often made in bright-colored leathers. Some were stamped with stripes or small repeating designs (see figs. 58, 59), and plain leather or silk shoes might be embroidered with silver thread and sequins, or cut out and backed with contrasting silk. Fringe, silk ruching, and rosettes were also common decorations. After 1815, there was a very gradual trend toward more conservative colors and less decoration in shoes (see plates 2 and 3).

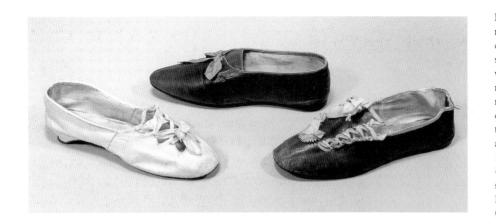

Slippers first acquired ribbons in the 1790s in imitation of the classical sandal, and pictures of them circa 1800 show elaborate methods for tying them round the leg (see fig. 32). Acknowledging their origin as a blend of slipper and sandal, the *Lady's Magazine* of January 1802 called them "sandal slippers" and reported that they were worn "in the morning by the pedestrian fashionables." At this early date, neither the pattern of lacing nor even the presence of ribbon ties was standard. Some surviving shoes have small tape loops sewn at intervals along both sides just inside the top edge through which the ribbon tie was threaded, allowing it to crisscross several times over the instep before passing around the ankle. What was to become the standard arrangement, a pair of ribbon ties attached near the side seams, then crossed and tied round the ankles, only took firm hold from the mid-1810s. These ribbon ties must very often have come untied from the brushing of the petticoats.

Tie Shoes: While the slipper was the most important low footwear in the first thirty years of the century, there were three other styles to choose from, all found chiefly in walking dress. The first, a low-cut shoe, had the top edge cut in a series of little tabs, each bearing a lace hole through which a ribbon was threaded to cross and tie on the instep. This style seems to have reached its peak about 1810 and passed out of use by 1815. The second was a more utilitarian shoe that covered nearly the entire foot and laced up the front. Versions of this simple shoe, called in this book a "slit vamp" shoe, persisted through much of the nineteenth century, eventually being replaced by the oxford tie. The last was a latchet-tie or "open tab" shoe that developed directly from the eighteenth-century buckled shoe. The quarters were extended into eyelet tabs called latchets that met without overlapping and tied over a tongue extension of the vamp (see fig. 35).

Boots: In this early period boots were not yet very common. One of the earliest and rarest styles is that which laces up the back. Back-lacing boots made of white silk heavily embroidered in gold and edged round the top with gold fringe are preserved from Napoleon's coronation in 1804. The style is shown in *Costume Parisien* in 1809[2] as a red walking boot with fringed top. The *Lady's Magazine* mentions the style in November 1812, "ankle boots of colored velvet or kid,

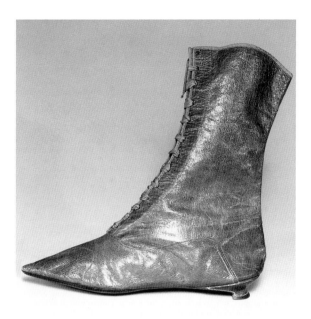

Fig. 36. This green morocco front-lacing boot of 1795–1805 may have been a display model; it has no mate and appears never to have been worn. Note the vestigial Italian heel. One side of the tongue is stitched to the boot all along the lace opening. Catalog #1952.50. *Courtesy Colonial Dames, Boston.*

to lace behind," but no evidence as yet suggests that this style was ever widely worn in America.

One of the earliest women's walking boots that does survive in America is in the collection of the Colonial Dames in Boston (see fig. 36). Made of green morocco, it has the long pointed toe and Italian heel typical of women's shoes in the late 1790s. It laces up the front and extends halfway to the knee. This is much higher than was fashionable again at any time until the 1870s. The midcalf height seems to have lasted into the first decade of the nineteenth century, although it is hard to be sure since so very few real examples survive, and in fashion plates the tops of the boots are obscured by the dresses. French plates of 1809 and the years following, however, provide occasional glimpses of boots that end just above the anklebone and are trimmed round the top with fringe. A pair of ankle-high, fringed, front-lacing boots in green silk said to have been brought from Florence, Italy, in 1818 is preserved in the Museum of Fine Arts, Boston. Two plainer versions from this early period, one in nankeen for summer, the other in utilitarian leather, are shown in figure 56.

Boots did not change very much through the 1820s, although, like 1820s shoes, they sometimes had a low, stacked heel. An example from this period at the Valentine Museum in Richmond, Virginia, has low heels and thick soles, with an upper of green kid trimmed with fringe round the top and down each side of the lace holes. Like nearly all other pre-1830 boots, it laces up the front (see plate 4).

1830–60 (Plates 5 and 6)

Heels and Toes: The narrow, square toe that had appeared in the late 1820s does not appear very frequently on surviving shoes. Those that do have it and have known histories cluster around the year 1830. The narrow, square toe probably continued for some years as an alternative style, but gradually through the 1830s, a broader, more sharply square toe shape took the lead, and this type survives in far greater quantity. In the late 1840s, the sharp square toe was itself replaced by a version with slightly rounded corners, and this rounded square toe was the norm for the next thirty years. Shoes and boots of the 1830s and 1840s are almost uniformly heelless, having not even the spring heel typical of shoes earlier in the century. Low, stacked heels are found on isolated examples in the 1830s and 1840s, and a Northampton, Massachusetts, advertisement lists "Ladies' leather strap'd and heeled Shoes" in 1840.[3] How common heeled shoes were in nonfashionable contexts is difficult to ascertain, but they returned to the world of fashion again in the 1850s, especially on walking boots. In the dressier shoes that tend to survive, there are few examples with heels until the early 1860s.

Slippers and Tie Shoes: Slippers changed little from the 1820s except for their square toes and narrower range of color and material, generally black or white satin, or black, white, or light brown morocco. Many were entirely plain once the skirt descended to obscure the shoe, but in the 1850s rosettes became fashionable again. The ribbon ties became quite narrow, and toward 1860 they were replaced with a thin elastic cord. Tie shoes became less fashionable as boots began to take over their role as walking footwear. Elaborate tie shoes were not unknown, but most were made in black or light brown kid with a simple slit in the vamp (see plate 5).

Boots: The side-lacing boot came into fashion in the late 1820s and probably replaced the older front-lacing style soon after 1830. As long as skirts were short in the early 1830s, boots extended high enough to fully cover the ankle and this height persisted into the 1840s (see fig. 60). But in the 1850s, boots were made lower than before, just barely covering the anklebone (see plate 6). While the front-lacing boots of the 1820s may have stacked heels and thick soles and be made of leather, the side-lacing boots of the 1830s and 1840s are usually heelless, thin-soled, and made in gaiter style; that is, with a wool or silk upper foxed with thin leather. All-leather boots became more common in the later 1850s and in the 1860s. Buttoned boots, like heels, are more typically found after 1865, but we know they existed earlier, and a careful look at fashion periodicals will turn up a few beginning in the late 1810s (see fig. 37).

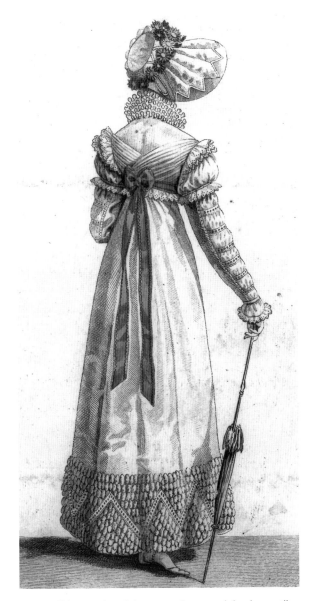

Fig. 37. Skirts continued short enough to reveal the shoe until about 1834, and in the 1810s could be short enough to reveal the ankle as well. Throughout the 1810s and 1820s, the eye was drawn toward the foot by masses of decorative trim on the hem of the skirt. This 1819 fashion plate shows the early-nineteenth-century version of the buttoned boot, with buttons straight down the side in the position later taken by side lacing. From *Costume Parisien*, plate #1818. *Smithsonian Institution Photo No. 76-14703.*

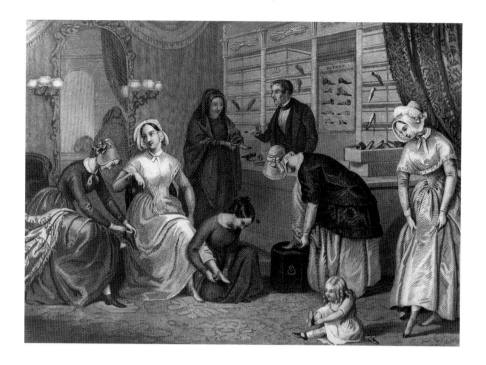

Every Lady Her Own Shoemaker provided a pattern for making one in 1856, noting that "these are very nice-looking gaiters, preferable to those that lace, and the uppers are less work to make"[4] (see fig. 262). The Society for the Preservation of New England Antiquities has a similar boot made of gray serge, but with six buttons, a scalloped fly, and deep foxings of black patent. It is said to have been worn by Elizabeth Sears Webb Farmer at her wedding, circa 1845–55.

The most important alternative to the side-lacing boot at this period, however, was one with gussets of elasticized fabric inserted on each side over the ankle-bone, a type known in the United States as the Congress boot. Elastic-sided boots were patented in England by J. Sparkes Hall in 1837,[5] but elasticized fabrics were not very satisfactory until the later 1840s, when the threads incorporated in the weave were vulcanized. The vulcanized version was introduced in 1847, and by September 1848 *Godey's* considered that "for promenading, the Congress boot is indispensable." *Every Lady Her Own Shoemaker* comments that "many ladies much prefer this kind of shoe; they will never wear slouching to the foot; the elastics always keeping them close to the foot, and there are no shoe lacings to be continually untying and getting under the feet"[6] (see figs. 38, 64, 281–283).

Changing Shoe Styles after 1860

Beginning in the 1860s, the pace of change in shoe fashions began very gradually to increase, a development reflected in the ever-decreasing number of years described in each of the following sections. By the 1920s, it becomes possible to see distinct developments with every new year in trade journals such as the *Shoe Retailer*. This quickened rate of stylistic change may have resulted in part from the mechanization and increased productivity of the shoe industry, but the same acceleration was occurring in other areas of dress as well. In the early twentieth century, competition among the shoe manufacturers did much to encourage the frantic development of new styles and variations upon styles, as did the shortened skirts of the mid-1910s and 1920s that fully exposed the feet. The race for novelty that characterized shoe fashions in the 1920s was an important phenomenon that reflected changing cultural and economic realities, but each little modification in itself rarely signified more than that the time had come for something new. Thus, once toes had been rounded for a few years, manufacturers tried out pointed ones. Once the public had had enough of pointed toes, fashion swung round to wider ones again. Likewise, deep, short vamps alternated with long, shallow vamps, and straight-sided heels with curved ones.

1860–80 (Plates 6–8)

Heels and Toes: The rounded square toe that had been standard for most shoes and boots since the later 1840s did not go out of style until the late 1870s. Before it disappeared, the sole became significantly broader across the ball of the foot while the waist became narrower, so that 1870s soles look very different from those of the 1850s and 1860s in spite of the similar toe shape. *Godey's* noted in 1877 that "each year brings into more general use comfortable broad shoes, that have full, wide soles, with extension edges."[7] This increased breadth in the sole is more obvious in walking shoes and boots than in slippers, which were still relatively narrow.

Although heels reappeared early in the 1850s, few examples clearly dating that early survive, presumably because in that decade they were more common in walking shoes than in the dressy footwear that is preserved. Judging from museum collections, one would think heels made their appearance about 1860 to 1865. The early heels one does find are either a low (half-inch), stacked leather heel (used in walking or day shoes and boots) or a one-inch wooden knock-on heel covered to match the upper (see plate 6, fig. 45). The latter style was used especially in light-colored dress shoes and boots to avoid the awkward conjunction of dark leather heel and white kid or satin upper. Heels of all types became somewhat higher in the late 1860s and 1870s.

In the late 1860s, the Louis heel with its curved silhouette and generally greater height reappeared for the first time since the 1790s. It was part of the renewed interest in eighteenth-century styles and a natural accompaniment to the startlingly shorter skirts worn for walking in 1867. The Louis heel is common in fashion illustrations in the 1870s and 1880s, and in collections that feature the clothing of the well-to-do. In middle-class collections one is more likely to find a covered wooden knock-on heel with a curved neck and straight breast. Louis heels were more difficult to make and added to the cost of the shoe (see plate 8, fig. 54).

Slippers: The rosette that had appeared on evening slippers in the 1850s grew gradually larger until by the late 1860s it was a very large oval that extended beyond the throatline to rest on and cover part of the instep. This style was known

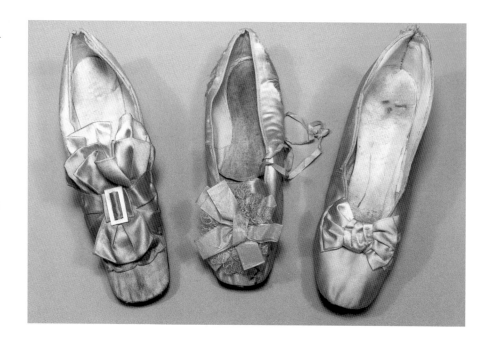

Fig. 39. White shoes with rosettes, 1868–80. *Left:* Low-heeled white kid wedding shoe of Agnes Laura Shaw, who married Erasmus Darwin Hudson in Plainfield, Massachusetts, on September 8, 1871. Catalog #66.671. *Center:* Heelless white satin wedding shoe of Mrs. Theodore Topping, 1868. In its mate is found the Henry H. Tuttle and Company label illustrated in fig. 6. Catalog #66.662. *Right:* Low-heeled white satin wedding shoe of Mrs. Frank N. Look, married in Northampton, Massachusetts, on October 20, 1880. Note the shorter vamp and simpler rosette. Catalog #66.672. *Courtesy Historic Northampton.*

in the 1870s as a Marie Antoinette slipper. It began to pass out of fashion about 1874, in favor of a simpler style with a rather short vamp that displayed pretty openwork stockings to advantage. The length of the vamp decreased to as little as 1⅜ inches by 1880. In that year, *Godey's* remarked that "these dainty [satin evening] shoes are so much open over the foot, that one might almost predict a return to the gilt sandals so much in vogue in the time of the Directoire"[8] (see fig. 39).

Shoes with Fastenings: Slipperlike shoes with a series of buttoned straps across the instep appeared in the later 1870s and set a new and lasting fashion. These multi-strap shoes (and their boot-high counterparts, which were equally popular) were meant to be worn with colored silk stockings (see fig. 54). The 1870s version often had three to five straps and was usually described merely as a slipper with straps, or as a shoe "barred across."

Shoes cut high enough to require fastenings other than straps also became more fashionable in the later nineteenth century. Some of these were made rather like a cut-down buttoned boot (see fig. 40f). Others had an elastic gusset on the ankle or instep. Occasionally a band of elastic over the instep was concealed beneath a very high tonguelike vamp. One of the most common types in the 1870s and 1880s was a latchet tie fastening with a ribbon over a prominent tongue. This style was often called a "Molière," since it was inspired by late seventeenth-century styles (see plate 7). Tie shoes are shown fastened with large ribbon bows in the 1870s, and with tasseled cords in the 1880s (see fig. 40).

Materials and Decoration: In the mid-1860s, the walking dress shortened to show the foot and ankle, and this encouraged a good deal more attention to be given to the footwear. "Now that the decree has gone forth in favor of short dresses, we must look to our boots. . . . One of the latest styles is of a bright cuir-colored

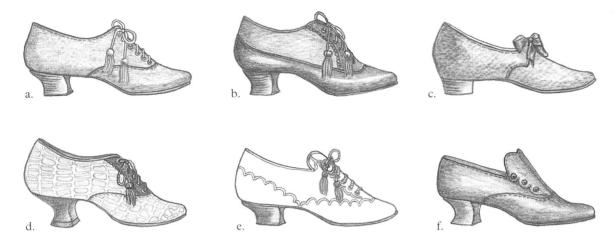

leather buttoned up the sides, made with very high Louis XV heels, and finished with tassels."[9] Even when the walking length dropped again to the top of the foot, the skirts still hung closer to the body in front than they had for many years, and shoes were far more likely to show in ordinary movement than they had been before 1865. As a result, both shoes and boots became rather exuberant in their color and decoration in the late 1860s and 1870s. Dark shoes were often embroidered with decorative curls and loops of machine stitching in a light-colored thread. The toe caps of boots were routinely edged with curlicues of white stitching, and braid and tassels were added to the tops of boots. Dressy daytime shoes might have holes cut in the vamp, edged with machine stitching and backed with contrasting leathers or fabrics. Sometimes heels and even entire boots were made of gilded leather, and even the soles were decorated with contrasting designs at the waist (see plate 7).

Boots: Side-lacing boots became less and less common throughout this period. Beginning in the 1860s, they were replaced for walking by front-lacing boots and for dressier occasions by buttoned boots. The elastic-sided boot suffered a similar slow extinction, although it was always more common than museum collections would suggest. All kinds of boots were somewhat higher in the 1860s than they had been in the 1850s, fully covering the ankle. By the

Fig. 40. Late nineteenth-century tie shoes. The closed-tab ties (a, b, d, e) and button shoe (f) were all illustrated on the advertising pages for the Jordan Marsh Boot and Shoe Department in the *Housekeeper's Friend*, an 1883 almanac published by Jordan, Marsh and Company of Boston, "Importers, Manufacturers, Jobbers and Retailers of Dry Goods," and until recently in existence as a department store. All were described as hand-sewn turn shoes, the oxfords being listed as "Edson Ties." Prices ranged from $2 (for the button shoe in the cheapest American kid) to $6 (for the alligator). (a) French Kid, Spanish Toe. (b) Mat Top, Patent Leather Foxed. (d) Alligator, Louis XV Heel. (e) Scallop Foxed. (f) French or American kid button slipper.

The open-tab tie shoe (c) was the type known as a Newport Tie, introduced about 1871 and advertised in Sears as late as 1907 in a modified version. This example is found with identical descriptions both in Montgomery Ward's catalog for 1895 (90 cents) and in Sears for 1897 (85 cents): "Ladies' Pebble Grain Newport Tie, all solid and well made, for rough wear." A very similar shoe with slightly higher and curvier heel was advertised as a "Fifth Avenue Tie" in Jordan Marsh's 1883 almanac.

1870s they could come halfway to the knee, as if to balance the higher heel. The top edges were often cut in fancy curved shapes, and as described in the preceding paragraph, they could be decorated with embroidery, gilding, and tassels (see plate 8).

1880–93 (Plates 7–9)

Heels and Toes: At the very end of the 1870s, a narrower oval toe replaced the rounded square that had been characteristic of the entire mid–nineteenth century. It continued with little change throughout the 1880s, becoming a little narrower and more pointed after 1890. Heels were in general lower than in the 1870s, with stacked heels continuing for walking, covered wooden knock-on heels for dressier occasions, and covered Louis heels in more sophisticated footwear.

Shoes: Short vamps continued to be fashionable throughout this period, although the most extreme examples tend to date from about 1879 to 1885. The elaborate cutouts and embroidery of the early machine period faded in the late 1870s, and by 1880 bows, strap effects, and beading were the rule in dressy shoes. Multi-strapped and tie shoes continued without much change through the 1880s, but from about 1890 a single strap (or occasionally a pair of crossed straps) took the lead, fastening with a button or a moderate bow (see figs. 132–134). Fastening shoes are rare in collections, but fashion commentaries suggest that they were becoming more and more important through this period (see figs. 40, 55, 66).

Boots: Front-lacing boots persisted as an alternative, but buttoned boots were far and away the most common style from the mid-1860s through the early 1890s. Side-lacing and elastic-sided boots were still made but were relatively rare. Very high boots and very high heels such as had been fashionable in the 1870s were rarely seen after 1880. After the rather delightful excesses of the 1870s, 1880s boots seem to embody no extreme at all. Except for the standard scalloped edge of the button fly, boots were generally made quite plain (see fig. 65). A fashion commentator in *Godey's* rejoiced in 1885,

> Nothing could be simpler, nor more absolutely unadorned than the foot covering *par excellence* of today. No fancy work, embroidery, stitching, beading, or even irrelevant fancy buttons are visible. The boot is ornamental only in its quality, which is of kid, the finest and softest. The toe portion is roomy yet shapely. The heel, with not a suggestion of the "French bend" about it, is yet graceful, and the sole of the foot is broad enough to allow of promenading without having to stop every few moments to give a rest to the pinched and rebellious foot.[10]

1893–1904 (Plates 10 and 11)

Heels and Toes: Reacting against the short vamps and moderate toe shapes of the previous twenty years, the mid-1890s saw the introduction of an extremely shallow and very long, pointed toe known in Sears catalogs as a "long drawn-out needle toe." This style must have ruined the feet of many a wearer who insisted on cramming her toes into the narrowed vamp rather than allowing the needle

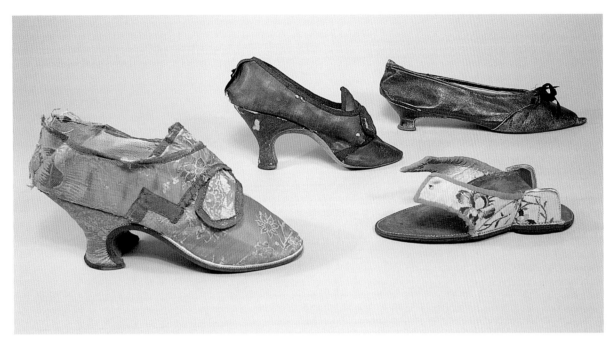

Plate 1. The transition from eighteenth-century styles was characterized by lowered heels, shortened vamps and tongues, and the replacement of buckled straps by latchet ties or no fastening at all. *Left:* Flowered-silk buckled shoe with oval toe, dogleg side seam, and long vamp with square tongue, typical of mid-eighteenth-century shoes. Possibly the 1765 wedding shoe of Elizabeth Foye Munroe. Its related clog is at right. Catalog #66.632A. *Center:* Buckle shoe of black glazed wool (less pretentious than silk) with the slender Italian heel, pointed toe, straight side seam, shorter vamp, and pointed tongue typical 1770–90. Catalog #66.633. *Right rear:* Dark blue-green morocco wedding shoe with pointed toe and low Italian heel worn by Anna Stoddard Williams in 1799. While cut as low as a slipper, it has one pair of lace holes tying over a vestigial tongue. Label: Sam Miller, Boot & Shoe Maker, No. 5 Cornhill [London]. Catalog #66.635. *Right front:* Clog of silk-covered leather and wood worn with ca. 1765 shoe at left. Catalog #66.632B. *Courtesy Historic Northampton.*

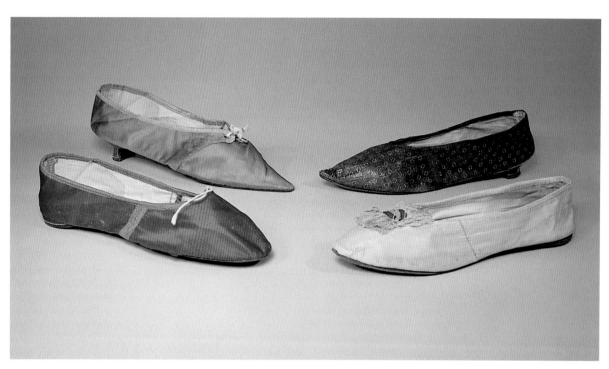

Plate 2. The heel continued to diminish from the 1790s to about 1815, and round or oval toes replaced pointed ones. *Left rear:* Blue satin latchet tie with pointed toe and low Italian heel typical of 1790–1800 (compare 1799 wedding shoe in plate 1). The stamp "Hon Sing" on the lining suggests it may have been made in Canton, China, either for export or for an American woman visiting there. Catalog #1948.50. *Right rear:* Slipper of purple kid stamped with tan rosettes, 1795–1805. The squat Italian heel is typical ca. 1800. Catalog #1952.7. *Left front:* Red satin slipper with minimal wedged heel covered in red satin and stitched in white, 1805–10. Short vamps and round toes are common in French fashion plates by 1804. Catalog #1952.533. *Right front:* Yellow kid slipper with spring heel, oval toe, and fringe and buckle on the vamp, 1805–15. Label: Jackson, Ladies Shoe Manufacturer, 54 Rathbone Place, Oxford Street, London (see fig. 4). Catalog #1952.532. *Courtesy National Society of the Colonial Dames in the Commonwealth of Massachusetts.*

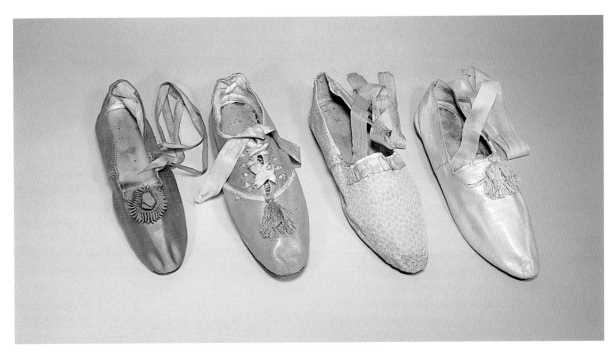

Plate 3. Shoes 1815–30 generally had an oval toe, long vamp, and narrow waist. Many, like those pictured here, had spring heels or no heels, but a significant number had low round stacked heels, as in plate 4. *Far left:* Beige wool serge slipper, right/left differentiated, lined with linen and leather. The slightly shorter vamp suggests a date of 1825–30. Catalog #71E. *Center left:* Closed-tab tie shoe of pumpkin-colored kid trimmed in blue silk, 1815–25. Made straight. Lined with linen and leather. Catalog #1952.105. *Center right:* Pale-green ribbed silk with amoeba-shaped woven figure. Long vamp, oval toe, pleated ribbon trim, and broad silk ribbon ties are typical 1815–25. Made straight. Lined with linen and leather. Catalog #1952.101. *Far right:* Pale-pink kid slipper with silk tassel, right/left differentiated, 1815–25. Lined with linen and leather. Catalog #1952.102. *Courtesy National Society of the Colonial Dames in the Commonwealth of Massachusetts.*

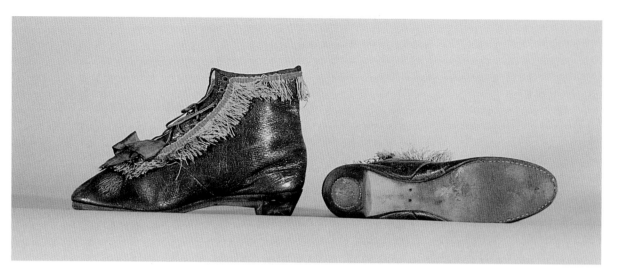

Plate 4. Green kid front-lace boot with cotton fringe, 1825–30. The small round stacked heel is typical of heels in the 1820s. The original lacing was probably a flat silk tape like those in plate 3. Right/left differentiated. In spite of its elaborate trim, the thick sole and leather upper make this the sort of practical boot an exasperated Mrs. Trollope thought American women should have been wearing in the late 1820s. Catalog #43.23.1. *Courtesy Valentine Museum.*

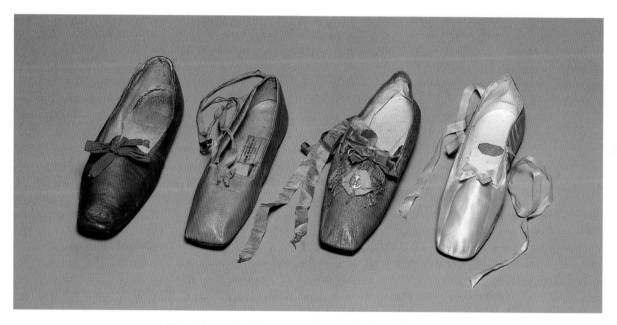

Plate 5. Square-toed slippers and tie shoes in shades of tan were common daytime wear in America in the 1840s. White satin was reserved for the very dressiest occasions. *Far left:* Tan kid slit-vamp shoe worn by Elizabeth T. Fisher Palmer at her wedding "about 1847." Catalog #122,427. *Center left:* Tan morocco slipper, 1835–50. Label: "Edward Haynes, Jr., 219 Washington St., Boston." Catalog #112,452. *Center right:* Beige glazed kid, slit-vamp tie shoe with rosette, fringe, and ankle ties, 1835–50. Catalog #133,695. *Far right:* White satin slipper with Esté label probably worn for a formal wedding 1845–50 (see also fig. 5). Catalog #136,315. *Courtesy Peabody Essex Museum.*

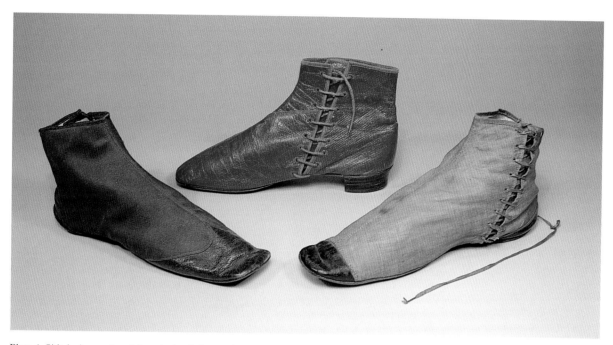

Plate 6. Side lacing replaced front lacing in boots about 1830. Side-lace boots were known as gaiter boots when made of fabric foxed with leather (common practice until ca. 1855). *Left:* Brown serge gaiter boot foxed with brown morocco. The sharply square toe suggests a date 1835–47. Worn by Jane Damon Smith of Northampton, Mass. Catalog #66.695. *Center:* Bright-red kid side-lace boot with small stacked heel, ca. 1860. Right/left differentiated. The all-leather upper, bright color, and small stacked heel are rare in side-lace boots much before 1860. Catalog #66.701. *Right:* Light-brown wool gaiter boot foxed with black patent. The rounded square toe with as yet no heel suggests a date 1850–55. Worn by Jane Damon Smith of Northampton, Mass. Catalog #66.698. *Courtesy Historic Northampton.*

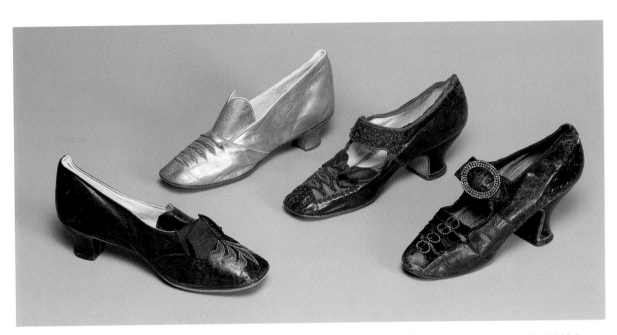

Plate 7. Dressy shoes 1870–90 could be brightly colored and decorated. *Front left:* Black kid shoe with knock-on heel, white leather lining and vamp cutouts backed in purple silk and outlined in white machine stitching. The silk ribbon bow is a functional tie, but the shoe slips on, adjusted by elastic goring on either side of the tongue. Made by the Goodrich and Porter Company of Haverhill and shown at the Centennial Exhibition in Philadelphia, 1876. USMC catalog #2287. *Center left:* Gold kid slip-on shoe with large tongue similar to the "Molière" style, knock-on heel, and vamp cutouts backed in purple silk. A purple silk tassel or rosette was probably once sewn at the juncture of vamp and tongue. The very high quarter is common in slippers 1870–90. Made by Bradley Goodrich of Haverhill and shown at the Centennial Exhibition in Philadelphia, 1876. USMC catalog #2296. *Center right:* Bronze kid shoe with Louis heel, single buckled strap, decorative beading, and vamp cutouts edged with buttonhole stitching, ca. 1880. Catalog #132,447.2. *Far right:* Black kid shoe with Louis heel and single strap fastened with concealed button and loop. The cut-steel buckles are all nonfunctional. The leather lining was once bright pink. Marked "Feris." 1880–90. Catalog #121,705. *Courtesy Peabody Essex Museum.*

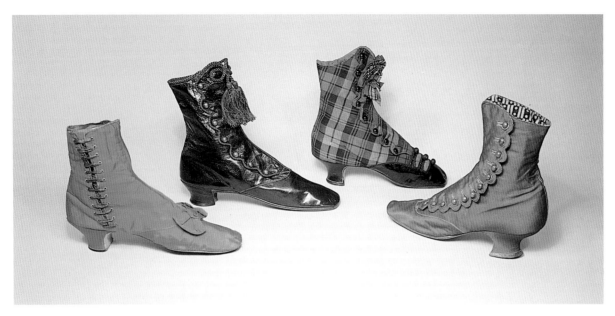

Plate 8. Boots were more likely to incorporate bright colors and trim from the 1860s, when walking skirts were made short enough to show the feet. *Far left:* Bright-green silk side-lace boot in the slightly higher style that appears in the early 1860s. The Louis heel, rare before 1865, and the fashionable shade of green suggest a date ca. 1865–67. Catalog #1960.169. *Center left:* Bronze kid buttoned boot with cord and tassel trim and welted sole, 1865–70. Label: Alexandre Sulzer, Cordonnier pour Dames, Rue du 29 Juillet, 7, Paris, Fournisseur de S. M. la Reine de Saxe. An inner lacing tightens the boot at the bend of the ankle so that it can be more easily and snugly buttoned. Catalog #1956.115. *Center right:* Blue-and-green plaid silk buttoned boot with black patent foxing cut to imitate buttoned straps and black patent-covered Louis heel, 1872–76. Catalog #1949.60. *Far right:* Rust-colored silk buttoned boots with Louis heel, top facing of black and yellow silk. The rounded toe, short vamp, and color suggest a date 1885–90. Catalog #1955.1. *Courtesy National Society of the Colonial Dames in the Commonwealth of Massachusetts.*

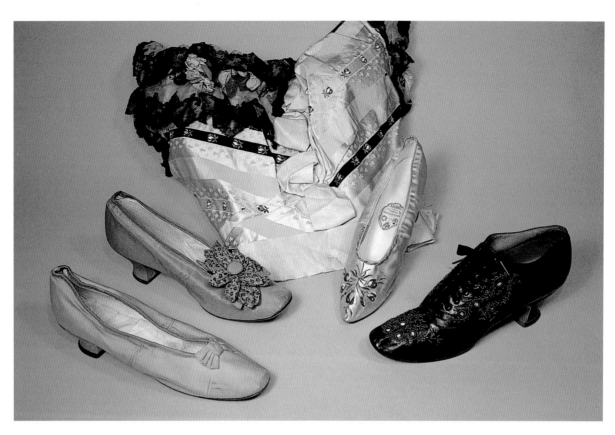

Plate 9. Except for the bronze oxford at right, all these shoes were made to match specific dresses, a refinement by which the upper class distinguished itself from those who were merely decently dressed. *Far left:* Chartreuse ribbed silk slipper with knock-on heel, ca. 1890. Worn by Mrs. Ernest Bowditch. Catalog #1938.97–8. *Center left:* Tan silk slipper with two bands of elastic under the figured silk rosette. Knock-on heel, 1878–80. Catalog #1949.45. *Center right:* The pink satin slipper with embroidered vamp matches an evening dress made for the trousseau of Mary Capelin Day in 1890 by the Paris designer Doucet (bodice shown in plate). While not made of the dress fabric, the shoe is embroidered to imitate the floral design in the dress. Shoe label: Hellstern, Paris, Droit (left shoe label: "Gauche"). The toe is somewhat more pointed than is typical of American shoes in 1890. Catalog #1961.32. *Far right:* Beaded bronze kid oxford shoe with Louis heel, leather lining, and silk laces, ca. 1885. Label: Stern Bros., 23rdSt., NY. Catalog #1961.23. *Courtesy National Society of the Colonial Dames in the Commonwealth of Massachusetts.*

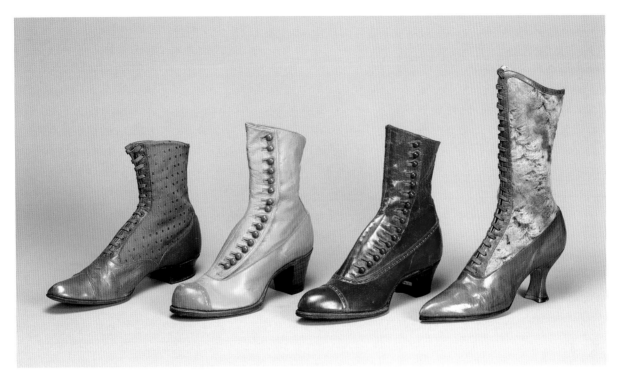

Plate 10. Walking boots, 1890–1920. *Far left:* Tan kid front-lace boot with figured half-silk vesting top, 1893–96. The long shallow toe, long pointed toe cap ("diamond tip"), and curved foxings meeting at the waist are typical of 1890s boots. USMC catalog #G387. *Center left:* Tan kid buttoned boot, now somewhat faded. The straight toe cap was common 1900–1930, but the very short vamp and high bulging toe were stylish only 1911–13. USMC catalog #2566. *Center right:* Red kid buttoned boot made by the A. E. Little Company (Sorosis label) of Lynn. In America a boot of this pattern (common after 1900) is described as "slipper foxed" or "whole foxed," while in Britain the "slipper" part is called a golosh. The still deep but lengthening vamp dates this boot to 1914–15. USMC catalog #2917. *Far right:* Front-lace boot of glazed brown kid with top made of fabric imitating haired kid. Made by John Cramer of Brooklyn in 1919. Boots were made taller as skirts became shorter in the late 1910s and front lacing replaced buttons as the preferred fastening. This is the last style for walking boots before they went out of fashion entirely. USMC catalog #1522. *Courtesy Peabody Essex Museum.*

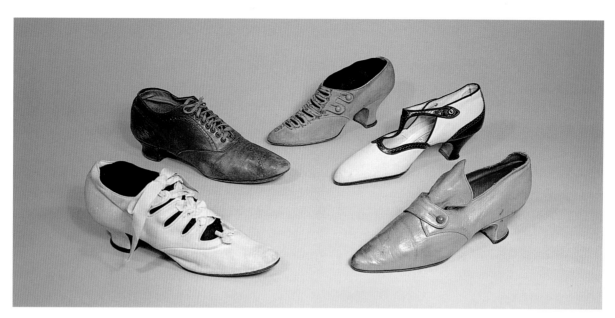

Plate 11. Among the new materials that became fashionable from about 1890 were tan leather, suede, and canvas. *Left front:* Cream suede "sandal" with knock-on heel and four straps tying over the instep, reviving a style worn ca.1805 (see fig. 35). Label: Henry H. Tuttle Co., Boston. 1900–05. Catalog #1989.22. *Left rear:* Tan leather oxford tie with stacked heel and diamond tip, suitable for summer walking, 1893–1900. Catalog #1952.189. *Center rear:* Gray suede buttoned shoe with cutouts, cut-steel beading, and Louis heel, a style named "Mazie" in Hazen B. Goodrich's ad for their 1916 line in the *Shoe Retailer*, September 18, 1915, p. 36 (see fig. 224). These bear the label of retailer Thayer, McNeil & Hodgkins. Catalog #1956.134. An identical pair in bronze kid is also in the Dames collection (Catalog #1956.139). *Right rear:* "Dressy sports" T-strap shoe of white canvas trimmed with black patent, 1924–30. Label: Thayer McNeil Company, Boston. Catalog #1956.138. *Right front:* Tan kid Colonial with buttoned strap over a large flaring tongue. Label: À la Gavotte, 26 Avenue de l'Opéra, Paris. This French shoe probably dates ca. 1900, although the last is not shaped quite like contemporary American styles, which had a shallower vamp and rounder toe. Catalog #1956.143. *Courtesy National Society of the Colonial Dames in the Commonwealth of Massachusetts.*

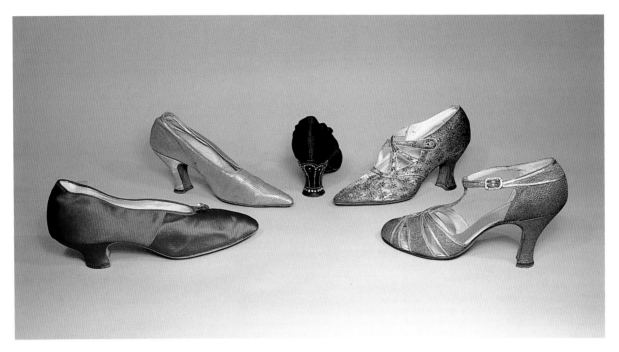

Plate 12. Once short skirts began to reveal the feet, there was every inducement to wear eye-catching shoes. *Far left:* Red satin slippers matching a dress worn by Mrs. Charles Dean of Weston, Mass, for her 40th ("ruby") wedding anniversary in 1915. Label: Connelley & Co., 31 Beacon St., Boston, Mass. The rather deep vamp, narrow throat opening, and tiny throat ornament are typical of the mid-1910s. Catalog #1965.188D. *Center left:* Silver brocade evening slipper with the very long vamp, pointed toe, narrow throat, and high Louis heel stylish 1917–21. Label: The H. H. Tuttle Co., Boston. Catalog #1947.1. *Center:* Black satin strapped evening slipper with celluloid-covered heel set with "brilliants" (rhinestones or paste jewels), 1924–26. While jeweled heels were briefly popular in 1913, they were more widely worn in the mid-1920s. Celluloid-covered heels were in common use by 1918. Catalog #x2000.1. *Center right:* Black-and-gold brocade slipper with cross strap and Louis heel, 1921–24. Catalog #1982.39. *Far right:* Evening sandal of purple and gold fabric trimmed with narrow gold leather straps and lined with pale-green satin, 1933. Uppers cut very low at the sides appeared in the later 1920s, but cutouts over the toes were rare until the 1930s. Catalog #1981.85. *Courtesy National Society of the Colonial Dames in the Commonwealth of Massachusetts.*

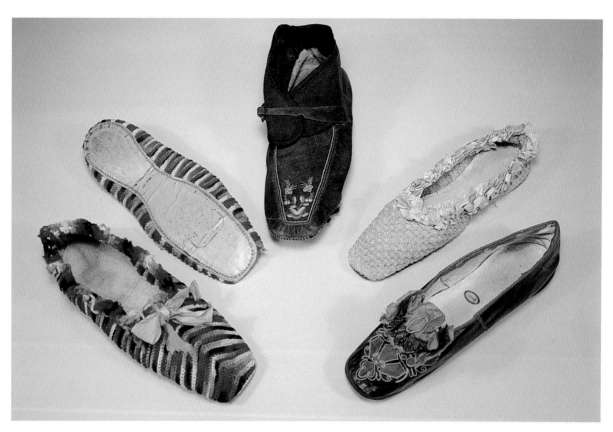

Plate 13. Bright colors and lavish ornamentation were acceptable in boudoir slippers in the 1840s and 1850s. *Left, above and below:* Boudoir slippers crocheted in shades of scarlet wool with a pink silk bow, stitched to a ready-made oilcloth sole lined with lamb's wool, 1855–70. Catalog #66.798. *Center:* Deerskin moccasin with chainstitch floral embroidery. Moccasins were made not only by American Indians for sale to tourists, but also by white Americans and worn by both men and women as boudoir slippers and carriage shoes. The lined ankle band and buckled strap are not traditional Indian features. Catalog #66.795. *Right, above:* Boudoir slipper of knitted pink and yellow silk trimmed with pleated pink silk ribbon, 1855–70. Catalog #66.799. *Right, below:* Bronze kid slippers with vamp cutouts backed with pink, red, blue, or green silk and edged with light-colored chainstitching were very fashionable ca. 1845–70. Fancy slippers were more formal than today's bedroom slippers but were still never appropriate outdoors, being more suitable for morning indoor wear with a fitted morning dress or dressy wrapper. This particular example is marked "Jolly 125" on the sole and "droit" in the sock lining and probably dates 1865–70. Catalog #66.659. *Courtesy Historic Northampton.*

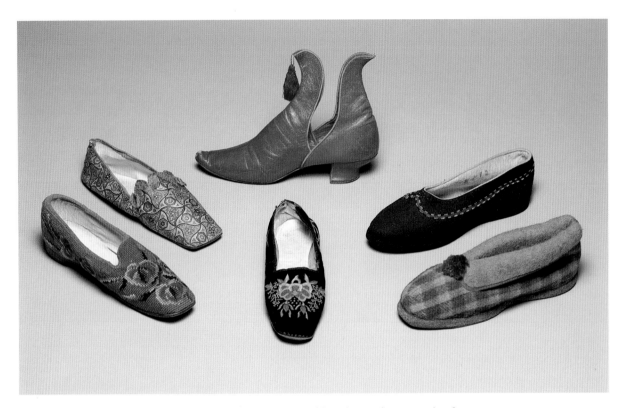

Plate 14. Boudoir slippers. *Center front:* Black embroidered velvet with oval toe and narrow waist of the 1820s, possibly as late as 1835. Catalog #132,109. *Far left:* Purple Berlin-work with tabbed throat line, 1860–65. Berlin-work slippers were extremely popular for both men and women, 1850–65, and were often made as gifts. Catalog #122,969. *Center left:* Unusual printed cotton slipper with square toe and dentate throat line edged with pleated purple ribbon 1835–50. Catalog #125,959. *Center rear:* Red kid "nullifier" or "Juliet," a style introduced for women in 1892. Nullifiers were made of felt as well as kid and often had fur trim. This one may date 1892–94, before fur trim became conventional. Marked "Wm. T. Ash, Shoemaker." Catalog #134,743. *Center right:* Navy-blue felt, 1912. A pompon is missing from the throat line. The plain round throat line is less common than a tabbed style among felt slippers 1890–1920. USMC catalog #2512 (G160). *Far right:* Brown-and-tan plaid upper of two-faced blanket material with McKay-stitched felt sole, 1912. The style appeared by 1891 and became common in the 1920s made in felt. USMC catalog #2504. *Courtesy Peabody Essex Museum.*

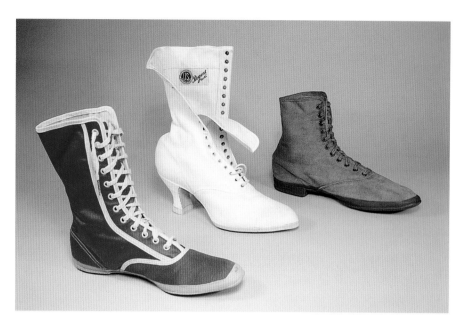

Plate 15. Shoes for sports. *Left:* Red satin bathing shoes with white cotton binding and laces and a white rubber sole, ca. 1920–25. Label molded into the sole: "Hood Seaview Bathing—Made in USA." Another example survives in green. Front-lace bathing boots of this type were worn in the 1920s just before bathing shoes and stockings went out of fashion entirely. Catalog #1976.121.1. *Center:* White canvas summer boot with rubber sole and heel, 1917–19. Label below top facing: "US Rubber System, United States Rubber Company and Associated Companies. Regent Keds." "Keds," a line of canvas shoes with rubber soles, was introduced in 1917. Boots were rarely worn in summer after 1919. Catalog #1976.121.2. *Right:* Brown canvas boots with rubber soles worn by Abia Stoddard Howland "to go walking, berrying, and to inspect fences and fields" in Royalton, Vt., in the 1920s. Catalog #1984.33.22. (See fig. 76 for brown canvas tennis shoes of this period.) *Courtesy Historic Northampton.*

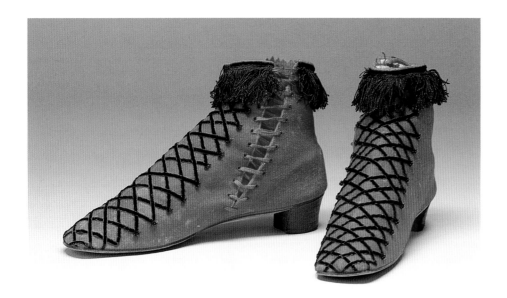

Plate 16. Side-lace boots of red wool with black velvet ribbon trim and low stacked heel. These boots were presumably considered appropriate for riding, as they were included with a saddle and riding whip as first prize for the "best and most graceful rider" in the ladies' equestrian competition at the Albany County Agricultural Society's Fourth Annual fair in September 1856. According to the *Albany Evening Journal*, the prize awarded "to Miss Catharine Fitch of New Scotland [was] a side saddle, valued at $50, and a pair of $12 gaiters." These expensive gaiters seem to have been purchased in advance without regard to the winner's size, and they show no significant wear. Census records indicate that Catharine was eight or nine years old when she won them. Catalog #1941.45A,B. *Courtesy Collection of the Albany Institute of History and Art. Gift of Margaret Boom, Slingerlands, June 13, 1941.*

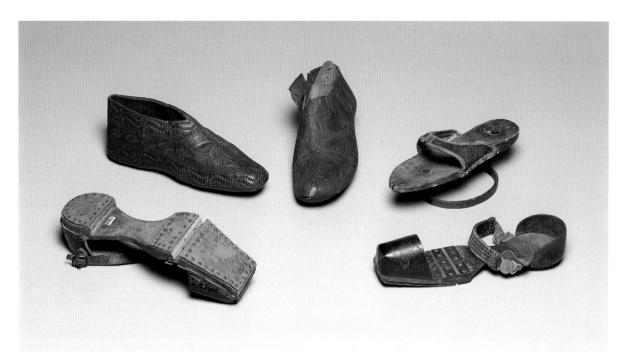

Plate 17. Overshoes were indispensable when fashionable shoes had thin soles and uppers and streets were awash with mud and manure. *Far left:* Clog turned sole upward to show the hinged wooden tread finished with a layer of sole leather nailed on, 1835–45. USMC catalog #860. *Center left:* Natural-rubber overshoe made by the Indians of the Amazon River valley, 1835–45. The leaf-shaped decoration may have been created with a small die, but the S-shaped dotted border units appear to be done freehand with a hollow reed. Catalog #112,846. *Center:* Natural-rubber overshoe on a wooden last made by the Indians of the Amazon River valley, 1830–50. The free-flowing hand-drawn floral design with a pinwheel-like center having wings ending in flower shapes is typical of the decoration on surviving rubbers. Catalog #101,657. *Center right:* Patten, a wooden sole raised on an 1 -inch-high iron ring and held on the foot with leather straps lined in white leather, covered in brown velveteen, and bound in red morocco. The flat sole and oval toe suggest a date 1810–30. (Compare fig. 78.) USMC catalog #1687. *Far right:* Clog with wooden sole hinged with leather, thick black leather toe cap and counter, 1835–50. The leather strap encloses four wire springs for elasticity. Catalog #112,455. *Courtesy Peabody Essex Museum.*

point to extend well beyond the foot. The new style was so exaggerated that for the first time alternative lasts (including one called "common sense") were widely advertised. Although rational people could avoid the needle toe, the shallow vamp was inescapably characteristic of all late 1890s footwear (see fig. 41).

The long, pointed toe went out of style about 1898, to be replaced by a rounded style called in the United States a "coin toe." The coin toe came in various widths but still all as shallow as before. One boot in the Sears catalog for 1900 is described as "the very latest, the toe being round, about the width of a quarter dollar." It wasn't much thicker than a quarter dollar either, but it was considered an advance in comfort after the needle-point toes of the 1890s. Along with the new rounder toes of 1900 came the extension sole, a sole that juts out slightly beyond the upper. The extension sole marked a new step toward substantial footwear (see fig. 28). Heels continued much as before, with stacked heels for walking and low covered wooden knock-on heels for dress. Louis heels were still a less common alternative, but they gained ground among stylish women in the years 1900 to 1905 and tended to be made somewhat higher than knock-on heels (see fig. 43).

Shoes: The plain "opera slipper" and the simple one-strap shoe with covered knock-on heel were the normal dress shoes of this period (see fig. 42). Occasionally there was a bow or rosette with an ornamental buckle, but the effect was relatively plain. Tie shoes were usually closed-tab oxford types with sensible heels and less sensible toes. Open-tab latchet-tie shoes were also worn, as were shoes with a patch of elastic goring on the instep instead of a tied fastening, a type more often advertised than surviving. Fastening shoes shared with boots a propensity for elaborate decoration during the 1890s, including pointed toe caps, curved and scalloped foxings, and perforated edges (see fig. 55). After 1900, the most elaborate examples employ the sinuous lines of art nouveau in their design. This period is notable for the introduction of russet (natural tanned leather color), suede, and white canvas to the materials used for footwear (see plate 11).

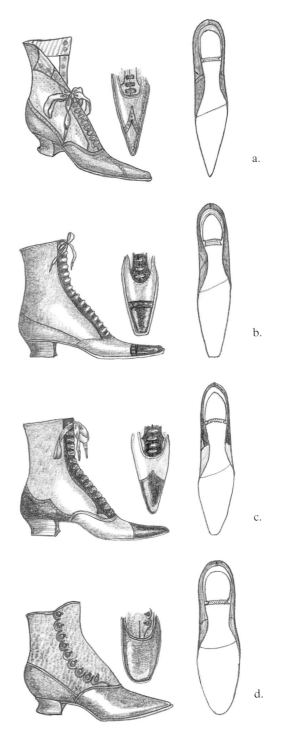

Fig. 41. Boots with alternative lasts from the 1897 Sears Catalog: (a) long drawn-out needle toe, chocolate color Dongola kid with tan cloth top; (b) imperial (square) toe, Vici kid with patent-leather tip and lace stays; (c) coin (narrow oval) toe, chocolate-color Vici kid with tan patent-leather tip; (d) common-sense toe, leather foxing with beaver felt top.

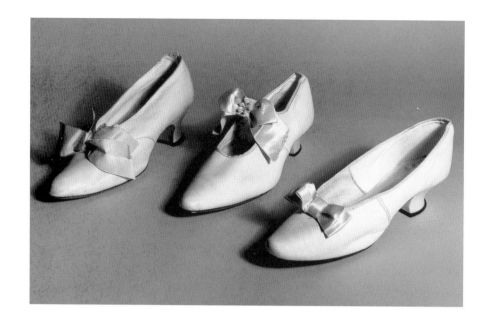

Fig. 42. White kid slippers with low knock-on heels. Note that while all three have pointed toes, the lasts over which they are made have subtly different shapes. *Right:* Wedding shoe of Annie Porter of Northampton, Mass., 1891. Catalog #66.675. *Center:* Wedding shoe of Gertrude Beckman Miller of Northampton, Mass., 1899. Catalog #1978.82.18. *Left:* Open-tab ribbon-tie shoe with porthole eyelets, a type worn for weddings and other dressy events, ca. 1908. Catalog #66.685. *Courtesy Historic Northampton.*

Boots: At the same time that pointed toes came into fashion, front-lacing boots superseded buttoned boots as the most fashionable style (see plate 10). Side-lacing boots continued to be advertised in Sears but were not fashionable. There was an attempt to update the Congress boot by making it over the new pointed-toe lasts and by adding a wavy decorative band up the center front seam, but it remained a minor style. After a decade of plainness in the 1880s, decoration returned to boots again in the mid-1890s. Along with the long, narrow, pointed toe, boots from the later 1890s typically have a peaked toe cap, and scalloped and perforated edges along the foxing and button fly (see fig. 41). After 1900, the toe cap is likely to be straight, though still perforated (see fig. 43).

1905–14 (Plates 10 and 11)

Heels and Toes: Beginning in 1905, the toe gradually became deeper, sometimes swelling into a noticeable bulge at the end of the toe in the years 1911 to 1913. The bulging toe is far more likely to appear in boots and high shoes than in the dressier slippers, but it is occasionally found even in them. In England this style was called a Boston or bulldog toe, but the *Shoe Retailer* calls it a "high toe," and American ladies' magazines rarely call it anything in particular, at best, a "full toe." During the same period the vamp gradually shortened, and it was rather stubby from 1910 to 1914 (see plate 10). In shape, the toe for evening slippers was usually a narrow oval, almost pointed, with broader shapes used for walking, especially in the early 1910s.

Even more conspicuous than the deeper toe was the adoption of the Cuban heel. At the turn of the century, rather curvy knock-on and Louis heels had been used for dressy shoes, and a low, broad heel called a military heel was universal for walking. Now both were replaced with Cuban heels, which were straight-sided but higher, narrower, and more tapered than the military heel. The shape was used in both stacked and knock-on types, for both walking and dress wear, and barely anything else was to be found from 1906 until 1913 or 1914 (see fig. 68).

Shoes: Slippers (now called pumps in contemporary documents) were quite plain, except for a very simple bow or a small, nonfunctional buckle and little, pointed tab at the throat (shoes with tab or tongue and buckle were now called Colonials rather than Molières). Strap shoes went out of fashion from about 1905 to 1909, replaced by the newer open-tab ties, but they did return slowly in the early 1910s. The new tie shoe (known in the United States as a "blucher oxford") had large "porthole" eyelets and was tied with broad silk laces or ribbons. If the toe cap was omitted, it was considered stylish enough even for brides (see fig. 42). Elastic and buttoned shoes, although far less common, were also available. By the mid-1910s, slippers became increasingly important, owing to the shortened skirt, the increased visibility of the foot, and the consequent desire to have it look as small as possible.

Boots: Boots nearly all had a straight, perforated toe cap, but otherwise the fancy seaming that had begun in the 1890s faded away. By 1909 or 1910, nearly all boots were "slipper foxed"; that is, the vamp extended in a single piece all the way to the back seam. When this foxing (known as a golosh in Britain) contrasted with the boot top, the result looked like a slipper with a gaiter above it. Buttoned boots began to gain importance early in this period, and from 1910 to 1915, nearly all fashionable boots advertised were buttoned (see plate 10). In the years around 1915, when short skirts encouraged variety in footwear, one could even find a few side-lace and elastic-sided boots.

1915–22 (Plates 10–12)

Heels and Toes: The bulge at the toe was no longer in fashion, but the toe was still a comfortable depth—nothing like the shallowness fashionable about 1900. The pointed toe returned, however, along with a lengthening vamp, which was quite drawn out

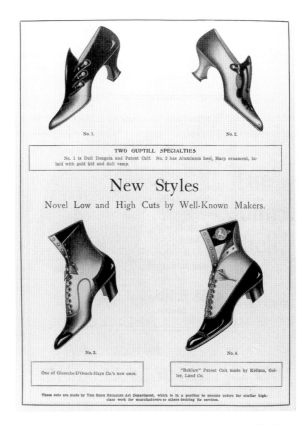

Fig. 43. New styles for the spring 1904 season previewed in the *Shoe Retailer,* August 5, 1903, p. 18. The vamps are still quite shallow but the right-hand boot has already begun to bulge upward slightly at the toe, a feature that will become quite pronounced about 1911–13. *Courtesy Lynn Museum.*

by 1917. Straight-sided heels might still be used for walking, but dressy shoes had high, curved Louis heels beginning in 1914. Even tie shoes and boots were frequently made with Louis heels in this period.

Shoes: Multi-strap shoes returned to fashion briefly in 1915 and 1916 (see plate 11) but the United States entry into World War I encouraged simpler pumps and oxfords. Slippers continued much as before except that the small tab on Colonial pumps grew again in 1917 into a large tongue that was often finished with a good-sized bow. The tie shoes of the late teens were generally oxfords (closed tabs) with either Cuban or high Louis heels. They were often made in dark brown or gray leather with perforations along the seams. After the war, sports oxfords could be made of contrasting materials such as white buck or canvas with brown or blue leather (see fig. 77). Relatively simple one-, two-, and three-strap shoes returned to style in 1921 and became the most characteristic style of the early 1920s.

Boots: In 1916, as a result of the shorter skirts, very high boots with eight- to nine-inch uppers came into fashion. These had the new longer vamp and pointed toe, high heels (Louis heels as often as not), and very often slipper foxing (see plate 10). This was the last period of the walking boot in fashion, and nearly all are front-lacing. Button boots became much less common once the height increased. The *Shoe Retailer*, reviewing fall styles in 1921, remarked, "The feeling continues that boots will be in little or no demand this fall except in the more Northern states."[11] Boots were rarely mentioned in the *Shoe Retailer* after that, and advertisements for boots no longer appeared in the *Ladies' Home Journal* after 1923. The demise of the boot seems to have been caused in good part by the ever-increasing price of leather, which made boots a more expensive option than low shoes, but also by the shortened skirt, which encouraged dressier and lighter types of footwear.

1923–30 (Plates 11 and 12)

Heels and Toes: The extremely long and pointed toe of the late teens gradually passed out of fashion beginning in 1921 in favor of a slightly shorter and more rounded toe. Manufacturers experimented throughout the twenties with short-vamped, square-toed lasts in the French style, but these seem to have been used chiefly in oxfords and other low-heeled informal shoes. Most dressy shoes still tended to have narrow, oval toes and higher heels, though a swing toward shorter vamps is noticeable toward the end of the decade. The curved Louis heel went out of fashion about 1923, and from 1924 nearly all heels had relatively straight sides, although they might have a Louis construction. Walking and day shoes had lower, broader heels, afternoon and evening shoes had higher, more slender heels, and by the later 1920s, heels could be as much as 2⅝ inches high.

Shoes: Slippers were still worn for afternoon and evening, but they were not nearly as fashionable as strapped shoes. In fact, the most remarkable characteristic of mid-1920s shoes is the use of complex strapwork, cutouts, and elaborate contrasting materials, including reptile leathers, gilded leathers, and gold and silver brocades. Fancy straps and cutouts were at their height from 1923 to 1925, but contrasting materials and dressy shoes cut down at the sides persisted into the late 1920s (see plate 12).

Tie or strap shoes were worn for walking (see fig. 44), since boots were no longer fashionable. Tie shoes for sports had low heels and more or less broad, squarish toes. They often incorporated contrasting leathers for the winged tips, foxing, and lace stays. Dressier tie shoes had a moderate Cuban or high Spanish heel, and three to six pairs of lace holes. The look of a high-cut shoe without the troublesome laces could also be achieved by insertions of elastic goring on each side of the instep. Gored shoes, like the strap shoes and oxfords, were generally embellished with contrasting strapwork and cutouts.

Boots: As far as fashion was concerned, boots barely existed after 1921. Winter walking boots continued to be worn by more conservative women for a few years, of course, but the occasional attempts made to revive them as fashionable walking footwear during the 1920s did not succeed. Plain front-lacing kid boots with low rubber heels did continue to be available throughout the twenties, but most were marketed as "comfort shoes" made only in wide widths. Other boots were designed only for specific uses. Stylish women did wear rubber overshoes with buttoned or zippered closures. Riding boots were worn as they had been for fifty years, while canvas tennis shoes with rubber soles were now available in high-tops as well as oxfords. Fleece-lined front-lacing boots were offered for utilitarian cold-weather wear and for winter sports.

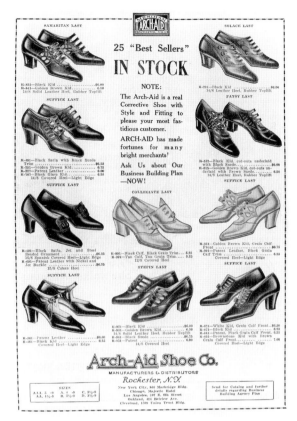

Fig. 44. A typical selection of late 1920s women's shoes, including strap styles, oxfords, and gored shoes, appears in this advertisement for Arch Aid Shoes in the *Shoe Retailer*, July 9, 1927, p. 21. *Courtesy Lynn Museum.*

CHAPTER FOUR

The Correct Dress of the Foot

We who look back at fashion as past history naturally find it useful to have a chronological summary of changing shoe styles such as was offered in the preceding chapter. What mattered to the woman who wore any of those transitory modes, however, was how to choose the right shoe from the range of alternatives allowed to her at that one particular time by the state of the industry, current fashion, her disposable income, and her position in society. In making this choice, she revealed her personal taste, perhaps her character, and very probably her class. To understand the messages conveyed by such personal choices in dress, it is necessary first to learn what alternatives were available at each period, and then which ones the conventions of etiquette considered suitable for each kind of occasion. Only when we compare individual choice against this standard of appropriateness (as it was understood in that time and place, not ours) can clothing begin to have for us the expressiveness that it had for the people who wore it.

Sartorial etiquette was no less complex during the nineteenth century than it is today. It can be difficult for us after so many years to discriminate the subtle distinctions within each category that were probably quite obvious to contemporary observers. In addition, what kind of shoe was considered suitable for walking or dancing or sports changed over time, and what constituted good taste at one period cannot be assumed to hold true in another. The requirements of etiquette became noticeably more demanding in the second half of the century, when fashion required different styles of clothing for different occasions during the day. In 1795, *Heideloff's Gallery of Fashion* was content to differentiate morning, afternoon, and evening dress with the odd mourning, riding, or court costume, and the shoes worn on any of these occasions might differ only in color. But by 1881, *Godey's* differentiated at least six occasions requiring a separate kind of shoe:

> In the street, on foot, ladies wear the rather high boot; at dinner semi-high shoes; in the evening, extremely low shoes, black, white, or colored, with semi-high heels and bows or open work straps in front; house shoes are also made of bronze kid, trimmed with satin bows and silk cord. Stuff or kid shoes are prettily embroidered with a bouquet of flowers in colored silk. The semi-high shoes, with open work bars, of kid or leather, are the most fashionable for the day time, to wear over colored silk or thread stockings. Boots for visiting and carriage are of fine kid or satteen, either black or of the color of the costume.[1]

And this enumeration does not even include utilitarian overshoes or special shoes for bathing or riding. If anything, the distinctions became yet more subtle in the early twentieth century, and it is clear that having a shoe specifically suited for the event, rather than an all-purpose shoe neutral enough to cover a variety of occasions, was one of the subtle ways used to express not only taste but status. Indeed, perhaps the most important function of clothing has always been to indicate class, and shoes are no exception. Status can be revealed through ostentation and display, but far more satisfying to the refined sensibility is knowing precisely what costume is appropriate for the occasion. A woman who wore light satin boots to do her shopping in 1870 might have succeeded in displaying an indifference to practicality only possible for the wealthy, but what would have struck everyone who saw her was how silly she looked in footwear suitable only for a ball.

The information presented in this chapter was gleaned primarily from fashion journals and etiquette books intended for middle-class readers. Such books may tell us a good deal about the standards prescribed for dress, but they cannot be assumed to describe what was actually worn any more than fashion magazines today describe what most women wear to do their grocery shopping. To discover what was really worn on ordinary occasions is not an easy task, especially before the twentieth century, when photographs were still likely to present their sitters formally posed in their best clothing. Nevertheless, it is important not to assume that most people, just because they were not rich, were ignorant of or were indifferent to fashion.

Most costume scholars now feel that at the top of the social pyramid, there was a very small group of extremely wealthy and urban women who could afford to represent every passing nuance of fashion in their wardrobes. At the bottom, there was a far larger group for whom any element of style in clothing was a luxury and whose real worry was obtaining food and shelter. The rules of etiquette in dress have nothing to do with either of these two extremes, but the large and broadly defined middle class in between seems to have taken these rules fairly seriously. What evidence is available suggests that the large majority of this middle group of women attempted (as far as their means allowed) to keep in step with current fashion and to dress appropriately for the occasion. But where a well-to-do woman could buy enough clothing to express many levels of formality, a poorer one made do with fewer. Perhaps she could afford only two pairs of shoes, but it was the rare American woman who made both of them utilitarian and then alternated them every day to make them last a long time, as pure practicality might suggest. Far more likely was that she would buy one sturdy pair to wear six days a week, and another light and dressy pair that she saved for church and other special occasions. Many hardworking women who dressed without pretension when working at home, with only the family about, would still attempt to observe more formal conventions when going to church, and rural families were more likely to adopt the standards of the etiquette books when they went into town. The prescriptions that follow are those that women who read the fashion journals would be aware of, whether or not they had the means to follow them in every detail.

The first and most basic distinction in nineteenth-century shoes is whether they were suitable for indoor or outdoor wear. This difference was far more strongly insisted on in the second half of the century, once boots became the rule for street wear, and it gradually faded in the 1910s, when boots began to pass out of fashion. By the 1920s, when low shoes were being worn for all occasions, they appeared in a great variety of cuts and materials, all of which implied gradations of formality to contemporary wearers. In general, it was permissible to wear outdoor shoes inside. What was frowned on was wearing indoor shoes outside, because wearing clothing defined by custom as private in a public setting violated strongly felt taboos. These conventions (as regards footwear) are much weakened today, but we demonstrate the shadowy persistence of this nineteenth-century attitude every time we feel faintly embarrassed at being caught outdoors in bedroom slippers.

Among indoor footwear, there were three main types: boudoir slippers, evening shoes, and general indoor shoes. Boudoir slippers were worn at home as a part of negligé dress—that is, with a dressing gown. They correspond with what we call bedroom slippers today, but many were not very "bedroomy," and they were not always clearly distinguished from general indoor shoes except perhaps by being worn in a more comfortable size. Evening shoes or boots were worn for the most formal of occasions, such as balls and evening parties, formal dinners, and the dressier theater parties. The less formal an evening event, the more likely the shoe worn would have been a general indoor shoe. These latter were shoes or boots worn chiefly indoors when a woman was fully dressed for an ordinary occasion, but in practice the type is not always easy to distinguish. They constitute the transitional category between indoor and outdoor footwear. While they might sometimes be worn to step outside, they were not considered heavy enough for serious outdoor walking. Shoes intended for wear indoors (or in a carriage) were typically made with turned soles, while shoes meant for walking outdoors or for general wear were made with welted or McKay-sewn soles. This distinction had almost the force of a rule, but apparently the infractions were widespread.

The walking or street shoe or boot is the main type of outdoor shoe. It can vary greatly in pattern and sturdiness, but in its day, each type was considered heavy enough for walking in paved towns. Lighter and more elegant versions of the street shoe were worn as part of an elaborate carriage, promenade, or visiting costume. The distinction between walking and carriage dress was that carriage costume involved an element of display. Nineteenth-century carriage, promenade, and visiting dresses were made of richer materials and were more elaborately trimmed, while walking dresses were supposed to be neat, plain, and practical. While one might set foot to earth in carriage dress, it was only under ideal conditions and for short distances. Thus the footwear could be made of silk or satin, materials that would be impractical for serious walking. The rough early-twentieth-century equivalent of carriage dress was afternoon dress, a term that denoted clothing for dressy daytime events like concerts and teas.

Walking shoes served most women as working shoes as well, although there were some heavier and more substantial alternatives specifically intended for heavy use in garden, farm, or factory. These utilitarian shoes, while they must have been common in their day, survive only rarely in museum collections, and while scattered references to them appear in written documents, they are more difficult to describe authoritatively than the more fashionable kinds of shoes.

Indoor Shoes
Evening Shoes

Evening Slippers, 1795–1870: It is ironic that of all early nineteenth-century shoes, the type that survives in greatest quantity is the very one that in its day was least worn: the thin-soled, white kid or satin slipper with ribbons to tie round the ankle (see plate 5). Although in the 1790s and very early 1800s, slippers both in white and in colors were appropriate both for walking and for evening, a division was soon made that limited colored shoes to walking and day wear and relegated white to the evening. Even by 1810, *Ackermann's* felt the need to comment that although the slipper represented with one evening dress is "of the same colour as the robe [blue], and is trimmed with silver, . . . those of white satin or kid are to be preferred."[2] After 1815 the colored shoe for full dress was almost unknown, and white predominated for evening wear in general. In the 1820s, black satin gradually began to encroach upon the domain of white slippers, being worn more and more for informal evening occasions and eventually for all but the most formal events. After 1830, white satin slippers were limited almost entirely to balls and weddings. This continued to be true through the 1840s and 1850s. *Godey's* tells a story in 1851 of a woman who was misled into overdressing for an evening party, "even to white satin slippers."[3] The white satin slippers we find so many of today were preserved as keepsakes of special occasions the wearers wished to remember, while other shoes, more characteristic of everyday dress, were thrown away without a thought.

These simple white slippers altered very little over the years. Although the toe shape changed subtly, the most remarkable development was the growing size of the rosette between 1855 and 1870. "For full toilet," *Godey's* wrote in 1855, "the prettiest dressing for the foot is a very thin embroidered thread-stocking and a white satin slipper, with a large rosette on the top of the foot."[4] Unlike the twelve dancing princesses, most women did not wear them to holes in a single night, and many a plain pair made in the 1840s was carefully packed away, to be brought out for service again ten or twenty years later, as good as new. They required only a rosette, easily stitched to the thin satin, to bring them up to date.

Sometimes an 1840s or 1850s slipper was modernized in the 1860s by adding a heel as well as a rosette, though the result was not by any means a graceful or well-fitting shoe (see fig. 344). What is more remarkable about 1860s slippers is how often the heel was omitted when the shoe was to be worn for a wedding, in spite of the fact that heels were nearly universal in other kinds of footwear. The Lynn Museum, for example, has an 1869 wedding slipper that was made in the entirely flat style that by that time was very old-fashioned. In 1869, there was certainly no dearth of white heeled slippers to choose from, so we must conclude that the bride made her choice deliberately. Perhaps she felt that the demure and ladylike heelless style her mother and grandmother had worn was more suitable for a wedding with its promises of wifely obedience than modern high-heeled shoes, even if she had no intention of continuing to wear such prim footwear after the wedding. Indeed, the Lynn wedding shoes have had heels added to them so they could be used again after the wedding (see fig. 45), and in this form they no longer fit into the triangular box in which they were bought. This persistence of the heelless slipper for weddings signals a drift in wedding garb away from contemporary fashions in dress and toward the highly symbolic archaic dress in which most brides get married today. The traditional relations between the sexes as expressed in the marriage ceremony have diverged so far from the realities of everyday life that to take those vows apparently requires putting on a sartorial identity that is entirely divorced from the way we normally present ourselves. The first steps on this road were already taken by the time the Lynn bride bought her wedding shoes in 1869.

Not all brides were as concerned with tradition as the Lynn bride seems to have been. A wealthy Chicago girl who married in 1863 seems to have cared

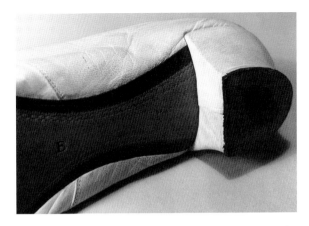

Fig. 45. Wedding shoe of Addie Smith, married June 2, 1869, in Lynn, Mass., showing the knock-on heel that was added to the original heelless shoe, presumably to make the shoe suitable for wear after the wedding. Note that the decorative edging continues beneath the heel, which would not be the case were the heel original to the shoe. The shoe was made by S. P. Driver and Bros. of Lynn and survives with its original labeled triangular white box, into which the shoes no longer fit because of the added heel. Catalog #5554. *Courtesy Lynn Museum.*

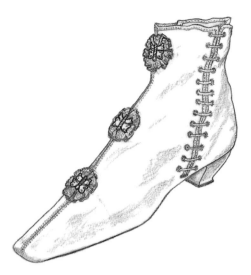

Fig. 46. White silk wedding boot of Frances Julia Tucker, who married Henry Alonzo Huntington in Chicago on July 23, 1863. The wooden heel is covered with gilded kid, and the tongue is lined with pink silk. The butterflies were a stylish motif in the early 1860s. Label: Cantrell, Maker, 813 Broadway, Between 11 & 12 St., New York. Historic Northampton catalog #1979.30.86.

less about the heritage of her grandmothers than reflecting every nuance of current fashion. She chose to wear white silk side-lacing boots with three lace rosettes down the front (see fig. 46). In the middle of each rosette a beautifully detailed gold butterfly alights (butterflies were the latest fad), and rather than proclaiming her wifely modesty, when this bride lifted her hem to ascend the church steps, the lucky observer glimpsed a flirtatious pair of little gilded heels.

Evening Boots, 1830–85: As boots became more fashionable through the 1840s, 1850s, and 1860s, they began to be appropriate for a wider range of occasions, and by the 1860s they could be worn even for formal evening occasions if they were made of silk or satin. One very early reference (assuming that the French word *bottines* is not being misused) appears in the English periodical *La Belle Assemblée*, reporting dress in Paris in September 1830: "*Bottines* of *gros de Naples* are the *chaussure* most generally adopted even in full dress. They are square-toed: some are laced before, others are fastened by small rosettes of ribbon." Fashion plates of evening dress in the late 1820s and 1830s show slippers, not boots, but by the 1850s evening boots are mentioned as if they were no longer a novelty. In November 1855, *Godey's* informed readers that "white or light-colored satin boots, with light heels, are still seen in ballrooms. . . . Those for dancing have the soles as thin as possible." Gradually through the 1860s, boots became the norm for evening wear, often being made of satin to match the color of the dress. By November 1862, *Godey's* opined that "for evening dress, though boots are in the ascendant, black satin slippers are the most suitable and becoming, as they reduce the apparent size of the foot. With dress slippers, stockings with colored silk clocks should be worn."

Boots became increasingly common in the later 1860s and early 1870s, and in February 1871 *Godey's* reported that "evening boots are invariably gaiters, slippers being confined to morning negligé. White satin or kid boots are most used, as they will suit any dress." The practice of wearing boots for evening persisted at least until 1880 (*Godey's* illustrates a pair in pale blue satin embroidered with flowers in that year) and probably a few years longer still, at least for weddings (a Montpelier, Vermont, bride wore a pair as late as 1884[5]). Other remarks in *Godey's*, however, indicate that the fashion for wearing boots with formal dress had begun to fade as early as 1873 and 1874. "Clocked stockings, open worked like lace . . . are again worn with full dress. In consequence of this, very low slippers take the place of gaiters."[6]

Evening boots can be distinguished from day boots in several respects. First, while day boots may have welted soles, the evening boot always has a turned sole, and through the 1850s and early 1860s has side lacing. The material will be satin or perhaps ribbed silk, usually white or black, but occasionally a color, and there is rarely any foxing on the heel or toe (though a contemporary American lithograph of a dance does clearly show foxing on the women's boots). Foxed satin boots would have been more appropriate for visiting or carriage dress. Although side lacing persisted occasionally into the 1870s, by the late 1860s buttoned fastenings were more usual for evening (both patterns are also found in contemporary walking boots). Front-lacing and elastic-sided boots, however, seem to have been primarily day or walking footwear. The "ball boot of white *gros grain*, embroidered with white cordon; satin knots and white cord tassels" pictured in *Godey's* in October 1870 is unusual in having elastic side gussets. A surviving boot made of white linen with white elastic side gores and turned sole (see fig. 287) may perhaps have been worn for less formal evening events or with the organdy dresses fashionable at this period.[7]

Evening Slippers, 1870–1930: Slippers began to replace boots for evening wear beginning in the mid-1870s. *Godey's* reported in 1874 that "low slippers, of black or white satin, are worn on full dress occasions by young ladies, instead of the buttoned gaiters formerly worn. The slipper is simply shaped, not covering the instep in the Marie Antoinette fashion, and displaying to advantage the elaborately embroidered and openwork stockings that are again in vogue."[8] Short-vamped slippers with low knock-on heels continued to be the typical evening shoe through the 1880s and early 1890s. Fashion illustrations often show 1880s slippers with rather complex rosettes and embroidery not all that different from shoes of the 1870s, but these were apparently noteworthy exceptions that required illustration in order to be understood rather than the normal choice (see figs. 476, 486). Fashion commentators are more likely to remark on the plainness of 1880s shoes. "Fine slippers are absolutely without ornaments, even a bow or tie for those low cut. They are of very fine kid, and the intent in effect is to make them so close fitting and plain that it is difficult to tell where stocking and slipper meet."[9] To ensure the desired effect, stockings were worn to match the shoes. Surviving slippers are found in both styles, either quite plain or with a bow or rosette. Shoes in white satin or ribbed silk, and in white, black, or bronze kid are common survivors, but shoes were also made in silk to match the color of the dress (see plate 9). Dinner and evening dresses of the late 1870s and 1880s were often made in rich, dark tones, and many surviving shoes are in shades of dark red or brown.

Beaded and embroidered vamps were a particularly fashionable choice in evening shoes of the late 1880s and early 1890s. In 1894 we are told that "evening shoes are very dainty, and often very elaborate. . . . White and black kid slippers are, of course, in great favor, and the toes of most evening slippers are embroidered in silk or beads to match the trimmings of the gown for which they are intended. With a light colored ball or evening gown a dark shoe is not in keeping, unless it be of tan-colored kid to match the shade of the gloves [although in 1892 the verdict had gone against tan shoes and gloves and in favor of white shoes with light evening dresses[10]]. Black satin or kid slippers should be worn with a black evening gown."[11] Surviving slippers from the early 1890s are often found in soft shades of off-white, yellow, gray, or pink satin to match the dress, but velvet and moire are also mentioned.

By 1899, dark shoes were more acceptable with light dresses than they had been previously. "If one can afford slippers and stockings to match the gown in point of color, it is always well to wear them, but not necessary. Handsome black slippers and stockings are always good form, and at the moment a severe black slipper of soft kid, set off by a single handsome plain gold or jeweled buckle, is considered quite smart with light gowns."[12] Exactly this state of affairs is reflected in the mail-order catalogs of the 1890s that catered to a middle-class clientele. Slipper choices were mainly white or black kid, either plain or with a single strap that was often entirely covered by a satin bow with a buckle in the center (see fig. 134). Only one style (a buttoned one-strap) was offered in satin in a choice of colors (black, blue, pink, red, white, Nile green, lavender, lemon, canary, or brown in the 1897 Sears catalog). At a price of $1.98 the pair, these were more expensive than kid slippers, which ranged from $1.00 to $1.65.

As low shoes, including pumps, began to be more and more worn for walking, evening shoes could not be distinguished by their slipper cut alone. After 1900, one finds that evening shoes generally have higher and slimmer heels than day shoes, and at periods where day shoes may have rounded toes, the toes of evening shoes will be narrower and more nearly pointed. When strapped patterns became fashionable for all kinds of occasions in the 1920s, the evening shoes were differentiated by having the sides cut down all the way to the sole. The small paste ornaments and satin bows that had been used as well as beading in the early 1890s continued in favor into the new century. Nineteen thirteen was a big year for shoe ornaments, often of cut steel or rhinestones in a buckle shape. These were sold separately, so that the customer could match the slipper of her choice with an ornament to her taste.

Evening shoes were also distinguished by their fabrics. They continued to be made in satin to match the dress (an advertisement in the *Shoe Retailer* in 1915[13] lists nearly the same colors for satin evening shoes as were available from Sears in 1897). A preference for light, neutral colors rather than black is often mentioned from the 1910s. For example, silvery gray satin slippers with matching hose were recommended in 1920 for evening frocks of every color.[14] By the mid-1920s, this neutral, all-purpose color was likely to be gold or silver, carried out in either kid or brocade. Metallic fabrics had appeared shortly after 1910, although they were not as common in that decade as they came to be in the 1920s. The *Ladies' Home*

Journal noted in 1913 that "silver and gold slippers made of the silver brocaded tissues are charming for dancing gowns, but are fragile, as they easily tarnish and it is difficult to clean them."[15] Throughout the teens and twenties, except for a flurry of popularity about 1921–22, all-purpose black had become a safe choice rather than a stylish one (see plate 12).

No account of early-twentieth-century evening shoes would be complete without mentioning "tango shoes." These shoes with their long ribbons crisscrossing several times across the instep and up the ankle were almost certainly among the "extreme novelties" that "a wise woman will hesitate before venturing to wear," according to the *Ladies' Home Journal* in June 1913. But somebody must have dared, because examples do survive. The Peabody Essex Museum has a pair in blue velvet with rhinestones set in the heels (see fig. 494). How practical they were is open to question. The *Shoe Retailer* noted, when describing this fad, "an objection offered by a prominent Philadelphia manufacturer is that in lacing this shoe and in fastening the ribbon around and half-way up the calf of the leg, in the manner shown in many of the illustrations of this novel form of shoe fastening, is that it will be impossible to keep the lacing from coming loose and sliding down the leg."[16]

Boudoir Slippers

Boudoir slippers (also known as toilet slippers and morning slippers) were roughly equivalent to bedroom slippers today. They were an element in negligé dress, of which the main garment was the wrapper, or alternatively, the sacque worn with a skirt or petticoat. Wrappers came in many variations and under many appellations, including dressing gowns, peignoirs, morning gowns, tea gowns, bathrobes, and housecoats. Sacques were also called matinées, bedgowns, combing jackets, and short gowns. The defining characteristic of all these garments was that the bodice was unfitted, or only loosely fitted, so that it could be worn without a corset. Negligé footwear, like the gowns it was worn with, was supposed to be loose, comfortable, and convenient to put on and off. In mail-order catalogs at the turn of the century,

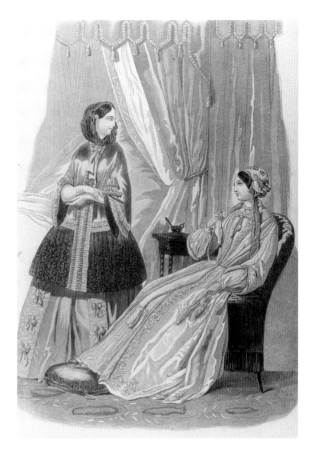

Fig. 47. "I am sorry you cant go," from *Godey's Lady's Book*, January 1850. The seated lady in this fashion plate is not feeling well enough to attend a party. She is wearing an elegant embroidered version of the loose, open robe known as a wrapper. Such garments were suitable only for the boudoir and the breakfast table (note, nevertheless, that the lady is shown wearing gloves), and were worn with decorative boudoir slippers.

most shoes are advertised in several widths, but most boudoir slippers are listed only as "full width."

Negligé dress was worn before getting dressed in the morning and could be retained through breakfast with the family and sometimes until noon, depending on its cut and material. Utilitarian versions of it were worn by women while working, but not ordinarily with boudoir slippers. It was also worn as a matter of course when one was sick or convalescent and confined to bed or to one's room, and by most women during the later stages of pregnancy.

In the middle of the nineteenth century, particularly in the 1850s, dressing gowns became very elaborate and were permitted in slightly more public indoor settings. One elaborate sacque and petticoat illustrated in *Godey's* in 1857 "is intended for a bride, a fashionable hostess receiving morning calls, or for a watering place later in the season."[17] Toilet slippers also stepped out into a world beyond the boudoir—although of course only when they were made in styles to accord with the pretty gowns. Dressing slippers were considered appropriate while inside a train, ship, or hotel, but they were never to set foot outdoors. "Dressing-slippers are well in their way, and often daintily becoming. It is never well to be without a pair, in your bag or basket, for your state-room or the hotel; but a slippered foot, descending from a rail car, or promenading a deck, however pretty and attractive, would be very likely to subject the owner to impertinent, if not unkind remark and criticism."[18]

In the 1850s, at least, boudoir slippers were permitted even in the public dining room of one's hotel during breakfast. In an illuminating article about the clothing a woman should wear during a trip to Washington, D.C., *Godey's* advised in 1853 that "a morning dress, particularly at a public table, cannot be too simple. Dressing-gowns are allowable; but it is best not to have them too elaborate. . . . Slippers are part of a morning toilet, and just now one [finds them] of every variety and style, from the plain black kid or morocco to the elegantly embroidered or quilted Paris tie, worn with white English cotton hose."[19]

Warm boudoir slippers made high on the foot, wadded with cotton or wool and quilted, were often recommended for the sick and the old who might suffer from poor circulation, and also for people traveling in cold carriages or trains. *Godey's* was talking about shoes of this type in 1859 in a small paragraph titled "Shoes for Invalids.—If the difficulty is chronic, and the feet seldom, if ever, a natural warmth, quilted silk buskins, or ties, often give relief. They are well suited to a sick-room, and excellent for a long, cold drive, where artificial warmth cannot be secured."[20] Another example was described in 1854 as "black silk, quilted in diamonds, the sole also lined with cotton wadding. For invalids or old persons, they are the best shoes we know"[21] (see figs. 25, 49).

Knitted and crocheted slippers were also recommended for this purpose and many were made at home. In one form or another, they have never gone entirely out of use. The *Ladies' Home Journal* extolled their virtues in 1892:

> The woman who knows how to knit slippers has it in her power to give comfort to many of her friends. The knitted slipper with its comfortable lambs'

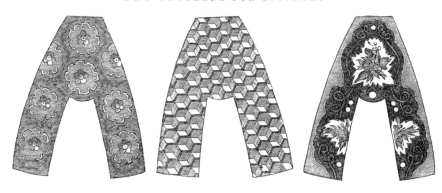

wool sole, is not only desirable as a bed-room slipper, but may be worn in bed by an invalid or one who suffers from cold feet. They become specially valuable to those who travel much in sleeping cars where the draughts are many and chances for catching cold are more than merely many. In pink or blue wool, in bright scarlet or scarlet and brown these slippers are oftenest noted. A rosette or bow of satin ribbon that is in harmony, gives a dainty finish to them.[22]

Historic Northampton has a charming if not very practical pair of pink and buff knitted silk edged with pink silk ruching dating from the 1850s or 1860s[23] (see plate 13).

Other homemade slippers were of silk or velvet that was then braided, appliquéd, or embroidered with colored floss or chenille, or even gold and silver thread. Canvas uppers were covered with needlepoint in brightly colored Berlin wools (see fig. 48, plate 14). The braided and Berlin-work styles particularly seem to have been equally suited for men or women. Many patterns for making slippers at home were given in ladies' magazines of the 1850s and 1860s, and one reader was told in 1856 that "the slipper pattern she inquired for] could not be found, being entirely out of date. She may not be aware that every year has its own special styles. Braiding is more used than the past year, but the favorite patterns are for canvas to be closely filled up."[24] When the uppers were complete, some women may have taken them to a local shoemaker to attach leather soles, but in the later nineteenth century, if not earlier, soles for slippers could be bought ready-made. In 1889, *Godey's* directed that "slippers are completed by a pair of soles lined with scarlet lamb's wool, which are sold for the purpose at shoe-stores."[25] Sure enough, search turns up a tiny advertisement in the *Ladies' World* in October and November 1899 for "Wiley's 'Capitol' Lambs-wool Soles. For Crocheted Slippers for gifts or home use. 25c." Other sets of slipper directions refer to "a strong pair of cork soles lined with flannel."[26] Berlin-work slipper uppers with the needlework done but never cut out or sewn to the soles survive in museums, their unshoelike shapes perplexing many a curator whose specialty does not happen to be costume (see fig. 48). Their numbers are perhaps explained by the *Ladies' Home Journal* columnist, who in discussing handmade gifts for men friends in 1901, recollected "as a child hearing of the revolt of men against embroidered slippers. They used to tell of how many superfluous pairs a popular man would possess. The unfortunate recipient was expected to have them made up by a shoemaker, which was costly, and it was apparently considered a delicate compliment to his foot to make them too small."[27]

Boudoir slippers tend to fall into three types: mules, slippers proper, and ankle-high shoes. Mules may or may not have heels but they have no quarters (in other words, no back half above the sole). Slippers are simply shoes cut low enough to slip on. The higher a shoe is cut, however, the more necessary some adjustment will become to get them on and off the foot. Since the whole point of boudoir slippers is not to have to bother with laces and buttons, they often incorporate distinctive methods to accomplish this. If the slipper need not be very high, the vamp can simply be extended into a tab. The tab covers and warms most of the instep, but the low sides make any fastening unnecessary. Another high form, known as a nullifier, has both a high front and high back, but there is a deep forward-slanting slit on each side, allowing the foot to be slipped in. A very similar shoe replaces the side slits with U-shaped insertions of elasticized fabric that provide the necessary ease (see figs. 51, 236).

Another solution is to make a high upper out of knitting or crochet that will stretch enough to allow the foot to get in and out. When the upper material does not have sufficient elasticity, like felt, a high shoe can be made with a wide pass line; that is, an enlarged opening. This type can never fit snugly to the ankle but it can be slipped on and off easily. Occasionally one finds a slipper that creates the wide pass line not by loosening the opening over the instep but by cutting down the quarter. The result looks very much like a mule with a little ledge around the back half (see fig. 50).

1795–1850: To find information in fashion plates about boudoir slippers before 1850 one must examine the figures wearing negligé dress, since there are almost never individual plates of footwear alone. Fashion plates of negligé dress are rare to begin with, and few of those that do exist either show the shoes clearly or describe them in the text. Museum collections contain few examples that are clearly boudoir slippers and also clearly belong to the period between 1795 and 1850. However, allowing for the limitations of the evidence, one can reasonably deduce the following:

One option was the mule. Heeled mules had been worn for negligé in the eighteenth century, and enough survive so that we have some idea what they were like then. *Heideloff's Gallery of Fashion* says that the lady in the fashion plate for November 1794 is wearing "white mules or slippers" with her dressing gown. Unfortunately, they are invisible beneath her petticoat, but at least we know they existed. A heelless mule with the throat finished with little toothlike points is clearly shown in the French periodical *Petit Courrier des Dames* for November 1829.[28] A similar pair with dentate throatline is shown in January 1833, but it is not clear whether they are mules.[29]

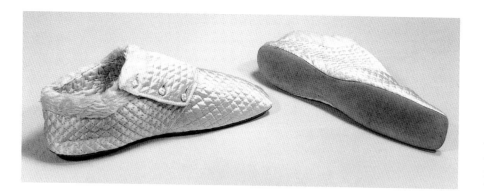

Fig. 49. These quilted white silk buttoned shoes edged with silk to imitate swansdown were preserved with the white satin slippers worn by Unis Mary Taylor Lovering at her wedding about 1844. Family history says the quilted shoes were worn over the slippers, but this would have been a tight fit as both are the same size. They might have replaced the slippers during the carriage ride to the church, but they were probably merely elegant and warm indoor shoes bought as part of the trousseau. Whatever their original purpose, it is rare to find women's buttoned footwear dating earlier than the 1860s. Catalog #122,803. Compare fig. 25. *Courtesy Peabody Essex Museum.*

Many fashion plates of negligé dress in the 1830s simply show the plain black satin slipper with ankle ties that was standard with any indoor and much outdoor dress of the period. But a few show a fancier slipper without any ties. The *Lady's Magazine* for April 1835 describes a pair with a peaked throatline as "wadded silk shoes." *Petit Courrier des Dames* for December 1831 shows a pair of long-vamped slippers embroidered with flowers, with a very low quarter, topline trimmed with fur (presumably), and a large bow. A pair of high quilted shoes with two bows on the vamp appears in *Petit Courrier des Dames*, July 1836, but the means of fastening is not shown—they could be mules. A pair of elegant white silk quilted shoes survives at the Peabody Essex Museum, but these are not technically boudoir slippers since they do not slip on and off. They are cut nearly high enough to qualify as a boot, and they fasten with three buttons. Their thin soles are slightly wadded inside, and the top edges are trimmed with silk meant to imitate swansdown (see fig. 49). They were certainly meant to wear indoors with an extremely elegant winter dressing gown, or possibly in a carriage on the way to a winter party. They are said to have been part of the trousseau of Mary Taylor Lovering in 1844.[30]

Another important kind of indoor shoe available during the early nineteenth century (and earlier) was the moccasin. This, of course, was borrowed from Native Americans, and some were still made by the Indians as tourist items at places like Niagara Falls and Saratoga. Many, however, seem to have been made by non-Indians. In 1836, Pamela Brown of Plymouth, Vermont, mentions in her journal trimming moccasins, including a pair for her mother.[31] Moccasins were worn by men as well as women. A pair at Historic Northampton is said to have been worn by a man who, after a serious accident, lived for many years as an invalid. These have the vamp plug, or apron, made with the narrow square toe fashionable in the early 1830s. The traditional drawstring ankle fastening is replaced with a side-buckling strap high across the instep (see plate 13).[32] Moccasins were also worn as overshoes for the carriage (see fig. 83).

1850–70: It sometimes comes as a surprise to modern students of costume that the most highly decorated shoes during the 1850s and 1860s were not worn for evening (those were likely to be plain white satin, as described above), but in the morning as boudoir slippers. The fashion for wearing colorful and elaborate morning slippers seems to have been a new one in the late 1840s, and *Godey's* early descriptions of them charm the reader today as much as they clearly delighted the writer over a century ago.

> The inimitable articles which we have pictured are so lovely, comfortable, and becoming, that we almost hesitate to offer them to our readers, lest many, whose distant or inaccessible residences may render their procurement impossible, will sigh for them. Designed expressly for the boudoir, they are constructed of delicately tinted silks or satins—the particular ones here delineated being respectively a rose-hued satin and pea-green silk of the richest description. They are ornamented with rosettes and that loveliest of all trimmings, the snowlike swan's-down, or equally pure ermine, which is set off by the needleworked lining, which like the outside, is of taffeta, and also quilted in exquisite workmanship. The inside soles are cushioned, so that the fair wearer may as softly tread as we would have each footstep of a beloved friend—and we mean each and all of our subscribers by that word—through this not-carpeted-with-velvet world.[33]

Of course not all boudoir slippers were quite so sumptuous. In April 1850, *Godey's* reports that "embroidered slippers, now so fashionable for a morning dress, are also cheap as well as comfortable. Some very pretty ones are made of plain cloth, bound with a ribbon that contrasts in color; with rosettes of the same." And, of course, simpler slippers meant more for warmth and comfort than for elegance were crocheted or knitted of wool or silk at home (see plate 13). But the pleasure in elaborate morning slippers persisted through the 1860s. "Toilet slippers are this season [autumn 1862] more fanciful than ever, being made of red, green, and violet morocco, with heels to match, and ornamented on the toe with velvet bows full three inches long, and wide, in the centre of which are huge buckles of steel, gilt, jet, or variegated."[34] Others in 1858 were made of "bronze, prunella, or kid . . . trimmed by ribbon a full inch broad, quilled on the outside of the opening for the instep, and running all around it, finished by a flat bow on the top of the foot."[35] This quilled ribbon running around the top of a slipper is a detail found quite often among surviving shoes during these decades.

1870–85: The period after 1870 was one of continued elaboration in boudoir slippers, but it was also characterized by the frequent use of high heels and the growing fashion for wearing mules. *Godey's* had illustrated a heeled mule as early as May 1856, and two heelless examples appeared in 1863 and 1867, but they became quite common in the 1870s and early 1880s, both with and without heels.

The upper of the boudoir slipper during this period was occasionally kid, but more often silk, velvet, or quilted satin. Many of them were elaborately trimmed (see fig. 50). Contrast appliqué, embroidery, puffy bows, rosettes, ribbon ruching, fur, and feathers were all used with abandon. One bride's slipper of 1873 was made of quilted satin edged with the eyes of peacock feathers.[36] But this delight in decoration faded in the early 1880s and by 1883, *Demorest's* reported that "for toilet and morning wear the plain fine kid slipper, without garniture of any sort, seems to be the favorite. This is a great improvement on the old fashion of bows and buckles and lace. . . . Bedroom slippers still take a wide range of styles. Fancy kid, bronze, gilt and bright colors abound, also seal leather and alligator tops."[37]

This 1883 reference is the earliest noted to "bedroom" slippers. *Godey's* had routinely referred to toilet, boudoir, or dressing slippers through the 1850s and early 1860s, and then to morning slippers from about 1870 to 1884. The change in terminology in the mid-1880s signals a change in the categories of the shoes themselves. The 1883 reference quoted above is not perfectly clear even in context, but it appears that a distinction was now being made between "bedroom" slippers, with their wider range of color and material, and "toilet and morning" slippers, more quiet in color and style. What happened over the next thirty years was that morning slippers slowly lost their special name along with their boudoir connotations and were increasingly worn indoors (and eventually even outdoors) instead of boots, as boots slowly receded in fashion. Meanwhile, bedroom slippers became far more distinctly differentiated from "public" footwear than they had been at midcentury.

1885–1910: In the late 1880s, the elegant boudoir or "morning" slipper faded from fashion and the homely bedroom slipper familiar to us today came in. Instead of feather-trimmed, high-heeled satin mules, we find low-heeled slippers made of soft leather or felt, lined with fleece, and trimmed with fur on the edges. Felt seems to have been a newly fashionable material for house shoes of all types in the early 1890s, and felt shoes were heavily advertised by Daniel Green and Company, who in 1892 claimed to be "sole agents" for "Alfred Dolge's Felt Slippers and Shoes."[38] By the late 1890s other makers had entered the market, and Daniel Green dropped the Dolge name soon after 1900.

The new, comfortable slippers were made in several styles. The simplest were low-cut, usually with

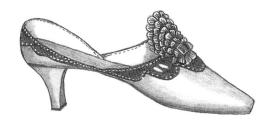

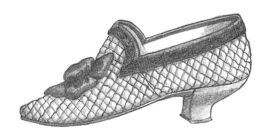

Fig. 50. Boudoir slippers typical of those illustrated in fashion magazines of the 1870s and 1880s. *Above:* "Morning slipper of bronze kid, with velvet scallops on top, edged with gold thread. Bow of velvet and gilt buckle." From *Godey's Lady's Book*, May 1870. *Below:* "Lady's morning slipper made of blue quilted satin, trimmed with a band of velvet and velvet bow." From *Godey's Lady's Book*, October 1883.

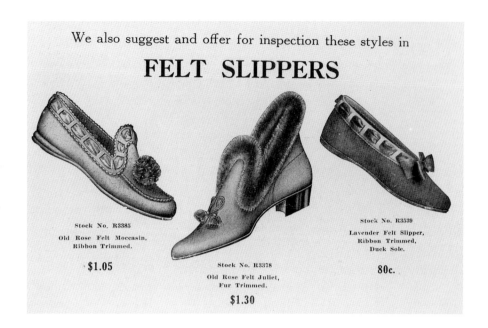

We also suggest and offer for inspection these styles in

FELT SLIPPERS

Stock No. R3385
Old Rose Felt Moccasin,
Ribbon Trimmed.

$1.05

Stock No. R3378
Old Rose Felt Juliet,
Fur Trimmed.

$1.30

Stock No. R3539
Lavender Felt Slipper,
Ribbon Trimmed,
Duck Sole.

80c.

round throatline (often fur-trimmed in the 1890s) and a low heel (see fig. 52a).
Mules also continued as an option, though less often illustrated than in the 1870s.
More common than either of these styles were slippers with the vamp extended
into a high tab to provide extra warmth and coverage over the instep.

Another type advertised in the mail-order catalogs by the early 1890s was
called a "buskin," but now no longer meaning what it had when *Godey's* used the
term in the 1850s and 1860s (see the glossary for information about this perilous
term). By the 1890s a buskin is a high-cut slipper, usually with a "gypsy" seam;
that is, one that runs from the tip of the toe straight up the instep. Inserted at the
top of this seam is a small triangle of elastic goring that provides just enough
expansion to allow the slipper to be gotten on. The goring is generally covered by
a rosette. Turn-of-the-century buskins were rather utilitarian affairs made of black
serge or occasionally an inexpensive kid, sometimes flannel-lined. Their toes had
a rounded square shape that recalled pre-1880 styles (see fig. 52b).

The most important new style was the "nullifier," also called a Juliet (the equivalent masculine style was of course a Romeo). This style seems to have been introduced for women in 1892. "The red Romeo shoe divided in the center and having
no heel has been, in the past, dedicated to gentlemen for house wear, but an enter-
prising shoemaker has discovered that they look pretty and picturesque on the
feminine foot in the house, and so they are offered for this purpose."[39] Typically,
the openings at the sides slanted forward and all the edges were lined with fur (see
plate 14; figs. 51, 52c).

There was a brief fad in 1891 for Turkish slippers. "They are all leather and are
shown in all the colors of the rainbow, heavily embroidered with either gold, silver
or white; are heelless, and have their pointed toes turned up in that coquettish
fashion which tends to make the feet look small. They are extremely comfortable

for bedroom slippers and as they are not expensive [the price is given elsewhere as $1], almost every woman who desires can have a pair."[40]

1910–30: An even wider variety of styles was offered in the 1910s and 1920s. Low-cut slippers, tabbed slippers, and nullifiers all continued in use, although the fur trimming on nullifiers became distinctly less common. One important new variation of the nullifier was similar in cut but rather than being trimmed with fur, it had satin ribbon run through slits bordering the top edge. This ribbon trimming was also used in lower tab-front styles (see fig. 51). The updated "Juliet" of the 1920s had plain edges, and, instead of a forward slanting opening, the sides were cut down in a U-shape that was filled with elastic goring (see fig. 294).

The ugly black serge buskin of the previous period died out and was replaced by another "gypsy" style. This new version was made high enough to cover the ankle, but the gypsy seam was left open far enough to allow the shoe to slip on. Like moccasins, the high tops could be turned up for warmth, or folded down, showing a decorative contrast lining. Slippers with such turndown collars were illustrated at least as early as 1891,[41] but they became a staple style in the 1920s (see plate 14).

Another newly fashionable type was the Indian moccasin, advertised in "buck, squaw and papoose sizes." These could be constructed like real moccasins, where the soft sole curls up around the foot and is sewn to an "apron" over the instep, but some also had hard soles. Most had a tabbed throatline, and many had a collar around the backpart, sometimes fringed. Naturally, moccasins were provided with "Indian" trimmings such as beadwork or images of deer heads or of Indians in feathered headdresses. Indian moccasin slippers are particularly common in advertisements in 1911 and 1912 (see fig. 52d). The apron characteristic of moccasin construction was incorporated into ordinary felt slippers as well.

While warm, comfortable felt slippers continued to reflect the "bedroom slipper" conventions of the 1890s and early 1900s, there was also a strong return of interest in lighter and more traditionally feminine

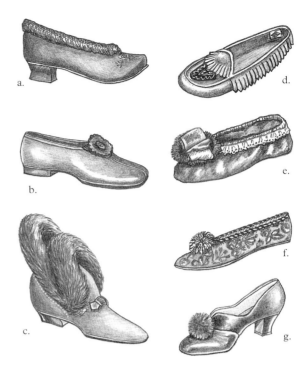

Fig. 52. Boudoir slippers, 1890s–1930s. (See also plate 14.)

(a) Felt slippers embroidered on the vamp, lined with flannel, and trimmed with plush. Made over a distinctively early-1890s last. From the Montgomery Ward Catalog of 1895.

(b) Serge buskins with a rosette hiding the small triangle of elastic goring inserted at the instep. Buskins were made in pebbled goat, serge, and felt and cost about $1. This example is from the Sears Catalog of 1902.

(c) Nullifiers were often called Romeos and sometimes Juliets and were advertised from the early 1890s to almost 1920. Other versions had decorative stitching on the vamp rather than the bow. This example, made by the Daniel Green Felt Shoe Company was advertised in *Delineator*, December 1905.

(d) "'Yipsi' Silent House-Shoes," made by the Ypsilanti Indian Shoe Company, from an advertisement in *Ladies' Home Journal*, March 1912.

(e) Slippers and mules that could be made at home from fabric scraps were frequently illustrated in the *Ladies' Home Journal* in the 1910s. They were made in a variety of styles and materials but always with flat soles, which could be bought in the local five-and-ten-cent store. This pair appeared in December 1914.

(f) Cretonne boudoir slippers advertised by the K. M. Stone Importing Company in the *Shoe Retailer*, September 20, 1919. Patterned fabrics were common in the 1910s.

(g) Bridge slippers appeared by the late 1920s. This pair was illustrated in Sears 1932 Catalog.

"boudoir slippers" after 1910. Simple, thin, round-throated slippers in a wide variety of light materials including kid, figured silk, corduroy, cretonne, crepe, and flannel were worn throughout this period. They usually had a rosette of some sort on the vamp (see fig. 52f). The *Ladies' Home Journal* included many suggestions in the 1910s for making slippers at home out of scraps of satin, ribbon, or flannel. "These lace and rosebud-trimmed satin mules may be bought ready-made, or [readers] may duplicate them on heelless soles."[42] Many of these home-made versions look as if they had elastic through the top edge to keep them on the foot (see fig. 52e). Mules returned to fashion, at first in flats, but by the end of the 1920s in heeled styles that were similar in character to the boudoir slippers of the 1870s. One Daniel Green mule of 1929 was made of rose-colored satin trimmed with maribou. A new marketing technique of the late 1920s and early 1930s was to call the dressier boudoir slippers "bridge slippers," which pegged them as suitable for home entertaining. Bridge slippers were usually made of kid or of a satinlike fabric over a stiff lining. They had high heels and leather soles (sometimes hard). One typical example was cut high on the instep but slit an inch or so to allow them to slip on. A pompon obscured the base of the slit (see fig. 52g). This renewed interest in the symbols of feminine frivolity lines up neatly with the renewed emphasis on femininity and domesticity that prevailed at the same time in women's magazines.

Indoor Day Shoes

The category of general indoor shoe is most meaningful at periods when boots were considered necessary for the street. When this was the case, it was natural to desire a lighter and lower shoe for the house, yet one that was not as loose and informal as a boudoir slipper. These indoor shoes could be either fastening shoes (ties, gores, straps, or buttons) or slippers, but when they were slippers, the distinction between them and evening shoes on the one hand and boudoir slippers on the other could be difficult to draw, especially in the period before the 1880s. After that, boudoir slippers were often made of felt or in distinctively bedroom cuts like the nullifier or the mule, so there is little confusion. But in the middle of the century, the distinction was not clearly made even by contemporary fashion commentators.

Before 1830, when boots were rarely worn and there was in general less differentiation in shoe styles, both slippers and tie shoes might be worn indoors and on the street. In the early 1830s, when shoes were still visible beneath the dresses, indoor and afternoon dresses were usually shown with black slippers, presumably satin or kid, although cloth-topped boots were not unknown. But as skirts got longer and then fuller, obscuring all but the tip of the toe, one cannot tell in a fashion plate whether a boot or a shoe is being worn. Unfortunately, footwear was rarely described either in the descriptions to the plates or in the general commentaries. But at some time in the period 1835–50, behind the mysterious curtain of ladies' skirts, the transition was made toward wearing boots at nearly all times of the day after the dressing gown was laid aside for a fitted dress (see fig. 53). About 1850, when the commentary in *Godey's* becomes more comprehensive, we find that elastic-sided boots were the norm for everyday wear both at home and on the street, although this could have been only a recent development since elastic-sided shoes were not widely introduced until 1847. Presumably they were preferred as a more convenient alternative to side-lacing boots, which with their minute handworked lace holes were rather troublesome to fasten.

Although boots could be worn indoors, women still had an alternative in low shoes. In the 1840s, black or tan slippers and slit-vamp ties were available. The most commonly surviving type of indoor day shoe from the 1850s and 1860s is usually made of bronze kid, the vamp cut out in fancy shapes and backed with rose or blue satin and chain-stitched in fancy looping designs (see figs. 54a, 467, 468; plate 13). With the many types of elaborate low shoes of this period, it can be difficult to decide how far from the boudoir any one example might be permitted to travel. Presumably the homemade versions in knitting, crochet, or Berlin work were for negligé only, while kid shoes with leather soles were admissible even when the lady was more fully dressed.

In the early 1860s, *Godey's* was still recommending "for house wear Congress boots with a half double sole and moderately high heel."[43] But by 1870, low shoes began to supplant boots for indoor wear and even sometimes for walking, at least in the summer. In 1872, we are told that the "Marie Antoinette slipper [that is, having a high tab and large oval rosette on the instep] is still retained for the house"[44] (see fig. 54b). In August 1875, a shoe that buckled over a tongue was described a suitable "for house or street wear." The practice of wearing boots indoors did not change all at once, however, and buttoned boots were very often worn, especially by women who could not afford a different shoe for every hour of the day. In 1875, "buttoned boots of French kid are the handsomest shoes for general wear."[45]

A new development in the mid-1870s was a "buttoned sandal slashed to display the color of the hosiery," that is, a shoe or boot with slots cut out down the entire front to suggest straps. This style was recommended for moderately dressy occasions in the 1870s and 1880s. "For home receptions, dinners, and

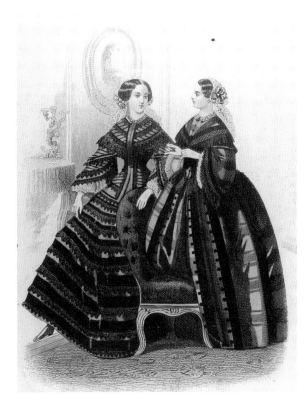

Fig. 53. From 1834 until the early 1860s, skirts rarely revealed more than the tip of the shoe, unless a lady, like this one, lifted her skirt intentionally. This plate provides evidence of the trend toward wearing boots indoors. From *Peterson's Magazine*, December 1857. *Courtesy Colonial Dames, Boston.*

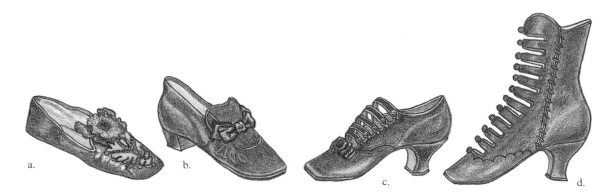

Fig. 54. Indoor shoes in the period 1850–90 tended to be somewhat more elaborate than those intended for walking.

(a) Bronze kid slipper with vamp cutouts backed with rose-colored satin, ca. 1855–65. The cutouts are edged with chain stitching and a rosette is added at the throatline. Shoes of this type may have appeared in France before 1850 and were worn in America through the 1850s and 1860s. This example contains the label "J. B. Miller & Co., Ladies' French Shoe Store, 387 Canal St., N.Y." Peabody Essex Museum catalog #123,789.

(b) Kid slipper of the type *Godey's* referred to as a "Marie Antoinette," having a high heel and a tabbed throat covered with a large rosette. These were fashionable from about 1869 to 1874. Historic Northampton, catalog #66.670.

(c) Multi-strapped shoes appeared occasionally from the 1850s but became an important indoor style in the late 1870s. *Harper's Bazar,* March 4, 1876, p. 149.

(d) Boots of the 1870s and 1880s were also made with strap effects. They are occasionally mentioned for street wear, but most were clearly intended for rather dressy indoor wear and were particularly handsome when worn with colored silk stockings. The type reappeared about 1901. This example is from *Godey's,* December 1877.

small evening parties [in 1880], the shoe with open work stripes in the upper part of stuff, dull kid, shagreen, or bronze kid, is that most generally adopted; with very light colored dresses it is also worn in white kid."[46] These multibarred shoes and boots were worn with fancy colored stockings, and must have been quite showy (see figs. 54c, 54d).

During the 1880s and 1890s, dark kid slippers and strap shoes were appropriate for indoors and dressy day wear, and they could be worn into the evening if they had a little decoration and if the heels were just slightly higher and more curved. Among black shoes, patent leather was a degree dressier than kid. Closed-tab tie shoes in the 1890s followed by open-tab ties in the 1900s became increasingly popular for wear indoors year-round, and for walking during the summer months (see figs. 55, 178, 198).

The slow but persistent inclination to limit the wearing of boots to the wintertime outdoors naturally broadened the role of the low shoes whose main sphere had previously been inside the house. This trend began in the mid-1870s and gathered speed after 1905 with the rage for tie shoes in open-tab patterns. By the early 1920s the habit of wearing low shoes was so fully established that boots were almost nonexistent, even for winter, and the difference between indoor and outdoor shoes disappeared with them. Instead, there were gradations of formality, from true evening shoes, to those suitable for formal day events, down to the most casual of sporting wear. These distinctions in formality are discussed below in the section on outdoor shoes.

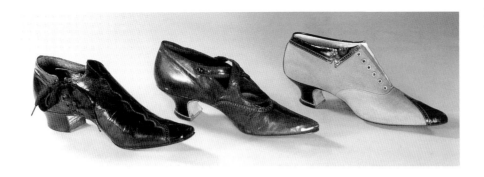

Outdoor Footwear

The Decline of Low-Cut Walking Shoes, 1795–1860

In the first quarter of the nineteenth century, most walking shoes were either slippers or tie shoes, the ties being either open-tab with one or two pairs of lace holes, or slit-vamp. While slippers tended to gravitate toward the dressier end of the wardrobe, tie shoes drifted in the other direction, losing fashionable ground especially after boots became important for walking. One finds tie shoes dating circa 1800 made in colored satin, demonstrating that the style could be quite dressy at that period (see plates 1, 2). By the 1820s, satin is no longer typical, but tie shoes do appear in fashionable shades of kid and serge probably bought to match dresses, gloves, and shawls (see plate 3). By the 1830s and 1840s, they are found in a more limited range of colors, notably fawn or golden-brown morocco, or in a beige or black patterned wool serge, foxed with morocco. Shoes of this type survive with wedding histories, but would have been appropriate only for an informal morning wedding in which day dress was worn (see plate 5). In the 1850s, when gaiter boots really took hold, tie shoes sank further down the scale of formality, and, for city walking at least, gaiters were always preferred (see figs. 60, 274, 275). As *Every Lady Her Own Shoemaker* noted in 1856, "Gaiters give the foot a much smaller and more genteel appearance than a kid walking shoe; they are easier to the foot, and if the wind blows one's skirts away from the feet, one's ankles are not so much exposed."[47] But leather tie shoes (known in *Godey's* at this period as buskins) were still permitted when cloth-topped boots were impractical. *Godey's* allows in 1857, for example, that although one really ought to put on side-lacing boots to step from a train to the platform, "those who object to gaiters as a hinderance, where a rapid toilet is necessary, may substitute a morocco buskin, neatly laced on the instep, especially if worn with a dark thread or cotton stocking."[48]

The Rise of Walking Boots, 1795–1860

American women seem to have been slow to adopt boots. "Half-boots," as the ankle-high version was called in the early nineteenth century, were worn in both England and France, but they appear to have been more particularly an English style (see fig. 56). What at first look like boots in French fashion plates before 1815 usually turn out to be a nankeen gaiter buttoning at the side and worn

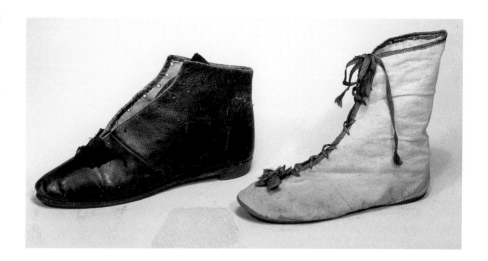

Fig. 56. In the first decade of the nineteenth century, boots were not worn for walking as often as were tie shoes in the United States, but for women who followed the English fashion and did wear them, both thick-soled winter boots and thin summer versions were available.

Right: This boot was probably worn about 1805 to 1815 by Sally Peirce Nichols (1780–1835) or her sister Betsey (1787–1864), daughters of a wealthy Salem merchant. Made of nankeen lined with linen and bound with green silk, it has a spring heel and very thin, turned sole that would have been suitable only for summer wear. Catalog #123,580.

Left: With its thick, welted sole and sensible low heel, this black leather boot would have served for winter walking, ca. 1805–15. USMC catalog #880. Dressier boots of the 1810s and 1820s had fringe around the ankle (see plate 4). *Courtesy Peabody Essex Museum.*

over a low shoe (see fig. 88). During the Napoleonic wars, when English and French fashions diverged, more and more half-boots appear in English fashion plates for walking dress. For carriage and promenade dress, however, low shoes were equally appropriate. In 1814, when fashion communication was reestablished across the Channel, one finds half-boots (identified as "brodequins à l'Anglaise") appearing more frequently in French plates, while the English abandon the half-boot in favor of French slippers with ankle ties ("sandals"). *Ackermann's* noted in 1815 that "the length of the walking petticoat continues to meet the top of the sandal, which appears in more estimation than the boot."[49]

So few boots survive in America from the period before 1835 that Mrs. Trollope's sweeping remark in 1830 that American women "never wear muffs or boots" becomes almost credible.[50] Between 1835 and 1860, however, gaiter boots (side-lacing cloth boots with a leather foxing at heel and toe) became an ever more important part of a woman's wardrobe. In the early 1830s, when skirts were still short enough to show the feet, fashion plates of walking dress show both side-lacing boots and black slippers with ribbons crisscrossed round the ankles (see fig. 57). No hard and fast rule seems to have been followed in this early period, but shoes are shown most often in summer or with carriage and promenade costume, and boots in winter or for walking. By the late 1840s, however, boots seem to have taken over as normal walking wear. They were made chiefly in black or brown wool serge, foxed in morocco to match. Brown linen was sometimes used in the summer, but the all-leather boot was not a fashionable choice from the 1830s until the late 1850s (see plate 6). Black gaiters were recommended for traveling in 1848 "as light hues are easily discolored—and the chief aim and charm of a proper traveling dress should be *neatness.*"[51] Colored boots made to match the dress were fashionable for carriage and visiting, but not often worth the expense when the feet could hardly be seen.

When elastic-sided Congress boots were introduced in the late 1840s, they began to supplant the side-lacing boot both at home and on the street (see figs. 38, 64, 283). Side lacing seems to have continued in fashion, however, with dressier costumes for visiting, the carriage, and the promenade. The fact that elastic-sided boots survive less frequently also supports the idea that they were perceived chiefly as walking and everyday wear. Slippers are rarely mentioned as street wear in the mid–nineteenth century, and when they are, they are clearly the exception rather than the rule. They appeared, for example, when the skirt in front shortened briefly in the late 1840s, but they seem to have been associated with the dressier forms of outdoor dress. By 1849, "slippers, as we have before said, threaten to supersede gaiters [cloth boots] for the street,"[52] and in 1855, "slippers, with strings and large bows, are now occasionally seen in carriages and on the public promenades."[53]

Leather Shoes for Work and Country Wear, 1795–1860

Mrs. Trollope was impressed by American women's unwillingness to wear warm stockings and practical walking shoes or boots in 1830, and in 1845, *Godey's* story "The Cheap Dress" (which is briefly excerpted in chapter 2) implies that really substantial outdoor shoes were hardly to be found in America. The narrator's English friend felt it necessary to send her heavy boots all the way from England "on the hypothesis that the slight, pretty articles manufactured for our use on this side of the ocean, were the cause of a national tendency to consumption."[54] Were substantial shoes really as rare as these references seem to indicate? Certainly, most of the women's shoes surviving in museum collections are "slight, pretty articles," but this is only natural. Wedding and ball slippers were treasured and saved while everyday footwear was worn out and discarded. While it is just credible that urban ladies who could rely on having carriages and paved sidewalks might manage in thin kid slippers and prunella gaiters, it is not credible that country ladies could do the same. What did real working countrywomen do who every day contended with muddy country lanes and feculent barnyards?

In the early part of the nineteenth century, country shoes do not seem to have been very different from city shoes, except in their materials. Leather slippers

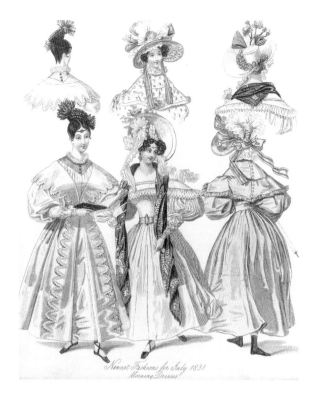

Fig. 57. After 1828, skirts were made of straight ungored panels pleated into the waistband. They were still short enough in the early 1830s to reveal the simple black slippers with ribbons crossed on the ankles and the side-lacing gaiter boots that were becoming increasingly fashionable. From *World of Fashion*, July 1831. In this transitional period, slippers were more likely to be worn in the summer and boots in the winter. *Smithsonian Institution Photo No. 77-2684.*

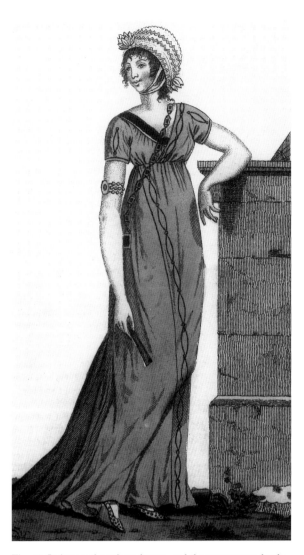

Fig. 58. Indoor and outdoor dresses and shoes were not clearly distinguished at the beginning of the century, and even walking dresses could have trains. Even when skirts were trained, they were skimpy enough to reveal the feet, and shoes were often decorated with fringe, cutouts, or embroidery, or were made of attractive stamped leathers, as in this example and in the very similar shoe illustrated in fig. 59. From the *Lady's Magazine,* August 1800, which copied the figure from a plate in the French fashion magazine *Le Journal des Dames. Smithsonian Institution Photo No. 76-16474.*

and low tie shoes were fashionable when the leather was kid or morocco, and such shoes were worn both indoors and out (see fig. 58). The 1806 wedding slipper with the double hearts incised on the sole (see fig. 59) has an upper made of fine white kid, stamped all over with a delicate black design. These shoes were not enshrined after the wedding, but were walked in until the owner wore holes through the edges of the upper where her foot overspread the narrow sole. Clear traces of straw and mud still cling to the bottoms. Rural people seem to have worn shoes very similar to these in shape, only with thicker, welted soles and heavier uppers. There are two pairs of women's substantial leather slippers in a private collection, one with the pointed toes of 1795–1810 (see fig. 358), the other with an oval toe perhaps dating from just slightly later. Few examples have survived that date clearly from the 1820s and 1830s, but we know that slippers and low ties continued to be made in calf and split leather, presumably differing little from the earlier examples except in toe shape.

There is very little evidence that countrywomen wore boots as practical footwear in the early part of the century. Boots were rare before 1830 even in fashionable circles, and although those that survive are sometimes made of leather and have reasonably thick soles (see fig. 56, left) they do not seem to have made headway in rural areas as utilitarian country wear. After 1830, boots were even less likely to be adopted in the country as a practical alternative, because they were by then usually made with thin turned soles and cloth uppers supplemented only by a leather toe cap and heel foxing. These new side-lacing gaiter boots were perceived as both ladylike and extremely flattering, because they covered the ankle and made the foot look smaller, but not as particularly sensible. They were introduced as fashionable footwear suitable for people who could afford fashionable lives (see fig. 60). In urban areas, gaiters gradually took the place of the kid slippers or ties that had been commonly worn for walking before 1830, and by the late 1840s, leather ties were closely associated with country wear.

Shoe-store advertisements in small-town newspapers suggest that slippers (often referred to as "slips") and tie shoes made of kid and morocco were the staple articles of women's footwear in the 1830s, with prunella (wool serge) and calf being mentioned occasionally as well. An advertisement in the *Maine Farmer and Journal of the Arts* of December 28, 1833, lists the following stock for the Winthrop Boot and Shoe Store.

> Josephus Stevens would inform his friends and customers that he has received his winter Stock of BOOTS & SHOES, consisting of
>> Gentlemen's thick and thin Boots and Shoes,
>> Ladies Gaiter Boots,
>>> Kid and Morocco Walking Shoes,
>>> Kid and Morocco Slippers
>>> India Rubber Over Shoes, lined and bound,
>>> Plain Rubber Shoes,
>>> Gentlemen's Rubber Over Shoes,
>>> Children's Shoes of all sorts and sizes.
> All of which he will sell as low as can be bought elsewhere.
>> N.B. Will be kept constantly on hand Shoe Nails, Thread, Pegs, Binding, Lining, &c.[55]

In the same issue, Chandler and Pullen also advertised shoes, having "just received a large and prime assortment of Ladies' Prunella, Kid, Morocco and Calf SHOES—Men's thick and thin Boots and Shoes, and youth's thick Boots. Also, Ladies' and Gentlemen's INDIA RUBBER OVER SHOES. All of which they offer very low." Chandler and Pullen evidently kept a general store, since in the same advertisement they also mention textiles, crockery, axes, and iron-hooped pails.[56] Where the Winthrop Boot and Shoe Shop advertised a more fashionable range of women's footwear, including only kid and morocco slippers and walking shoes, with the addition of gaiter boots, the general store offered shoes made of calf (more practical for the farm) and of prunella (cheaper for indoors), but apparently did not carry the more stylish but less practical gaiter boots. These differences suggest that the Winthrop Boot and Shoe Store may have catered primarily to an in-town clientele, while Chandler and Pullen dealt with people coming in from the countryside to shop.

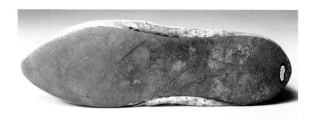

Fig. 59. Low-cut kid slippers were worn for walking in the early nineteenth century. This very stylish pair, very similar to those shown in the fashion plate illustrated in fig. 58, was worn in a wedding in 1806, and that date is incised in the sole along with a pair of overlapping hearts. Unlike the white satin wedding slippers common in the mid–nineteenth century, these were put to repeated use. Not only are the hearts nearly worn away, but since the wearer's foot was wider than the shoe, she has dirtied and even worn holes into the edges of the stamped kid uppers. Proof that they were worn for outdoor walking exists in the traces of mud and straw that still cling to the sole. Catalog #2973. *Courtesy Lynn Museum.*

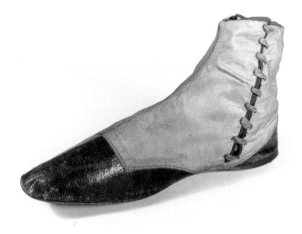

Fig. 60. Side-lacing "gaiter boot" of tan-colored silk with bronze morocco foxing, with the date "1838" written on the lining. The date is plausible. The color and quality of the silk used in this boot was common in American dresses of the late 1830s. Boots of this type became popular about 1830 because they made the foot look small and neat. They were considered suitable for paved sidewalks, not country roads. Catalog #1088. *Courtesy Lynn Museum.*

An advertisement placed by Moses Mandell for the Barre Shoe Store in the *Barre (Vermont) Gazette* in 1839 suggests the variety of shoes then being offered in some country towns. At the dressiest end of the spectrum, Mandell offered "bronze slips and double satin French slips . . . splendid articles for particular and important occasions." Moving down in formality, women could also buy "superior kid slips" and "superior kid ties," and they could choose between "elegant kid walking shoes" and "stout undressed kid walking shoes." Winter elegance called for the "ladies' French morocco fur lined walking shoes, a superior article for the coming season." For more workaday occasions, "stout calf-shoes" were available. The only women's boots listed were still cloth-topped gaiter boots, and it sounds as though they were far outnumbered by kid ties. Both India-rubber overshoes and "sole leather over shoes" are also listed.[57] The sole leather overshoes have no gender identification, but what may be an example of these is illustrated in figure 81.

The following year, in February 1840, Rufus Sacket, who sold shoes in Northampton, Massachusetts, advertised in the *Hampshire Gazette:*

Gent's calf and thick Boots and Shoes.
    do. calf and thick Brogans and Pumps.
Ladies' French Kid Slippers,
    do. kid and leather Vil. [sic] Lace and Ties.
    do. leather strap'd and heeled Shoes.
Children's Shoes, all descriptions.
             —Also, a large assortment of—
Ladies' and Gentlemen's RUBBERS, lined and bound, and plain.[58]

The "ladies' leather strap'd and heeled Shoes" were almost certainly open-tab latchet ties with one or two eyelets. The other possibility, that they were strapped slippers, is very doubtful, since strapped slippers were in general wear only before 1815 and after 1875 and at both periods they were considered dressy footwear and were made in fine materials. Sacket's strapped and heeled shoes are described as "leather," implying calf or side leather, which was suitable for workaday footwear, rather than as the dressier "kid," which seems always to have been specified by name. They probably looked like the latchet ties illustrated in figures 169 and 171, but they may have been similar to the three-eyelet brogans men were wearing for work at the same period (fig. 170). The 1840 Sacket advertisement, like that of Chandler and Pullen in 1833, lists shoes clearly meant for work, but lists no women's boots at all, even the gaiters that were coming into fashion for dressy occasions.

Perhaps by the later 1840s, gaiter boots began to be worn more generally in country neighborhoods than is suggested by these 1830s advertisements. At any rate, *Godey's* felt called upon to object to the practice in an 1849 article called "Dress in Rural Districts." Instead of consulting cheapness, durability, comfort, and health (the qualities most appropriate for country dress), *Godey's* complained, rural women insisted on aping city fashions, wearing silk mantles too heavy for the summer heat, fashionable bonnets that failed to shade the face, sunshades so stylishly small as to mock their purpose, and serge gaiters that were no match for either the mud or the dust of country roads. "Morocco walking-shoes, high in the instep, no matter what is worn on Chestnut street or Broadway [the fashionable promenades in Philadelphia and New York, respectively], are the things for country wear."[59] Two years later, "buskins," meaning leather tie shoes for walking, are again advised. "We would recommend the [buskins] for country wear, as a gaiter is folly in the extreme the moment the foot is off the pavement."[60]

The morocco shoes *Godey's* recommended as sensible for the country may have been less permeable than cloth gaiters, but they hardly qualify as thick and heavy. Morocco is one of the lightest leathers suitable for shoes, and the thin turned-sole morocco tie shoes that survive from the early nineteenth century are hardly our idea of work shoes. The more practical examples, however, are made with a welted sole rather than a turned sole, and it is probably this welted sole that distinguishes the "buskins" and "walking shoes" so often mentioned in *Godey's* in this period from otherwise similar indoor shoes. Even heavier shoes were made of calf, which itself was the lightest and finest of the leathers made from cattle skins. The "thick leather shoes" occasionally mentioned for women were presumably made from kips or from side leather, which can be split to make it as thin as calf, but which is coarser than calf in texture.

The shoe stores in larger cities offered a variety of footwear similar to that in the smaller towns, including heavy leather shoes for working women. "Ladies' kid, Prunella and Calf Shoes" were sold at the Worcester Boot and Shoe Store in 1834, along with "women's thick leather shoes."[61] It is curious that the lighter varieties of shoes were advertised for "ladies," while those expected to buy the "thick leather shoes" were "women."

Evidence for leather boots, as opposed to gaiters, is very limited before the late 1840s, but they were probably available. In a Hartford paper of 1840,

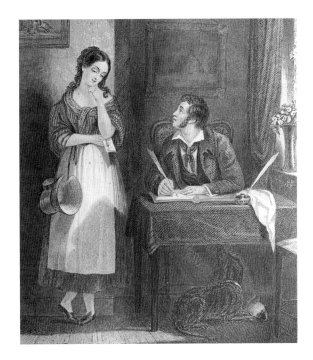

Fig. 61. "The Village Amanuensis," from *Godey's Lady's Book*, June 1842. The young girl, a model of rural innocence and virtue, is dictating a letter to her brother. The well-to-do young man who is writing it for her eventually teaches her to write and marries her to boot. Notice her laced leather shoes, probably slit vamp but possibly latchet tie. *Courtesy Heidi Fieldston.*

the Brimfield Boot and Shoe Store (apparently located on State Street in the city of Hartford, not in the town of Brimfield fifty miles to the northeast) advertised a new shipment of assorted footwear including:

1000 pr ladies' sewed and pegged boots	[16.4%]
1000 pr ladies' sewed and pegged shoes	[16.4%]
1000 pr ladies' kid walking shoes	[16.4%]
1000 pr ladies' kid slippers and pumps	[16.4%]
1000 pr ladies' cheap slips and ties	[16.4%]
500 pr ladies' morocco walking shoes	[8.2%]
500 pr ladies' gaiter boots	[8.2%]
100 pr ladies' fancy colored slippers[62]	[1.6%]

Even in this city shoe store, gaiter boots constituted less than 10 percent of the footwear offered to women in 1840, and only 25 percent consisted of any kind of boot, suggesting that most women were still wearing slippers and tie shoes for most occasions. Since cloth gaiter boots are listed as a distinct category, and pegging is not typically the way cloth footwear is constructed, it is reasonable to think that the sewed and pegged boots mentioned were made of leather. This is important evidence, considering the extreme rarity of women's leather boots surviving from the period 1830 to 1850.

Unfortunately this advertisement does not make clear how large a proportion of the "sewed and pegged" footwear in the first two categories was pegged. Few tie shoes or boots having pegged soles that seem clearly to be women's survive from the 1830s and 1840s, a fact that makes it difficult to judge how common they really were. Perhaps stiff pegged shoes were the "noisy shoes" that one 1838 etiquette book damned as being in the worst taste.[63] Pegged shoes were almost exclusively sturdy utilitarian affairs. As pointed out by Saguto, the rigid vertical attachment of the peg prevents the easy flexing of the sole and as a result the shoes are rather stiff. This was acceptable when stout, hard-wearing shoes or boots were wanted, and therefore it is in men's and boys' boots and work shoes that pegging is most commonly found. Pegging was not suitable for women's dressy slippers where the sole must be flexible and the foot must appear small and light, but if seven-eighths of American-made shoes were pegged (which was reported to be the case by 1860), then some of them must have been for women.[64]

Heavy shoes made in distinctly women's closed-tab or slit-vamp styles are rarely represented in museum collections, but they can be seen at the Peabody Essex Museum in the United Shoe Machinery Corporation collection.[65] This kind of shoe must have been worn far more commonly by women who had to work in the house, garden, and factory than the minute sample left in museums would indicate today (see fig. 62). It is also possible that the thick leather shoes and pegged shoes listed in all these advertisements were essentially identical to the heavy open-tab brogans that men and boys wore, and in that case, surviving women's heavy shoes will be indistinguishable from those worn by boys (see fig. 170).

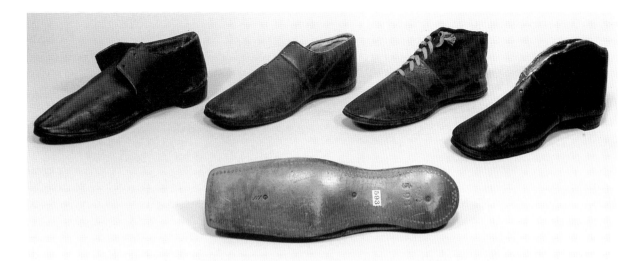

Certainly, slaves in the South wore heavy side-leather brogans when they had any shoes to wear at all, and the evidence does not suggest that there was any difference between men's and women's versions. An illustration in *Harper's Weekly* in 1856, for example, shows an African American cook in heavy open-tab brogans of the type typically worn by men (see fig. 63). Often these brogans were made in New England, but some slave memoirs describe brogans made by slave shoemakers using both pegging and stitching techniques (pegging was faster) and working with hides tanned on the plantation. The tanning was not always very thoroughly done, and slaves rubbed their shoes with soot to improve the appearance of the leather. When Mollie Dawson recollected her days in slavery for the Federal Writers' Project in the 1930s, she was recorded as saying,

we did't wears no shoes only in de wintah time and on special occasions, and de was made on de plantation too. Dey sho' was ugly lookin' things, dey was made outten hides dat was tanned on de plantation, what dey calls rawhide and when dey gits wet dey was like tryin' ter hold a eel, sho' did feel messy and look messy too. When de slaves was gittin' ready ter goes ter a dance er church you could see dem all gittin' soot outten de chimney and mixin' it wid water der shoe polish, and

Fig. 62. It is not always possible to distinguish men's or boys' shoes from women's shoes when they are made of heavier leathers and cut high on the foot as these are, but in general, slit-vamp styles seem to be associated with women and open-tab "brogans" with men. These shoes are about 9½ to 9¾ inches long, plausible women's sizes.

Far left: Black leather latchet-tie shoe with welted sole and a stitched and pegged heel. The oval toe and sole shape suggest a date ca. 1815–30, a period at which the open-tab pattern is more likely for women than it is later in the century. USMC catalog #1391.

Center left: Black calf slit-vamp tie shoe lined with coarse linen. Spring heel and pegged sole with second row of pegs in waist area, ca. 1850–60. USMC catalog #1959.

Center front: Pegged sole of a black leather slit-vamp shoe, ca. 1835–50. USMC catalog #593.

Center right: Black kid shoe bound with black silk, lined with twilled cotton and with a welted sole, ca. 1850–60. The leather is lighter in this example than in the others shown. USMC catalog #584.

Far right: High-cut shoe of heavy and stiff black leather lined with twilled cotton with a three-quarter-inch stacked heel. The pegged sole is a quarter-inch thick at the tread and has a second row of pegs at the waist. Only one pair of lace holes has been punched at the bottom of the slit opening. The shape of the sole, with its broader tread and narrow waist, and the presence of the heel suggest a date ca. 1865–75. USMC catalog #1807. *Courtesy Peabody Essex Museum.*

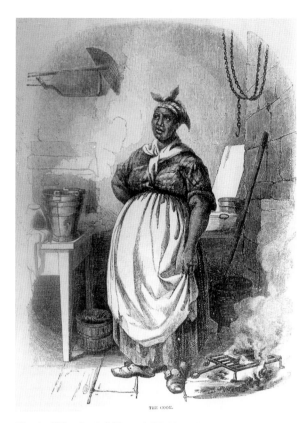

THE COOK.

Fig. 63. "The Cook," *Harper's Weekly*, vol. 12, no. 68 (1856). This black woman is wearing what passed for decent clothing for slaves. Her dress is made of colored, patterned fabric rather than plain unbleached cotton, she has head- and neck-kerchiefs for ornament, and she wears a pair of shoes, probably without stockings. The shoes are heavy leather open-tab brogans with two pairs of lace holes. The laces (which are missing) would have passed through the two holes visible in the tongue of her left shoe as well as through the latchets.

dis is what dey all polish der shoes wid. It didn't look nice and slick like it does now, but it made dem ole buckskin shoes looks a lot bettah though.[66]

Technically, "rawhide" refers to untanned leather and "buckskin" to deerhide, but Mollie Dawson seems to be using both terms to try to convey the poor quality of the finished product and the fact that the leather was left in its natural (but at that period unfashionable) tan color rather than being dyed black. Another former slave recalled that the plantation shoemaker "tanned de leather and made brass-toe broughans [brogans]. A lot ob times we wo'e shoes wid tufts of hair still in de toe paht! Sometimes we blacked our shoes by goin' to de wash-pot and takin' a rag, we'd rub it against it and den put the blacknin' on our shoes. We'd also smear tallow on de shoes to make 'em shine."[67]

Urban working women would not necessarily find thick stiff shoes an advantage, but those who stood all day at their work would have appreciated more cushioning than could be provided by the one thin, heelless piece of leather that constituted the sole of a turned shoe in the 1830s, 1840s, and 1850s. One young woman describing her life in the Lowell textile mills in 1844 said, "It makes my feet ache and swell to stand so much but I suppose I shall get accustomed to that too. The girls generally wear old shoes about their work, and you know nothing is easier [i.e., more comfortable]; but they almost all say that when they have worked here a year or two they have to procure shoes a size or two larger than before they came."[68]

An interesting sidelight on this question is shed by a pair of cut-down 1820s or 1830s man's Wellington boots preserved in the Old Stone House Museum in northern Vermont. These boots have a history of having been worn by a "schoolmarm in Browning-ton" in the 1840s.[69] Early nineteenth-century country schoolteachers often boarded for one or two weeks at a time with each of their pupils' families and might well have had to walk some distance to school through dew-laden grass or adverse weather. Owning a pair of ankle-high leather boots would have its advantages under such circumstances. Perhaps the teacher who wore them was too poor to buy substantial women's shoes and turned to second-hand boots from a brother or neighbor, but judging from the Barre advertisement of 1839, which listed no women's boots other than cloth gaiters, it seems at least plausible that no more appropriate alternative was available.

All-leather boots were probably gaining wider acceptance throughout the 1840s, as they would be a good deal drier and warmer than cloth in the winter. *Godey's* quotes Hall's *History of Boots and Shoes* in an 1848 article, noting, "For the little toe-caps and golashes of ladies' Congress boots, [the enamel or varnish leather, commonly called patent] answers admirably, and as it requires no cleaning, always looks well. The upper part of the boot is constructed variously of morocco, prunella, cloth, silk or satin, according to the season."[70] This implies that morocco was accepted first as an upper material for winter boots. Some of the earliest all-leather boots that survive from this period are Congress boots dating from the early 1850s (see fig. 283). After 1860, all-leather boots became far more common and are frequently mentioned in contemporary sources. Even when the uppers were made of serge with only a patent toe cap, the thicker soles fashionable in the 1860s would have made them more practical for country wear (see fig. 64). Once all-leather boots had become widely available, both as a practical and a fashionable choice, they were worn by women in rural areas all over the country, and continued to be the standard choice into the twentieth century.

Part of the answer to the question of what countrywomen wore before substantial boots came into use must lie in overshoes. From the mid-1820s, rubbers made in Brazil were being imported, and most advertisements mention them, in both plain and lined versions, throughout the 1830s and 1840s (see plate 17). By the late 1840s, vulcanized rubber overshoes were made in the United States (see fig. 85). The styles that nearly covered the foot, although too clumsy-looking to be much relished by young women, would have protected shoes from pouring rain or long wet grass. Another alternative, mentioned above in the Barre advertisement of 1839, may have been "sole leather over shoes," that is, overshoes made of thick side leather (see fig. 81).

Another important country overshoe in the early nineteenth century was the clog, which was essentially a sandal with a wooden sole. A broad leather strap tied over the instep, and there was a stiff leather counter or sometimes a leather-covered spring at the back to keep the clog from slipping off (see plate 17 and chapter 6). The thick wooden sole raised the shoe above the wet and mud, and would have carried women into their dooryards, vegetable gardens, and barns in comfort and safety. Under ordinary circumstances, women probably did not expect to cope with really deep mud. Even today, when main roads are paved, the two- or three-week period following the spring thaws is known in rural areas as "mud season," and town folk delay visits to their country friends until it is over. When all country roads were unpaved and wagon wheels stirred up deep muddy ruts in the spring, only real necessity would have made it worth the trouble to walk any distance. And at home on the farms, menfolk in high leather boots

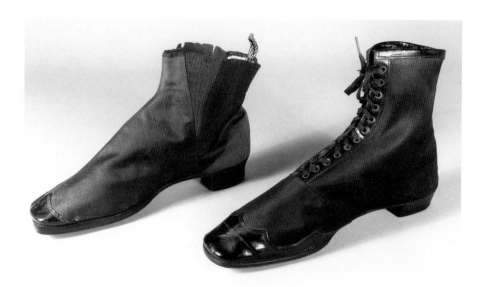

Fig. 64. Everyday walking boots of the 1860s and 1870s had heavier soles than those of preceding decades. Machine-made boots of this type were probably the most common type of everyday footwear worn just after the Civil War.

Left: A typical Congress boot of the period 1865–75. On the bottom of the heel are the remains of the numbered paper stamp that shows that the shoe was made legally, using the new McKay Sole Sewing Machine, patented August 1860 and in common use after 1864. Catalog #3147.

Right: The characteristic front-lacing walking boot of the 1860s, made of black serge with foxing, lace stay, and binding of black patent. The sole is almost entirely covered by two licensing labels, varnished over to preserve them. The first reads "Patent July [6?], 1864. Warranted. The C.O.D. Man." The second reads "Pat. Jan. 26, 1864 and June 13, 65. Bancroft & Purinton. Warranted. Lynn, Mass." Catalog #3146. *Courtesy Lynn Museum.*

would have been better prepared than long-skirted women, no matter what they had on their feet, to walk into the churned-up mud of the pigpen.

Walking and Working Boots, 1860–90

In the early 1860s, the front-lacing boot began to replace the side-lacing boot for both walking and the promenade. At first these front-lacing boots could be quite elaborate. *Godey's* reports in 1864, "Polish boots are now worn both by young and old. They are generally of black morocco, laced up in front quite high on the leg. They are bound with scarlet leather, and trimmed with scarlet tassels; some are tipped with patent leather. Lasting boots [lasting is a wool fabric used for uppers] are frequently trimmed with velvet rosettes. Boots matching the dress are considered in very good taste."[71] Swann shows an elaborate British example of this period in green satin trimmed with gold braid.[72]

In the United States, however, front lacing seems very quickly to have been relegated to utilitarian walking boots (see fig. 64). As a result, like most other everyday clothing, the front-lacing walking boot of the 1860s is sadly underrepresented in museum collections except in the USMC collection at the Peabody Essex Museum. Here, gazing at whole shelves of brown pebble-grain or black serge boots with foxing and lace stays of black leather and low stacked heels, one can begin to grasp what everyday footwear really looked like in the early machine-made period.

As soon as fashionable boots began to be made in leather rather than serge, a development that gained momentum in the 1860s, they became a much more practical choice for country wear than they had been in the earlier part of the century. At the same time, walking boots in general acquired thicker soles and low heels, which made boots more widely practical even when the uppers were still made of serge. Thus from the 1860s on, boots were more and more likely to be worn by those classes of rural women who had been wearing leather tie shoes in the 1830s and 1840s. An illustration titled "The Quarrel," published in *Peterson's* Magazine in April 1863, shows a young woman standing in a barn wearing working clothes, including thick, front-lacing boots.

As front lacing subsided into a utilitarian style in the later 1860s, it was the buttoned boot that came to the fore for all dressy and many ordinary outdoor occasions. *Demorest's* admitted in 1879 that a walking boot "laced up the front in the old-fashioned way . . . gives a better support to the ankle and waist of the foot than is possible if the boot is buttoned, but there is little likelihood of any style superseding the buttoned boot, which is considered the most elegant for all purposes of promenading, visiting, shopping and house wear."[73] Not only did buttoned boots make the foot appear smaller, but they may also have been less troublesome than laced boots, since the brushing skirts would have been less likely to undo the fastenings. In 1880, "the city *chaussure* is ever the high boot, either buttoned all the way up or cut out in open work straps over the instep to make it lighter."[74] The open straps over bright stockings seem rather showy for the street, and they were probably worn more for the promenade than ordinary walking. By 1883, *Demorest's* stated categorically, "Buttoned boots are the undisputed rulers of the shoe kingdom. Front-laced shoes made a long and desperate struggle for a permanent appointment, but finally went down under the frowns of their brethren of the buttons, and have gone to weep their eyelets out in the obscurity of dusty boxes, or as solitary prisoners of war in plate-glass Bastilles. Side-laced shoes are occasionally made to order, but mostly for conservative elderly ladies, and younger ones who want a change; but no stock of them is kept by the average dealer."[75]

While front lacing was usually associated with utilitarian boots in these decades, buttoned boots were also offered in practical calf and less expensive split side leather (the latter usually described as "thick" or "grain" leather). These heavy buttoned boots were cut just like the dressier boots made of kid (see fig. 65). Their thick soles were welted or McKay-sewn, or more rarely pegged or screwed. Pegging was in decline by 1880 because of the introduction of other bottoming machines that could compete in speed, including the McKay (1860), Standard Screw (1875), and Goodyear welt machines (1877).

Out of a total of sixty-three women's boots in the spring/summer catalog for 1895, Montgomery Ward offered thirteen in leathers heavier than kid or pebble goat. Of these, none of the eight buttoned boots (in glove grain, cordovan, bright grain, kangaroo calf, calf, and oil grain) had pegged soles, while four out of the five front-lace styles (in calf or oil grain) were pegged. Sears offered a similar range in its 1897 catalog, but included one buttoned boot that was "pegged or screwed." Pegged front-lacing boots were among the cheapest boots offered by Montgomery Ward, at $1.10 the pair (the most expensive boot offered cost $4.25). In comparison, the cheapest of the buttoned boots was $1.25, a "Ladies' Glove Grain Button . . . specially constructed for general wear, with good plump uppers, soft and pliable, and also solid bottoms and counters, thereby making a

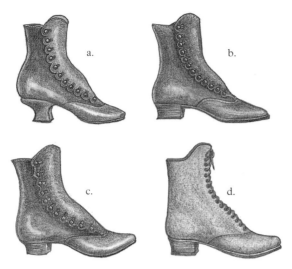

Fig. 65. The differences between elegant and working boots in the 1880s and 1890s were more a matter of material than of upper pattern, and therefore catalog illustrations all look very much alike, even when quality and price vary dramatically. Thicker soles and lower and straighter heels characterized expensive walking boots as well as farm boots. In 1895, the date of the working boots illustrated here, more stylish lasts with long pointed toes were available, but conservative lasts that had been in use for about fifteen years were still being used both for light kid boots and heavier working boots like these. These conservative styles of 1895 thus look very little different from the Jordan Marsh boots of 1882.

(a) Ladies' French kid buttoned boot with turned sole and Louis heel, advertised for $8.25 by Jordan Marsh in the fall of 1882. The high Louis heel and thin, turned sole made this boot more suitable for indoor or carriage wear than for serious walking.

(b) Ladies' goat buttoned walking boot with welted sole and low, broad heel, advertised by Jordan Marsh for $4.50 and $5.00 in the fall of 1882.

(c) Calf button boot, machine-sewn, field and farm brand, advertised for $1.90 in Montgomery Ward, 1895.

(d) Oil grain front-lace boot with double soles, pegged, field and farm brand, advertised for $1.15 in Montgomery Ward, 1895.

shoe that will give abundance of service for a little money." The same boot cost $1.75 when made with half-double soles, worked buttonholes, and a leather that was oil tanned to make it more waterproof.

Besides material and fastening, the choice of the heel was the most important element in distinguishing walking from promenade boots. In the 1860s, in the first rush of enthusiasm for high heels, high curved Louis heels were used on all kinds of boots. But by 1874, the arbiters of good taste ruled against Louis heels for walking: "Ladies' walking boots are made with thick projecting soles, like those worn by the gentlemen, and with low, broad heels. The high French heel is entirely out of fashion. Dull, unpolished kid is chosen for street boots, and the favorite shape remains the buttoned boot."[76] Five years later, *Demorest's* wrote, "French heels are, of course, the standard for sandals, slippers, and boots for all dressy occasions, but for ordinary use they evince lack of good taste and refinement in the wearer."[77] For walking, it is clear, one ought to have the sense to wear a stacked heel (see fig. 65).

Unfortunately, not everyone was sensible enough to choose boots appropriate for the occasion, and *Godey's* felt it necessary to remind readers in 1877 that "a sensible woman will always travel in thick boots to avoid the danger of wet feet, if, as must often be the case, she has to get out at an uncovered station in the rain, and will also realize that high heels, dangerous under any circumstances, are absolutely perilous when brought in contact with carriage steps, rough platforms and railway crossings."[78]

The Revival of Low Shoes for Fashionable Walking, 1870–1900

In the first half of the century, fashionable boots had not been suitable for wear in the country because they were made of cloth, and the dust sifted right through them. Leather tie shoes called buskins were preferred instead. After 1860, there were plenty of leather boots to choose from, and contemporary illustrations suggest that countrywomen had begun to wear them.[79] However, the tradition of tie

shoes for the country did not die out entirely. Indeed, perhaps once real countrywomen no longer
wore them, ties could be seen as a piquant asset to
the fashionable wardrobe. At any rate, as early as
1872 we hear of "the garden shoe, a low buskin, tied
over the instep like the brogans worn by gentlemen.
This is similar to the Newport tie of last summer. It
is made of kid or morocco."[80] Other references in
the 1870s suggest the growing use by fashionable
women of shoes rather than boots in the summer
and in the country. In 1875, a shoe that buckled over
a tongue was described as suitable "for house or street
wear."[81] In 1877, the reader is told, "buttoned boots
of French kid are preferred for dressy walking shoes
[but] in the warm weather, low shoes are worn both
in the house and street. The Newport buttoned shoe
of French kid, and the buttoned sandal, slashed to
display the color of the hosiery, will be the favorite
styles."[82] The name "Newport" suggests that these
low walking shoes first returned to fashion in the famous Rhode Island seaside resort town of that name.
Open-tab, two-eyelet tie shoes identified as "Newports" survive in the USMC Collection[83] and are
illustrated in Sears as late as 1907 (see figs. 40, 172,
179). In 1883, *Demorest's* predicted that "the leading
style of foot wear for street use in warm weather will
be the French kid seamless Oxford tie. The lacings
will be of fine silk braid, the ends carefully tucked
out of sight. They will cost $4.50. Black silk or Lisle
thread stockings will be arbitrary with this style."[84]

Some of the lingering ambivalence about wearing
shoes rather than boots outdoors is conveyed by the
careful delimitation of their proper use in an article
on traveling in *Mme. Demorest's What to Wear* for
spring/summer 1883. While recommending "common-sense" boots for traveling, worn with heavy Lisle
thread or cotton stockings, the writer adds that "it is
well to have a pair of Oxford or Newport ties in the
hand baggage, as in an all day ride the boots grow
tiresome; and with black stockings the low shoes are
admissible for a walk during a long wait, or change of
cars, a run across the station to meals, or a moment's
pause on the platform if the conductor and brakeman

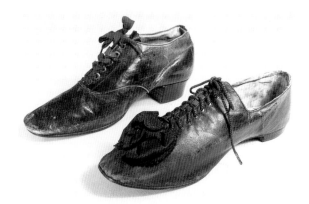

Fig. 66. Tie shoes became increasingly important for summer
walking from the late 1870s. *Right:* Unusual black kid shoe with
low heel and slit vamp, serge rosette at the toe, and cord lace,
said to have been made by Eben Brown, probably in Lynn, ca.
1877–85. Catalog #1735. *Left:* Black kid oxford tie, said to be a
sample shoe from Dole and Whittredge Shoe Company, Willow
Street, Lynn, which was in business at that address from 1882
to 1887, going out of business entirely in 1887. Catalog #4179.
Courtesy Lynn Museum.

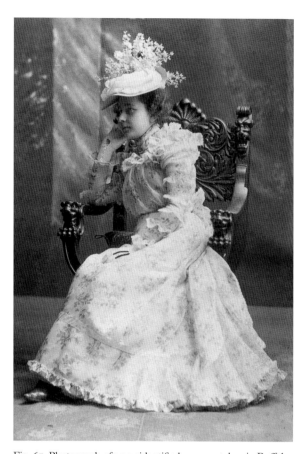

Fig. 67. Photograph of an unidentified woman, taken in Buffalo, New York, about 1899. Black shoes were considered perfectly appropriate to wear with light dresses at the turn of the century. *Courtesy Nen Rexford.*

will allow it, as you dash by some point of historic interest, or some unusually attractive bit of mountain scenery."[85]

The habit of wearing boots for winter and more formal walking occasions and shoes for summer continued into the late nineteenth century. The standard all-purpose color for both winter and summer in the 1890s and early 1900s was black leather with a black stocking, even with white summer day dresses (see fig. 67). In an article on summer shoes in May 1891, the *Ladies' Home Journal* reports that "the low shoe that is laced, with a high vamp of patent-leather and an upper of kid, a medium high heel and an arched instep, is given the preference in black; and unless one is going to have a great many shoes, that would be the wisest to choose. . . . One never errs in wearing black shoes and stockings." While that general rule was enough to guide the woman of limited means, her more affluent sister might own several varieties of walking shoe and several carriage shoes as well. A July 1894 article in *Godey's* lists the alternatives:

Almost all women hold strong opinions upon the subject of suitable foot gear, and to be *bien chaussée* simply means that the shoes and stockings should never be out of keeping with the rest of the attire. Much attention to detail is necessary to attain this end. Walking boots, for instance, should be stout and strong, so as to resist dampness, and the heels should be square and low with medium toes. For country wear and rough usage laced boots and cork soles are in order. For ordinary use in the country russet [natural brownish-tan color] boots or Oxford ties will be popular. They have indeed already made their appearance in the city, and many women find them, of all foot wear, the most comfortable. Russia leather, with its deep reddish color, is the handsomest material for Bluchers and ties, and although expensive at first is the cheapest in the end. Suede walking shoes are not so much worn this year, Russia and the various russet leathers taking their place. . . . For ordinary wear low shoes have taken the place of boots, and, although the French models are very graceful, English lasts are the most in vogue. All the French shoes have very pointed toes.

No walking boot or shoe should be made with Louis Quinze heels. For carriage wear these heels are quite proper, and give a distinction to the foot which is very fetching. Black patent leather ties, with Louis Quinze heels, are suitable for carriage wear. . . . Many well-dressed women who require boots to support their ankles have them made of black or bronze French kid with thin soles and high heels, and these are suitable for carriage wear. Some modish women have thin carriage boots of satin, either black, or to match the color of the gown. A black satin boot, with Louis Quinze heel and jet buttons, is a very dainty affair, and nothing prettier has ever been devised in the way of foot-wear.[86]

New Materials, New Distinctions, 1890–1910

Introduction of Tan Shoes: The "russet" shoes and boots that *Godey's* mentioned were perceived as a new fashion in the 1890s, although, in fact, a careful look at the preceding decades will find a scattered history of russet shoes, especially among the slit-vamp ties of the 1840s (see plate 5) and the utilitarian front-lace boots of the 1860s. In shoe parlance, "russet," also known as "tan," means the natural yellowish-brown color of tanned undyed leather. In its 1894–95 catalog, Montgomery Ward advertised a $2.75 front-lacing boot in "russet or tan colored Dongola. . . .This shoe requires no blacking or dressing and will be all the rage for the coming season." It appears that at first brown leather shoes were permitted for a wide range of informal occasions. In 1892, "fashion has decreed that soft, undressed leather shoes in the natural russet shade may be worn all day long, unless, indeed, one is gotten up very gorgeously for some special occasion."[87] And in 1896 we read that "tan ties and hose are cooler looking and very stylish with thin street or house gowns."[88] However, in May 1901, the *Ladies' Home Journal* warned that "russet shoes are reserved for country and seashore use," as if the arbiters of taste had had second thoughts (see plate 11).

The issue of when to wear russet shoes was settled in the first years of the twentieth century. Sears' selection of tan shoes in 1906 still shows all of them with utilitarian ties and stacked heels for walking. But by 1908, the maker of Red Cross Shoes was announcing that "tan pumps and oxfords will be worn more than ever. The correct shades are a golden brown or a rich tan."[89] The fact that pumps (slippers) were now being made in natural brown leathers is a clear sign that russet has moved up in the scale of formality. By 1913, "for general street wear the russet and black shoes and slippers are preferred, worn with buckles covered with the kid to match the shoe, or with very plain steel or gilt buckles."[90] Nevertheless, of two shoes identical in all respects except color, the black one would always be considered a bit dressier than the brown (see fig. 68).

Suede Shoes: In 1908, in the same advertisement that announced the correctness of tan pumps, Red Cross also noted that "suede, both in tan and black, will also be worn, chiefly in tops," the part above the foxing in either shoes or boots.

The following spring, American Lady Shoes advertised "swell new Suedes—London smoke, black and tan."[91] Suede was by no means a new technical development—it simply had not been fashionable in the nineteenth century. Swann says that it was reintroduced in 1865 by White Brothers and Company of Lowell, but that it did not become popular until the 1890s.[92] The earliest reference I find to suede shoes is in the *Delineator* in November 1891, which notes that "both Suede and glacé kid ties and Cleopatra slippers or sandals are presented in colors to match the gowns. The glacé foot-wear, however, is newer than the Suede." By 1894, *Godey's* remarks that "Suede walking shoes are not so much worn this year."[93] Suede was particularly useful as a leather of contrasting texture in boots and shoes through the nineteen-teens and -twenties, though all-suede pumps and boots are also advertised (see plate 11). "Suede holds its own in popular favor. This model [an all suede button boot in 1913] is correct for either street or dress wear."[94]

Canvas Shoes: Another important new material that appeared as a major fashion in the 1890s was white canvas (see plates 11, 15). Like russet leather, canvas was considered suitable only for informal wear. In 1896, "white ties . . . in canvas are worn with white hose at summer resorts and chiefly with white suits. They are certainly entirely out of place on the streets of a large city."[95] Nevertheless, they did accustom the eye to seeing white shoes with summer costumes. By 1906, we are told that "every careful dresser will have at least one pair of white shoes. No doubt of it, every ultra dresser will have several pairs of colored shoes repeating the colors of as many frocks."[96]

Canvas shoes continued to be worn in the summer. Canvas shoes with rubber soles were recommended for boating in 1915, and in 1917 the U.S. Rubber Company began to market its version as "Keds," a name familiar today as a brand of "sneakers." Rubber-soled canvas shoes were not at this period limited to sports. The first style advertised as Keds was a simple slipper with a very low heel and a tailored bow at the throat, and the description makes clear they were intended for general informal wear:

> The tops of Keds are of the firmest and finest of cool canvas, giving these shoes full elastic support. They have rubber soles which make them delightfully flexible and durable. No shoes are more comfortable or prettier for warm-weather wear.
>
> Keds for you will cover all daytime occasions—home wear; golf, tennis and all other outdoor games; for ordinary walking or 'hikes'; for yachting and riding wear; and plenty of other styles just as prettily suitable for wear with morning frocks and daintiest house gowns, at home or on the country club porch.[97]

New Developments in Walking Footwear, 1910–30

Increase in Lighter-Colored Footwear: The role of black shoes became somewhat more limited in the 1910s than it had been at the turn of the century, when they were worn with everything. Black was still in good taste for street wear, especially in winter, and it was considered an acceptable, if conservative, choice for afternoon and evening. But white and light neutral colors were more and more worn in the warmer weather and to carry out fashionable colors in the rest of the costume. In 1913 "light-colored slippers are the prettiest to wear with thin clothes for summer. Champagne-colored kid proves useful to wear with gowns of many colors. The lighter-toned shoes are pretty with silver buckles to match for day wear."[98]

Light shoes continued to be an important choice for day wear in the 1920s, but in the enormous variety of shoes and materials available it was difficult even for contemporary observers to discern trends that lasted for more than a few months, and references to black making a comeback seem to occur almost every year. For example, in 1923 the *Shoe Retailer* reported that "somewhat of a surprise element has entered the women's style note for the immediate future, . . . in that all-over black pumps came into strong demand almost over night." The trade journal reassured its readers, however, that "there will be an active demand from two distinct classes of customers; those who will wear the modish woody shades of costumes and those who will fall into the black class. There need be no fear that the sudden sale and call for all-over blacks will kill the sale for light colors in suede because costumes shown in the woody shades of fabrics will be in great quantity and these costumes will of necessity need shoes to match or harmonize."[99]

Footwear never returned to the days when almost all shoes were black, but black continued to form a very important part of the fashion scene, especially for women who could not afford colored shoes to match every outfit. Considering the coverage given in magazines to passing fashions in colors and materials, it is worth reading the first fall sale reports for 1926 in the *Shoe Retailer*, which revealed that while both light and dark browns sold in both suede and kid, black—and especially black patent—were the biggest sellers all around the country. Cincinnati: "75% patent leather." Cleveland: "blacks in turn types 95%." Richmond: "patent leather is leading." Chattanooga: "women's patent out in front." Dallas: "patents plain and trimmed best." Portland: "women's patent leather 70%." Omaha: "looks like a big black season." Philadelphia: "patent and black satins have been the outstanding materials."[100]

The Disappearance of Boots: The trend toward wearing low shoes instead of boots was confirmed in the early twentieth century. Boots were advertised chiefly in the fall, and to a lesser extent in the late winter, as they were more and more relegated to cold weather walking. Tie shoes and slippers (now called pumps) were advertised in the spring for walking, indoor and evening. In the spring of 1917, however, it was predicted that "high shoes [boots] will be in vogue even during the summer in white, gray and brown shades"[101] as if this were rather an oddity. Presumably, the prediction proved correct, since Historic Northampton does have a high boot of this period made in white canvas that must have been intended for summer wear (see plate 15).[102]

After some fifty years of substantial boots on the street, the trend toward wearing turned-sole low shoes struck some observers as nearly indecent. The

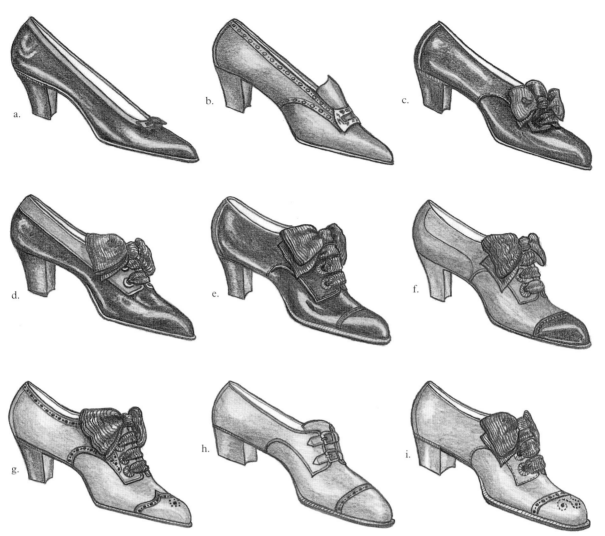

Fig. 68. These shoes are all drawn from an advertisement for Red Cross Shoes in the *Ladies' Home Journal*, April 1908. In spite of their overall similarity, they evince subtle variations in formality. They are drawn roughly in order from most dressy to least dressy:

(a) "Patent Colt Pump with narrow dull leather collar and bow $3.50. Also made in tan suede with calf collar $4.00." The low slipper cut, high narrow heel, and patent leather offer the dressiest option.

(b) "The lower the cut—the more fashionable." Puritan pump, tan calf or kid. Tan calf makes a sportier shoe than patent, as does the broguing, but the low cut and thin sole still suggest indoor occasions.

(c) "Just a little higher than a pump—clasps the foot closely." Two-eyelet patent colt oxford. Also made in tan. The relatively low cut (only two eyelets), thin sole, the use of all patent, and the lack of any toe cap make this the dressiest option among the ties.

(d) "Always a correct model—modified along the newer lines." Three-eyelet blucher, patent colt with dull mat top. The thin sole, the choice of patent, and the absence of any toe cap keep this shoe on the dressy side.

(e) "An attractive model that is always correct." Patent colt oxford. Just a bit more utilitarian than (d) because while it is entirely of patent, the sole is thicker and there is a simple toe cap.

(f) "A serviceable oxford for all occasions." Blucher oxford, glazed black kid with patent tip. The use of a duller leather is more practical than patent, and therefore less dressy.

(g) "This new 'shield' tip shortens the appearance of the foot." Tan blucher oxford. The tan leather and broguing make this a sportier model.

(h) "A new idea already a favorite with college girls." Buckle oxford, tan calf or patent colt. The buckle fastening is not a standard style, but the extension sole, perforated toe, and low, blocky heel put this firmly into the sporty end of the spectrum.

(i) "The greatest walking shoe ever built." Blucher oxford—tan calf, gun metal, glazed kid or patent colt. The low, blocky heel; broad, round toe; extension sole; and broguing make this an informal outdoor shoe.

1916 edition of the *Shoe and Leather Lexicon* allowed itself the following comment in its definition for "STREET SHOES. Especially in women's wear, boots or low-cuts of solid construction, suitable for street use, as distinguished from more delicate varieties of boot, or from most slippers. Women have shown a tendency in late years to wear on the street shoes suitable only for indoor use; that came about partly because women are much accustomed to follow fashions set by those who desire to drag boudoir suggestiveness through the streets, not only in shoes but in all their attire."

Variations in Formality in Twentieth-Century Low Shoes: The distinctions in formality among the myriad styles of slippers, strap shoes, and ties are difficult to discriminate now and must have been a challenge even when they were in fashion. But the following guidelines cover many of the options for the period 1905–30 (see fig. 68):

(1) Shoes that covered most of the foot (including most ties and multi-strap shoes) were less dressy than those that exposed the instep (including slippers and the lighter strap shoes). In the 1920s, shoes cut down to the sole at the waist were suitable only for evening.

(2) Stacked leather heels were less formal than Louis or covered wooden knock-on heels.

(3) The thinner and higher a covered wooden heel, the dressier the shoe (the distinctions can be quite subtle).

(4) A shoe with a plain toe was dressier than one with a toe cap.

(5) Among shoes with toe caps, additional fancy seaming made a shoe more dressy, not less, unless it was perforated. Perforations along the seams (broguing) always made the shoe look sportier.

(6) A tie or multi-strap shoe for indoor use had a turned sole where one for street wear had a welted sole (though turned shoes were increasingly common for street wear after 1910).

(7) Fabrics were in general dressier than most leathers. Among the fabrics, satin and gold and silver brocade were dressier than moiré. The metallic brocades were recommended for use with plain evening dresses. Black satin could be worn in the afternoon as well as in the evening. Canvas was for informal summer wear.

(8) Among the leathers, gold and silver kid were for formal evening wear only, and very fashionable in the 1920s. Black patent was otherwise the dressiest (but still entirely appropriate for street wear). Kid in white, black, or colors might be worn at any time, depending on the shoe's cut and decoration. However, after about 1905 kid was rarely used for evening except in gold and silver, or in white as part of wedding ensembles. In the 1920s, suede and reptile leathers were very stylish, but only for day. Brown ("russet") leathers in various shades were suitable for the city street from about 1908 but never quite as dressy as black, and browns were also used for the most active sports.

In September 1926, the *Ladies' Home Journal* took it upon itself to sort out all these alternatives and explain what kinds of shoes were really essential for its middle-class readers:

"Suppose a woman could afford four pairs of shoes," I said; "what would be her best choice?"

"She must have a one-strap or two-strap pump in tan or black, or a plain oxford for general service, averaging in cost about $12. Next she will require for sports wear a white oxford of buckskin or white linen, with low heels, crepe or rubber soles, white, patent leather or tan saddles, costing about $12. Her third pair, for informal [i.e., afternoon] wear, will be of patent leather or black or blond satin or kid, simple in design, with few trimmings, and costing from $15 to $20. For formal wear, gold or silver kid, gold or silver brocade or plain satin will be suitable with any gown. The satin will be about $15, the brocade about $20, the kid about $25."

"Suppose a woman's dress allowance did not permit even four pairs of shoes," I suggested. "What then?" . . .

"It is quite simple. One pair would have to be for general wear, the other for dress. The first will see hard use and should be of dull leather or tan Russia in a one-strap pump or plain oxford. I have them as low as $10 or $12 in excellent models. The dress shoe shows more variety. It may be of patent leather or black suede or satin. They can all be purchased for $12 and should be of conservative design without cut-outs. . . . If she goes to more evening functions than afternoon, the satin pump is suggested. If on the other hand, afternoon teas and bridge overtop the dances, patent leather or suede is better. The suede is a little more durable than the patent, and harder service would definitely call for the suede. . . . Formerly, two pairs of shoes a year were enough. Their cost was $3 or $3.50, and $5 was almost an extravagance. Do you know the highest price paid by a customer this summer? . . . The slippers were jewel-trimmed and cost $165, and the hose to match were $50."

In September 1928 the *Ladies' Home Journal* offered advice on "Planning the College Girl's Wardrobe." The list compiled would cost one thousand dollars if everything were to be bought new, but the writer assumes that some clothing would already be on hand, and that many items on the list would last the entire four college years. The list included five coats, seventeen dresses, and seven pairs of shoes, one pair each of evening slippers, afternoon slippers, street shoes, oxfords, sports shoes, bedroom slippers, and mules. This was not very different (except for the bedroom slippers and mules) than the list described in more detail two years earlier.

Many American women, however, do not seem to have thought the subject out quite so carefully as the *Journal,* and apparently had some difficulty negotiating the subtleties of taste when presented with such a tempting array of choices. In 1925, a writer for the *Ladies' Home Journal* described a young European whose

American contacts "had been limited to a series of dinners, luncheons, teas and dances. He had been dazzled by varicolored, highly ornamented, gorgeous footwear on display." But the *Journal* writer, while waiting for a train, "had taken occasion to note how the American woman was expressing herself in traveling footwear. I had not been edified. The feet that I saw were pudgy, gaudily bedecked, wabbly, bulging over satin and brocade and soft leather in a thousand unbecoming curves. They were the feet of women trimly tailored, smartly hatted, otherwise satisfactorily groomed."[103] Certainly the bulging instep overbrimming a too small shoe is a distressing feature also visible in many 1920s photographs. It seems that in some ways American women had not changed so much after all. In spite of their advances in education, employment, and physical activity—advances that brought with them more substantial shoes and shoes more sensibly adapted to the variety of endeavors women were now involved in, American women still betrayed a predilection for wearing shoes too thin, too small, and too elaborate for the occasion. The women whose feet bulged out over satin shoes in a train station in 1925 are the direct descendants of the ladies Mrs. Trollope had seen a century earlier stepping to their sleighs in miniature slippers "incapable of excluding as much moisture as might bedew a primrose."[104]

CHAPTER FIVE

Shoes Adapted for Sports

Shoes adapted particularly for active sports, like the sports themselves, were not widely adopted by women until the latter part of the nineteenth century. Although women had been riding on horseback for centuries and had occasionally worn special boots for the occasion (Samuel Pepys disapproved of them in 1666), only the most avid riders wore anything other than ordinary walking shoes or gaiters until the 1870s. Bathing shoes were barely differentiated from ordinary slippers, and other than these two activities, most women pursued little in the way of active games that required special footwear until the 1860s. But from that date, the century saw a series of sports fads in which women participated as well as men: croquet in the 1860s, tennis in the later 1870s, hiking in the 1880s, and bicycling and golf in the 1890s. By 1900, the value of taking active outdoor exercise had become firmly established in popular thinking about women, and by the end of the First World War, rubber-soled canvas shoes were well on their way to becoming the all-purpose sports shoe we continue to wear today.

Riding

Women had worn riding boots at least occasionally since the seventeenth century,[1] and when boots came into fashion for women's general wear in the late eighteenth century, they were still associated with the equine sports. Swann says that boots were "worn by women . . . from 1778, though chiefly for riding and driving, calf-high kid, front lacing, with fashionable toe and Italian heel."[2] But until the early 1800s, shoes, even very low-cut heelless slippers, were also still worn for riding. In June 1795, *Heideloff's* describes a figure in a scarlet riding

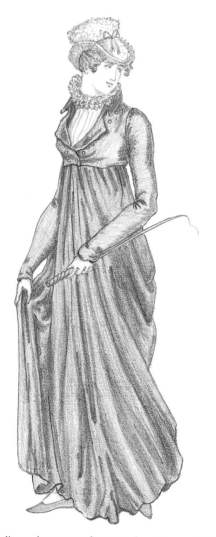

Fig. 69. Ordinary shoes were often worn for riding, as is clear in this fashion plate from *Le Journal des Dames*, 1803, where apparently identical red kid slippers are worn with both the walking dress and the riding habit.

habit as wearing "purple Spanish leather spring heel slippers." In the French series *Costume Parisien*, a woman on horseback is very clearly shown wearing white stockings and red slippers with pointed toes in 1801,[3] and similar slippers appear regularly in plates showing riding costume through 1804 (see fig. 69). In that year, however, one figure in a gray trained habit is described as wearing "souliers d'homme." These "man's shoes" are black and a shade too long in the vamp to be slippers. The details are unclear, but a latchet-tie shoe is probably intended (a small black blob over the instep may be the bow the ribbons are tied in).[4]

Women continued to wear slippers for riding in Mexico and probably also in Spanish California through the first half of the nineteenth century. Fanny Calderón de la Barca recalls meeting during her travels in Mexico in 1840 "the prettiest little *ranchera*, a farmer's wife or daughter, riding in front of a *mozo* [manservant] on the same horse—their usual mode—dressed in a short embroidered muslin petticoat, white satin shoes, a pearl necklace and earrings, a *rebozo*, and a large round straw hat."[5]

In European centers of fashion, however, boots quickly replaced slippers for riding. The *Lady's Magazine* reported in January 1803 that in Paris "gaiters [i.e., over-gaiters; not gaiter boots] are as much worn as boots" for riding. Three years later a French equestrienne is shown in blue front-lacing boots of uncertain height—the skirt obscures the tops—and half-boots for riding are mentioned in an English periodical that same year.[6] Blue kid half-boots are shown in 1817,[7] and slate-colored leather boots in 1818.[8] Brown or black half-boots are mentioned as a Paris fashion in 1829,[9] and dark-colored bootlike objects peep out from beneath the skirts from time to time through the 1830s and 1840s.

While women's boots were often made of leather before 1830, after 1830 the commonest walking boot was a cloth gaiter with leather added only at the toe and heel, and presumably it was these flimsy cloth boots that were worn for riding in the 1830s and 1840s. In an 1844 series on "Horsemanship" in the *National Magazine*, footwear is not even mentioned in the section on attire, suggesting that specialized garb was not required. In 1848, *Godey's* advised that "dark boots should be worn for riding. Ladies who ride much will find the advantage of having a neat kid or morocco boot,"[10] suggesting that women did not ordinarily own all-leather boots and that cloth gaiter boots were considered good enough for occasional riding. In that same year, the British periodical *La Belle Assemblée* reported that "the *chaussure* is always *bottines*, either of rich black silk, or else corresponding with the colour of the habit; they are buttoned at the side, and are made with small heels."[11] Neither buttons nor heels are very common in walking boots of the 1830s and 1840s, and it is not clear whether they were standard for riding or whether they were mentioned in 1848 because they were new.

The Gallery of English Costume includes in its booklet *Costume for Sport* a photograph of a solid leg boot that it dates 1830–50.[12] However, I find no evidence of women wearing leg boots without lacing in America at this early date. When riding footwear is described in 1851, the choice is still not between cloth gaiters and leather leg boots, but between gaiters and slippers. "Gaiters are indispensable, as a slipper could not bear the strain of the foot in the stirrup, or are liable to be 'cast' by the wayside by the breaking of a very slender string."[13] Indeed, the prize offered in a ladies' equestrian competition in Albany, New York, in 1856 consisted of a saddle, riding whip, and pair of red wool side-lacing boots trimmed with black fringe and velvet ribbon (preserved at the Albany Institute of History and Art). Given the context, these boots were presumably considered suitable for riding (see plate 16). It is not until June 1854 that a tasseled leg boot is illustrated in *Godey's* and then it is described as a novelty (see fig. 70a).

> We are at pains to present our friends with every *recherché* article that can contribute to their welfare; for this purpose, we illustrate a pair of riding boots for ladies, which, in addition to their ostensible purpose, are admirable for damp or muddy walking, especially in locations where vegetation renders protection desirable. . . . They are made of patent leather, of a rich, lustrous black hue, the upper portion of fancy colored morocco, purple, maroon, green, or bronze, and bordered with silk galloon, finished with neat tassels. Excepting in their elegant proportions and ornamental appearance, they are essentially similar to the dress boots of the sterner sex; and we are gratified to observe this move in the right direction. This fashion is in accordance with sound sense and comfort.

It is doubtful that leg boots were widely adopted immediately. Footgear is rarely mentioned in descriptions of riding dress in the 1850s and 1860s, as if it were of less interest and variability even than gloves, cravats, and whips. When shoes are described, it appears to be only for the sake of completeness, not because there is anything new to say about them. Thus in 1861, "gaiters or morocco boots with heels, and long stockings, of course, will complete the footgear."[14] Presumably, no revolution had yet taken place.

Fig. 70. Ladies' riding boots:

(a) Riding boot (see description in text), *Godey's Lady's Book*, June 1854.

(b) "Riding-boot of kid, with patent leather top and toe-cap, ornamented with a black gimp tassel," *Godey's Lady's Book*, November 1869.

(c) Riding boot, not described, but visible beneath the lifted hem of a riding habit, *Godey's Lady's Book*, June 1870.

(d) "Ladies' riding boot with spur; cord and tassels ornament it," *Godey's Lady's Book*, October 1877.

(e) Riding boot, not described, illustrated with other riding accessories, *Godey's Lady's Book*, May 1881.

(f) Riding boot, not described, illustrated with other riding accessories, *Harper's Bazar*, May 25, 1889, p. 384.

(g) "Extra High Cut Shoe. Ladies' Glazed Dongola Kid Button, opera last, high heel and pointed toe, extra high cut tops, with tassel, attractive and dressy, flexible soles, very desirable as a riding boot," advertised in Montgomery Ward's 1895 catalog.

(h) Walking boots worn with puttees for riding, Franklin Simon and Company catalog, 1914.

(i) Walking boots worn with leather leggings for riding, Franklin Simon and Company catalog, 1914. The same arrangement was illustrated in the *Ladies' Home Journal*, Summer 1927.

(j) Boot of the type shown in most riding illustrations of the 1920s, this one drawn from the *Ladies' Home Journal*, September 1920.

(k) Riding boot made to order in the 1920s for Mrs. Paul T. Haskell by Peal and Company, of London. The lacing arrangement allows for a tight, slim fit at the ankle. Peabody Essex Museum catalog #135,574.

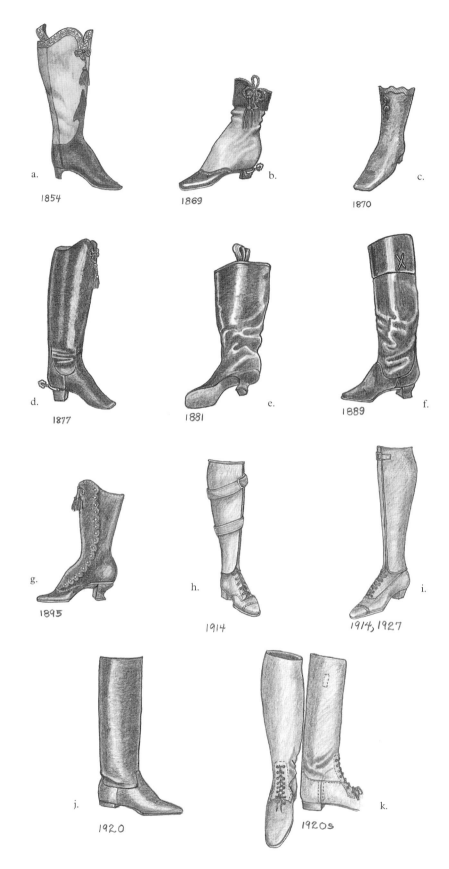

a.   1854

b.   1869

c.   1870

d.   1877

e.   1881

f.   1889

g.   1895

h.   1914

i.   1914, 1927

j.   1920

k.   1920s

Then in 1869, a "riding-boot of kid, with patent leather top and toe-cap, ornamented with a black gimp tassel" appears in the November issue of *Godey's* (see fig. 70b), and in June 1870 one fashion-plate lady lifts her skirt expressly so that we may see her high scallop-topped and tasseled boot (see fig. 70c). Neither of these boots has any obvious fastening. They are almost certainly solid leg boots. Although an etiquette book of 1876 still says only that "the boots must be stout" with no further description,[15] it seems likely that leg boots for riding came in as part of the renewed interest in footwear that accompanied shorter walking skirts in the 1860s. A very high and mannish version with blocky heel, spur, and tassel is shown in *Godey's* in December 1877 (see fig. 70d), and the trend is confirmed in 1879 by the backhand remark that "loose top-boots are never worn by ladies unless for equestrian exercise, but a very high top laced or buttoned boot may be worn with perfect propriety for walking excursions."[16] Although the basic style for riding boots seems to have been set for the next fifty years by 1880, there was still some variation in practice. *Harper's Bazar* notes in 1888 that with riding habits "the trousers [are] long enough to strap under the feet or else short knee-breeches are used with top-boots."[17] The implication is that the longer trousers were chosen when ordinary street boots were worn riding. As late as 1895, Montgomery Ward advertised a buttoned boot not much different from any other walking boot except for its slightly higher cut and ornamental tassel as "very desirable as a riding boot" (see fig. 70g).

An alternative style does appear in the mid-1910s. "Riding togs for cross-saddle riding in the open country" in 1915 included "either riding boots or puttees of leather, or stiffened leggings of the same brown corduroy as the suit"[18] (see fig. 70h, i). The puttees are shown as separate stiff leggings worn over a pair of front-lacing boots and strapped and buckled round the leg. During this same period, boots may be designed to allow a few inches of lacing at the ankle only. This arrangement provided ease when putting boots on and off and allowed a slimmer ankle once they were laced (see fig. 70k). But the older solid leg boot continued to be worn as well. "The fashions in sidesaddle habits are definite and standardized, but there are still divergent opinions on what women should wear when riding cross-saddle, since this practice is a development of recent years. . . . The same difference in detail arises concerning boots; although many people wear black boots with patent-leather cuffs, it is generally considered more correct for dress occasions to wear a black boot without a cuff. Another example of the stress laid upon correctness of detail."[19] Of four habits illustrated in this 1927 article, both the informal cross-saddle and side-saddle habits were worn with tan boots. The formal cross-saddle habit (worn on dress days for fox hunting) is shown with black boots, the formal side-saddle habit with black boots with patent-leather tops. These elaborately correct costumes, of course, belong to that world in which riding is indeed a sport, not a means of transportation. They were most likely to be worn by wealthy women who had houses in the country where they could keep saddle horses, or who lived in a county that enjoyed hunting. Special riding habits and boots were not worn by farm wives who kept a nag to pull the wagon.

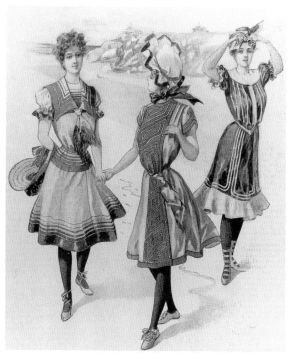

Fig. 71. Once knee-length rather than ankle-length bloomers came into use for bathing in the later 1870s, stockings were usually added to cover the legs, and from the 1890s stockings might provide the only foot covering worn. Nevertheless, bathing shoes continued as a fashionable option right through the 1920s. The figure at left in this 1903 plate wears the most often illustrated style, with tapes crossed on the instep and tied around the ankle. The low tie shoes at center were a less commonly shown option, and the high strapped boots at right are quite unusual. However, high bathing boots did become common from 1915, only with lacing rather than straps (see plate 15). From the *Designer* (a publication of the Standard Fashion Company, a New York pattern maker), July 1903. *Courtesy John Burbidge.*

Bathing

About the same time as specialized riding boots reappeared in the nineteenth century, we find evidence of shoes especially adapted for bathing. Bathing shoes were always optional, depending on how rough the terrain was and how tender the feet. They could be worn into the water if desired, but many were probably worn chiefly on hot sand and sharp stones. Kidwell[20] notes a reference to "gum overshoes for tender feet" in *Peterson's*, August 1856. Gum overshoes are rubbers, which were available as a natural rubber product from Brazil from the late 1820s, and from about 1845 of vulcanized rubber made into shoes in America (see chapter 6). Patterns for needleworked mules suitable for wearing on the beach were published in the 1870s, one embroidered in colored wools and edged with scarlet braid,[21] the other of gray linen embroidered in red, white, and blue cotton.[22] Both were sewn to cork soles covered with linen (see fig. 72e). According to Swann, rubber-soled shoes were in use in England by the mid-1870s for the seaside and for summer wear.[23] It seems likely that rubber soles were also used in the United States, but when the soles are specified in the sources I have seen, they are either cork or hemp.

The most common bathing shoe at all times is a low slipper fitted with tapes that cross over the instep in varying arrangements and tie round the ankle. These are shown as early as 1867 with small rosettes at the throatline (see fig. 72a). Very similar shoes appear in the 1880s, except that since the bathing drawers are now shorter, the crisscrossing tapes come higher on the leg[24] (see fig. 72g). In July 1872, *Godey's* illustrates two styles of canvas bathing shoes with soles of thick plaited hemp (see fig. 72b, c). The bare-toed style never became standard.

As long as bathing garments covered most of the legs, that is until the late 1870s, stockings were not considered absolutely necessary. There seems to have been a transition when both stockings and long trousers were worn, since we are told in 1876 that "full trowsers gathered into a band at the ankle . . . and merino socks of the color of the dress complete the costume."[25] The first mention in *Godey's* of bathing

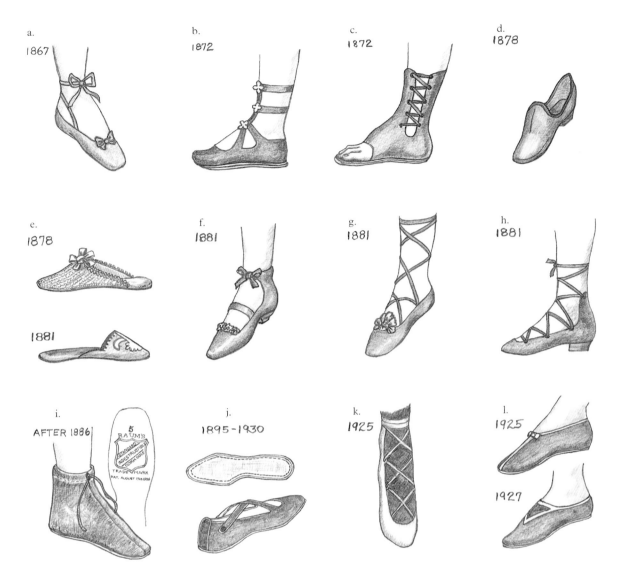

Fig. 72. Bathing shoes, 1860 to 1930 (also see plate 15).

(a) Typical midcentury bathing slippers with ribbon ties, from *Godey's Lady's Book*, July 1867.

(b, c) Two examples from *Godey's Lady's Book*, July 1872, described as "Different styles of bathing shoes, a sole of thick plaited hemp is placed at the bottom of foot, and the upper is made of canvas."

(d) *Ehrlich's Fashion Quarterly*, Summer 1878.

(e) Two bathing mules, the upper one made of gray linen cloth embroidered in red, blue, and white, also considered suitable for a bedroom slipper, from *Peterson's*, June 1878; the lower one from *Harper's Bazar*, July 2, 1881, p. 429.

(f) Strapped high-back bathing shoe from *Harper's Bazar*, July 2, 1881, p. 429.

(g) Cross-laced bathing shoe from *Godey's Lady's Book*, July 1881.

(h) Laced high-back bathing shoe from *Peterson's*, July 1885.

(i) Bootee-type bathing shoe of black cotton knit, with cork soles covered with canvas and stamped "RAUH'S Standard Indestructible Cork Soles, Trade Mark, Pat. August 17th, 1886." Natural History Museum of Los Angeles County catalog #A.10030-82.

(j) Cross-strap, black cotton sateen bathing shoes bound with white cotton bias binding, cotton covered cork(?) sole, probably McKay-sewn, ca. 1895–1930. Connecticut Historical Society catalog #1959-72-20.

(k) Typical bathing shoe of 1910s and 1920s, this one drawn from a Skinner Satin advertisement in the *Ladies' Home Journal*, May 1925.

(l) Simple bathing shoes in a dark color with white trim, the upper one from the same Skinner Satin advertisement referred to above, the lower one from a figure in the *Ladies' Home Journal*, Summer 1927.

stockings appears in July 1880. "All ladies now wear stockings while in bathing, the color to contrast with, if not match, the suit. Some also wear sandals, which they fasten on with braid in the same style as those worn for morning toilets." The braid is a woolen tape about half an inch wide.

In the late nineteenth and early twentieth centuries, black stockings were very often worn for bathing without any shoe at all. The *Ladies' Home Journal* advised in August 1892 that "long black woolen stockings are in order, and if you are going to bathe much, and wish to keep them from wearing out, it will be wise to get them a size larger, and to insert in their feet the soles sold in the stores for knitted slippers." When bathing shoes are shown, they are usually lighter than the stocking (Kidwell notes that they were often white canvas), and the commonest style is still the low slipper, presumably cork-soled, with tapes to cross once or twice and tie round the ankle. This ankle-tie bathing shoe continued right through the 1920s. An example in black canvas is preserved at the Peabody Essex Museum.[26] Another black canvas bathing shoe in the same collection is a simple front-lacing style—no ankle ties at all. Occasionally they were made with straps across the instep instead of ties around the ankle. The Connecticut Historical Society has a pair in black cotton sateen with white bindings, a white cotton sole and cross-over straps[27] (see fig. 72j). A similar style in black satin sold in 1918 for $1.75.[28] Yet another alternative has a cotton-covered sole, but the upper is made of black machine-knitted wool and simply has a drawstring run through the topline to keep it on, like an infant's bootee[29] (see fig. 72i).

About 1915, a new style of bathing footgear appeared, a mid-calf-high boot, solid on the sides and back of the leg, but open down the front and laced across the opening (see fig. 72k). A solitary early version of this illustrated in 1903 had instead of laces a series of straps buttoning across the open front much like the barred shoes of the late 1870s (see fig. 71). In the 1920s, instead of being open beneath the lacing, they were often made to lace closely over a tongue, and in this version they were very little different from the high walking boots of the period 1916–23, except for the materials and their lower heels. A surviving pair of this last type is made of bright red satin, with white trim and a rubber sole marked Seaview Bathing (see plate 15).[30] A similar pair at the Kansas City Museum is of black canvas with black rubber sole, and a collar and lace stay of white canvas, with white laces.[31]

Kidwell points out that the acceptance of real swimming (as opposed to splashing in the waves) brought about changes in bathing costume.[32] Women like Annette Kellerman, the Australian diver, both popularized the sport and campaigned for more sensible costume. "Don't wear any more clothes than you need," Kellerman advised in 1915. "They hinder your movements and make the body much heavier. Many of the costumes I have seen along the shore are inspired more by vanity than modesty."[33] Closer-fitting knitted suits appeared in the 1920s, and gradually the long black stockings were discarded (the last fashion picture I find including them is from 1922). In the late 1910s and early 1920s, short stockings were worn gartered someplace below the knee, but soon even these disappeared, and bare legs began to appear in the early 1920s. Bathing shoes were still worn over bare feet when rough ground made them desirable, but they were a matter of utility, not modesty.

Bicycling

The next addition to the sporting wardrobe was the bicycling boot. This was a knee-high front-lacing boot in black or natural russet leather with a low, stacked heel. The high boot covered and protected the leg when short skirts or bloomers were worn. While these boots laced in the ordinary way at the foot, the upper leg was fitted with lace hooks of the type still used on ice skates. Surviving examples show signs of having been grooved on the sole, presumably to keep the foot from slipping off the pedal (see fig. 74). Bicycling boots can be seen at the Chicago Historical Society, Connecticut Historical Society, the Peabody Essex Museum, and the Old Stone House Museum.[34]

Boots specially adapted for bicycling seem to have been first offered in 1896. Boots, leggings, and other bicycling paraphernalia were widely advertised in that year and to a lesser extent to 1900. Thereafter, one is likely to find clothing advertised as adapted for active sports in general rather than just cycling. In 1900 Sears advertised a "Ladies' Storm or Skating Boot . . . made from box calf stock, which is slightly pebbled, as near waterproof as leather can be made. . . . Being a very sightly shoe it is also suitable for street wear, and many of our patrons use it for bicycle riding." This boot is a good deal higher than others in 1900, and the text notes, "The latest styles in skirts for street wear are cut about six inches from the ground and are intended to be worn with this style of boot." The implication that specialized sports boots were going out of fashion about 1900 is corroborated by a remark in the *Shoe Retailer*, which in 1901 interviewed a department store buyer who reported that tan "oxford ties for women have almost entirely taken the place of sporting boots for golf and outing wear."[35]

An alternative to the high boot was an ordinary walking shoe worn with a gaiter or legging that buttoned up the side to the knee. Leggings were available ready-made (they appear regularly in Sears catalogs) and they could also be made at home, if desired.

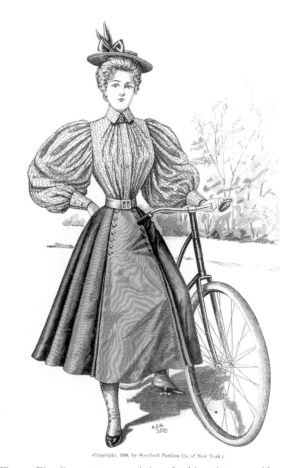

(Copyright, 1896, by Standard Fashion Co. of New York.)

Fig. 73. Bicycling costume consisting of a shirtwaist worn with a skirt that is combined with trousers in a single garment. The bicyclist is shown wearing cloth gaiters over ordinary shoes, a choice far more commonly illustrated than special bicycling boots. From the *Ladies' Standard Magazine* for April 1896, p. 5. *Courtesy Heidi Fieldston.*

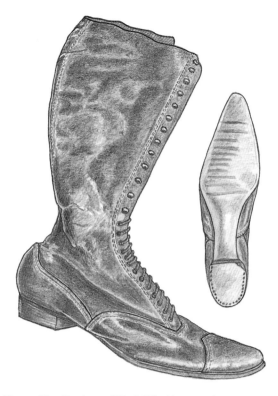

Fig. 74. Bicycling boot of black kid with grooved ("corrugated") tread, and lace hooks on the upper leg, ca. 1896–1900. Donor's history said that it was worn by Miss Rose Morgenthaler of Westmore, Vermont, for horseback riding. Although riding boots at this period are normally solid leg, high laced boots of this type were advertised for general outdoor activities, including skating, golf, and storm wear as well as bicycling, and they could easily have been worn for horseback riding as well. Old Stone House Museum, Brownington, Vt., catalog #T-321.

Patterns for them are common in contemporary catalogs such as Butterick's. Wearing leggings did away with the need to purchase a separate pair of boots just for cycling and they must have been adopted by many, if not most, bicycling women. They are the only thing recommended in the *Ladies' Standard Magazine*'s special April 1894 issue on cycling dress (see fig. 73), and considering the depth in which cycling clothing is discussed there, it is fair to assume that special boots were not yet available. The shoes recommended for cycling are described only as low and broad-toed.

General Sports Shoes

Rubber soles proved to be useful in many of the sports shoes that developed in the later nineteenth century. Not only were bathing shoes often provided with them, but they were also recommended for boating and for tennis. The earliest women tennis players did not play a very vigorous game, and many found it possible to play in the trained and bustled dresses and high heels that were fashionable in the late 1870s and 1880s when the game was becoming popular. The tennis court was for most women merely a new place in which to be charming, but a few women took the sport up seriously for its own sake, and they knew the value of a more practical kind of attire, including sensible shoes with rubber soles. *Demorest's* recommended in 1883:

> The skirt should be short and not tied back, and the shoes low, with low, square heels. French heeled shoes are incompatible with good tennis playing. The real lawn-tennis shoe for ladies is of black French kid, laced on the instep with any colored ribbon to suit the costume, and with India Rubber soles. While this style of shoe is most becoming with the costumes worn, it most effectually preserves the feet from dampness, cannot possibly injure the lawn or tennis court, as the shoe with a high French heel is sure to do by cutting into the turf, and the danger of slipping when the grass is damp is entirely avoided.[36]

Judging from Horace Partridge and Company's 1887 *Illustrated Catalogue of Lawn Tennis,* women's tennis

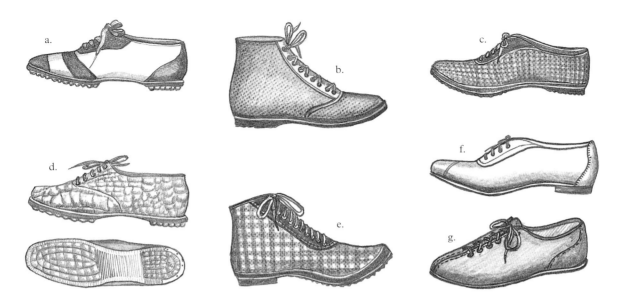

shoes were almost indistinguishable from men's except that there was a smaller variety of styles offered. For instance, Partridge offered spiked leather soles only for men, while alligator-skin uppers seem to have been an option only for women. Otherwise the differences were minimal (see fig. 75). Tennis shoes were offered in brown, black, and white canvas, terra-cotta goatskin, russet calf, white buck, and black kangaroo, with black or red rubber soles. The tennis shoes advertised in Montgomery Ward in 1895 show this same indifference to gender labeling, being made in high or low styles and in black or checked canvas for both men and women.

By the 1890s, when tan leathers and canvas had come into fashion for general summer informal wear, ladies' magazines recommended these materials in comfortable styles for most outdoor activities. The *Ladies' Home Journal* advised in 1892 that "for mountain wear you must give a great deal of thought to your shoes; well-fitted, comfortable russet ones are most desirable for all the day."[37] An 1902 article in *Good Housekeeping* on "Dress for Camping" listed the clothing essential for a vacation spent "tramping" in the country.

Comfortable shoes are the greatest essential to a pleasant trip, and these should be tried some

Fig. 75. Tennis and general sports shoes.
  (a) "Ladies' Low Cut, Brown or White Canvas Shoes with wine colored leather trimmings and patent red rubber soles." From Horace Partridge and Company's *Illustrated Catalogue of Lawn Tennis* (Boston, 1887). The sole appears similar to the sole for (b).
  (b) "Ladies' Low Cut Selected Alligator Skin Shoes, hand sewed, with patent tournament soles." From Horace Partridge and Company's *Illustrated Catalogue of Lawn Tennis* (Boston, 1887).
  (c) Black canvas Tennis Bals [balmorals], corrugated rubber soles, with leather insoles. Montgomery Ward Catalog, 1895.
  (d) Ladies' Check Tennis Bals, corrugated rubber soles, with leather insoles. Montgomery Ward Catalog, 1895.
  (e) Ladies' Check Canvas Tennis Shoes, with corrugated rubber soles. This style also came in plain black canvas. Montgomery Ward Catalog, 1895.
  (f) Ladies' Wigwam slippers, "with sole leather soles and heels. These slippers are made throughout with leather, making the most durable and comfortable foot covering for house, lawn and camping out purposes." Montgomery Ward Catalog, 1895.
  (g) Gym shoes, soft black kid with the gypsy seam characteristic of this kind of shoe, ca. 1895–1915. Kansas City Museum catalog #76.121.5.

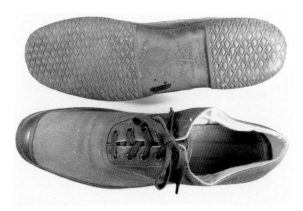

Fig. 76. Brown canvas tennis shoes worn by Alice P. Chase in the 1920s, marked "Goodyear's Glove M'f'g. Co. Naugatuck, CT, USA. Keds." While the tennis racket molded into the sole identifies this as a tennis shoe, shoes of the same type were worn for boating and other sporting activities as well as general outdoor wear. These have a leather inner sole. Catalog #6842. *Courtesy Lynn Museum.*

days before leaving home. There are fine boots now made just for tramping, but we like best the lighter ones that our feet have grown used to. Just before starting we have a heavy sole put on and Hungarian nails fixed in both soles and heels. Unless they are nearly new, two pairs of tramping shoes should be taken, as the stitches in old shoes are soon loosened by moisture. A lighter pair for resting in camp is necessary to keep the feet in good condition.[38]

Other activities called for other specialized shoes. Soft leather tie shoes with a gypsy seam and flexible leather soles were considered appropriate for gymnastics (see fig. 75g). "Russet shoes with hobnails or bits of rubber on the soles are worn to prevent slipping" when playing golf,[39] but for canoeing, "nailed boots of any sort are taboo."[40] Canvas shoes with rubber soles were far safer and more appropriate for boating because they dried out quickly. The combination of canvas and rubber quickly became characteristic of sports shoes (see plate 15). The rubber-soled canvas "Keds" introduced in 1917 were meant to be worn for "golf, tennis and all other outdoor games; for ordinary walking or 'hikes'; for yachting and riding wear" but also for general summer wear indoors and out.[41]

By the 1920s, as outdoor activities became an ordinary part of most women's lives, the less-specialized kinds of "sports shoe" began to merge with the walking shoe in the form of the sports oxford (see fig. 77). In 1919, the *Shoe Retailer* noted the elaboration of the sports shoe beyond practical requirements.

The sport oxford is somewhat of a revival of a style popular a few years ago, although, like all revivals, it does not reappear just as it was. There are many styles of sport oxfords, some combining leather toe caps and fancy foxings with white leather, also with white canvas. There are some fancy lace stays and—well, the variety of patterns is as wide as the imagination. The sport oxford bids to be popular the coming year, due largely to the revival of interest in tennis, golfing and other games that young—and some middle-aged—folks indulge in, and which lagged in interest during the war. Color combinations, and some startling ones, are seen in this style of shoe for women. Green, blue and even red and orange leather are offered with white as the background. Few all-leather sport shoes are shown.[42]

By 1926, oxfords were being defined outright as sports shoes, and the sports category had expanded to include what were known as "dressy sports" shoes. "Oxfords, by their nature belonging to the sports type, are often rather fancy in treatment and are used more than ever before for actual sports and as dressy-sports footgear. For actual sports, buckskin with ap-pliqued bands of tan leather makes the majority of shoes, and the heels are of the low spring variety. For semi or dressy sports, the heels range all the way from 1¾ to 2 or even 2⅜ inches high, usually of the Cuban wood kind."[43]

Elsewhere, the term "dressy sports" was explic-itly equivalent to afternoon costume.[44] In 1928 the same shoe could be proper for both 'spectator sports' or summer street wear,[45] and a pair of high-heeled single-strap shoes are "of the sports type and are suit-able for afternoon as well as street wear."[46] It is clear that in the mid and late 1920s, sports, walking, and afternoon wear had become difficult even for con-temporary writers to distinguish clearly and that sports clothing had infiltrated all but the most for-mal of occasions. The backlash arrived in 1929, when the *Ladies' Home Journal* warned of "the passing of sports-clothes-all-around-the-clock, [and of] the in-creased formality of this winter's mode" that would require afternoon footwear more ceremonious than what had for the last few years been known as "dressy sports."[47]

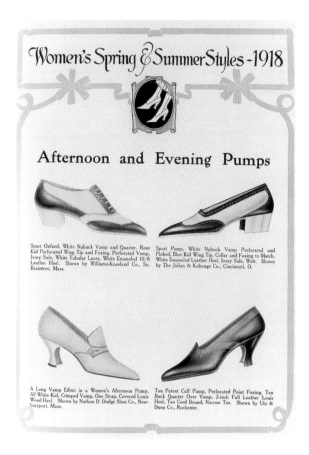

Fig. 77. New styles for spring and summer 1918, illustrated in the *Shoe Retailer* for September 22, 1917, p. 51. The upper two shoes are sports types, characterized by their use of decorative perforations and two colors. The oxford at left is white Nubuck and rose kid, and the pump is white Nubuck with blue kid. After World War I, green, blue, red, and even orange were mentioned as possible colors for use with white in women's sports shoes. *Courtesy Lynn Museum.*

CHAPTER SIX

Shoes Adapted for Protection

Overshoes are any kind of shoe or boot worn over another shoe or boot in order to protect the foot and under-shoe from cold, inclement weather, or slippery floors. This category includes clogs, pattens, rubbers, and carriage boots. The term "carriage boot" may refer simply to an ordinary dressy boot worn as a part of carriage dress as described in chapter four, but often it means a boot-style overshoe worn over evening shoes when driving to and from evening entertainments. Overshoes that were carriage boots in all but name were also worn indoors to protect the feet from cold and these are closely related to the warmer varieties of boudoir slippers. This chapter also describes the fleece-lined winter boots and wooden-soled shoes that were not overshoes but that were worn in much the same way for protection against bad weather or adverse working conditions.

Clogs and Pattens

In the early nineteenth century, when even walking shoes and boots were made of thin leathers and lightweight fabrics, overshoes of some sort or another were an absolute necessity. One time-honored choice both for the country and for wet pavements in town was the clog. The word clog has several definitions, but for the purposes of this book clogs are wooden-soled overshoes, secured to the foot by a leather strap over the instep, sometimes supplemented by a toecap. In the early nineteenth century they could also have some arrangement to secure the heel, either a stiff counter, a leather-covered spring or both. Because of their inflexibility, wooden-soled shoes are awkward to wear. To solve this problem, many from the nineteenth century were constructed with a sole in two pieces, the

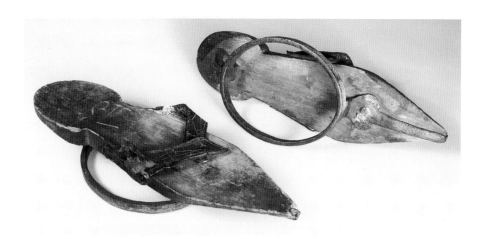

Fig. 78. According to the history that came with them, these pattens (marked "S.L." on the sole) were "presented to Susannah Meacham Lewis by her son, Captain Thomas Lewis in 1804. Captain Lewis was lost with all his crew on his next voyage, foundered at sea." Had these pattens not been the gift of a lost son, it is unlikely that they would have been preserved, much less preserved with a date. They were made to fit the pointed toes and flat soles fashionable in women's shoes in 1804. The straps are of calf lined with white kid and covered with red morocco, the layers stitched through with white thread. The iron ring raises the wooden sole an additional 1⅛ inches off the ground and is designed to provide reinforcement at the pointed toe of the sole. Catalog #118, #119. *Courtesy Lynn Museum.*

break coming beneath the ball of the foot and joined with a leather hinge. This allows the foot to bend while walking (see plate 17). The patten, like the clog, has a wooden sole, but it is never hinged. Instead, it is raised on an iron ring (see fig. 78, plate 17).

Clogs and pattens were cut to match the fashionable shoe shape. If made to wear with a heeled shoe, they will have a step at the back to accommodate the heel. These are likely to date from the eighteenth century. The most common kind of surviving eighteenth-century clog consists of nothing but a thick leather sole with straps, the wooden element being reduced to a mere block supporting the arch of the shoe in front of the heel. Clogs and pattens with flat soles and sharply pointed toes probably date before 1810, those with oval toes from circa 1800 to 1830, and those with square ones from 1830 to 1850. From about 1850, pattens would have been superseded by rubbers.

Pattens were more useful in town than in the country. The ring would have sunk deep into a muddy road, but it carried the wearer safely, if noisily, through the puddles on a paved surface. In Jane Austen's *Persuasion* (1817), Mrs. Russell enjoyed "the ceaseless clink of pattens" in the English city of Bath as one of the "noises which belonged to the winter pleasures."[1] Clogs, however, had a wider range of usefulness and could be worn wherever it was desirable to protect the shoes from mud and wet. Elizabeth Simcoe found them convenient even on board the ship that carried her and her husband, the British lieutenant-governor of Upper Canada, from England to Quebec in 1791. "The floor of my Cabbin is scarcely ever dry and the Baize with which it is covered retains the wet, therefore I always wear clogs."[2]

Another kind of wooden-soled shoe that turns up in American collections is not a sandal-like overshoe but a true shoe with a complete leather upper (see fig. 79). Most shoes of this type seem to have been brought back as souvenirs from the north of England, where they were worn well into the twentieth century. They typically have iron bands called clog irons edging the bottom of the sole, very much like a horseshoe. These served to keep the wood from wearing out too quickly. Those most often preserved here as souvenirs have leather uppers in an open-tab pattern that fastens with a fancy clasp over the tongue extension of the vamp. No doubt this style was chosen by tourists as the most quaint and attractive, but in England clogs were made in a variety of patterns and fastenings. They were worn by the working classes, men, women, and children, both on farms and in factories, and not just for the actual heavy work, but for everyday at home and at school as well.[3]

Clogs with irons on the sole in the English style seem to have been worn only rarely in America. However, wood-soled shoes without irons were apparently worn with increasing frequency from the mid-1890s. The *Shoe Retailer* describes these American shoes as having "a heavy basswood sole and heel . . . made somewhat attractive by receiving the usual contour of leather bottoms and with the inside so shaped as to conform to the anatomy of the foot. The upper is cut in buckle or congress pattern and is made from serviceable oil grain." The A. H. Reimer Company, of Milwaukee, began to make wood-soled shoes in 1895, and shoes of this type were advertised in the 1895 Montgomery Ward catalog as useful in laundries, dairies, and on the farm, being very light and durable. By 1900, the factory was planning to produce forty-five thousand pairs as wooden-soled footwear began to find uses in an increasing variety of settings. They were worn by workmen in ice-cream factories, creameries, breweries, and by the barkeepers in "beer saloons where the floors are kept constantly wet from drippings from the beer glasses." When made with a rubber upper, wood-soled shoes were found useful in tinplate and enameling works because they resisted the action of acid. A version produced especially for miners had an iron rail added to the outer edge of the wooden sole, presumably producing something close to the English style of clog.[4]

Wooden-soled shoes were also used for dancing. Montgomery Ward advertised "Men's Dancing Clogs" (Sears called them "Professional Clog Shoes") in its 1895 catalog. Made of "red, blue or black morocco leather, wood soles, all one piece," they sold for $2.50 the pair, brass jingles twenty-five cents extra. These were oxford ties. Shoes made entirely of wood (looking much like traditional Dutch shoes) were described in the same catalog as "wooden shoes for clog dancers and comedians, also extensively used in dyeing establishments, laundries, cellars, dairy farms, etc." These were the only style available in women's as well as men's and boys' sizes. Otherwise, wooden-soled shoes, like most other heavy work shoes, were normally intended for men.[5] However, women did occasionally wear them when they worked in wet or slippery settings that made such footwear practical. A young woman who worked at Armour and Company in Chicago and was interviewed by the Federal Writers' Project during the late 1930s reported that "most of the girls in Casings [the department where pig guts are cleaned out] have to wear wooden shoes and rubber aprons. The company doesn't furnish them. They pay three dollars for the shoes and about a dollar and a half for the aprons."[6] The Lynn Museum has a pair of wooden-soled leather shoes that are very similar to the men's dancing clogs advertised in Montgomery Ward, but in a size plausible for a woman. These could also have been intended for industrial use, possibly in one of the many leather factories associated with the shoe industry, which was centered in Lynn (see fig. 80).

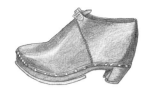

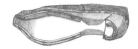

Fig. 79. Clogs of this general type with a complete upper and a wooden sole reinforced with grooved iron bands were worn in a variety of patterns and fastenings for all kinds of occasions by people in the north of England well into the twentieth century. They were brought back to the States as souvenirs and occasionally appear in American collections without being identified as foreign shoes. This pair is from the Peabody Essex Museum, USMC catalog #596.

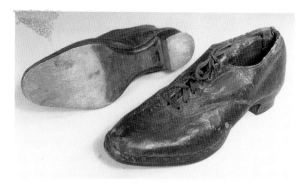

Fig. 80. This wooden-soled shoe, ca. 1900–1910, does not survive with a history, but it could plausibly have been worn in one of the leather factories in the Lynn area. Leather factories had some very wet and sloppy work areas (see fig. 13) where protective footwear would have been necessary. This shoe is small enough to have been a woman's. It has been slit across the vamp to allow a bit more room for the left foot. Catalog #6377. *Courtesy Lynn Museum.*

Leather Overshoes

Less commonly recognized than clogs and pattens are leather overshoes. According to an advertisement in the *Barre Gazette* for November 11, 1839, "sole leather over shoes" both "lined" and "plain" were sold by Moses Mandell of the Barre Shoe Store.[7] Unlike other entries in Mandell's list, these overshoes are not described as "gents'," or "ladies'." Perhaps they were worn by both sexes. Two pairs of leather shoes that are thought to be overshoes are in the collection at Old Sturbridge Village. They are cut much like a slipper, but are of heavier leather with a heavier sole, and they do appear long and wide enough to wear over another lighter shoe (see fig. 81b).

Occasionally one finds a nineteenth-century descendant of the eighteenth-century clog having a leather rather than a wooden sole. One survives with its matching shoe at the Museum of Fine Arts, Boston (see fig. 81a). The clog consists of a forepart only, held on by a leather-covered spring that passes round the low heel of the shoe. This heel is hollowed slightly on the sides and back to keep the spring in place.

Carriage Shoes

Clogs and pattens, however useful they were on wet pavements, were no help to a woman faced with a deep snow, and early diaries and letters refer to women staying indoors because roads and walks were impassible or being carried from place to place by convenient young men. Anna Green Winslow, age twelve, writing to her parents in December 1771, recounts how returning from a visit to friends, "the snow being so deep I was bro't home in arms. . . . The snow is up to the peoples wast in some places in the street."[8]

A decade later, young women seem to have been no better provided for dealing with adverse weather. Eliza Southgate Bowne wrote about her difficulties getting to and from an evening party in Portland, Maine, in 1802:

> Thursday it snowed violently, indeed for two
> days before it had been storming so much that the
> snow drifts were very large; however, as it was the
> last Assembly I could not resist the temptation of

going, as I knew all the world would be there. About 7 I went down-stairs and found young Charles Coffin, the minister, in the parlor. After the usual enquiries were over he stared awhile at my feathers and flowers, asked if I was going out,—I told him I was going to the Assembly. "Think, Miss Southgate," said he, after a long pause, "think you would go out to meeting in such as storm as this?" Then assuming a tone of re-proof, he entreated me to examine well my feel-ings on such an occasion. I heard in silence, un-willing to begin an argument that I was unable to support. The stopping of the carriage roused me; I immediately slipt on my socks and coat, and met Horatio and Mr. Motley in the entry. The snow was deep, but Mr. Motley took me up in his arms and sat me in the carriage without difficulty.[9]

The storm continued through the assembly and when the coach brought her back, "The gentlemen then proceeded to take us out. My beau, unused to carry-ing such a weight of sin and folly, sank under its pres-sure, and I was obliged to carry my mighty self through the snow which almost buried me."[10] The next Monday, after several more days of snow, Eliza decided to try to get home to her sister's house. The poor horse finally came to a standstill in the midst of a huge drift not far from her destination. Stepping into the breach, "the gentleman took me up in his arms and carried me till my weight pressed him so far into the snow that he had no power to move his feet. I rolled out of his arms and wallowed till I reached the gate."[11] For Eliza this was all a lark and she was none the worse for wear. One wonders, however, about the unspecified "gentlemen" who never even got their names mentioned for their trouble.

A lady like Eliza Southgate Bowne in "feathers and flowers" on her way to an evening party in winter did not want to put on awkward wooden clogs or pat-tens or the ugly rubbers of later times to protect her dancing slippers from the snow. Eliza says she put on "socks," presumably nothing more than thick stock-ings pulled on over her light shoes to keep her feet warm in the carriage since she did not expect to do

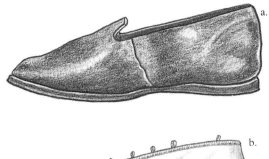

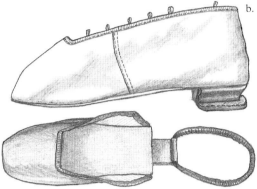

Fig. 81.

(a) Overshoe, ca. 1810–20. According to June Swann (*Shoes*, p. 30), "In 1785 Alexander Gillies took out a patent for sprung clogs: a toe cap with forepart sole, with or without latchets, and a kid-covered spring loop to hook round the heel." This example fits Swann's description. It is made to fit an unusually high-cut shoe of purple silk whose top edge is fitted with eight pairs of loops through which a lacing tie passes. The kid-covered wooden heel juts out in a lip around the bottom in order to hold the spring of the clog in place. Museum of Fine Arts, Boston, catalog #43.1737.

(b) Leather overshoe: This slip-on shoe may perhaps be an overshoe. It is made of thick, unlined leather with no binding at the top edge and has a heavy, pegged sole. The shape of the sole suggests a date of 1835–50. Another similar shoe, machine-made, has a somewhat lower throatline cut into three scallops. Old Sturbridge Village catalog #12.14.116.

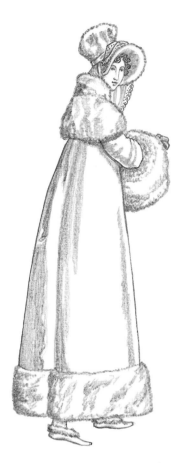

Fig. 82. This elegant figure in her pink pelisse trimmed with white fur is also wearing fur-trimmed shoes, very possibly overshoes. Similar shoes, red with black fur edging, are shown in Rolinda Sharples' 1817 painting *The Cloakroom, Clifton Assembly Rooms* (reproduced in Swann, *Shoes*, on page 33) and are unmistakably overshoes—one has been taken off, revealing the white evening shoe worn underneath. From *Le Journal des Dames*, 1817.

any walking. The use of warm stockings as carriage overshoes continued to be a cheap and practical alternative right through the nineteenth century. In *These Happy Golden Years*, Laura Ingalls Wilder recounts how she put woolen stockings on over her shoes when riding in an open sleigh in the intense cold of a South Dakota winter about 1883.[12]

While American ladies counted on being carried to their carriages by helpful young men, the British lady Elizabeth Simcoe (the same who sensibly wore clogs on board her ship to Canada) seems never to have been deterred from walking by cold, wet weather, or rough country. Upon arriving in Canada, she described walking from Quebec to Cape Diamond in her diary for November 18, 1791, remarking that "it seemed very perilous walking over acres of ice, but cloth shoes or coarse worsted stockings over shoes prevents slipping."[13] On another occasion that same winter, having traveled by sled to make her calls, she walked the two miles home through the snow, noting that "it is fatiguing to walk on snow when not perfectly frozen & my half boots were heavy with Icicles."[14] Her half-boots may simply have been walking boots, which were occasionally worn at this period (see fig. 36). However, considering the amount of snow, she may have been wearing some sort of warm overshoe, perhaps similar to a pair preserved at the Society for the Preservation of New England Antiquities (SPNEA). SPNEA's red morocco ankle-high boots have sturdy leather soles suggesting a date circa 1805–15, and they show the remains of a woolly lining. They do not lace in the ordinary way through eyelets but tie with three pairs of silk ribbons (once red) over a tongue. They have low, stacked heels and appear large enough to go over another pair of shoes.[15]

Though having a much heavier sole, SPNEA's red morocco boots are very similar in pattern to the carriage boots worn over evening slippers on the way to and from parties later in the century. Traditionally made of velvet and lined with fur, carriage boots were dressy overshoes, soft and thick enough to keep the lady's feet warm in the carriage and just sturdy enough to take her from the carriage to the door. Boots of this type were available throughout the nineteenth century. Swann points out a pair in an 1817 painting by Rolinda Sharples of *The Cloakroom, Clifton Assembly Rooms*.[16] Similar fur-trimmed shoes appear in French fashion plates of the same year (see fig. 82). It is possible that some of these French pictures are of walking shoes rather than overshoes. "Ladies' French morocco fur lined walking shoes, a superior article for the coming season" are mentioned in a newspaper advertisement in Barre, Vermont, in 1839.[17]

In North America, women seem to have worn Indian moccasins as overshoes from at least the eighteenth century. A letter written by Elizabeth Russell of York (Toronto), Ontario, to a friend in England in November 1797 refers to the practice. "I wish I had anything to send you worthy of your acceptance, but the Indians here do not make anything but common kinds of baskets and brooms. . . . Some of them make mawkinsons which all the Indians wear instead of shoes and they ornament them very nicely with beads, ribbons, and porcupine quills. . . . I had a squaw spoken to make me some but I have not heard any more of her. As soon as I can get any made I will send them to you. Mrs. Simcoe used to wear them over her shoes and she looked very smart."[18] Apparently the idea took hold in England, since in May 1828, the English periodical *La Belle Assemblée* mentions wearing moccasins as overshoes, when during one cold April, muffs and fur mantles "were yet prevalent, as were the furred boots lined with flannel, and the Indian mocasins [*sic*] drawn over the dress shoe." A "carriage shoe" described in *Godey's* in January 1861 is probably an overshoe. It is made like a moccasin "of black or any dark-colored velvet, richly embroidered, and bound with satin ribbon. The sole is of stout wash leather, wadded and lined with satin." In December 1866, *Godey's* offered instructions for knitting an ankle-high "winter boot . . . suitable for wearing over a thin shoe, or they may be used for sleeping socks, omitting the cork sole." Directions for a similar boot in crochet had been given in October 1850, with the note that adding a gutta-percha sole to the cork sole would make it "an admirable snow boot,"

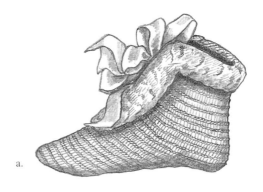

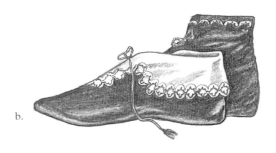

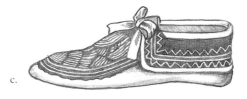

Fig. 83. Three mid-nineteenth-century carriage shoes:

(a) Crocheted "carriage slipper" illustrated in *Godey's Lady's Book*, October 1850, pp. 245–46, with directions for making of drab or stone-colored Berlin wool with a fluffy trimming of black and white sheared loops, a lining and bow of cerise silk, and a sole of cork. "With the addition of a gutta percha sole to the cork, this will make an admirable snow boot."

(b) Boots "designed more especially for the carriage, in order that the passage to and from it may not allow the feet to become chilled; as well as for persons who suffer with cold extremities. The material is black velvet, lined with taffeta, which is embroidered upon the edge with delicate needlework. The shoe is confined with cords, which are finished with tassels." These were sold by E. A. Brooks, 575 Broadway and 150 Fulton Street, New York City, and illustrated in *Godey's Lady's Book*, April 1855.

(c) "[Moccasin-style] carriage shoe . . . made of black or any dark-colored velvet, richly embroidered, and bound with satin ribbon. The sole is of stout wash leather, wadded and lined with satin. It is a warm and handsome carriage shoe." Illustrated in *Godey's Lady's Book*, January 1861.

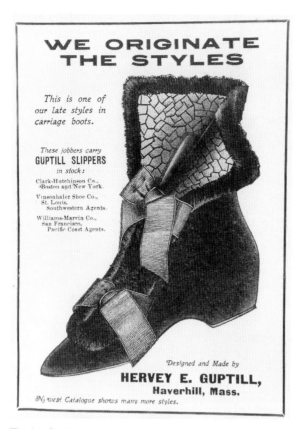

WE ORIGINATE THE STYLES

This is one of our late styles in carriage boots.

These jobbers carry
GUPTILL SLIPPERS
in stock:

Clark-Hutchinson Co.,
Boston and New York.

Vinsonhaler Shoe Co.,
St. Louis,
Southwestern Agents.

Williams-Marvin Co.,
San Francisco,
Pacific Coast Agents.

Designed and Made by
HERVEY E. GUPTILL,
Haverhill, Mass.
Newest Catalogue shows many more styles.

Fig. 84. Carriage boot, probably of velvet, trimmed with fur and tied with two pairs of broad grosgrain silk ribbons, made by Hervey E. Guptill of Haverhill, Massachusetts, and advertised in the *Shoe Retailer* for September 21, 1904. Late-nineteenth-century versions look very much like this one, except that the toe shape varies to conform with the squarish or oval toe shapes of nineteenth-century slippers. *Courtesy Lynn Museum.*

an assessment that hardly seems plausible by today's standards (see fig. 83). A surviving example dating from the early 1850s is made of knitted scarlet and white wool in a crossbar pattern. It laces up the side, has an oilcloth sole, and a felt sock lining.[19]

The evening overshoes most likely to survive in shoe collections, however, date from the last third of the nineteenth century. Many are black or brown velvet or plush and are trimmed with fur, but some are made of lighter-colored silks, brocade, or suede. They cover the ankle and are tied with pairs of broad ribbons over a tongue. A look at the inside will reveal a lining of quilted silk and a depression in the sole designed to receive the heel of the evening shoe. *Godey's* may be referring to overshoes of this type when it notes in February 1862 that "carriage boots of velvet, fancifully trimmed with fur, are among the novelties" of the winter season. They are advertised in the *Shoe Retailer* in 1904 (see fig. 84), and a picture appears of them in the *Ladies' Home Journal* as late as November 1914. A version with rubber soles was worn into the 1940s.

Rubbers

Clogs and pattens gradually went out of use with the advent of vulcanized rubber overshoes in the late 1840s. But even before vulcanization, natural rubber overshoes were worn in the United States. Early white explorers had reported the existence of rubber in the Amazon valley, but because Brazil was permitted to trade only with Portugal, its "mother country," only small quantities in the form of rubber bottles found their way into the hands of curious scientists. Bits of these bottles were found handy to rub out pencil marks (hence the name "rubber"), but until 1808 rubber was really little more than a curiosity outside its natural habitat. In that year the king of Portugal, fleeing the aggression of Napoleon, took refuge in Brazil and opened Brazilian commerce to friendly nations, including the United States and Great Britain. According to Howard and Ralph Wolf (whose 1936 history *Rubber: A Story of Glory and Greed* provides perhaps the most complete account of the early rubber trade and industry), the first pair of rubber shoes—gilded and with long, pointed toes—arrived in the United States from Brazil in 1820.[20] The first significant quantity of rubbers, five hundred pairs, was imported in 1823 by Boston merchant Thomas C. Wales and sold for $3 to $5 a pair. This first lot was sufficiently profitable that Wales sent back wooden lasts so that the shoes could be made in sizes more suitable for the American public.[21] This began a trade in Brazilian-made rubber shoes that increased to five hundred thousand pairs a year by the late 1840s.[22]

These early Brazilian rubbers can still be seen today, the best selection being at the Peabody Essex Museum in Salem. Surviving examples are distorted and even crystallized with age and repeated heating and cooling, but they seem originally to have been of varying thickness up to a quarter-inch, crudely shaped, with round toes. They are an uneven smoky brown or black in color and usually have stylized flower designs incised on the vamp. Most of these surviving Brazilian rubbers are unlined, but advertisements of the 1830s and 1840s mention others that were "lined and bound." One of these is preserved at the Peabody Essex Museum with an old label describing them as "Para Rubbers first lined." They are shaped like a slit-vamp shoe, lined with kid in the quarter and a felt material in the vamp, bound with black galloon, and decorated with floral designs in the Brazilian Indian style. Lined and unlined rubbers seem to have been offered side by side in the 1830s and 1840s. The Brimfield Boot and Shoe Store in Hartford listed in 1840 a shipment of three thousand pairs of men's and women's rubber overshoes, "plain and figured," and one thousand pairs of men's and women's rubbers, "lined and bound, plain and figured." The "figured" presumably refers to the Indian floral designs. In 1833, the *Maine Farmer and Journal of the Arts* carried two advertisements mentioning rubbers. The first was for Chandler and Pullen's general store, which listed only "Ladies' and Gentlemen's INDIA RUBBER OVERSHOES." The second was for the Winthrop Boot and Shoe Store, which appears to have carried a slightly more elegant range of goods. It listed both "Ladies' Plain Rubber Shoes" and "Ladies' India Rubber Over Shoes, lined and bound" as well as "gentlemen's Rubber Over shoes." Presumably the lined and bound rubbers were somewhat more expensive than the plain ones, and perhaps more comfortable. They certainly look more like ordinary shoes.

Brazilian-made rubber shoes were made by pouring successive layers of the liquid latex over a last, and curing each layer carefully with smoke from a fire of urucuri nuts. According to the Wolfs, the completed rubbers were exposed to the sun for a day or two, remaining soft enough to be decorated with a pointed stick. The designs the Indians put on them often had a radiating figure somewhat like a pinwheel centered on the vamp, with flowerlike elements at the end of each arm. Others incorporated little circles probably made with the end of a hollow reed, and a few look as if parts of the design may have been created with a stamp or die (see plate 17). In at least one example, the design is a ship in full sail. The Wolfs explain that the rubbers remained too soft to be packed for some time. Therefore, they were suspended from long poles to keep them from sticking together during the trip by foot or canoe to the port of Para, and once there, they were stuffed with grass so they would keep their shape until they were sufficiently hard to withstand the export voyage. Portuguese merchants paid the Indians ten to fifteen cents a pair, but on a credit system that made virtual slaves of the Indian producers.[23] An 1876 article in the *Scientific American* suggests that at least sometimes in this early period, leather boots made in the United States were sent to Brazil to be coated with the liquid latex. Boots of this type were shown at the Fair of the American Institute in 1833 by J. N. Hood of New York, and men's rubber-coated leather boots that appear to fit the description survive at the Peabody Essex Museum.[24]

Rubbers were also made in the United States beginning in 1832 by several companies clustered in the Boston area. The raw natural rubber could not be imported as liquid latex—the latex solidified on exposure to air and spoiled if it had not been properly cured. So at first the early manufacturers used as their raw material rubber bottles formed over gourds by the Indians; later they were sent seventy-pound balls of layered cured rubber. Most American rubber makers in the 1830s dissolved the rubber in turpentine so that it could be spread on cloth or leather, and from the rubber-covered material made objects such as shoes, life preservers, or wagon covers. Unfortunately, rubber dissolved in turpentine always remained tacky and had to be sandwiched between two layers of cloth. Even when the turpentine was omitted and the spreading done mechanically, this natural crude rubber had serious defects. When the weather got very hot, it melted and stank, and during the cold New England winters, it turned brittle and cracked.[25] The Roxbury India Rubber Factory "turned out large numbers of shoes in the winter of 1833–34 and then had $20,000 worth of goods returned the following summer, half melted and emitting so villainous a smell that they had to be buried."[26] Under the circumstances, it seems unlikely that any of these very early nonvulcanized American-made rubbers survive.

Charles Goodyear picked up the problem of curing rubber in 1834 and worried at it for five years, in spite of great financial hardship and even imprisonment for debt. In 1837, he obtained a patent for treating rubber with nitric acid. This did cure the surface and although it left the rest of the rubber unchanged, rubber shoes were apparently made using this "acid gas process" in Providence, Rhode Island, until vulcanization proved a better solution. Whether any of these shoes survive is not known. Finally, in 1839, Goodyear discovered that heating rubber with sulfur would prevent stickiness, brittleness, decomposition, and loss of elasticity. He was so poor, however, that he was unable to patent his process in the United States until 1844, and by that time the British rubber manufacturer Thomas Hancock had seen a sample of Goodyear's cured rubber and, smelling the sulfur in it, figured the process out in time to get the English patent for himself. Even the English name for the process, "vulcanization," became the standard term.

Only after vulcanization could practical rubber shoes be made successfully in the United States. The first shoe manufacturer legally to make shoes of vulcanized rubber was L. Candee and Company, of New Haven, incorporated in 1843. Vulcanized rubber overshoes at first competed with the natural rubber overshoes imported from Brazil, but eventually supplanted them. Rubbers that may date from the postvulcanization period survive at the Connecticut Historical Society, lined with flannel and shaped to imitate a slit-vamp tie shoe (see fig. 85a). An early pair of men's vulcanized rubber oveshoes, low cut with one strap, is preserved at the Albany Institute of History and Art.

Judging from the few examples surviving, early American-made rubbers are distinguished from the Brazilian product in several ways. While Brazilian rubbers were formed in one seamless piece, American rubbers were made of several pieces cut from flat sheets of prepared rubber and then glued together with rubber cement. Because they were made of several pieces like any other shoe, American rubbers tended to imitate contemporary shoe patterns and the stiff counter can be felt inside the quarter. They also lack the characteristically Indian floral decoration. In order to strengthen the shoe, American manufacturers used heavy calender rollers to press the flat sheets of prepared rubber against a cloth backing under great pressure. This bonded the two layers together so that no cloth binding galloon was necessary. In contrast, Brazilian rubbers were either totally unlined but rather thick, or else had a lining added after they were made by stitching lining and rubber together with a galloon binding around the top edge. Most American manufacturers seem to have added lampblack to the rubber to produce a black color, while many (but not all) Brazilian rubbers are brown. See appendix C for more information on the early history of rubber and a more complete description of how rubbers were made.

Rubbers inevitably made the feet look big, and in an age when small feet were admired, no girl wanted to wear them. "India rubbers are odious-looking things, to be sure, and many a lovely girl has sacrificed her health, life even, rather than put them on,"[27] warned *Godey's* in 1847. One Lowell mill girl was perhaps thinking how reluctant she and her fellow boarders were to wear them when she compared a good boardinghouse keeper in 1844 to the virtuous woman of Proverbs, "'She is not afraid of the snow for her

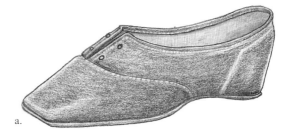

a.

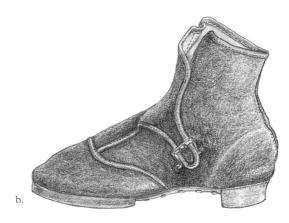

b.

Fig. 85.
   (a) Rubber overshoes probably made in the United States ca. 1845–60 of vulcanized rubber lined with brown twilled cotton with a soft brushed surface. They imitate the cut and shape of ordinary walking tie shoes, and tie with brown twilled laces. Connecticut Historical Society catalog #1963-33-1&2.
   (b) Overshoe, ca. 1865–75. The upper is made of a cotton foundation fabric coated with some sort of rubber (now flaking off), and lined with flannel. It has a low, stacked heel and leather sole doubled at the tread. A strap, now missing, probably originated at the waist just above the sole and passed through the buckle. The strap closure, as well as the rubber coating, suggests that this was an overshoe rather than a walking shoe, which would have had a full laced or buttoned closure. Connecticut Historical Society catalog #1960-37-14G.

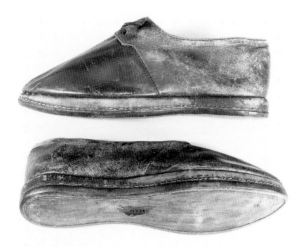

Fig. 86. Cork-soled shoe, ca. 1810–30. The thick outsole and extra layer of cork in this black kid tie shoe would have made it a reasonably practical defense against cold and wet pavements. Catalog #1423. *Courtesy Lynn Museum.*

household,' for she maketh them wear rubber over-shoes, and thick cloaks and hoods, and seeth that the paths are broken out."[28] The writer of *Every Lady Her Own Shoemaker* (1856) advised that "cloth gaiters should not be worn on the damp ground without India-rubbers, as the mud will soil the cloth. . . . Besides, health requires that the feet should be protected from the ground, when it is damp and cold. If heavy rubbers are an objection, get some India-rubber sandals."[29] These sandals were described in *Godey's* three years earlier as "rather ornamental than disfiguring to the foot, if inclosed in a gaiter. They come a little above the patent leather tip, and are confined across the instep by a light strap of the same. Price $1. They would not answer very well, however, for *wet* country walking."[30]

Another clue to midcentury overshoes survives in a rare boot dating from about 1865 to 1875.[31] It is made very much like any ordinary walking boot of the period, with a low, stacked heel and leather sole doubled at the tread. But the upper is made of a flannel-like material that has been coated with some sort of rubber compound that is now flaking off. The coated fabric was then cut out, stitched, and bound just like any boot of serge or leather. The fact that the center-front opening laps over and fastens with a single buckled strap suggests that it is an overshoe rather than a regular walking boot, which would normally have a full laced closure (see fig. 85b).

When walking shoes became more substantial in the later nineteenth century, overshoes became less important for most women. Winter walking boots especially were made with thicker soles and linings to protect the foot from cold and wet. *Demorest's* reported in the fall of 1879 that "dryness is secured by the cork soles that are now used in all the best grade of winter boots. Since the introduction of cork soles, many people dispense entirely with rubbers for ordinary occasions, using them only if compelled to be out in a 'driving rain' or 'deep slush.'"[32] Cork soles were not as new an invention as this suggests. A pair that may date as early as 1810 is preserved at the Lynn Museum (see fig. 86), and another from the 1860s is in the United Shoe Machinery Corporation collection at the

Peabody Essex Museum. In these examples, it is not the actual walking surface that is made of cork. Rather a layer of cork three-eighths to one-half an inch thick is inserted just above the outsole, and the edge is covered with leather so that the cork itself cannot be seen. The term "cork sole" was also used to describe welted shoes that used a layer of cork to fill the hollow between the outsole and the insole. In this latter type of shoe, the presence of the cork is not detectable from the outside.

By the late nineteenth and early twentieth century, as low shoes were more and more often worn for walking in the summer, leather boots came to be seen as the thing to wear when the weather turned bad. In Gene Stratton Porter's 1909 novel *Girl of the Limberlost,* when Margaret and Wesley Sinton buy Elnora a pair of stylish low shoes for school in September, they also buy "a pair of top shoes for rainy days and colder weather. . . . 'About those high shoes, that was my idea,' said Wesley. 'Soon as it rains, low shoes won't do, and by taking two pairs at once I could get them some cheaper.'"[33]

The turn away from rubbers may have resulted partly from adulteration of the common product. *Mme. Demorest's What to Wear* noted in 1883 that "rubbers are a necessity with fine shoes in wet weather, but they have lately been of such poor quality that the wearer never felt certain whether they would not part at the next step, and prove worse than nothing. This vexation has given rise to the attempt to put a new rubber on the market, which is warranted nine-tenths pure rubber. They will be very light and fine, low cut in front, and high at the back. They will be somewhat expensive, about $1.25, but will outlast three or four pairs of ordinary rubbers, and will not therefore prove an unprofitable investment."[34] By the 1890s and early 1900s, it was standard for rubber companies to sell two or even three grades of goods known as firsts, seconds, and thirds, each being sold under a different trade name. The firsts were the longer-lasting but more expensive pure rubber described in *Demorest's.* A list of these trade names as provided in the *Shoe Retailer* is given in appendix C.

Few late-nineteenth-century, adult-size rubber overshoes survive, but advertisements and mail-order catalogs suggest that four staple styles were available by at least the 1890s and right through the 1920s: footholds, croquet sandals, storm rubbers, and solid leg boots (see fig. 87).

The foothold, also known as a sandal or a heelless rubber, consisted of a fairly low-cut forepart with a sling across the back of the foot to keep it on. This was the most fashionable alternative because it avoided the problem of fitting the rubber over the high heel, but it provided a good deal less protection than the other styles and was suitable only for the lightest rain (fig. 87a).

Croquet sandals and "imitation sandals" were rubber overshoes with a complete sole and relatively low-cut upper with a round throatline much like a pump or slipper. Croquet sandals seem to have been somewhat lighter and dressier in effect, while imitation sandals (or just plain "sandals") are sometimes described as "medium weight . . . made especially to fit heavy shoes and for hard wear. Medium toe only" (fig. 87b).

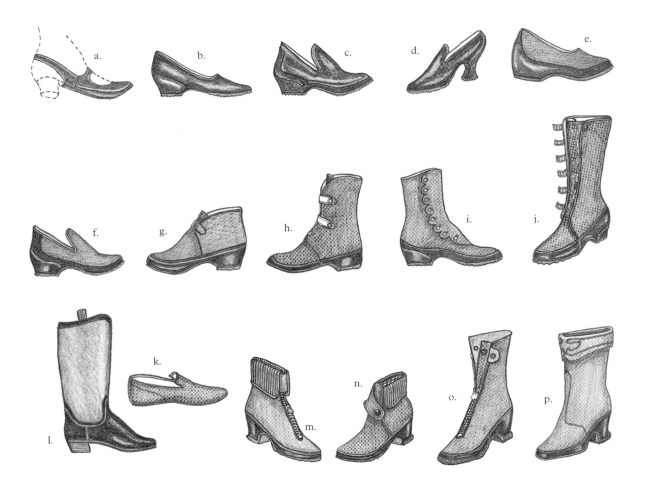

Fig. 87. Rubbers and winter overshoes. Most of these styles were made over a long period of time, but the toe and heel shapes varied to fit currently fashionable lasts. Nearly identical illustrations of these overshoes appear in the catalogs of several mail-order companies through the 1890s and early twentieth century.

(a) Foothold, made of net-lined rubber.

(b) Croquet rubber, also known as a croquet sandal.

(c) Storm rubber, also called an Instep Over.

(d) Storm rubber designed to fit over the higher Louis heels worn from the late 1910s. *Ladies Home Journal*, April 1920.

(e) Croquet alaska: overshoe with rubber bottom, wool cloth top, wool fleece lining, and choice of toe shapes.

(f) Storm alaska: slightly higher overshoe with rubber bottom, wool cloth top, and wool fleece lining.

(g) Buckle arctic: rubber bottom, heavy cloth top, fleece lining; described in the 1890s as suitable for heavy wear.

(h) "High cut Buckle Gaiter, made from first quality pure gum, Jersey cloth top, and wool fleece lined . . . in regular, opera and piccadilly toes." Advertised in Sears, 1897.

(i) Cashmerette high-button overshoe, wool lined, a style available in a higher version in the early 1920s.

(j) Extra-high six-buckle gaiter with fine black jersey cloth top. Advertised in Sears, 1922. These buckles were available in the 1890s, normally three to a boot.

(k–l) The most typical style of women's fleece-lined solid-leg rubber boot, offered from the 1890s through the 1920s. Wool felt slippers worn inside for comfort.

(m) "Low arctic or ankle type golashe" with zipper fastening made by the Goodrich Company (*Shoe Retailer*, October 8, 1927, p. 40).

(n) "Among the latest patterns from the line of the United States Rubber Co., New York is the Streak, a low jersey cloth Gaytee of the Kwik fastener type, made with black, tan and gray corduroy cuff or plain cuff as ordered" (*Shoe Retailer*, October 8, 1927, p. 41).

(o) The "Zipper," a high arctic or gaiter made by the Goodrich Company, gave the common name to the hookless fastener. *Shoe Retailer*, October 8, 1927, p. 41.

(p) "Cap'n Kidd Boot," Cambridge Rubber Company ("Camco"). Not described, but appears to have a felt or cloth top, rubber bottom, and decorative chainstitching. *Shoe Retailer*, October 8, 1927, p. 41.

Storm rubbers (sometimes called storm slippers or instep overs) covered nearly the entire foot and shoe and were cut with a tonguelike tab on the instep. Occasionally storm rubbers were fleece lined. The instep overs illustrated in the Jordan Marsh catalog for fall 1893 are described as "Something new. They give full protection against wet skirts. A great convenience" (fig. 87c).

By the early twentieth century, rubber manufacturers faced the challenge of designing rubbers that would fit neatly over higher heeled shoes and an ever-changing stream of toe changes, a problem apparently only indifferently solved. Advertisers in the 1920s worked hard to combat the image of rubbers as clumsy and awkward, claiming that their rubbers did not share the usual defects of wrinkling, bulging, bagging, sagging, and gapping, a list of ills that would discourage any stylish woman. But other than the changes in toe and heel shapes, the rubbers advertised in the *Ladies' Home Journal* in the early 1920s look very little different from those illustrated in Sears in the 1890s (fig. 87d).

Rubber overshoes were also made with warm linings to wear in cold weather. For wet winter days and light snow, manufacturers offered low-cut overshoes called "alaskas." These looked much like storm rubbers or croquet sandals except that they had wool cloth tops and wool fleece linings. Only the soles and lower edges were made of rubber (see fig. 87e, f). Heavy snow, however, required "arctics," which Swann mentions were available by 1872.[35] Arctics (sometimes called "snow excluders") were ankle-high overshoes usually made to buckle over a bellows tongue. Like alaskas, they had rubber soles and foxings, wool cloth tops, and wool fleece linings (fig. 87g).

Calf-high winter overshoes often referred to as "gaiters" were also advertised in the 1890s and early 1900s. These were, like the lower arctics, rubber soled, cloth topped, and fleece lined, and they came in buttoned and buckled styles. The women's buckled versions had three buckles down the center front over a bellows tongue, while men's boots had four buckles (fig. 87h). The buttoned versions echoed contemporary walking boots in style (fig. 87i). Fleece-lined, calf-high, solid-leg rubber boots were also available, but in fewer styles for women than for men. Fleece slippers might be worn inside for warmth (fig. 87k, l).

By the 1920s, as skirts rose, leaving the legs exposed to the cold, the ankle-high arctics lost ground to the taller gaiter, which was now sometimes called a high arctic. In contrast to the three-buckled version worn at the turn of the century, those made in the 1920s could have from two to six buckles (fig. 87j). Sears' 1922 catalog shows them worn buckled, unbuckled, and even with the tops flopping down (one story claims that the flapping boot tops affected by young women in the 1920s was the origin of the name "flappers").

By the late 1920s, there were attempts to make rubber overshoes look a little more stylish and a little less utilitarian. Rubber now came in a narrow range of colors, including black, brown, and tan (tan had been introduced by 1908 for use with tan shoes), and was available with flowered or moiré surface patterning. In 1927 a new ankle-high type of overshoe for rain came into fashion. This had rubber soles and edges, but the tops were made of wool jersey, cotton jersey, or "rayton," presumably an early rayon fabric. In most styles, the tops could be turned down to form a cuff around the ankle, often displaying a facing of contrasting color or pattern (fig. 87m, n).

The *Shoe Retailer* pointed out in 1927 that improvements in clasps, fastenings, and other formfitting devices "have been in a large measure responsible for the increased demand for such footwear [rubber-soled overshoes]."[36] While many were still fastened with buckles, buttons, or the newer snaps, some featured B. F. Goodrich's "hookless fastener"—that is, a zipper. Zippers were not actually new, having been patented in 1893 by Whitcomb L. Judson, but they were rare before the late 1920s. By 1927, zippers were widely used in both high arctics and ankle-high rain boots (fig. 87m, o). Solid leg boots also continued to be available, now in slightly more stylish and decorative forms (fig. 87p).

Some women made their own warm winter overshoes. Three examples survive at the Society for the Preservation of New England Antiquities, all consisting of a hand-knitted upper part stitched onto an ordinary rubber overshoe.[37] One of these, knitted in a heavy ribbed pattern in dark green wool, is shaped like a calf-high sock. This sock is placed inside a rubber of the croquet sandal type, and a separate knitted border covers the stitching that joins the sock to the top of the rubber. The sock itself is made with a hole in the bottom so that the heel of the shoe can pass through it and fit neatly into the heel of the rubber. The donor described these as a pair of "Finneys" made about 1890, "sort of homemade arctics." The uppers of a second pair, from about the same period, are knitted in brown wool with a bushy edging of cream-colored yarn loops. These are open down the front like carriage boots and tied with three pairs of brown satin ribbons. The donor described these as "Mother's knitted-top rubber driving shoes."

Gaiters

Gaiters (also known as spatterdashes or spats) are separate coverings for the ankle and top of the foot, worn over a shoe or boot. They are usually made of cloth, fastened with buttons, and kept in place either by a buckled strap or an elastic band that passes beneath the waist of the shoe. The fashion for wearing gaiters for walking led to the development of the gaiter boot with its cloth top and leather foxing that imitated the appearance of a separate gaiter over a leather shoe. Gaiter boots are referred to as early as December 1802, when the *Ladies' Magazine* reports that in Paris, "to satisfy the petit maîtres [dandies] who are attached to gaiters, we have a late invention of gaiter boots, which resemble leather and stuff." Gaiter boots were worn so much more often than true gaiters in the mid–nineteenth century that the term "gaiter" began to be used to refer to the boot, and it became necessary to say "over-gaiter" when the real thing was meant.

Gaiters for women appear as early as 1813 in a charming plate in the series *Costume Parisien* (see figs. 88, 89a, b). The figure is shown raking the grass wearing a rather short white percale dress and black leather shoes that are mostly covered by a pair of "guêtres de nankin." They continue to be mentioned from time to time in the late 1820s and early 1830s. *La Belle Assemblée* refers to shoes of black kid with pearl-gray gaiters in December 1827 and to black kid shoes with blue gaiters the color of the dress in August 1828. In *Godey's*, October 1833, an article on fashion in the guise of a letter from Paris reports "instead of buskins, which are only worn of a morning, I have had laced gaiters of bronze gros de Naples to wear with English leather shoes of that colour."

By the 1840s and 1850s, the prevailing fashion for gaiter boots made separate gaiters superfluous, but a related garment known as an anklet was available in the early 1860s (see fig. 89c, d). This fastened round the ankle above the boot, essentially serving to extend the boot higher on the leg. *Godey's* illustrated a version in 1862 made of patent leather and fastened with "steel clasps with elastics. . . . Every one must see at a glance how useful they must be in wet weather. They will prevent a lady from taking cold, and from the excessive unpleasantness of the wet skirts coming in contact with the stockings. John W. Burt, 27 Park Row, New York, is the manufacturer."[38] In 1863, *Peterson's* offered a pattern for one that could be made at home "of kid, lined with flannel, the whole bound with galloon. Where it fastens on the outside of the ankle, it may either have eyelets put in, and laced, or buttons and loops of gum elastic."[39] Both versions were longer in front and back than they were on the sides, the *Peterson's* pattern giving a length of seven inches up the back. By the later 1860s, the boots themselves began to be made higher, as if to answer the need the anklet had attempted to fill.

When gaiters were made long enough to cover the calf or even the knee, they were usually known as "leggings" (see figs. 89g–j). Patterns for leggings were advertised in Butterick catalogs by 1879, and both leggings and gaiters were routinely offered in Sears through the 1890s and the early twentieth century. In the 1890s, leggings were very commonly worn over shoes while bicycling rather than permitting the gap that would have been left between the top of an ordinary boot and the shortened skirt or bloomers. Calf-high leather leggings (sometimes fastened with wraparound straps and called "puttees") were also an option with riding dress. They were probably cheaper than solid leg riding boots and had the advantage

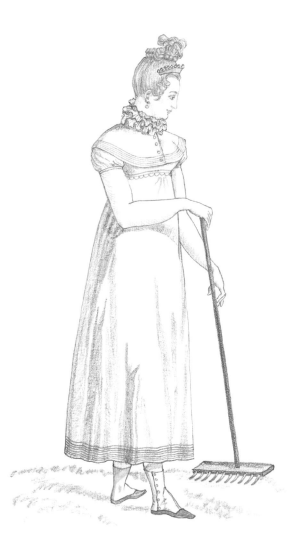

Fig. 88. This fashionable lady playing at yard work is wearing a pair of buttoned "guêtres de nankin" over low black shoes that are probably made of kid. From *Le Journal des Dames*, 1813. A pair of nankeen gaiters very similar to these survives at the Connecticut Historical Society, catalog #1963-8-6. They are lined with linen and have a leather strap to go under the foot.

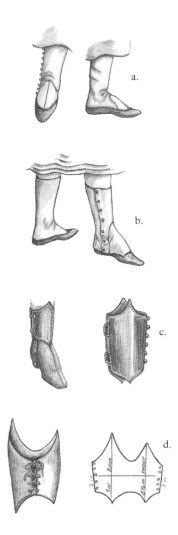

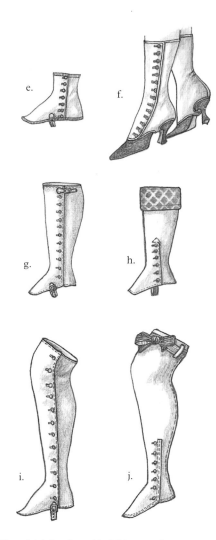

Fig. 89. Gaiters, anklets, and leggings:

(a) "Guêtres de nankin" shown over red shoes in an 1808 plate from *Le Journal des Dames*. Note that the seaming of these very early gaiters is entirely different from those of the later nineteenth century. Compare it, however, to side-lace boots of the late 1820s (see figs. 271, 272).

(b) Close-up of the "guêtres de nankin" from *Le Journal des Dames*, 1813, illustrated in fig. 88.

(c) This anklet was illustrated (upside down) in *Godey's Lady's Book* in November 1862. Made of patent leather with steel clasps and elastics, it was manufactured commercially by John W. Burt of New York.

(d) This anklet, shown in *Peterson's Magazine* for March 1863, was an adaptation that could be made at home, substituting a simple lacing for the elastic and clasps.

(e) Seven-button gaiter with straight opening and buckled strap, the type advertised from the 1890s through the 1910s. They were made of broadcloth in a range of neutral colors. Slightly longer gaiters in this same style were made into the 1930s.

(f) Fourteen-button gaiter with forward-curving opening and no buckle on the strap. This type was made in the late 1910s and early 1920s by the Tweedie Boot Top Company.

(g) Knee-high legging with full button closure, a type made from at least 1879 into the late 1910s. This style is described in Sears 1897 catalog as "Ladies' bicycle leggins," made either of wool jersey cloth or of corduroy in black, brown, or blue.

(h) Knee-high legging with half button closure, a type advertised in the 1890s and 1900s. This particular example, drawn from the 1897 Sears catalog, is described as "Ladies' bicycle leggins. Made from the very finest imported all wool Jersey cloth, cut golf style, the tops being turned over, and of fancy figured patterns. The Jersey Leggin fits like a stocking, and is the coolest and most comfortable bicycle leggin made. Colors black with gray mixed top, blue with fancy top, and brown with fancy figured top."

(i) Thigh-length legging with full button closure, a type available from at least 1879 into the 1930s. Sears examples are described as being made of black wool jersey.

(j) Thigh-length legging with partial button closure at the bottom and ribbon or elastic garter at top, a type advertised in the 1890s and 1900s.

of creating a slimmer looking ankle. Otherwise leggings do not seem to have been fashion items, but to have been worn instead for warmth. They are usually described as being made of black wool jersey with buttons up the side. The longer versions may have a ribbon at the top to act like a garter (see fig. 89j). Two pairs of wool leggings survive at Historic Northampton. One is hand-knitted in green and dark gray. The other is machine-knitted in plain black and is said to have been worn by a schoolteacher in the 1850s.[40]

Shorter calf- or ankle-high gaiters of broadcloth or similar heavy wool are mentioned as fashionable gear throughout the 1890s and early 1900s and they seem to have been related to the growing tendency to wear low shoes rather than boots for walking in the summer. "The grey, mode or white 'spats' worn last summer over low shoes are no longer counted good form, and in their place the solemn black rules. Spats, by-the-by, to look well, must fit like the proverbial glove, and when they wrinkle, or do not adapt themselves closely to the ankles, they are to be cast to the winds" (1892).[41] In 1907 Sears advertised sixty-five-cent over-gaiters in alice blue, brown, pearl gray, and tan, which it claimed "are all the rage in the large cities and will be worn extensively this spring." Documented gaiters are rare, but the mail-order-catalog descriptions suggest that men's gaiters usually had five buttons only, while women's gaiters or spats had seven or more (see fig. 89e).

The last and most important episode of gaiters came in the late 1910s and early 1920s, when the shortening skirt caused the gaiters to be made longer, about mid-calf in height, with eight to fourteen buttons. One brand-name maker of this period, the Tweedies Boot Top Company, held patents dated 1915 and 1918 on their spats, perhaps for leaving off the buckle that had previously adjusted the strap that passed under the shoe. Their gaiters also featured a curved rather than a straight button line (see fig. 89f). "Spats, retailers say, will be popular again this fall [1917]. These are not sold as a means to economy, but chiefly from the standpoint of style. Overgaiters at $5 a pair find ready purchasers. Fawn, gray and white are popular numbers."[42] Nevertheless, gaiters would have been a sensible and economical style for women who were accustomed to wearing boots in colder weather. The shortened skirts had caused boots to lengthen and the high price of leather made them so expensive as to depress sales. Although at five dollars, spats cost as much as a pair of shoes in fashionable shops, any woman who could sew could use a pattern offered through the *Ladies' Home Journal* to make gaiters that would provide a neat and inexpensive substitute for boots. As boots went out of use, spats may have cushioned the transition, but as skirts continued to shorten in the 1920s and lighter shoes with elaborate and bumpy straps came into style, spats no longer fit with current fashions. The last year that they are advertised as a fashionable garment is 1921, but both gaiters and leggings were advertised in Sears at least as late as 1934.

PART TWO

Dating Women's Shoes, 1795–1930

What does it mean to date a shoe? Is the date meant to indicate when the shoe was made? When it was fashionable? When it was worn? Dating may not be an exact science, but if it is to be meaningful at all, it is necessary to answer these questions. In this book, to date a shoe means *to offer an educated opinion as to when that particular style of shoe was being made and sold as a general fashion in the United States.* This is likely to correspond with the date at which the shoe was worn, but not necessarily. Unless a shoe comes with a credible history, no scholar can ever be perfectly certain when it was worn. It may have been worn by a trend-setting lady two years before shoes in that style were generally adopted. Or it might have been worn from time to time by some frugal lady over a period of twenty years. Or perhaps it was found hideously uncomfortable the first time it was put on and was never worn again. The best one can say of an undocumented shoe is that the style in which it was made was generally fashionable, say, from 1870 to 1874, and that it was during those years that the shoe was most likely to have been bought and worn.

But this still leaves a problem. How does one decide at what point a shoe becomes "generally fashionable"? New styles do not spring up without warning and flood the market overnight. At one end of the fashion cycle, there are precursors a year or more ahead of every style, while at the other a style may continue a thin existence for years after other styles have overtaken it. Do these extremes count?

It depends on the evidence. In the early nineteenth century, when surviving shoes and separate illustrations of shoes are comparatively rare, it is not always clear precisely when a fashion was rising, or at its peak, or in decline. Therefore, the date offered simply spans all the examples known. The style may in fact have been worn longer than this range suggests. But as the quantity and quality of evidence about shoes increases after 1860, it becomes possible to be more focused in dating, and with material like the *Shoe Retailer* to consult in the twentieth century, dating can be reasonably precise, since the wealth of material makes it obvious which style elements are dominant in any one year.

How one dates a shoe depends in part on where it has come from. How well-to-do and how fashion-conscious was the family who owned it and where did they live? Were they buying their shoes in Paris, New York, or Milwaukee? New styles were generally tried out by those manufacturers in Brooklyn and Philadelphia who catered to wealthy, urban, and stylish women. If a new style caught on, a few samples would be added to the lines of manufacturers serving a middle-class clientele. If these found a market, more were made in that style the following season, and eventually the new style, if successful, would crowd out the old standard, which would be made in decreasing numbers until it was entirely discontinued. The whole process might take several years.

As a sort of coda to the normal cycle of fashion, once a style had won wide acceptance and then "gone out of fashion," it might very well continue to be made for some years in small quantities to meet the demands of a conservative clientele (these late examples can sometimes be identified if they are made over a newer last, or incorporate some later detail). For example, side-lace boots of the general type fashionable in the 1870s still show up in mail-order catalogs in the early 1890s, especially for women whose swollen ankles made button boots hard to fit. It is also important to remember that in some cases, one particular class or geographical region showed a preference for a last or pattern not particularly favored elsewhere, as the East Coast clung to narrow toes in the 1920s when the rest of the country enjoyed the comfort of broad square ones.

The date given with the illustrations in Part II may be (1) the date in which the shoe is known to have been worn, as in the case of a documented wedding shoe; (2) the date in which the specific shoe was illustrated in a fashion or trade journal; (3) the period during which shoes of this style were generally advertised and described, if the shoe is from an era rich in documentation; or (4) a range of years that roughly spans all the examples known in a particular style, if the shoe is from an era from which evidence is less abundant. The specific information about each shoe, including the periodical source, or in the case of a surviving shoe, the name of the museum that owns it, the accession number, and a brief history (if any), is given in "Credits for Illustrations in Part II" following the appendixes.

The reader should be aware that in trying to draw attention to one important detail (slipper foxing, for example), it is still necessary to illustrate it with some particular shoe whose other styling details will almost certainly have been of different duration than slipper foxing. The captions attempt to clarify such discrepancies, but a reading of the accompanying text is advised.

The chapters in Part II are intended as a reference guide for dating surviving shoes or shoes that appear in photographs, paintings, or other graphic media. They are organized to lead the reader from simple observations about upper patterns that any novice can make with confidence to the more subtle comparison of detail about soles, heels, lasts, and materials that is necessary for establishing a date. Beginners are recommended to work through the following steps in order.

(1) Decide whether the footwear in question is a boot (which covers at least the ankle) or a shoe (which doesn't cover the ankle). If it is a shoe, observe how it fastens and turn to the section in chapter 7 dealing with that kind of shoe. If it:

    (a) has no fastening* .... see pages 169–77
    (b) straps over an open instep .... see pages 169–75, 177–82
    (c) ties on the instep .... see pages 183–91
    (d) laces on the side .... see page 192
    (e) buttons (but has no straps) .... see pages 192–94
    (f) has elastic insertions .... see pages 194–96

*Includes shoes with ribbons stitched to the sides (as opposed to being laced through eyelets).

If it is a boot, observe how and where it fastens and turn to the section in chapter 8 describing that kind of boot. If it:

    (a) laces down the front .... see pages 198–202
    (b) buttons .... see pages 202–4
    (c) laces on the side .... see pages 204–5
    (d) has inserts of elastic fabric .... see pages 206–10
    (e) fastens across an open front ...... see pages 211–12
    (f) has no fastening (solid leg) .... see page 212

Chapters 7 and 8 describe upper patterns only. Some of the more complex categories, such as shoes that tie on the instep, are divided into smaller groups of related shoes, but any such divisions are explained at the beginning of each chapter. Within each section, the illustrations are given in chronological order. Skim down the illustrations to find one that appears similar to the shoe in question. The related text describes the details critical for dating and will help identify shoes that are less typical than those illustrated. Make a note of the most likely date span.

(2) After reviewing the sections on upper patterns, turn the shoe over to see the bottom, and turn to chapter 9, "Looking at the Bottom: Heels and Soles." Heels are made in four basic ways. To learn how to identify the difference between them, consult the beginning of chapter 9, where all four types are defined and illustrated. If the shoe or boot to be dated has a:

    (a) Louis heel .... see pages 216–17
    (b) spring or flat heel .... see page 218
    (c) knock-on heel .... see page 219
    (d) stacked heel .... see pages 220–21

Make a note if this alters the probable date.

(3) Next, turn to the second half of chapter 9, "Looking at Soles," and compare the sole of the shoe to be dated with those illustrated. Check first those soles from the period that seems likely for the shoe in question. If they do not clearly corroborate the initial date, skim over all the illustrations to find a plausible candidate. The text will point out the details to watch for. Make a note of the revised date.

(4) After examining the bottom, it is time to consider subtleties produced by the shape of the last, such as toe spring, the depth of the vamp, the height of the instep, and the degree of swing in left/right shoes. These are discussed in chapter 10, "Variations in Lasts." Determine whether any of these variations relate to the shoe in question and whether they suggest a different date from that already arrived at.

(5) The date may seem clear by this time, but it is still often helpful to consider what the shoe is made of, its color and ornamentation. Ornamentation in particular can be an important clue to date. Chapter 11, "Materials and Decoration," is divided into two parts, the first dealing with shoes, the second with boots. Each part is divided into chronological sections so that it is possible to refer immediately to the section most likely to contain information about the shoe to be dated.

(6) Once the date of the shoe is ascertained, chapter 4, on the etiquette of shoes, may provide further information of interest. Note that if a shoe is a slipper or mule made in a soft material or with bright colors or unusually elaborate decoration, it may be a boudoir slipper, and information about this class of footwear will be found in chapter 4. If it has a rubber sole and/or canvas upper, it may be a sports shoe (see chapter 5), and if it is entirely or partly of rubber and/or appears to be an overshoe, detailed information will be found in chapter 6. Even though these shoes were intended for a specialized use, many were made over currently fashionable lasts, and therefore much of the information in Part II, especially that found in chapter 9, will be relevant in dating them.

If the dates suggested by analyzing upper pattern, sole, heel, last, material, and decoration do not corroborate each other, there are a number of possible explanations:

(a) It may be an unusual shoe not represented in this book.

(b) It may be a large child's or small man's shoe. Both had their distinctive styles, and cannot be accurately dated from descriptions of women's footwear.

(c) It may be a foreign shoe. French and English shoes are superficially like American shoes, but subtle differences abound, making dating tricky. Obviously, this book makes no claim to date shoes outside the western European/American tradition.

(d) More care may be required in the visual analysis; dating shoes takes practice.

CHAPTER SEVEN

Upper Patterns in Shoes

For the purposes of this book, a shoe is defined as any footwear that does not cover the ankle (specifically the knobby bone on each side of the ankle). Shoes cut low enough to slip on and off without any fastening are called slippers or pumps. Because such shoes were likely to slip off when they weren't supposed to, ribbons were often stitched to the sides, crossed over the instep, and tied around the ankle to keep them on, but these are still slippers in their basic cut. After the 1860s, the problem was solved by adding straps over the open instep. When a shoe is made with several straps or with straps linked together to cover most of the instep, it falls into a border area between slipper types and higher-cut fastening shoes.

When a shoe is desired that fits closely and covers most of the foot, there has to be some means of loosening it to get it on, and then fastening it again to keep it on. This element is called the adjustment. Laces provide the greatest degree of play in the adjustment. Buckles have less flexibility, and buttons can be adjusted only by resetting them. Shoes with elastic gussets slip on and off like slippers, but they do adjust and they relate in their high cut to other fastening shoes.

This chapter is divided into three main sections based on these distinctions. The first deals with slippers, slippers with ribbons, and shoes that have straps added over an open instep. The second deals primarily with tie shoes, dividing them into open-tab, closed-tab, and slit-vamp types. Shoes with straps that buckle or tie over a tongue are a category of open-tab shoe and are discussed in that section. The third section describes the less common kinds of shoe that lace on the side, button, or have insertions of gored elastic.

Slippers and Strapped Shoes

This section deals with slippers—that is, shoes that slip on and off without fastening—and with two other related types: slippers with ribbons stitched to the sides, and shoes with straps. Strapped shoes are an important category in themselves, but because they share so many characteristics with slippers, it is more efficient to consider them together. The initial sections on seam placement and vamp length apply to all these groups. The section on throatline shape applies chiefly to plain slippers and to those with added ribbons. Slippers with tongue and buckle effects are also described here, although they are similar in appearance to open-tab shoes in which the buckle is a functional fastening.

One important category of slip-on shoe is the bedroom or boudoir slipper, and specific information on its history may be found in chapter 4. Boudoir slippers can often be recognized by their material (felt, knit, crochet, quilted, or needlework uppers, fleece linings, and soft leather or cork soles) and unusually elaborate and colorful decoration (feather, fur, or plush trim, heavily embroidered vamps). In cut, boudoir slippers may be similar to ordinary day or evening slippers, but many are cut to cover as much of the

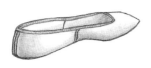

Fig. 90. Pattern 1: Vamp/quarter pattern typical 1800–1900 and common later. Sometimes no back seam ca. 1830–75. Heels usual after 1865.

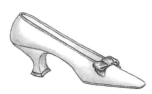

Fig. 91. Pattern 2: Whole-vamp slipper (back seam only) appeared by 1895, continued through twentieth century. This example 1901.

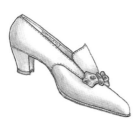

Fig. 92. Pattern 3: Curved side seam appeared in slippers imitating latchet ties by 1890, common from 1907. This one 1908. Some tongues and bows smaller.

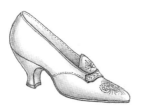

Fig. 93. Variation of Pattern 3 with sham buckled or buttoned latchets also common from ca. 1907. This example 1911. See also fig. 504; compare figs. 111, 487.

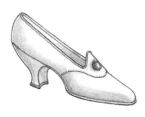

Fig. 94. Curved side seam with vestigial tab and ornament of the midteens. This example 1915. See also figs. 123, 505.

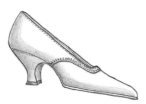

Fig. 95. Curved side seam paralleling the throat with no tab or ornament appeared by 1917. This example 1918. See also fig. 117.

foot as possible without requiring a fastening. Typically, these have a high tabbed vamp, or come high on the foot in front and back with a forward-slanting slit on the sides. Mules (slippers without quarters) are generally boudoir slippers, but some were made for bathing (see chapter 5). Some warm slip-on shoes were used as carriage overshoes, while others having very heavy leather soles and uppers might be utilitarian overshoes (see chapter 6 for protective shoes, including rubbers). In addition to reading these specialized chapters, consult chapter 9 on soles and heels, since the toe and heel shapes of special-function shoes tend to reflect contemporary fashions.

Seam Placement

Since slippers have no fastening and must be low and open enough to slip on the foot, they can be very simply cut. There are three major patterns for slippers. The first, most typical in the nineteenth century, has three pieces, a vamp and a pair of quarters. This results in a center back seam between the quarters and a pair of side seams joining the quarters to the vamp (fig. 90). The back seam may be omitted from about 1830 to 1875 in imitation of French-made shoes. This pattern is also common for one-strap shoes, the strap rising from the quarter (figs. 134, 158).

The second common pattern is known as a whole vamp; that is, an upper made in one piece with just one seam, usually at the center back. What appear to be whole-vamp slippers are advertised in the 1895 Montgomery Ward catalog, but the pattern becomes increasingly common after 1900 (fig. 91).

The third important slipper pattern has a side seam that curves forward to meet or parallel the throat edge. Such curved seams had become fashionable in front-lacing boots during the 1860s (fig. 251) and in the new strap and tie shoes that appeared in the 1870s (figs. 131, 172–74) because they have the advantage of allowing the straps or latchets to be cut as part of the quarters. Straps cut as part of the vamp cannot overlap each other or the tonguelike tab of a high-cut vamp. Among slippers, this seam pattern first appeared in those that imitated buckled and latchet-tie shoes about 1890,[1] becoming more common after 1907. The normal pattern was for the throat to be extended into a tonguelike tab, the curving seam to imitate the line of the latchet, and an ornamental bow or buckle on the instep to replace the functional buckle or tie of the true Molière (fig. 92). In some the buckle or bow was technically functional but the shoe was cut so low that it was unnecessary to use them (fig. 93). By the midteens, the nonfunctional buckle was shrinking (fig. 94), and the first slippers having a curved seam but without even a vestigial tongue or ornament appeared in 1917 (fig. 95).

Beyond these three basic patterns, one finds far more variety in the cut of low shoes after 1900 than before. Extra pieces such as collar, toe cap, and heel fox (fig. 96) may be added, although these are often only imitated with perforations. While there is evidence that these elements were used earlier, they became common in slippers only from 1908, when they result from the desire to make slippers look suitable for wearing outdoors by incorporating style details from boots.

Other variations in pattern were tried in the late 1910s. The first, appearing in 1915, was a heeled slipper made with a gypsy seam, a detail that had hitherto been confined to very cheap and plebeian comfort shoes. It was illustrated in the *Shoe Retailer* but whether it ever caught on is doubtful (fig. 97). For a year or two about 1918, slippers were made in which the side seam curved forward and then cut back abruptly toward the throat edge, imitating latchets that did not meet each other on the instep (fig. 98). Another variation had a separate piece inserted at the throat of a whole vamp shoe. This throat piece, often tongue-shaped, was generally made of a contrasting color or texture. A version called a wing throat is illustrated in figure 99.

During the 1920s, further mutations in slipper patterns developed as ways of incorporating two contrasting materials (fig. 100). In the mid-1920s, ornamentation often filled the broad space between the forward-curving side seam and the throatline of a high-cut shoe (fig. 101). When a shoe was cut very high, slips of elastic goring were inserted on the instep to provide sufficient ease for getting it on and off. The elastic was sometimes hidden beneath the ornament, making the shoe look like a slipper (fig. 125).

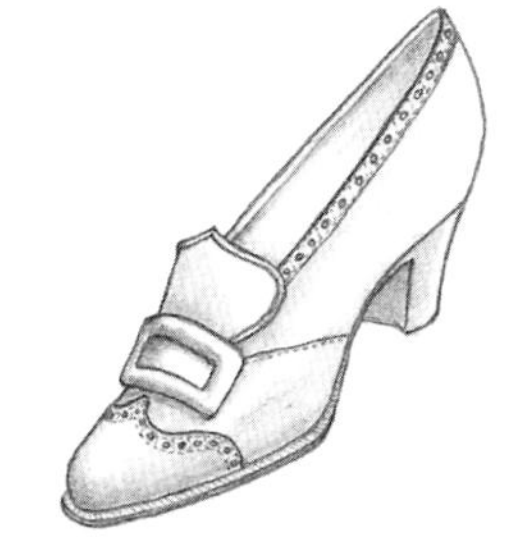

Fig. 96. Perforations, toe caps, collars, and extension soles made slippers look more suitable for walking after 1908. This example 1912. See also figs. 502, 503.

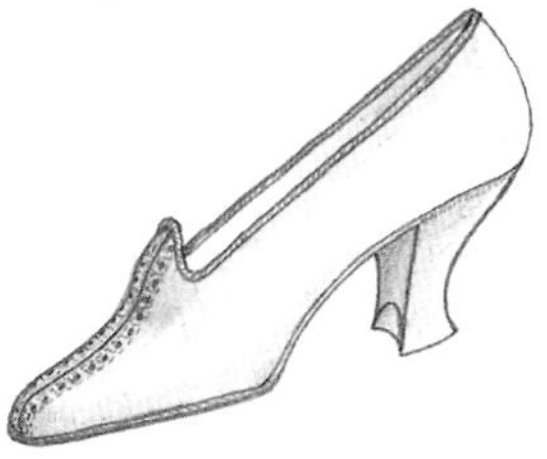

Fig. 97. Slipper with "gypsy" seam (from toe tip to throat) was tried out in 1915–16 and again in spring 1920. This one 1916. Compare gored shoes, figs. 228, 234.

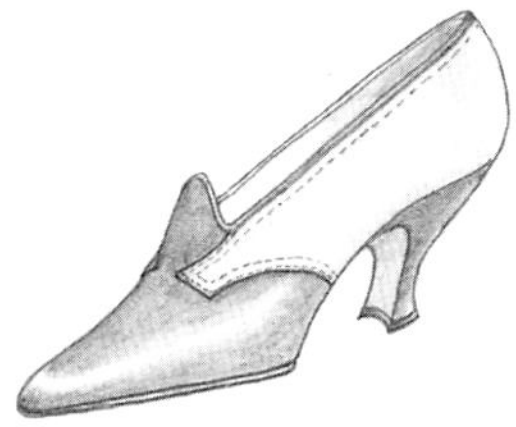

Fig. 98. Quarters extended to suggest incomplete latchets were fashionable in 1918.

Fig. 99. Whole-vamp slipper with wing throat was advertised from 1918 to 1920. This example spring 1920.

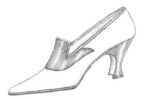

Fig. 100. Slippers were less stylish than strap shoes in the 1920s. Some late 1920s slippers had inlays of contrast leather in novel patterns. This example 1928.

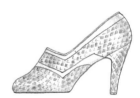

Fig. 101. Slippers of the 1920s often filled a broadened area above the vamp with decoration. This example 1930. See also fig. 119; compare fig. 237.

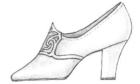

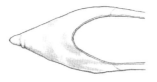

Fig. 102. Long vamp (some are shorter after 1800), pointed toe, round throat of 1790–1805. This one ca. 1800. Compare figs. 112, 117; see also figs. 355–58, 439–41.

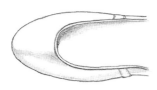

Fig. 103. Short vamp, round toe, round throat in style 1804–15. Vamp slightly longer in the 1810s. This example 1805–10. See figs. 359–62, 443–44.

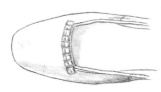

Fig. 104. Medium vamp, round toe, 1810–15. A transitional example with square throat, 1815. See also figs. 363–65, 442, 445–47.

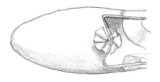

Fig. 105. Long vamp, oval toe, and square or peaked throat worn 1815 to 1830. Some shorter vamps from 1823. This one ca. 1820. See also figs. 366, 368–70, 449–53.

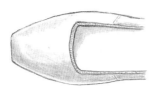

Fig. 106. Medium short vamp, narrow square toe, and square throat in style by the 1830s. This example 1830. See also figs. 371–72, 374–75, 448.

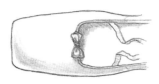

Fig. 107. Medium vamp, broad square toe, and square throat in style 1835–50. This example 1837. See also figs. 373, 376–77, 423, 454–57.

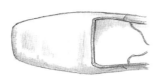

Fig. 108. Medium vamp, rounded square toe, and square throat (or more rarely round) in style 1847–73. This one 1845–55. See also figs. 378–85, 458–68.

Vamp Length

Because the cut of slippers varies so little, especially in the nineteenth century, it is helpful when trying to date them to measure the length of the vamp from the tip of the toe to the throatline. The following measurements indicate the typical range of vamp lengths in slippers.

ca. 1795–ca. 1805, pointed toes: 3⅜ decreasing to 2⅞ inches (fig. 102). A clear decrease in vamp length is visible in French fashion plates in the years 1800 to 1802.

ca. 1804–ca. 1815, round toes: 1⅞ to 2⅝ inches. The *Lady's Magazine* reported in December 1803 that in London high-fashion circles, shoes "are so extremely long-quartered as to but barely admit the toes." Surviving shoes show this to have been true (fig. 103).

ca. 1815–ca. 1830, oval toes: 3½ to 4⅝ inches. About 1815 (earlier in France) the vamps became a great deal longer, and they stayed fairly long at least through the early 1820s. Because of the fashion for shoes that covered the foot, there was also an increase in tie shoes (generally slit-vamp) in this same period. By March 1823, *La Belle Assemblée* was noting that "the slippers are of white satin, and are made more long-quartered [that is, with shorter vamps] than formerly so as to discover the beauty of the instep." Although dated American shoes show the very long vamp continuing in use until at least 1828, it seems likely that some shoes of the later 1820s were made with shorter vamps since by 1830 vamps could be as short as 2¾ inches (figs. 104, 105).

ca. 1830–ca. 1835, narrow square toes: 2¾ to 3½ inches. This is a transitional period before shoes settle down in the proportions of the mid–nineteenth century (fig. 106).

ca. 1835–ca. 1870, broad square or rounded square toes: 3⅛ to 3⅝ inches. Slippers are fairly consistent in vamp length in the mid–nineteenth century (figs. 107, 108). However, in boots, whose vamp lengths usually parallel the changes in slipper vamps, a few slightly longer vamps appear in the later 1860s (fig. 251).

ca. 1870–ca. 1880, rounded square toes: 3¼ tending to decrease to about 2½ inches. In the early 1870s, the actual vamp length may be extended by a tongue or obscured by a long rosette that extends above the throat (fig. 479), but these went out of fashion in the mid-1870s. *Godey's* noted in 1874 that "low slippers, of black or white satin, are worn on full dress occasions by young ladies. . . . The slipper is simply shaped, not covering the instep . . . and displaying to advantage the elaborately embroidered and open-worked stockings that are again in vogue"[2] (fig. 109).

ca. 1880–ca. 1894, oval toes: 1⅝ to 2¾ inches, the shortest usually appearing in the early 1880s. "These dainty shoes are so much open over the foot [in 1880], that one might almost predict a return to the gilt sandals so much in vogue in the time of the Directoire"[3] (figs. 110, 111).

ca. 1895–ca. 1905, pointed or oval toes: 3⅛ to 3¾ inches. Very long vamps became a necessity in the later 1890s with the new style for an extremely pointed and shallow toe. These needlepoint shoes were made to extend beyond the end of the foot—indeed, no toe could possibly fit into the narrow shallow end. Occasionally at the height of this style, about 1897–98, vamps passed four inches in length, but 3¼–3½ inches is more typical of the period as a whole. The extremely pointed toe passed out of fashion about 1900, replaced by an oval shape, but relatively long shallow vamps continued in use through about 1905 (figs. 112, 113).

ca. 1906–ca. 1913, pointed or oval toes: The vamps in high-style shoes had begun to change in 1904, becoming slightly shorter, more pointed and deeper at the toe. This tendency was quite marked by 1906 and continued through 1910 (fig. 114). The years 1911 through 1913 saw rounder toes coupled with even shorter vamps and higher toes, but the extremes in this style appeared more often in boots than in slippers. It was felt that a very short vamp in a slipper produced a poor fit. "However, as the woman of fashion 'wants what she wants when she wants it,' she becomes totally oblivious to her impending discomfort when she has served up to her a pump with an extreme high heel and an equally extreme low vamp, a combination in pumps, that neither by argument nor mechanical ingenuity could ever be made a perfect fitting shoe"[4] (fig. 115).

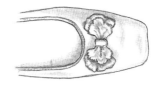

Fig. 109. Medium vamp, rounded square toe persisted to ca. 1880. Round throat became the norm in the early 1870s. This early example, 1869. See also figs. 386–91.

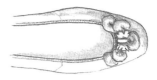

Fig. 110. Very short vamp, rounded oval toe, and round throat characteristic of 1880–85. This example 1885. See also figs. 392–95, 477, 482–86.

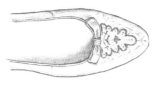

Fig. 111. Short or medium vamp, narrow oval toe, and round throat in style 1885–93. This one ca. 1890. See also figs. 396–99, 478, 487, 489.

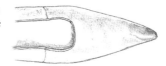

Fig. 112. Long vamp, with a narrow, pointed, shallow toe and round throat in style 1894–99. This one ca. 1898. See also figs. 400–401, 488.

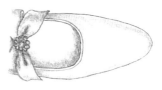

Fig. 113. Long, shallow vamp with shallow oval toe and round throat in fashion 1900–1905. This example 1902. See also figs. 91, 402–3, 490, 500.

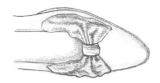

Fig. 114. Medium-length, deeper vamp with pointed or narrow oval toe typical 1906–10. This example 1909. See also figs. 92, 404, 491, 493, 501–2.

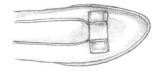

Fig. 115. Short, deep vamp and rounded toe in style 1910–13 but rarer in dressy shoes and on the East Coast. This one 1912. See also figs. 96, 405–6, 492, 503–4.

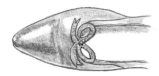

Fig. 116. Vamp became longer, narrower, and more pointed in transitional period 1914–16. See also figs. 407–9, 494, 505.

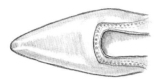

Fig. 117. Very long vamp with pointed toe and round throat characteristic 1917–21 and sometimes later. This example 1918. See also figs. 410, 412, 434, 506.

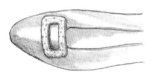

Fig. 118. Short "French" vamp worn occasionally from 1922. This example made on a stage last in 1922. See also fig. 411.

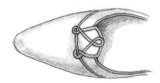

Fig. 119. Medium vamp with narrow oval toe appears throughout the 1920s. This example 1926. See also figs. 150–57, 413–14, 495.

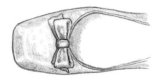

Fig. 120. Shorter, square-toed vamps were common in the Midwest and on cheaper shoes by the later 1920s. This one 1930. See figs. 415–17, 435, 496–98, 507–8.

1913–16, round or oval toes: These were transitional years between the extremely short vamp of the beginning of the decade and the extremely long one fashionable at the end of it. Small-town and western buyers tended to like the short, deep rounded toes, while big eastern cities preferred the longer and more pointed ones, and the latter gained ground everywhere in the years 1914 to 1916. "The samples [for spring 1914] show all lengths of vamps, from the extreme 4-inch vamp and very narrow toe for the large city trade to the short vamp and modified high toe for the middle western trade. What the manufacturers called their long vamp pump a year ago [fall 1912] has really a short appearance as compared with the vamps in the new styles. . . . In all styles of low and high cuts vamps are gradually lengthening."[5] The standard length for spring 1916 was 3 to 3½ inches (fig. 116).

ca. 1917–ca. 1921, pointed toes: 3½ to 4¼ inches. "Vamps [for spring 1920] show no great change over those of last season. Those manufacturers who went the limit and featured the extreme long vamps of four and a quarter inches and over have come back to the standards of good shoemaking and are now sticking close to the four-inch mark. Brooklyn manufacturers [style leaders in the United States] are making their new styles with vamps ranging from three and three-quarters to three and seven-eighths and four inches"[6] (fig. 117).

ca. 1922–ca. 1930, oval or rounded toes: 1922 was a transitional year with some new styles experimenting with the very short French vamp, about 2½ inches long (fig. 118), while others did not depart very far from the long vamps of the late teens. The average seems to have been 3 to 3½ inches. Two years later, in descriptions of new shoe styles for spring 1924, the vamp length is often specified, and it ranges from 2½ to 3¼ inches, suggesting a slow shift toward shorter vamps in the mid-1920s. Meanwhile, the French had apparently abandoned the short vamp. The *Shoe Retailer* reports in the fall of 1923 that "extremely long foreparts and raised narrow toes, now shown in Paris, will be followed this fall with slightly rounder toes and a little shorter forepart."[7] Evidently, while France influenced American shoe styles, the two were by no means synchronized. By the late twenties, there was no one standard length, longer vamps with narrower toes (as in fig. 119) appearing along with short vamps with broad squarish toes (as in fig. 120). The significance of this range is revealed in the regional reports from midwestern cities in the *Shoe Retailer*. In December 1927, for example, Cincinnati reports "narrower toe on better shoes; wider toe on cheaper," and the following February, Omaha reported "short vamps on cheaper shoes; long vamp in better."[8]

Throatline Shape

Another detail helpful in dating slippers is the shape of the throatline, which may be round, square, peaked, or tabbed (refer to figs. 102–26 for illustrations). In nearly all examples noted from the 1790s to 1814, the throatline is round. It is perhaps a little narrower with pointed toes than it is with round and oval toes. Beginning with documented examples of 1815 and 1816, and continuing into the 1870s, the throatline is square. Sometimes there is the barest rounding off of the corner, but not much. The most important exception is that from about 1845 to 1855 one finds a few clearly round throatlines with long vamps. They look awkward compared to other shoes of the same period. In the 1820s the throatline is quite likely to be peaked because the peak added a degree of apparent length to vamps already fashionably long, and one finds occasional peaks in the 1840s, 1850s, and 1860s, especially in boudoir slippers.

The 1870s were a transitional period with square throatlines persisting occasionally through at least 1873. The new narrow round throatline appeared by 1869 and became the rule by the late 1870s. The shape of the throatline in the transitional period was very often obscured by the practice of sewing on separate tongues and rosettes that considerably increase the apparent length of the vamp.

From 1880 through the 1920s, almost all slippers had a round throatline. This was often quite narrow, especially in the 1910s. The narrow throat was a feature of the new pump last that the *Shoe Retailer* considered a major achievement in 1911:

The most pronounced effect in lasts is the improvement of the pump last with a *tendency to straighter lines, wider bottoms and more wood over the toes. . . .* Manufacturers have studied the fitting problem until they feel competent to guarantee the fitting qualities of pumps and Colonials. Indeed, some shoe manufacturers openly aver that they are but just learning to make pump lasts correctly, and add that on the right pump last they can also make any other style shoe from button boots to oxfords.

Pump lasts show a hollowing out at the side of the foot, wrought by the last makers in their successful efforts to *give pumps better fitting qualities* by crowding the fatty portion of the foot towards the bottom of the shoe and drawing the throat of the pump across the instep and at the side so as to obviate gaping as the wearer steps. The progress made in this direction during the last year has done more towards stapleizing the pump last than any other move. . . . The introduction of lasts that produce good fitting pumps and oxfords has removed the necessity, and discomfort, of high back shoes, and some of the most progressive shoe manufacturers are sending out their new samples, with the back line of a 4B pump or oxford measuring two one-half inches from the sole to the top.[9]

In the 1920s, plain formal pumps were still made with the narrow round throatline, but the presence of complicated strapping often produced variations. When the quarters were cut down to the sole at the sides, of course the throatline was entirely altered.

Very occasionally a slipper will be found with a dentate (toothed) or scalloped throatline. These are usually variations of the square throat fashionable between 1815 and 1870. Most seem to be boudoir slippers, but one, made of heavy leather and preserved at Old Sturbridge Village, may possibly be an overshoe (see chapter 6, fig. 81).

Tabbed throatlines: A tabbed throatline is one with a tonguelike extension, whether square, pointed, or curved. The earliest ones likely to show up in American collections are from the 1780s and 1790s. Their pointed tabs are the last vestige of the eighteenth-century tongue, but the buckled latchets have now entirely disappeared. One pair of these slippers is said to

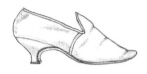

Fig. 121. Slipper with pointed toe and pointed tab gradually came into use from 1780. This 1798 shoe, a late example, has ribbons added to the sides. Compare fig. 167.

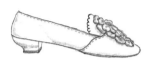

Fig. 122. Slipper with square or scalloped tongue, elongated rosette or bow, most stylish in 1869–74 but some into the 1880s. See also figs. 479–81; compare figs. 173, 174.

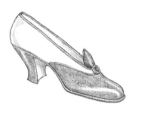

Fig. 123. Colonial pump with small pointed tab and throat ornament in style 1915–17. This example 1915. See also figs. 94, 97, 503–5; compare figs. 96, 177.

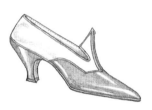

Fig. 124. "Tongue pump" of 1917–21 has no throat ornament to make it a Colonial. This example for spring 1920. See also figs. 98, 99, 506.

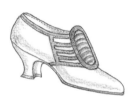

Fig. 125. Gored pump in style 1923–26. Buckle conceals elastic. This one advertised as an upcoming style in September 1923. See also fig. 495.

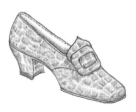

Fig. 126. Colonial pump with the broad square toe of late 1920s. This example advertised for winter 1927–28. See also figs. 507–8.

have been worn at the wedding of Sophia Wadsworth in Hartford, Connecticut in 1798 (fig. 121).

In the early nineteenth century, tabbed throatlines were rare except on boudoir slippers or as an unobtrusive peak (fig. 105). True tabs returned about 1870, at first covered by a long rosette (fig. 122). In the 1870s, tabbed slippers were worn side by side with shoes having functional straps that buckled or tied over a tongue. These fastening shoes were known as Molières in the 1870s and 1880s (figs. 173, 174), and they were revived about 1900 under the name Colonials (fig. 177). As pumps became ever more fashionable toward 1910, Colonials, too, were often made low enough to slip on and off. The straps and buckles of such "Colonial pumps" did not need to be functional, but sometimes a piece of elastic was added beneath the tongue to help the shoe cling to the foot.

Between 1906 and 1915 both the tongue and the decorative buckle of the Colonial decreased in size and importance, and the straps were stitched down to the vamp. By 1915 all that was left in many Colonial pumps was the curving seam connecting quarters and vamp, echoing the shape of the old buckled straps. The throatline was cut into a peak or tab, an atrophied version of the earlier tongue, and the space just above the seam on the instep was frequently embellished with a tiny decorative buckle (fig. 123). One advantage of this simplified cut was that when the quarter was made of a contrasting material, as it often was from 1914 to 1916, it was visible on the front of the shoe where the contrast could have more decorative impact. In its form as a slipper in the 1910s, the Colonial was also advertised as a Puritan, Priscilla, or Mayflower pump.

The decorative buckle characteristic of the Colonial shoe was sometimes omitted in the late teens, but the peak, tab, or tongue at the throat was generally retained because it added even greater length to the fashionably long pointed vamp. This style was known as a "tongue pump" (fig. 124). In some of these shoes, the latchet strap that formerly would have carried a buckle was now finished with one or two decorative buttons, although these had no real function (fig. 93).

In the mid-1920s, high pumps were made in which a buckle or other similar ornament was placed on the instep to conceal the slip of goring that provided the essential adjustment (fig. 125). Colonial shoes with both buckle and tongue (functional or not) returned to fashion only in the late 1920s (fig. 126).

In addition to these fashionable kinds of tabbed slippers, bedroom and boudoir slippers could be made at any period with a tabbed throatline in order to cover as much of the foot as possible without requiring a fastening. See the introduction to this chapter for the criteria by which to determine whether a shoe is likely to be a boudoir slipper, and then refer to chapter 4.

Slippers with Stitched-On Ribbons

Included in the slipper category are shoes cut exactly like slippers but having ribbons stitched or looped to their sides. These are present in fashion plates by 1797 and by 1802, "almost all slippers have coloured ribbands, which are crossed upon the leg."[10] These ribbon-tied slippers, like strapped shoes, were inspired by classical footwear and were often called sandals or sandal slippers. By the 1820s, fashion writers refer to "black satin slippers tied 'en sandales,'"[11] and in the 1830s, "sandals" came to mean the ribbon ties themselves.

Some of the earliest versions had complex lacings that extended some distance up the leg (see fig. 32), the ribbons first crossing the instep through several pairs of tape loops spaced along the top edge of the shoe. By 1815, as the interest in literal imitations of classical dress faded, ribbons were usually attached at but one point on each side, crossed over the instep, passed round the ankle, and tied in back or front (see fig. 57). Through the 1820s, the thin silk ties were usually about an inch wide. By 1830, they were closer to half an inch; by 1840 a quarter inch; and in the later 1840s and 1850s three-sixteenths or even one-eighth inch wide. By the 1860s, one-eighth-inch bands of elastic were used instead of silk, and wedding slippers with elastic bands survive from as late as 1872. Half-inch elastic straps with bows were used on some slippers after 1870 (fig. 226). Ribbon ties were never universal, but it is worth checking

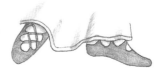

Fig. 127. Sandal with tabs for lace holes, *Costume Parisien,* 1803–4. See also figs. 35, 128, 443.

for old stitch marks or tape loops to determine whether an apparently plain slipper once had sandal ties.

The slipper with ribbon ties reappeared briefly circa 1900–1905, and then as the tango shoe in the 1910s. The tango was introduced as an exhibition dance in 1912, and beribboned shoes appear in the *Shoe Retailer* in 1913 and beneath many dancing frocks illustrated in the *Ladies' Home Journal* in 1914. The Peabody Essex Museum has one in blue velvet with rhinestone-studded heels and blue satin ribbons stitched at two places on each side. Some tango shoes had tabbed sides for lacing the ribbon, in the manner of figure 136.

Canvas slippers with rubber or covered cork soles, and woolen tapes stitched on to tie around the ankle, are bathing slippers (see chapter 5).

Strapped Shoes

Except that one or more straps are added over the open instep, strapped shoes are very similar in cut to slippers, and the information provided above on vamp length and throat shape applies to them just as it does to slippers. The straps themselves are made in three basic styles:

(1) Tablike straps, too short to meet each other, but whose ends each have a lace hole through which a ribbon lacing is drawn. This type is noted in French fashion plates as early as 1804, and reappears in the early twentieth century, most memorably as the tango shoe.

(2) Straps long enough to meet end to end, each end having a lace hole through which a ribbon tie is drawn. This type appears in French fashion plates by 1806 and recurs occasionally in the late nineteenth and early twentieth century.

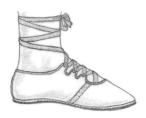

Fig. 128. Sandal with tabs for lace holes, ca. 1805. Ribbons cross and lace over foot and ankle. See also figs. 35, 127, 443.

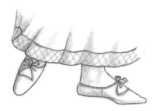

Fig. 129. One-strap yellow slipper, probably kid, *Costume Parisien,* 1807. This type noted through 1815. See also fig. 130.

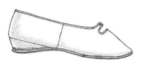

Fig. 130. Rare surviving black kid one-strap shoe with wedged heel, ca. 1805–10. See also figs. 315, 361.

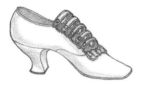

Fig. 131. Multi-strap shoes were most stylish 1875–80 but were also worn through the 1880s. This example 1876. Compare figs. 138, 218, 224, 230.

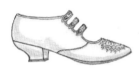

Fig. 132. Black kid beaded three-strap shoe, ca. 1885–90. In the 1890s one-straps were more common than multi-straps. Compare figs. 138, 141, 143.

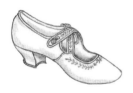

Fig. 133. Cross-straps are noted occasionally in 1890–1920 and commonly in the 1920s. This beaded, white suede wedding shoe 1891. Compare figs. 147, 148.

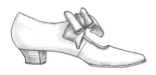

Fig. 134. Kid or satin one-straps (sometimes with a bow on the strap) were worn for formal events from 1890 on, the heels and lasts varying. This example 1895.

(3) Straps long enough to overlap each other across the open instep, fastening with either a buckle or button. This is the normal form of strapped slippers from 1870 through the 1920s.

Note that sandal-like wooden-soled shoes with a strap over the instep are a kind of overshoe and are discussed in chapter 6, under "Clogs and Pattens." Strapped shoes of black or white canvas with heelless or very low-heeled soles of rubber or covered cork are probably bathing shoes and are discussed in chapter 5.

Early-nineteenth-century strapped shoes seem to have been inspired by Roman sandals. The pattern was of the first type described above, much like a slipper, but with the sides extended into tabs, usually three to a side, each tab bearing a lace hole. Sometimes a pair of holes were also placed at the center-front throat-line. Thin silk ribbons or tapes were laced through in a crisscrossing pattern, and might continue crossing round the ankle as well. Sandals clearly of this type appear in French fashion plates by 1804, the year of Napoleon's coronation (fig. 127). A number of related examples survive in American museums (see figs. 35, 128, 443). Shoes like these may have been made in the 1790s, but shoe ribbons in 1790s fashion plates appear to be either threaded through loops sewn to the sides or stitched to the sides directly rather than laced through eyeleted tabs cut as part of the upper. In 1806–7, French fashion plates show a simpler version with one pair of straps that meet on the instep and tie with a ribbon (fig. 129). Similar shoes survive at SPNEA and the Lynn Museum (fig. 130).

A slipper with cutouts on the vamp to imitate straps was illustrated in the October 1855 issue of *Godey's,* but shoes with real straps did not return as a significant fashion until the middle 1870s. In this decade, both boots and shoes appear in styles that were described as "barred across" or having "open-work stripes." From the beginning, varying numbers of straps were used, so the number is not a sure guide to date. In the simplest version the single strap rises from the quarter and the side seam is fairly straight, just as in a traditional pump. When there are more straps, the side seams curve forward, sometimes meeting the throatline, sometimes passing in front of it across the vamp, a point at which there is likely to be some decoration. The side seam that passes across the vamp may have a square corner where it turns to follow the throatline. Any of these patterns may be found in strapped shoes from the 1870s on.

There was a predilection for three to five parallel straps in the late 1870s (fig. 131), but this tended to be reduced to one, two, or three in the 1880s (fig. 132). By 1890, one strap was the rule, the strap often being nearly obscured by a ribbon bow. Beneath the bow, the actual closure was usually a button, but sometimes the strap itself was made of elastic, and in other cases the strap ends met on the instep and tied with ribbon, the bow being functional. This is the most common kind of wedding shoe surviving from the period 1890 to 1905, and it appears as late as 1908 (fig. 134).

Multiple straps had never gone entirely out of fashion, but they did not again become a major fashion until the early 1900s, when "sandals" with two to four straps were popular (fig. 138). A few slippers had been made with a pair of crossed straps in the 1890s (fig. 133), and a T-strap said to have been worn in 1896 is in the USMC collection (fig. 135). Another early T-strap is illustrated in the *Shoe Retailer* among shoes for the spring of 1905.[12] Occasionally a group of straps were connected together at the buttoning end, a style that merges with the button shoe (fig. 137). At this same period, it was also fashionable to make dressy shoes with multiple cutouts that often imitated straps. These were frequently beaded (see button shoes below). One shoe depicted in the *Shoe Retailer* in 1901 was made with short, eyeleted tabs and laced with a ribbon, a style reminiscent of the sandals of the early nineteenth century (fig. 136) and much like the tango shoes that were to become fashionable in 1913 and 1914.

But from about 1906, strapped shoes became less fashionable than plain pumps. Perhaps the most important new strapped style of the next few years appeared in 1909–10, a single nearly horizontal ankle strap starting from near the back rather than the side seam (fig. 139). A few one- and two-strap shoes were shown in those years as well (fig. 140), but by 1911, when manufacturers prided themselves on producing a pump last that produced a snug fit, straps were

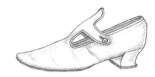

Fig. 135. Figured-silk T-strap shoe worn in 1896. A similar shoe noted in the *Shoe Retailer* in 1900. Compare figs. 144, 146, 150, 156.

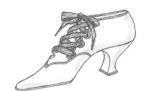

Fig. 136. Ribbons were again added to slippers 1900–1905, or laced through scalloped sides as here, 1901. Tango shoes of 1913–14 were similar but had deeper toes.

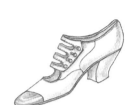

Fig. 137. Shoe with linked straps, a type noted in 1900–1902, 1910, 1917, 1918. This one 1902. Compare figs. 148, 217, 218, 224, 225.

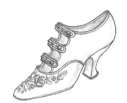

Fig. 138. Three-strap, often beaded, was stylish in 1900–1905, occasionally worn later and stylish again in 1915–16. This example 1904. Compare figs. 132, 141, 218, 224.

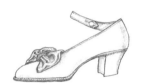

Fig. 139. Straps attached near the back were new in 1909–10. Mary Janes, babyish low-heeled shoes with strap attached at center back, worn 1914–18. Compare fig. 146.

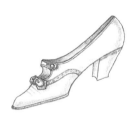

Fig. 140. One-strap shoe in short vamp style of 1910–13. This one 1910. Straps 1910–22 often flare out at end; 1920s straps do not. Compare figs. 134, 142, 153, 154.

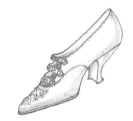

Fig. 141. Three-strap beaded shoe with longer vamp of 1914–16. This example spring 1916. Compare figs. 132, 138, 224.

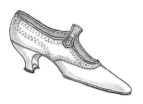

Fig. 142. One-straps often have contrast color stitching and low Louis heel in 1921–23. This example autumn 1921. Compare figs. 153–55, 158.

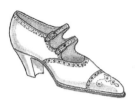

Fig. 143. Less dressy two-strap of 1921–23 with Cuban heel and perforations. This example 1921. Compare figs. 153, 154.

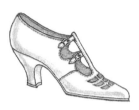

Fig. 144. T-strap with vamp cutouts typical 1921–22. This example spring 1922. Compare figs. 135, 146, 149, 150, 156.

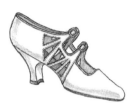

Fig. 145. Branching cutouts at base of straps were tried out in 1915, revived in spring 1922. Side cutouts continued in use through the 1920s. Compare figs. 147, 150.

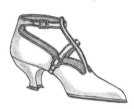

Fig. 146. New ankle-strap with higher heel than the Baby Doll of the midteens was advertised for 1921–23. This one 1922. Compare fig. 139; see also fig. 306.

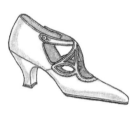

Fig. 147. Cross-straps, found occasionally from 1890 (see fig. 133), were common by 1923. Straps with cutouts were tried in 1915 and revived in 1923–24. This one autumn 1923.

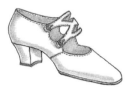

Fig. 148. Straps linked by cutout bands evolved about 1916 from shoes like fig. 137 and became common in 1923–27. This one 1923. Compare figs. 157, 238.

no longer considered as necessary as before. However, strapped styles became more important in 1915–16, when shortened skirts encouraged renewed attention to shoes. Two- and three-strap shoes were offered, some with beaded vamps (fig. 141), as well as cross-straps of varying styles and button shoes with additional cutouts imitating straps, a style very similar to the beaded and cutout shoes made about 1902–4. But under the sobering influence of World War I, straps went out of fashion during the late 1910s and did not return as a force in fashion until 1921.

From 1921 through the end of the decade, straps were the single most important fashion element in shoes. The first styles offered were relatively simple one-, two-, or three-strap patterns trimmed with contrast stitching and perforations (figs. 142, 143). But even as early as the fall of 1921, when the spring 1922 styles were being described, the *Shoe Retailer* found that "patterns run literally into the hundreds, perhaps thousands."[13] The most important new development of the early 1920s was the T-strap, with either one or two horizontal straps (fig. 144). Cutouts on the vamp were designed to mimic extra straps, while those on the sides just above the waist made the instep straps appear to branch and spread out toward the sole (fig. 145). In one new style that was at its height in 1921 and 1922, the quarter was extended up the back of the ankle to form a kind of back strap and to this was fixed one or two straps that passed horizontally round the narrow part of the ankle (fig. 146).

The interest in strap styles was given a boost by the discovery of Tutankhamen's tomb in 1922 and by 1923, Egyptian-style "sandals" were inspiring Paris modes. The *Shoe Retailer* adds a wry footnote to the King Tut fad, however, remarking in September 1923 that "smart dealers say . . . that they are all through with crazes and mob tactics in style. They are not paying much attention to the various motifs or periods, one reason because a good many took considerable losses on account of the King Tut vogue."[14]

The branchlike cutouts sprouting downward from the instep straps continued in 1923 and beyond, and the technique was also applied to cross-straps (fig. 147). In this year the idea was revived of connecting a pair of instep straps with branching bands (fig. 148). Most dramatic of all the innovations of 1923, the T-strap was elaborated by making the vertical strap splay out broadly at the bottom and filling it with cutouts, forming a "cutout apron" (fig. 149). These complex patterns were now set off by being edged with contrasting colors or textures of leather.

In 1924, contrasting materials became even more important while the cutouts became somewhat less elaborate, although most of the designs described for 1923 continued. The cutout aprons disappeared or shrank to a few little cutouts at the base of the T-strap (fig. 150). Some new designs featured a point of focus at the throat with straplike bands streaming out from it toward the waist (fig. 151). A few complex new designs of intertwining straps defy attempts to categorize them (fig. 152). Another feature of this year was the gore pump, a high shoe with gussets of elastic goring inserted in the instep. The cutouts embellishing these shoes may take on straplike effects, although none of them actually fasten (fig. 237).

During all these years, fairly plain one-, two- or three-strap shoes much like those fashionable in 1921 continued to be made (figs. 153, 154) and probably in more quantity than the elaborate designs described above. As the *Shoe Retailer* had noted as early as 1921, "Strap patterns are more ornate than ever in their design, but the plainer varieties will outsell the more expensively cut types. It does not require much fancy cut-out work, stitching and trimming to make shoes cost a dollar a pair more, and dollars count heavily to-day in selecting shoes."15

By 1926–27, cutouts were less often featured. When they did appear, they were likely to be on the sides, at the base of the straps, and in this position they were found right through the end of the twenties. The one-strap was the standard style. It was recognized that a very narrow strap would cut into the flesh, and therefore some broader straps were offered (fig. 155), but dainty narrow straps were still typical for dressy shoes. Evening shoes were increasingly cut

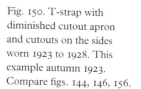

Fig. 149. T-strap with large cutout apron in contrast material was most stylish in 1923–25. This example autumn 1923. See also figs. 150, 151.

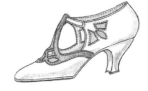

Fig. 150. T-strap with diminished cutout apron and cutouts on the sides worn 1923 to 1928. This example autumn 1923. Compare figs. 144, 146, 156.

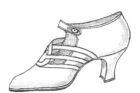

Fig. 151. Straplike cutouts streaming from a central focus, 1923–26. This example autumn 1923.

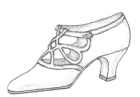

Fig. 152. Radiating strap design, an example of complex patterns of 1923–24. This example autumn 1923.

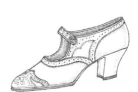

Fig. 153. One-strap trimmed in contrast material appeared by autumn of 1923 and continued to 1930. This one 1923. Compare figs. 134, 140, 142, 154.

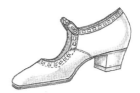

Fig. 154. Shoes illustrated in catalogs catering to middle-class women tend to have rounder toes, lower heels. This one is from the Charles Williams Catalog, 1925.

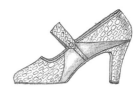

Fig. 155. Straps got skinnier on dressy shoes by the later 1920s, but broader ones like this were also available. This example 1926. Compare figs. 142, 156.

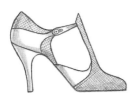

Fig. 156. T-strap, 1928, with narrow straps of 1926–30. Sides cut down to sole appear by 1926, but open toes and sling backs belong to the years after 1935.

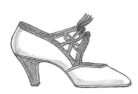

Fig. 157. Semi-oxford's broad cutout straps tie over an open instep. Most stylish 1925–27 but worn to 1930. This one spring 1928. Compare figs. 148, 184, 207, 209.

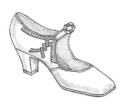

Fig. 158. Fancy buckles, small slips of contrast material, and square toes are typical by 1928. This example is from the Sears Catalog, 1930. Compare figs. 153, 154.

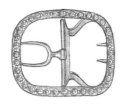

Fig. 159. Typical eighteenth-century buckle with chape (loop and tongue beneath the ornamental oval). See figs. 166, 167.

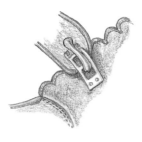

Fig. 160. Fold-down buckles were common on overshoes by the 1890s, but this one appears on a dressy bronze T-strap of the early 1880s.

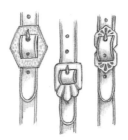

Fig. 161. Buckles of the late 1920s and early 1930s were made in Art Deco shapes with ornamented surfaces. Early 1920s buckles were thin and plain.

down to the sole at the sides, with a single thin strap extending nearly horizontally from the quarters, as high as possible. T-straps, which became even more important in 1928, were also very thin and came high on the foot (fig. 156). Open toes did not appear until the mid-1930s.

Single straps and T-straps continued to be the major styles through the end of the 1920s, but in these last years they were increasingly fastened with buckles rather than buttons. The sense of complexity created by straps and cutouts in the earlier 1920s was now created by using contrasting leathers in fancy bands, patches and inlays, often in rather small bits (fig. 158). Another new style of the mid- and late 1920s was a broad cutout strap that tied with ribbons over an open instep (fig. 157), a style discussed with the other "semi-oxfords" of the 1920s under closed-tab tie shoes.

Strap fasteners: Removable buckles were used to fasten eighteenth-century shoes (fig. 159), and again in the late nineteenth century for some Molières and Colonials, though the later buckles often had only a crossbar rather than a chape. Most nineteenth-century buckles were purely decorative and were stitched in place.[16] An unusual strapped slipper from the 1880s having a fold-down buckle survives at the Peabody Essex Museum (fig. 160), but by far the vast majority of strapped shoes made from the 1870s through the 1920s fastened with buttons. The most common alternative to buttons was to make each pair of straps meet on top of the foot and tie them together with ribbon. Functional buckles did not appear again in force until the late 1920s.

The typical 1920s buckle, rather than being removable, is permanently sewn to one strap, while the other strap, pierced with a series of small holes to receive the tongue, is threaded through it (fig. 161). When straps were first reintroduced in 1921, stylish shoes often had buckles, normally rectangular and rather plain. But after this initial experiment, buttons appeared far more commonly than buckles until 1927, when buckles gradually returned. By 1930, buttons were no longer stylish. The buckles of the late 1920s and early 1930s were sometimes oval, hexagonal, or had differently shaped ends. Little jeweled buckles for the thin straps of evening shoes became particularly popular in the years around 1930 as did buckles incorporating art deco designs.

Shoes That Tie or Buckle on the Instep

This section is divided into two parts based on the distinction between open-tab and closed-tab shoes.

In open-tab shoes the quarters are extended into narrow or wide straps that meet on top of the foot, usually over a tongue that is an extension or addition to the vamp. The characteristic detail of all open-tab shoes is that the quarter extensions bearing the lace holes are not completely stitched down to the vamp, but can be lifted up slightly at the bottom of the lace opening.

When the straps of an open-tab shoe are relatively narrow and bear only one or two pairs of lace holes, the shoe may be called a latchet tie, and the straplike extensions of the quarters are called latchets (fig. 162). If the latchets are long enough to overlap they can bear a buckle, the fastening technique used in the eighteenth century. Very occasionally a latchet will button at one side over a tongue, but this is normally a decorative detail on what is really a slip-on shoe (fig. 93; but see fig. 217 for a functional example). Broader extensions of the quarter can bear from three to six pairs of lace holes, and shoes of this type are known as bluchers (fig. 163).

In classic closed-tab shoes, the seam joining the vamp with the quarters passes over the instep and the vamp is fully stitched down over the quarters, so that the quarters cannot flap at all loose at the base of the lace opening as they can in open-tab shoes. This style is known as an oxford when it has three or more eyelets (fig. 164). Buttoned shoes, which are sometimes classed as closed-tab shoes, are discussed in section 3 of this chapter.

A slit-vamp shoe is a variation of the closed-tab type in which the opening for the lacing consists in whole or in part of a slit into the vamp (fig. 165). This kind of shoe was very commonly worn by women and children well into the 1860s. By the 1870s, however, the slit vamp was rarely used. Instead, the side seam curved far enough forward before crossing the instep

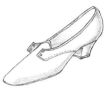

Fig. 162. Open-tab shoe (latchet tie) with one or two eyelets.

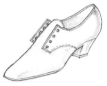

Fig. 163. Open-tab shoe (blucher) with three or more eyelets.

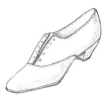

Fig. 164. Closed-tab shoe (oxford) with three or more eyelets.

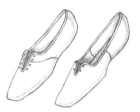

Fig. 165. Slit-vamp shoes. In the left-hand shoe, the opening passes between the quarters before slitting the vamp.

to allow sufficient opening without slitting the vamp, resulting in the classic oxford pattern.

Both closed-tab and open-tab shoes may date from any part of the nineteenth and early twentieth century, but there are periods where one is more likely than the other. Latchet ties with one or two pairs of laces were worn throughout the period while slit vamps were rare after 1865. Oxfords (closed-tab ties with three or more pairs of lace holes) became important from the 1870s, while bluchers (open-tab ties with three or more pairs of lace holes) seem to have become fashionable only in the 1890s.

Open-Tab Shoes (Latchet Ties and Bluchers)

1790s–1860s: The open-tab shoes of the nineteenth century developed directly from the buckled shoes of

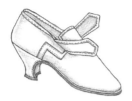

Fig. 166. Buckled shoe with stepped side seam and square tongue, a type found ca. 1700–1775, this one with oval toe, 1760s.

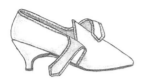

Fig. 167. Buckled shoe with pointed tongue and straight side seam placed nearer the toe, 1770–90.

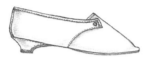

Fig. 168. One-eyelet latchet tie noted occasionally in the 1790s. This one in pink satin. See also plates 1, 2. Compare figs. 169, 171.

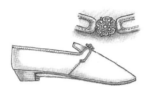

Fig. 169. Latchet shoes still worn by women in the 1820s. This one of cream serge has a round ornamented silver clasp, ca. 1825. Compare figs. 168, 171.

the eighteenth century. For most of the eighteenth century through the 1780s, women's shoes had straps that extended from the quarters and buckled with a separate functional buckle over a tongued vamp. The seam connecting the vamp to the quarters was stepped (dogleg) from the early eighteenth century until the 1770s, when it became straight and was placed very far forward. At the same time, the tongue, which had been rectangular, became pointed (figs. 166, 167).

From about 1785, the latchets and buckles began to be omitted from women's shoes, resulting in a high-heeled slipper with a rather long vamp and pointed tab throat. These were worn through the 1790s. Sometimes, however, the buckles were replaced by ties (a change also characteristic of men's shoes of the

1790s). These women's latchet ties have short and inconspicuous tongues and a single pair of lace holes. From a distance they look very much like an ordinary slipper with a ribbon bow at the throat. Surviving examples include a dark greenish blue morocco wedding shoe of 1799[17] and two similar undated shoes in pink and in blue satin (fig. 168, plates 1, 2). The seam connecting the vamp and quarters arises at the waist and slants toward the toes, curving slightly before letting the latchets go free.

The side seam that slants or curves forward and then makes a square corner going into the latchet became the usual nineteenth-century pattern. An alternative design appears in a mid-1820s cream serge latchet shoe that has a stepped side seam, a detail more typical of the eighteenth century. This 1820s shoe was designed as a tie shoe, but instead of being punched with lace holes, the latchets are fastened by means of a round decorative clasp stitched to their ends (fig. 169).

Latchet-tie shoes were quite stylish early in the nineteenth century, but once side-lacing boots came into use in the 1830s, they seem to have lost status and been relegated to work or unfashionable country wear. By 1840, latchet ties were described as made of "leather," implying calf, kip, or split side leather rather than the more fashionable kid (which was usually specified). While women's heavy leather slit-vamp shoes do survive from the mid–nineteenth century, leather latchet ties in women's sizes from that period are rare, and there is some reason to think that latchet ties gradually came to be thought of as masculine and slit-vamps as feminine footwear. Working men in this period wore a higher version of the latchet tie called a brogan, a heavy, ankle-high, open-tab work shoe that by midcentury was likely to have a pegged sole. While it survives in smaller sizes, it is hard to ascertain whether these were worn by women or boys. They are rarely preserved in good condition with a history but show up, dirty and misshapen, in archaeological finds, discarded in old barns, and occasionally concealed in the walls of old houses[18] (fig. 170). Dressier latchet ties also exist, such as the black patent-leather shoe Lyman Blake sent to the U.S. patent office in 1860 to represent the work of what would become known as the McKay sole-stitching machine (fig. 171). Most of these, however, are ten inches or longer, sizes that we cannot feel certain were worn by a woman.

1870s–1920s: In the 1870s, when shoes began to supersede boots for walking, at least in the summer and on informal occasions, the latchet tie began to return to fashionable notice. "For country wear is the garden shoe, a low buskin, tied over the instep like the brogans worn by gentlemen. This is similar to the Newport tie of last summer [1871]. It is made of kid or morocco."[19] Newport ties dating from the 1870s survive by name in the USMC collection. They are made in substantial grained leather with low, stacked heels, and one pair has pegged soles. The latchets have rounded ends with two pairs of lace holes (fig. 172). A nearly identical shoe was advertised as a "Ladies Pebble Grain Newport Tie, all solid and well made for rough wear," for ninety cents in Montgomery Ward in 1895 and for eighty-five cents in Sears in 1897. Sears was still listing them as late as 1907. By that time, a more up-to-date last was being used, and, since latchet ties were becoming quite fashionable again, the Newport was perked up with a high peaked tongue, gypsy seam, and slightly broader latchet (fig. 179).

The Newport, however, was never a dressy shoe. That role among open-tab shoes was taken in the 1870s by the Molière. The quarters of the Molière shoe were extended into straps that buckled or tied over a vamp with a large flaring tongue (figs. 173, 174). It was not essentially different from the Newport except in being made of dressier materials such as kid or black patent, and in having a higher heel. The buckle of course added a decorative touch, and if it were a tied version, the laces used were broad ribbon. Up through the early 1890s, these shoes tended to be cut rather high at the center back seam, sometimes just enough to be noticeable but sometimes creating a pronounced peak (figs. 172, 175). The side seams curve forward before releasing the latchets, and a square corner is made where the latchet begins to cross over the vamp. The same style was revived about 1900 as the Colonial (fig. 177). Molière and Colonial shoes were known as Cromwell shoes in Britain.

An elaborated version of the latchet tie called the "Empress tie shoe" is illustrated in the 1890 catalog of Hirth, Krause and Wilhelm, a company making

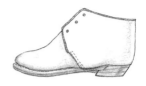

Fig. 170. Brogan, a heavy leather open-tab work shoe usually worn by men. This example is small enough to be a woman's or boy's, ca. 1840–60.

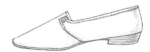

Fig. 171. Latchet tie (probably a man's dress shoe), sample made in 1860 for the U.S. patent office on the McKay sole-sewing machine by inventor Lyman Blake.

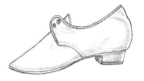

Fig. 172. Woman's two-eyelet tie, known as a Newport, this one of grained leather, 1870s. Similar shoes appear in catalogs, 1890s–1907. See also figs. 179, 425.

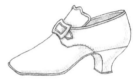

Fig. 173. Molière with working buckle over tongue, 1875–80 and then rarely until 1900. This example 1875. Compare figs. 166, 177.

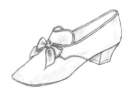

Fig. 174. Molière with ribbon tie over tongue, 1870–80. This example 1876. Compare figs. 122, 179, 181.

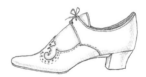

Fig. 175. An elaborate perforated version of the Newport called the "Empress Tie" in an 1890 catalog. See also fig. 216.

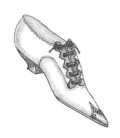

Fig. 176. Open-tab with more than two eyelets was worn 1894–1900 with pointed toe, diamond tip: Montgomery Ward's "Blucherette oxford," 1895. Compare figs. 178, 180.

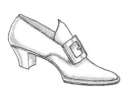

Fig. 177. Buckle/tongue style was called a Colonial by 1900. Some functional buckles 1900–1902; later buckles mostly for show. Compare figs. 500–501 to 503–5.

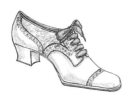

Fig. 178. Blucher tie for street wear returned to wide use about 1906 with straight tip and heel foxing. This one Sears 1906. Compare figs. 176, 180.

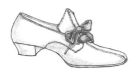

Fig. 179. Late Newport tie with gypsy seam, 1907 Sears Catalog. Its side seam is more curved and its tongue higher than 1870s Newport (fig. 172).

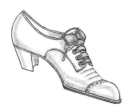

Fig. 180. Open-tab tie with deep toe typical of period 1906–15. Note curved side seam. This example 1908. Compare toes in figs. 176, 178.

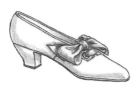

Fig. 181. Two-eyelet open-tab shoe now called a sailor tie. Made in white kid with satin ribbon, it was worn by brides 1906–10. This one 1908. See also fig. 502.

uppers in Grand Rapids, Michigan. Its decorative perforation and fancy seaming are closely related to some of the "gents' shoes and gaiters" shown in the same catalog (fig. 175).

The higher open-tab tie shoe with three to six pairs of laces did not come into fashion until the mid-1890s. Until that time, stylish high tie shoes were closed-tab. Montgomery Ward advertised a "Blucherette Oxford" as "the very latest novelty in footwear" in 1895. This had the long pointed toe that was fashionable in the 1890s, and a contrasting peaked toe cap and lace stay for decoration (fig. 176).

The open-tab tie shoe, or blucher-cut oxford, as it was known then, became a major style by 1904 and was extremely popular from 1906 to 1909. These new open-tab shoes were characterized by a side seam that began perpendicular to the sole but then curved sharply forward, turning a square corner where the stitching stopped. The inner corners of the eyelet tabs were rounded off. The tongue was just long enough to clear the top of the quarter, and was not conspicuous in wear (fig. 180). With three or four pairs of lace holes and a moderate Cuban heel, these shoes were suitable for street wear. Many had straight toe caps, usually perforated. A black patent vamp with a dull quarter and very large metal eyelets (called "porthole eyelets") are also characteristic features, and in the more informal examples, a curved heel fox might be added as well (fig. 178). In the lower versions with one or two pairs of eyelets, these shoes were considered dressy enough to wear with a wedding dress, when made in fine white leather without a toe cap. This seems odd at first, especially if one sees them without their broad silk laces, since the eyelets are very large, almost clunky. But the eyelets would have been covered when the shoe was tied, so the effect was that of a slipper with a large bow at the throat (fig. 181).

Replaced by pumps and Colonials, blucher ties went out of fashion in the 1910s. They reappeared in the early 1920s in rather mannish forms. They were a noticeable feature of spring 1922 styles, when some were made with three buckles rather than ties over the tongue (fig. 182).

About 1925, the blucher was updated. The more casual versions were made over a broad, square-toed last, and many were elaborately cut with underlays of contrasting material. It was common to include in this combination one or even two textured or patterned materials, typically an imitation reptile skin or a figured fabric. Contrast materials were often used to create a saddle effect across the instep, a detail that was to become even more important in the 1930s. The side seams of these newer bluchers rarely had the strong curve of earlier twentieth-century styles. Instead, most curved gently forward, and many ran straight from the sole to the inner corner of the eyelet tab without any curve or corner at all (fig. 183).

A new variation of the open-tab, the Dixie tie, had a broad tongue, often of contrast material to make it more conspicuous, that showed below the laced quarters (fig. 183). Sometimes this broad deep tongue was omitted, leaving an open space between the vamp and the eyelet closure, and resulting in a shoe similar to a strapped slipper (fig. 209). Another new type, sometimes called a Southern tie, continued the contrasting broad tongue as a narrow band of underlay down to the sole at the sides (fig. 184). Open-tab shoes generally had low broad heels in the 1920s, but there were higher versions for dressy street wear, and this type became more important in the early 1930s (fig. 185).

Closed-Tab and Slit-Vamp Shoes

1790s–1860s: True oxfords were rather rare in the early nineteenth century (but see fig. 189). Their place was taken by the slit-vamp shoe. Slit-vamp shoes come in two types. The simpler type is made with vamp and quarters like a slipper but is cut too high on the instep to slip on. To provide the necessary adjustment, the vamp is slit down the center, bound, and punched for lace holes. In fact, should a slipper be found too narrow for comfort, one way to provide a little ease was to slit and bind it at home and then wear it as a tie shoe (fig. 186). In the second type, the side seams slant forward and join over the instep. The natural division between the quarters at this point is lengthened by slitting the vamp, instead of stopping at the seam like a classic oxford (fig. 187).

The earliest noted nineteenth-century slit-vamp shoe appears in *Costume Parisien* in 1806.[20] While the details are unclear, the shoe has a narrow oval toe,

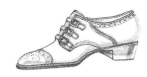

Fig. 182. Mannish buckled open-tab shoe with perforation and rubber heel, 1921–23. This example spring 1922.

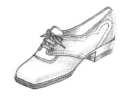

Fig. 183. Open-tab tie with wide tongue effect called a Dixie tie, worn 1925–30. This example Sears, fall 1927. Compare straight side seam to fig. 182.

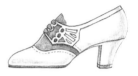

Fig. 184. Dressier open-tab with wide tongue extending to sole at sides, called a Southern tie, worn 1925–30. This one 1928. Compare figs. 157, 207, 209.

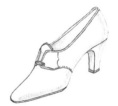

Fig. 185. Open-tab tie shoe with high heel for dressy day wear appeared by 1927, important in the 1930s. This one Sears, 1933.

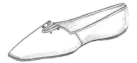

Fig. 186. First type of slit-vamp: side seams do not cross instep.

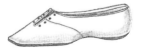

Fig. 187. Second type of slit-vamp: side seams meet and cross instep. Vamp slit continues the natural division between the quarters.

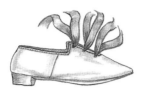

Fig. 188. Slit-vamp shoe with long vamp, oval toe, and small stacked heel of the 1820s. This one ties with three separate silk ribbons to form three bows, ca. 1825.

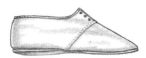

Fig. 189. Rare early oxford (opening does not slit the vamp) made as an exhibition shoe in 1839.

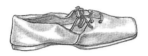

Fig. 190. Heelless squared-toed slit-vamp typical of women's shoes 1835–50. This heavy leather pegged-sole example suitable for work. Compare figs. 170, 171, 193.

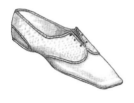

Fig. 191. Gaiterlike tie shoe with cloth upper, kid foxing worn in 1830s and 1840s. This wedding shoe, 1846, has front opening. Compare figs. 211, 273.

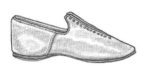

Fig. 192. Slit-vamp shoe with the long vamp and closely spaced lace holes occasionally found in the 1850s and 1860s, sometimes with a low heel. See figs. 66, 249.

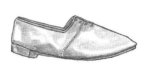

Fig. 193. Slit-vamp shoe of grained leather with typically awkward low, stacked heel of midcentury. For work or everyday wear, ca. 1855–70. Compare fig. 190.

comes very high on the instep, and has about seven pairs of lace holes. The number of slit-vamp shoes increased when long vamps became stylish about 1815. An early example is marked 1816, but in this case the slit was added or lengthened later (the silk binding of the slit does not match that on the rest of the top edge).[21] The most common type of slit-vamp shoe made between 1815 and 1860 has short side seams that do not pass over the instep and two to four pairs of lace holes (fig. 188). A few that appear to be from the late 1850s or 1860s have exceptionally long vamps and eleven to fourteen pairs of lace holes (fig. 192). Simple slit-vamp shoes were made over the prevailing lasts of the period, with oval toes between 1815 and 1830, square toes in the 1830s and 1840s, and rounded square toes in the 1850s and 1860s.

Slit-vamp shoes of the second type, where the opening passes through the quarters before slitting the vamp, were particularly common in the 1840s (fig. 190). Many survive from this period, most of them made of tan kid and having three to five lace holes. Some have wedding histories, confirming that slit-vamps with turn soles were suitable for dressy day wear in that decade (plate 5). Others, dating from the 1840s, 1850s, and 1860s, are made of heavier leathers with pegged soles, suggesting that they were worn for work (figs. 62, 190, 193).

During the 1830s and 1840s, front-lacing shoes were also made with serge uppers and leather foxings that mimic the appearance of gaiter boots. The center front seam, which would be closed in the side-lacing boot, is partially slit in these shoes to form the laced opening. One pair with a known history was worn by Mary Anna Warner at her wedding to Charles J. Pierpont in Waterbury, Connecticut, on April 20, 1846 (fig. 191; compare figs. 211, 273).

1870s–1920s: The slit-vamp style passed out of use in the late 1860s in favor of the classic oxford pattern in which the side seam slants or curves sufficiently far forward to clear the opening. This pattern was standard from the 1870s on and very plain examples can be rather difficult to date. Attention to changing fashions in lasts and toe shapes will help, but dating is easier when some distinctive decorative detail is present.

In the late 1860s and 1870s, that distinctive detail is likely to be decorative stitching in a light color that contrasts with the dark ground of the shoe. Swann illustrates an example from the *Englishwoman's Domestic Magazine* of 1867 with blue morocco quarters, blue decorative stitching on the dark calf vamp, and a blue silk bow.[22] A lovely example of this type is illustrated in figure 194. Note that the seam joining vamp and quarters springs from a point quite far forward on the foot, and although it is embellished with graceful curves, its basic thrust is straight forward over the instep. Similar seam arrangements appear in shoe illustrations from the late 1870s and early 1880s, and an even more striking version appears in a shoe said to have made for an 1894 wedding (fig. 195). Here the side seam nearly parallels the sole before turning upward to cross the instep, resulting in a very broad and short-looking vamp. Most of the details of this shoe could reasonably date any time from the late 1870s to about 1890, suggesting how little significant change there had been in well over a decade. Closed-tab tie shoes over that entire period are often shown with a fairly high Louis heel (especially in the 1870s) and a quarter that rises to a peak at the center back. In contemporary illustrations, contrasting foxing and trim are also apparent (fig. 196).

Closed-tab shoes changed radically, however, in the early 1890s. The most obvious difference was in the shape of the lasts with their shallow, pointed toes, which became very long in the second half of the decade (figs. 197, 198). Where earlier heels had often been high, now they were generally low and broad, and the side seams curved forward without any noteworthy exaggeration. Perforation became common from 1890 and lace stays and pointed toe caps in contrasting materials are characteristic 1890s details.

Oxfords were generally less fashionable than bluchers from 1900 to 1917 and less likely to incorporate high-style details. For example, the exaggerated curve that appeared in the side seams of open-tab shoes from about 1895 to 1910 is rarely so pronounced in closed-tab shoes, although when present it is a useful clue to the date. As in other footwear, straight toe caps outnumbered pointed ones after 1900, and perforations were common, the perforations being rather large in

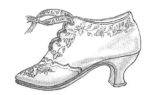

Fig. 194. Oxfords came into use for dressy wear by 1867. This one is black kid with colored embroidery, seams and vine design in white, red kid lining, ca. 1875.

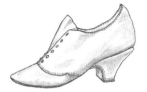

Fig. 195. White kid oxford, a bit old-fashioned when custom made for a wedding in 1894. Note similar side seam in fig. 194.

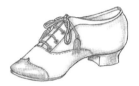

Fig. 196. Less dressy oxford with lower heel, tasseled cord lace. This one, with new perforated patent-leather shield tip, 1889.

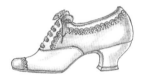

Fig. 197. Oxfords of the early 1890s still had a relatively short vamp. Scalloped and perforated tip and foxing typical of 1890s. This one exhibited in 1893.

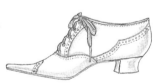

Fig. 198. Oxfords had long vamps and pointed toes, ca. 1894–1900. This one, 1897, also shows pointed tip, wave-shape foxing.

the early 1900s and sometimes cut in fancy shapes (fig. 199). In the late 1890s and early 1900s, many oxfords had a heel foxing that began near the sole at the waist, curved up and back and then up again where it met the center back seam (as in fig. 178), but the more dressy versions had no heel foxing at all (fig. 200). More rarely, a slipper foxing or vamp and heel foxing made of black patent to contrast with a duller top is found in oxfords from 1900 to 1915 (fig. 202), and a

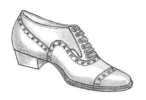

Fig. 199. Oxford with the low stacked heel, toe cap, and perforations characteristic of the mannish style 1900–1930. This example 1902.

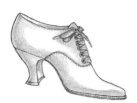

Fig. 200. Dressy oxfords more likely to have high Louis heel and no perforation. This example, 1902.

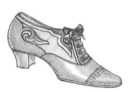

Fig. 201. Oxford typical of the years 1900–1908 except for the whimsical Art Nouveau fishtail foxing, a detail only rarely noted. This example Sears, 1906.

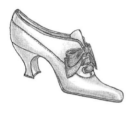

Fig. 202. Oxfords were less stylish than open-tabs, 1900–1917, and less quick to incorporate the new deep, narrow toe of 1906. Dressy slipper-foxed oxford, 1908.

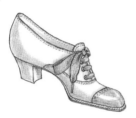

Fig. 203. Semi-dressy oxford with Cuban heel, patent toe cap, and moderate perforation. The deeper toe of 1906–13 finally appears in this example, 1911.

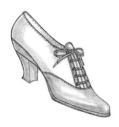

Fig. 204. Dressy oxford with shallow heel foxing of 1915–16. Heel is straighter, toe a bit longer and shallower than before. Compare figs. 200, 202, 205.

handful of novelty shoes incorporated fancy shapes inspired by Art Nouveau (fig. 201). In 1915–16, a brief period of experimentation, any heel foxing was likely to be quite shallow and to meet the vamp at a very wide angle (fig. 204).

After 1900, closed-tab shoes were made in several degrees of formality. At one extreme were "mannish" oxfords with low, broad heels, thick extension soles, and decorative perforations (figs. 199, 206). At the other were dressy oxfords with high, slender heels, thin turn soles, and little or no ornamentation (figs. 200, 202, 205). In between were oxfords with medium high Cuban heels, welted soles of ordinary thickness and some perforation or fancy cutting (figs. 203, 208). All three grades were available from 1900 to 1930, though they were not always equally stylish or numerous. The dressiest oxfords with high, curvy heels, for example, nearly disappeared from 1908 to 1917, but returned in 1918, when all kinds of oxfords came back into fashion and the Louis heel was revived as well.

It is the prevailing opinion of shoe manufacturers and shoe merchants that 1918 will see a strong revival in the popularity of oxfords. This type of shoe has been at low ebb for a number of seasons. This paper for months has made its readers aware of the renewed interest in this type of shoe and it is not surprising to see so many beautiful patterns among the 1918 samples. While the Blucher pattern [open-tab] is shown to some extent, it may be conceded that the Balmoral pattern [closed-tab] is decidedly the neater and will have the greater sale. The types of oxfords which have met with the greatest amount of favor up to this writing are the four and five eyelet patterns, blind eyelets prevailing, while the lacings are small and neat.

As oxfords will be worn as street shoes, the popular type of heel is on the Cuban order, ranging in height from 10/8 to 13/8. An occasional oxford in the higher grades carries a 2-inch military heel and where the shoe is intended as a semi-dress affair the full or half-Louis heel also is shown[23] (fig. 205).

In the period 1918 to 1921, the side seams of oxfords and other shoes were sometimes made with a pronounced curve as they had been about 1900 (fig. 205). By the mid-1920s, however, the side seam generally straightened out, heading from the waist directly forward over the instep (fig. 207).

Casual oxfords with low, broad heels were still designed with wing tips, heel foxing, perforations, and contrasting materials (especially white buck with brown leather). Shoes of this type were worn for general walking and sports from the midteens through the 1920s (figs. 77, 206) and a version recognizable as a "saddle shoe" appeared by 1928. Less casual styles with higher, Cuban heels and unobtrusive perforation continued as a dull staple through the decade, changing very little from those introduced in 1918 or even from those worn before 1910 (compare fig. 208 with fig. 203, or even with fig. 201, omitting the fancy quarter foxing).

The dressiest oxfords continued to be made with high heels—Louis heels from 1918 to 1922, Spanish heels thereafter. High-heeled oxfords were suitable to wear with the new dressy "sports clothes" (worn by spectators, not participants). The most elaborate versions combined kid or suede with reptile leathers (fig. 210). When strapped shoes became popular in the early 1920s, oxfords were embellished with cutouts to bring them into harmony with prevailing taste. Typical modifications included putting a row of cutouts next to the lace holes (fig. 207), widening the laced opening, and omitting the tongue and cutting away the vamp just below the laced opening (fig. 209). Such changes made oxfords look very much like strapped shoes. "Semi-oxfords," as they were called, often had high heels and were particularly fashionable from 1925 to 1927. Oxfords with cutouts continued to the end of the decade, but the newer styles in tie shoes tended to be made in open-tab patterns.

Side-Lacing, Button, and Gore Shoes

Three minor kinds of fastening shoe are grouped together in this section. Most side-lacing shoes are closely related to side-lacing boots, as button shoes are to button boots. Button shoes include, however, hybrid styles that also relate to strapped shoes that

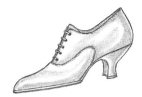
Fig. 205. Dressy oxford with high Louis heel was common 1917–21. This one, 1918, has extreme curve in side seam. Compare figs. 200, 202, 204.

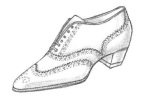
Fig. 206. Mannish perforated oxford with the long pointed toe of 1917–21. This example of 1920 has wing tip.

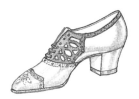
Fig. 207. From 1923, oxfords acquired cutouts to mimic fashionable strapped styles. This one 1924. Compare figs. 157, 184, 209, 225.

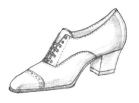
Fig. 208. Rather plain oxfords with Cuban heels (but some with more perforation than this) were staples from 1918 through at least the mid-1920s. This one, fall 1926.

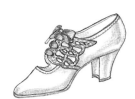
Fig. 209. Oxford ties with cutouts like fig. 207 might also omit the tongue, suggesting a strap or open-tab shoe, 1925–27. This one 1927. See also figs. 157, 184.

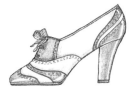
Fig. 210. Oxfords with high Spanish heels and contrasting leathers were stylish 1925–30 for dressy day wear. This example, of black patent and reptile skin, 1929.

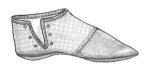

Fig. 211. A few shoes, 1835–50, were made like low side-lacing gaiter boots with serge tops and morocco tips. This one is an 1839 exhibition shoe.

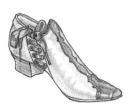

Fig. 212. Unusual side-lacing shoe in black kid with patent tip and front stay, almost certainly made for exhibition in 1893. Compare fig. 231.

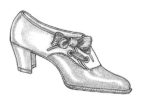

Fig. 213. Side-lacing shoe with off-center lacing, shown in catalogs in 1907 and 1908.

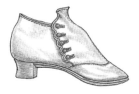

Fig. 214. Buttoned shoe made like a buttoned boot, a basic style in use ca. 1875–93. This example 1876. See fig. 265.

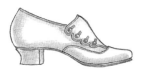

Fig. 215. Buttoned shoe without the center front peak, a second type in use ca. 1875–93. This example fall 1882.

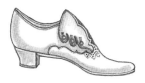

Fig. 216. Button shoe on new last of early 1890s, an early example with perforation, 1890. See also fig. 175.

fasten with buttons. A gore shoe is one that has an insertion of elasticized fabric, called "goring," to provide the means of adjustment. Some are very similar to elastic-sided boots (Congress boots) and in the higher cuts are nearly indistinguishable.

Side-Lacing Shoes

In the late 1830s and 1840s, some shoes were made exactly like side-lacing boots except that they stopped at the ankle. They simulated the effect of a cloth gaiter (often woven in a fancy pattern) with heel and toe foxings of morocco. The cloth top was seamed down the center front and back. Sometimes the join between cloth top and leather foxing was covered with thin silk tape rather than the customary double lines of stitching (fig. 211).

The side-lacing shoe was never very common (even examples from the 1840s are rather rare), but an example survives from the early 1890s at Lynn (fig. 212), and another appears as a novelty in the Sears 1907 and 1908 catalogs. The 1890s side lace is identified by the typically 1890s pointed toe cap that extends up the center front to cover the center seam (the same detail is found in elastic-sided shoes). The 1907–8 version is distinctive because the lacing is not truly on the side, but is placed where the buttons would be in a buttoned shoe or boot (fig. 213).

Button Shoes

Button shoes are a category of closed-tab shoe since the vamp is fully stitched to the quarters. But here the front edge of the inner quarter, instead of bearing lace holes, is extended with a reinforced strip (the button fly) that bears the button holes. The buttons are sewn to the outer quarter where the button fly overlaps it.

Button shoes appeared as a major style for women in the 1870s (but see fig. 49 for a rare early exception), and were made essentially like button boots except that they stopped short of the ankle. *Godey's* reported the "Newport buttoned shoe of French kid" to be one of the favorite styles in the summer of 1877.[24] A shoe exhibited at the 1876 Philadelphia Centennial Exposition is made of plain black kid with five buttons and a medium stacked heel, peaked front, high sides, and unusually deep button fly (fig. 214). A similar shoe appears in the 1883 Jordan Marsh Almanac, and another varies in not having the peaked front (fig. 215). A pair with purple brocade top and black kid vamp and heel is preserved at the Aldrich Public Library in Barre, Vermont. A more elaborate example from the 1890 Hirth, Krause and Wilhelm Catalog called the "Empress Button Shoe" has a scalloped vamp that extends as a stay up the center front seam, deep indentations between the button holes, and decorative perforations, a new feature of women's shoes in this period (fig. 216).

Laced shoes were more fashionable than buttoned shoes in the 1890s, but a new buttoned style did make its appearance by 1897 and was made through at least 1901. Rather than being designed like a cut-down buttoned boot, as had been the case before, this shoe had a broad strap with three buttonholes that passed over a prominent tongue high on the instep (fig. 217).

From 1902, this broad, buttoned strap was cut out to imitate narrower straps and the tongue was omitted, turning the buttoned shoe into a kind of sandal (see fig. 137). In other examples, the series of cutouts begun in the buttoned strap were continued down the vamp (fig. 218). This particular style enjoyed a revival in 1915–17 (fig. 224). These shoes are closely related to others made with several separate and functional buttoned straps that are described and illustrated with strapped shoes earlier in this chapter. Another buttoned style having a gypsy seam and leaf-shaped cutouts appeared in 1902 and again, slightly updated, in 1910 (fig. 222). Thus, sandal-like buttoned shoes were a novelty item offered throughout the early twentieth century until they were defeated in 1918, like other frivolities, by the practical oxfords designed when the United States entered World War I.

The older bootlike button shoe that had last been seen about 1890 returned by 1904, usually made of patent leather, or at least with a patent leather vamp and heel foxing (figs. 219–21). The button shoes of the twentieth century can usually be distinguished from those of the 1870s and 1880s by their straight-edged button flies (the nineteenth-century button flies were generally scalloped), and by the straight

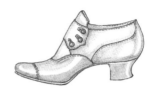

Fig. 217. Shoe with buttoned flap over a full tongue, a type worn 1897–1901, perhaps longer. This example 1901. See also fig. 137.

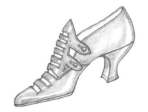

Fig. 218. Buttoned shoes took on straplike attributes ca. 1900–1905. This one with cutouts, 1903. See also fig. 137; compare figs. 222, 224.

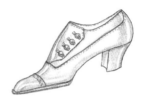

Fig. 219. Button shoe made like a button boot, 1904–14. Compare this one, 1904, with its straight button fly, to figs. 214, 215 (scalloped edge), 220.

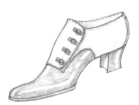

Fig. 220. Button shoe made like a button boot, but the button fly does not narrow at bottom, 1904–8. This example 1904. Compare figs. 219, 267.

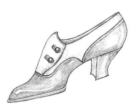

Fig. 221. Lower-cut two-button shoe, noted 1907–10. This example 1907. Compare fig. 215.

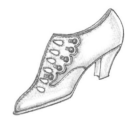

Fig. 222. Dressy button shoe with gypsy seam and cutouts, 1910. A similar shoe of 1902 had slanted cutouts pointed at both ends. Compare fig. 218.

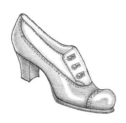

Fig. 223. Button shoe made like a button boot with whole foxing and distinctive full toe of 1911–13. This example 1912. See fig. 268.

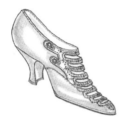

Fig. 224. Dressy button shoe with straplike cutouts, quite common 1915–17. This one spring 1916. Compare figs. 138, 141, 218, 222, 225.

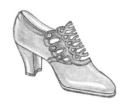

Fig. 225. Buttoned shoes with cutouts were closely related to oxfords, 1924–28. This example 1927. Compare figs. 207, 209.

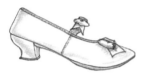

Fig. 226. Slippers with one to three elastic straps (not cords) trimmed with bows were worn in the 1870s and 1880s. This example is ca. 1883.

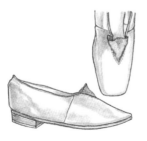

Fig. 227. Unusual shoe with elastic gore placed off-center on instep, ca. 1865–75, may be a forerunner of the gored buskin in fig. 235.

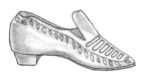

Fig. 228. Shoes with elastic goring became common in the 1870s. This 1876 exhibition shoe has a gypsy seam, two elastic gussets on the instep, and white stitching.

toe cap. In some button shoes in the period 1904 to 1908, the button fly was made in one piece with the quarter and did not narrow at the bottom where it met the vamp as was the traditional design (fig. 220). Most, however, were made in the standard pattern and varied only in their foxing, the number of their buttons (two to five), and the last over which they were made. Buttoned shoes enjoyed their greatest period of popularity from 1911 to 1913. The shoes of this period are likely to be slipper foxed and to be made over the mannish high-toed last (fig. 223). By the fall of 1913, the *Shoe Retailer* was remarking that sales of button oxfords had fallen off that summer and that very few were being shown in the samples for 1914.[25]

When strapped shoes became popular in the early 1920s, many fastened with buckles, but buttons soon became the preferred fastening until about 1928–29, when buckles supplanted them entirely. Shoes with buttoned straps are discussed with strapped shoes earlier in this chapter. It should be mentioned here, however, that some buttoned shoes in the mid-1910s and mid-1920s were elaborately cut out over the instep to suggest a series of narrow straps (figs. 224, 225). These shoes were similar to the multi-strap and cutout novelty shoes of the early 1900s and are closely related to the semi-oxford ties of the mid-1920s (fig. 209).

Gored (Elastic) Shoes

Unlike Congress (side-gore) boots, which appeared in the 1840s and remained in use in one form or another well into the twentieth century, shoes with inserts of elastic goring were never a prominent and long-lasting pattern. They did, however, have distinct moments of popularity.

Elastic was first used in low shoes in the 1860s, as a replacement for the ribbons on evening slippers. The stringlike elastic cord was made long enough to twist around the ankle. In the 1870s and 1880s, two or three half-inch-wide bands of elastic goring were sometimes placed across the instep, each one bearing a bow or large rosette (fig. 226).

Goring seems to have been first used to provide adjustment in a higher-cut shoe in the 1870s. One attractive shoe of black kid with cutouts backed with blue silk, is cut with a gypsy seam and has a small gusset of goring inserted on each side of its high tongue (fig. 228). This is in the USMC collection. Another, at the Valentine Museum, of black kid with ornamental white stitching, is similar in overall shape, but the quarters pass beneath the tongue and are joined by a band of elastic (fig. 229). In April 1881, *Godey's* illustrated a shoe with straplike cutouts and insertions of elastic on each side, a far more convenient arrangement than actually buttoning three or four straps (fig. 230).

It seems likely that elasticized shoes continued to be made in the 1880s and early 1890s, but the dearth of evidence suggests that they were not very common. However, when Congress boots were updated in the 1890s with a decorative front stay added to the gypsy seam, similar effects were also tried in shoes. By 1895, Montgomery Ward was advertising the "Ladies Prince Albert." This had the new fancy patent stay, but the elastic gore was placed closer to the front than it was in Congress boots (fig. 231). By 1897, this style was joined in the Sears catalog by a "Ladies Elastic Front Slipper," in which an elaborately shaped elastic gore was centered directly over the instep. This was described as "one of the leading novelties in low shoes, out this season" (fig. 232). A similar but somewhat simpler version was made by the Rich Shoe Company and was advertised from at least 1901 to 1908. In addition to this style, the Rich Company on October 23, 1900, patented a shoe that combined the elastic patch on the instep with a three-eyelet lacing above (fig. 233), along the same lines as the "Julia Marlowe" boot it had patented in 1896 (described with gored boots in chapter 8).

Instep goring was incorporated into many stylish shoes in the early 1900s. It was found particularly convenient when the look of several straps was wanted without the trouble of fastening them all. Several examples of this type were advertised in the *Shoe Retailer* in 1903 (fig. 234). At the opposite end of the fashion scale were the dowdy comfort shoes such as buskins and Juliets. The kid or serge buskin with its gypsy seam and instep gore concealed by a rosette

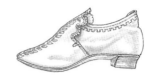

Fig. 229. Elastic was also used in the 1870s to connect the quarters beneath a tongue, as in this black kid shoe with white stitching, ca. 1875.

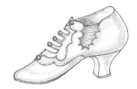

Fig. 230. Strap shoes were stylish in the 1870s and 1880s but troublesome to fasten unless made with elastic, like this one, 1881.

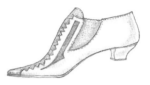

Fig. 231. The fancy stay over a gypsy seam was an important new detail used in gored shoes from at least 1892 to 1935. This one, 1895, has the 1890s long, pointed toe.

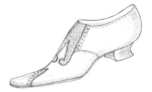

Fig. 232. Goring inserted at the top of the instep was a new development ca. 1897. Similar but simpler shoes were sold until about 1910.

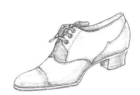

Fig. 233. Shoe patented by the Rich Shoe Company under the "Julia Marlowe" name has an instep gore below a front lacing, advertised 1900–1910. See also figs. 296, 297.

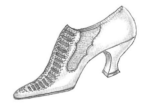

Fig. 234. Dressy gored shoe with cutouts and beading of 1903 relates to strapped shoes in fashion 1900–1905. Compare figs. 136–38, 218, 303–4.

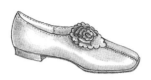

Fig. 235. Black kid or serge house shoe with elastic gore hidden under the rosette at the top of the gypsy seam, known as a buskin ca. 1890–1910. Compare fig. 227.

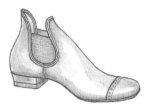

Fig. 236. Side-gore house shoe known as a Juliet, nullifier, or half-Congress shoe, is a lower version of the Congress boot. This example 1907. Compare figs. 240, 290, 294.

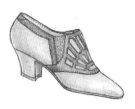

Fig. 237. Gored shoes were in style for general day wear 1923–26. The goring blended well with the cutouts. This one 1923. See also fig. 125; compare fig. 207.

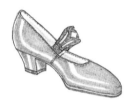

Fig. 238. Shoes made with wide cutout instep straps with elastic inserts are noted in 1925. Compare figs. 148, 157.

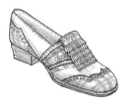

Fig. 239. This 1927 shoe with fringed fold-over "shawl" tongue has goring underneath, but a buckled strap passing over the fringe is more common by the 1930s.

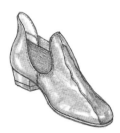

Fig. 240. This dowdy side-gore Juliet house shoe of 1934 is not much different from gored boots of the 1870s on. See figs. 287–94; compare figs 231, 236.

was a standard offering in mail-order catalogs in the 1890s and early 1900s (fig. 235). An extremely cheap and ill-made example from this period is preserved at the Peabody Essex Museum. It is made of crude black cotton with a barely finished sole and a rosette sewn on with a black four-hole button.[26] What appears to be an early (1865–75) example of the gored buskin survives in the USMC collection, this one made of leather and lacking the gypsy seam and rosette (fig. 227).

Once pumps and Colonials came to the forefront of fashion in the years around 1910, one rarely finds shoes that are overtly gored except for the persistent Juliet bedroom slippers (figs. 236, 240; see also the section on gored boots in chapter 8). But oftentimes, beneath the ornamental buckle or bow of a slip-on shoe, a band or insert of elastic goring would provide the cling to keep it on. Gored shoes returned to fashion quite suddenly in 1923 when they were made in elegant styles and became the recommended choice for informal day wear. The gored insertion seems somehow less awkward when incorporated in a shoe with other cutouts and insertions (figs. 237, 238). But even this successful gored shoe did not last very long, and few gored shoes are shown in later seasons, except, as before, occasionally concealed beneath the buckle, bow, or ornament of a high slip-on shoe. The "Latest Sport Shawl Pump" listed in Sears' 1927 fall/winter catalog, for example, had elastic goring under its fringed fold-over tongue (fig. 239).

CHAPTER EIGHT

Upper Patterns in Boots

This chapter is divided into sections according to the way a boot adjusts or fastens—whether with front or side lacing, buttons, elastic gores, straps or ribbons over a broad front opening, or no fastening at all (solid leg boots). Solid leg boots were very rare except for riding (see chapter 5) and appear for walking only after 1910. Boots with straps or ribbons over a broad open front were only a minor style found chiefly between 1870 and 1890. But front-lacing, side-lacing, button, and elastic boots all had rather distinct periods during which they dominated the fashions. In broad terms and ignoring the secondary styles that were always available, these were as follows:

1800–1830	front lace
1830–1865	side lace
1865–1875	front lace; buttons growing
1848–1875	elastic-sided boots important
1875–1895	button
1895–1909	both front lace and button
1910–1914	button
1915–1916	transition to front lace
1917–1923	front lace

Independent of the means of fastening, boots are cut according to several different patterns. While there may be extra pieces for reinforcement or decoration, these cutting patterns fall into three basic types:

The most common pattern has a seam that passes across the instep connecting the "circular vamp" with the two quarters, which extend high enough to cover the ankle. This type usually fastens down the center front by lacing or buttons. It is common from 1800 to 1830 and from 1860 to the 1920s (fig. 241). Many boots of this type have a "heel fox," a piece added around the heel as if the counter were put on the outside. When a heel fox meets the vamp at the waist, this pattern begins to merge into the next type (fig. 256).

In the second common pattern, the vamp extends back along the sides to meet at the center back seam, taking much the same shape as a slipper. Where the top edge would be in a real slipper, a seam running around the entire boot connects this lower part, called the "slipper foxing" or "whole foxing" (or, in Britain, the "golosh"), with the top. The foxing may have only a center back seam, or both back seam and side seams. The top typically has a back seam and a front-lace or buttoned opening that ends at the foxing (fig. 242). A toe cap may or may not be added (fig. 255). This style is found only occasionally from the 1850s through the 1890s, but is the dominant type from 1900 to the 1920s. In Britain this pattern is called a balmoral boot.

In boots of the third type, the upper is split into two sides by seams running up the center back and center front (gypsy seam). This is the pattern normally chosen for boots with a laced or gored side

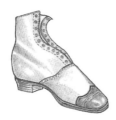

Fig. 241. Boot Pattern 1: side seam curves forward over the instep (circular vamp). The side seam of this 1865–70 example is almost straight. It also has a toe cap.

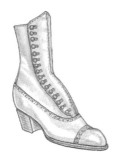

Fig. 242. Boot Pattern 2: the vamp extends to the back seam (slipper foxing; in Britain, a golosh). This example, ca. 1914, has a toe cap.

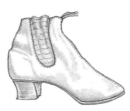

Fig. 243. Boot Pattern 3: a seam down the center front from top to toe (gypsy seam) is especially common in side-lacing and gored boots. This example 1876.

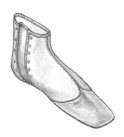

Fig. 244. Pattern 3 variation: has gypsy seam but leather tip is deep enough to resemble a vamp. This example ca. 1835–50.

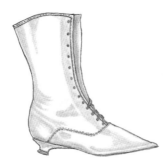

Fig. 245. Boots were available to women from the 1770s. This high example, green kid with pointed toe and tiny Italian heel, 1795–1805. See also fig. 36.

opening (fig. 243), and it also appears in some front-lacing boots of the 1860s. Common from 1830 through the 1870s, it continues in occasional use thereafter for Congress boots. When made with a deep toe foxing, as this pattern sometimes was in the nineteenth century, the foxing looks essentially like a vamp—indeed, the two words were nearly synonymous in American usage (fig. 244).

A boot's height, as measured between the heel seat and the top of the boot at the center back, can be a helpful indicator of date.

ca. 1790–ca. 1810	9–10 inches
ca. 1805–ca. 1840	4.5–6 inches
ca. 1840–ca. 1860	3–3.5 inches
ca. 1860–ca. 1870	4 increasing to 7.5 inches
ca. 1870–ca. 1880	6.5 inches (7.5 high-style)
ca. 1880–ca. 1913	5–6.5 inches
ca. 1914–ca. 1923	7.5–9 inches

Riding and bicycling boots, of course, can be knee-high.

Front-Lacing Boots

Both Swann and Cunnington note that women are known to have worn boots in the seventeenth and eighteenth centuries, chiefly for riding, and Swann says that women occasionally wore them for walking from 1778.[1] These late-eighteenth-century women's boots were calf-high, front-lacing, and had a pointed toe and Italian heel. A boot fitting this description and probably dating 1795 to 1805 survives at the Colonial Dames, Boston. It is made of green morocco with a long pointed toe, a low Italian heel that barely looks functional, and an atypical pattern in which the vamp extends along the sides as far as the heel. It has no mate and shows no sign of having been worn, suggesting that it may have been a display model (figs. 36, 245). A tiny picture in a London maker's label in another shoe dating 1805–15 shows a similar front-lacing boot, cut higher at the back of the leg and with a fairly high, perhaps stacked heel (fig. 4).

At some point during the first decade of the nineteenth century, boots ceased to be made calf-high.

"Half boots" are mentioned by Jane Austen in *The Watsons* in 1804 rather as if they were a novelty about which differing opinions might be expected. The *Lady's Magazine* refers to half-boots in October 1807 when discussing Parisian modes, and the earliest noted fashion plates that clearly show boots are in *Ackermann's* and *Costume Parisien* in 1809.[2] The plates show front-lacing boots with oval toes and no perceptible heel. How high they are is obscured by the skirt, but by 1811, when shorter skirts became fashionable in France, French plates occasionally show the entire boot. These end just above the anklebone and are trimmed around the top with fringe (fig. 247). Several of the boots surviving from this period have light uppers and turned soles, but some were made substantial enough for serious walking. A pair in the USMC collection is made of black leather with a reasonably thick welted sole and very low, stacked heel and may date as early as 1805–15 (figs. 56, 246). A similarly sturdy pair, but more gorgeous, survives at the Valentine Museum. This boot is also welted, and has a round, stacked heel of the kind often found in the late 1820s (plate 4, fig. 248). All these pre-1830 front-lacing boots have a straight, forward-slanting side seam connecting vamp and quarters. In most examples, the laced opening cuts slightly into the vamp rather than stopping at the seam, and in many the back of the boot is higher than the front.[3]

Side-lacing boots began to displace front lacing at the end of the 1820s, but front lacing returned to popularity about 1860. The pattern was not all that different from pre-1830 boots, although the toe was now squarish, the center back was rarely higher than the center front, and the lace opening did not normally slit the vamp. At first, as before, the seam connecting vamp and quarters might still be fairly straight, passing over the foot rather high on the instep. However, before long, the side seam began to curve forward toward the toe just enough to clear the opening slit (figs. 251–54). This curved seam helps distinguish most front-lacing boots of the later nineteenth century from those made before 1830. A less usual front-lacing boot that seems to date from the 1860s, or possibly the very late 1850s, was made

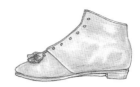

Fig. 246. Front-lace boots, less tall than fig. 245 and with rounded toes, worn 1805–15. Same black leather, low-heeled, welted boot appears in figs. 362, 509.

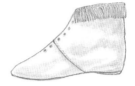

Fig. 247. Boots were made with oval toes and often had fringe edging the tops, 1815–25. This example is of purplish-brown kid with a thin sole.

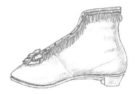

Fig. 248. Low, stacked heel is typical of footwear 1825–30. This green kid boot has a thick sole, cordlike fringe, and rosette. See plate 4.

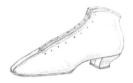

Fig. 249. Front lacing returns to fashion ca. 1860. One type is low cut, often white kid with low or no heel and a gypsy seam related to side-lacing boots. See fig. 192.

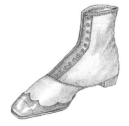

Fig. 250. Typical everyday front-lacing boot of black serge with black patent tip, foxing, lace stay, and binding, metal eyelets, low, stacked heel, 1865–75.

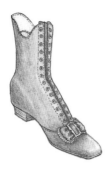

Fig. 251. Some boots were made quite high ca. 1864–80. This one of black serge with green kid facings, vamp bow, and buckle is ca. 1865–75. See also fig. 513.

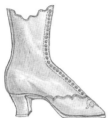

Fig. 252. In the 1870s, front lacing was becoming less stylish, but this tall 1876 exhibition boot has a fancy vamp/quarter seam and white machine embroidery.

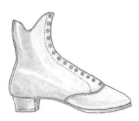

Fig. 253. Front lacing was out of style 1875–93. This rare utilitarian boot with heavy upper, low heel, and short vamp dates to the 1880s. Compare fig. 265.

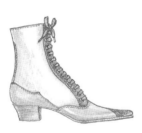

Fig. 254. Closed-tab styles predominated when front lacing came back into fashion ca. 1893. This one with long, pointed toe and diamond tip, 1897.

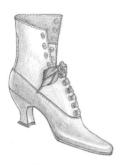

Fig. 255. Whole foxing was very common from 1900 on. Louis heels were an option in dressy boots through 1905 but far from universal. This example 1902.

in the third pattern described above, with a gypsy seam that was left unsewn at the top to form the laced opening. These were made both in the normal height of about five inches and in a short version that barely clears the anklebone, and they may appear with or without heels (fig. 249).

In the 1860s, front-lace boots could be quite dressy. They were made higher than the side-lacing boots of the period, rising to a peak in front, with tassels at the top and/or a rosette on the vamp (fig. 513). But soon after 1870, front lacing seems to have become more and more associated with practical footwear while buttoned boots replaced side lacing for dressy occasions. These everyday front-laced boots are often made of a textured leather (texturing hid imperfections), with a patent toe cap, sometimes straight, but often scalloped and stitched in white (fig. 241). Similar boots were made up in black serge (which seems to acquire a greenish cast with age) with black patent toe cap, lace stay, and binding (fig. 250). Nevertheless, some stylish front-lacing boots did continue to be made in the 1870s. Those shown in the Centennial Exposition in Philadelphia in 1876 are quite high, have wavy tops, and designs in white machine stitching. The seam joining vamp and quarters is sometimes scalloped or waved and the heels are higher than in the 1860s (fig. 252).

By the 1880s, however, front lacing seems to have lost the fight for a place in high-fashion footwear, and this fastening seldom appeared in that decade except in boots intended for rough wear. Those that survive are similar to contemporary buttoned boots in that they are lower than in the 1870s, have sensible stacked heels, a relatively short vamp, and a simple curve on the top edge. Utilitarian boots of this type were made well into the 1890s and advertised in Sears and other mail-order catalogs (figs. 65, 253).

Front lacing began to return as a point of fashion in the mid-1890s, and at first both closed-tab and open-tab (blucher) styles were tried. The closed tab proved the more popular; by 1897 it was established as the standard style. Boots of the 1890s have the long, shallow pointed toes characteristic of the period, and they are likely to be embellished with black patent-leather diamond tips, lace stays, and heel foxing, many with perforated edges. The heel foxing may be cut in wave shapes or scallops, and other seams are occasionally elaborated as well (figs. 254, 519).

About 1900 the fancy scalloping began to die out and pointed toe caps gave way to straight ones, but now the seam connecting vamp and quarter very often made a distinctive exaggerated curve in order to meet the sole at right angles (fig. 256). Heel foxings of several designs were used, including a kind of wave shape, another that mirrored the sharp vamp curve to meet the sole at a right angle resulting in a whole-foxed effect, and a gentler curved version. The true whole-foxed boot itself became increasingly common after 1900 (fig. 255), being fashionable enough even to be simulated in open-tab boots (figs. 257, 258). In spite of the awkwardness of reconciling whole foxing with the open tab, bluchers were successfully reintroduced beginning in 1904, and they became very fashionable from 1906 to 1909, although the older closed-tab styles continued to be made and worn right alongside them.

Buttoned boots had been growing in importance toward the end of the decade, and they were by far the dominant pattern between 1910 and 1914. Within the reduced field of front-lacing boots during these years, the bluchers steadily lost ground. When front lacing returned to fashion in 1915, the closed tab was nearly universal, the blucher becoming only a minor alternative. The shorter skirts of the midteens encouraged the adoption of higher boots, a trend that was fully established by 1917, when nine-inch tops became standard. The higher boot encouraged a return to front-lacing styles. In 1917, the *Shoe Retailer* explained that "just so long as skirts remain short, lace boots will hold the center of the stage. Shoemen all know that a nine or 10-inch boot must be in the laced pattern. Button boots, while genteel and modest, and preferred by many persons for dress wear, are not practical in a height above eight inches. In boots, therefore, the big demand will continue to be for lace styles."[4]

The increased visibility of the foot seems to have encouraged a flurry of experimentation and elaboration in American footwear designed in 1915–16. The front-lace boots were often made with a separate vamp and heel fox, which allowed more scope for variation

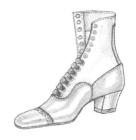

Fig. 256. An exaggerated curve in the side seam and fancy foxings were common 1900–1910. This boot still appeared in 1907 catalogs, though the shallow forepart was no longer in style.

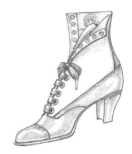

Fig. 257. Open-tab styles were very stylish 1906–10 although not easy to reconcile with equally stylish whole-foxed effect. This example 1908. See also fig. 258.

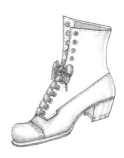

Fig. 258. A second technique for creating a whole-foxed effect in an open-tab, front-lace boot. This example 1913.

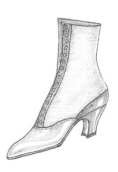

Fig. 259. The shallow heel foxing and contrast materials are common in boots 1915–16. See also figs. 269, 527.

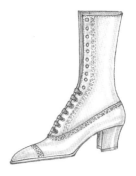

Fig. 260. Whole-foxed boots seven to nine inches high with pointed toes were typical 1917–23. Perforations and cloth uppers common. This one 1919. See fig. 270.

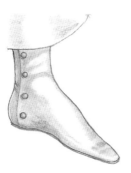

Fig. 261. Buttoned boot as it appears in fashion plates from 1817 to the 1830s. This example 1828.

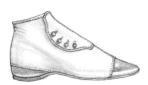

Fig. 262. Boot style for which pattern is given in *Every Lady Her Own Shoemaker*, 1856.

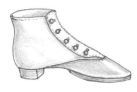

Fig. 263. *Godey's* called this an "English walking boot" in 1860. It came gradually into use after 1850.

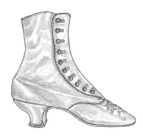

Fig. 264. Straight button flies, high Louis heels, and embroidered vamps were all options on 1870s boots. This black satin boot came from Italy, 1877–80.

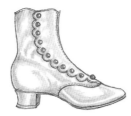

Fig. 265. Boots made ca. 1880–92 tend to have shorter vamps, lower heels, curved tops, and a scalloped button fly. This one 1885–90.

than the unified whole-foxed pattern. In reaction to the broad curves found in the previous decade, the typical pattern for the middle teens was to make the heel fox rather shallow so that the seams of vamp and heel fox now met the sole at an acute angle. Narrow, pointed tips, and contrasting light-colored heels and lace stays were other stylish details characteristic of these years (fig. 259). When the United States entered World War I, however, boots reverted to conservative patterns and colors. The front-lace boots that were standard from 1918 until boots went out of fashion entirely tended to be made closed tab with whole foxing, in utilitarian black or brown (fig. 260).

Buttoned Boots

Button boots seem to have grown out of the fashion for wearing a buttoned gaiter over a low shoe, a style illustrated in *Costume Parisien* as early as 1808 (fig. 89) and from time to time through the 1820s. True buttoned boots were mentioned by 1817, and an 1828 fashion plate shows "lapis colored boots of kid buttoned on one side, with mother-of-pearl buttons,"[5] where the buttons run vertically from the anklebone to the sole at the waist (fig. 261). In 1856, *Every Lady Her Own Shoemaker* offered a pattern for buttoned gaiter boots that were cut like a side-lacing boot except that the center front seam was left open partway. To one edge of this opening was sewn a flap (the button fly) that carried the buttonholes and lapped over the side bearing the buttons. The maker was directed to lap the button fly "towards the inside of the foot on each shoe, so that the gaiter will be rights and lefts. . . . These are very nice-looking gaiters, preferable to those that lace, and the uppers are less work to make"[6] (fig. 262). SPNEA has a boot of this type made in 1866 of gold ribbed silk with a white rosette on the vamp (fig. 512).[7]

Most surviving buttoned boots, however, date after 1860 and have the button fly beginning at the vamp/quarter seam. This pattern is illustrated in *Godey's*, June 1860, as an "English walking boot" (a front-lacing style shown in the same plate is called a "French walking boot"). It is essentially identical to the button boots that men had been wearing since the 1840s (fig. 263). By the time buttoned boots became the dominant style in the 1870s, fashion had decided to lap the button fly toward the outside of the foot, a pattern that became standard. SPNEA has a boot of this type in gray ribbed wool with patent foxings.[8]

The buttoned boots of the 1850s and early 1860s were quite low and cut straight across at the top. Those made from the mid-1860s on were higher, and until the mid-1890s, the top edge was generally cut in a graceful curve. Scalloped button flies were typical, but there were also waved or straight ones in the 1860s and 1870s (fig. 264). Other than subtle changes in toe and sole shape, there are few perceptible differences in button boots from circa 1865 to circa 1893. One of the few modifications in the upper was the tendency to shorten the vamp, which could be as long as 2¾ inches in 1870 and as short as 1⅝ inches in 1890 (fig. 265).

The first really dramatic change appeared in the mid-1890s with the arrival of the long pointed toe. Buttoned boots, like those with front lacing, acquired pointed tips and fancy foxings, and button flies were once again sometimes cut in pointed waves rather than scallops (fig. 266). But from about 1900, the lines were simplified. Straight top edges had come into use even in the later 1890s and were seldom challenged afterward (although they did slant upward in the front in the years 1909–13). Straight edges on the button flies gained strength about 1900, and after 1906 they were almost invariable (fig. 268). Straight toe caps replaced pointed ones about 1900, and plain whole-foxed styles became more common than those with separate vamps and heel foxing, especially at the period 1910–14, when button boots outsold all other styles (fig. 268). The most important exception came at the very end of the button boot's fashionable life, in 1915–16, when the button fastening was combined with the gypsy seam. In this brief style, the button fly was sometimes carried down to the sole. The toe was often covered with a pointed tip that merged into a narrow stay covering the gypsy seam (fig. 269). More conservative button boots in

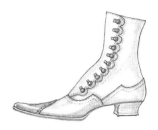

Fig. 266. Long, pointed toes, diamond tips, and wave-shaped foxings were usual in late-1890s boots. Scalloped button fly was also general. This one 1897.

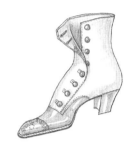

Fig. 267. Peculiar button fly in use ca. 1904–8. This example 1905. Compare more common tapered button fly, 1900–1920, fig. 268.

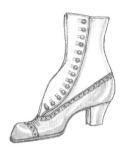

Fig. 268. A straight button fly tapered toward the bottom was the norm after 1900, as was whole foxing, but the high, short toe dates 1911–13. See figs. 223, 258.

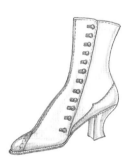

Fig. 269. Distinctive gypsy seam of 1915–16 was usually combined with a pointed tip and front stay. See also figs. 280, 293.

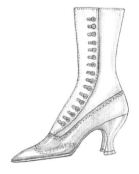

Fig. 270. High boot of 1917–21, when buttons were less common than front lacing, and whole foxing and high Louis heels were very stylish. This one 1918.

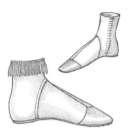

Fig. 271. Fashion plates of 1828–29 suggest that no one pattern was yet standard for side-lacing boots but that a seam often passed high across the instep.

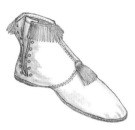

Fig. 272. An early side-lacing boot with a rather high side seam and fringe around the top. Made in tan cotton, left/right, ca. 1828–30. See also fig. 370.

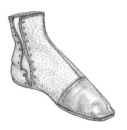

Fig. 273. Square toe and deep foxing, sometimes peaked (compare fig. 244), became standard in the 1830s. This dotted wool boot foxed in black kid, ca. 1830–35.

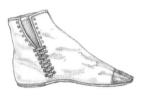

Fig. 274. Short, straight toe caps were typical of side-lacing boots by the 1850s. This one 1850–55. See also figs. 275, 277; compare figs. 273, 276.

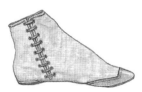

Fig. 275. The short toe caps of the 1850s were often augmented by shallow extensions along each side.

these years were either whole-foxed or had a shallow heel fox that met the vamp at the sides. A few button boots persisted to 1920, but they were considered impractical in the higher styles then worn, and as an important fashion they ended by 1917 (fig. 270).

Side-Lacing Boots

Side-lacing boots seem to have grown out of the fashion for wearing gaiters over shoes in the early nineteenth century. The gaiters first buttoned straight down the side, but side lacing began to replace the buttons by 1822. A French plate of that year shows what may be either gaiters or true boots and describes them as "guêtres lacées en dedans," that is, "gaiters laced on the inside."[9] In 1828, an English periodical notes that "there is a new mode of lacing halfboots and gaiters forming St. Andrew's cross: this lacing, as formerly, is on one side."[10] Pictures of side-lacing boots appear regularly from the latter year. They normally show a center front seam and a straight or peaked toe cap but occasionally display a variant pattern having a seam passing high over the instep (fig. 271). Another variation from this transitional period survives at SPNEA (fig. 272). Since skirts were short from 1828 to 1833, boots acquired decoration: fringe or frills around the ankle, or embroidery on the instep (fig. 511).

Side-lacing boots with the narrow, square toes that suggest a date in the early 1830s are quite rare (fig. 273). Possibly they were not yet widely adopted in America. It was, after all, the era in which Mrs. Trollope commented on American women's habit of wearing thin, tight slippers rather than sensible boots.[11] What evidence there is indicates that the side-lacing boots of the 1830s were very much like those of the 1840s. One example with an unexplained date of 1838 written in the lining in an old hand is 5½ inches high (fig. 60). This boot, along with those visible in fashion plates, suggests that the earlier side-lace boots (like the front-lace boots that preceded and overlapped them) may have been higher than those that came later, to harmonize with the shorter, scantier skirts of the first third of the century.

The typical side-lacing boot of the 1840s and 1850s measures only 3 to 3½ inches from the heel seat to the top edge, which is straight and plain. It has center back and front seams and generally a toe cap and shallow heel foxing. Deep peaked toe caps were common in the 1840s, and also, apparently, in the 1830s (fig. 244). In the 1850s, the typical pattern had a very short, straight toe cap that sometimes extended back in shallow wings on the sides (figs. 274, 275). Occasionally a side-lacing boot was whole-foxed. When textiles were used for walking boots, the leather foxing protected them from wear. Silk or satin boots that have no leather foxing were probably restricted to evening or the carriage (fig. 277). Side-lacing boots made entirely of leather were not very common until the early 1860s, but when they did appear, the toe cap was not essential and was often omitted. Most leather side-lace boots were cut without the center front gypsy seam and had instead a squarish gusset inserted at the top edge in front (fig. 276). Side-lace boots usually lace on the inner side of the foot (they are very awkward to lace otherwise). A separate tongue sewn on the inside covers any gap behind the lacing.

As front-lacing and button boots became increasingly fashionable in the 1860s, side lacing fell out of use, though it did not entirely disappear. In the 1870s, front lacing came to be used more for utilitarian boots, while button boots were worn for dressier occasions. Button boots, however, had no means of adjusting to minor changes in foot size as lacing boots did. Therefore, it is not surprising to learn in 1875 that "side laced gaiters are said to be coming into fashion again, as they give a perfect fit, and are easily adjusted to the foot when it swells from fatigue or over-exertion."[12] Many side-lace boots were shown in the 1876 Philadelphia Centennial Exhibition. At 6½ to 7½ inches high, they were significantly higher than the side-lace boots of the 1850s and early 1860s (three to four inches), and they also had higher heels. By this time, they seem to be limited to rather dressy styles and may be machine embroidered. Some are made with the traditional gypsy seam, but most have a circular vamp like contemporary front-lacing boots.

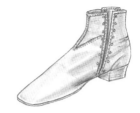

Fig. 276. When made entirely of leather, side-lacing boots had a squarish gusset at the top instead of a gypsy seam. Leather boots became more common 1855–65.

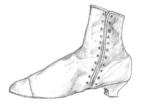

Fig. 277. Satin evening boots were often cut with a matching tip instead of having the seam go all the way to the toe. This French-made boot ca. 1865–70.

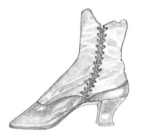

Fig. 278. Some 1870s side-lacing boots were made with a circular vamp instead of a gypsy seam. This one in black satin and kid with high, stacked heel 1876.

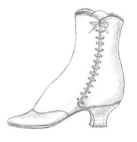

Fig. 279. This side-lacing boot was still being sold in an 1890 catalog when the style had long been out of fashion. The very short vamp fits with the late date.

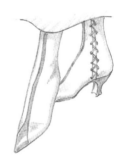

Fig. 280. In 1915 side lacing was revived briefly, and back lacing was also tried. This boot appears in a 1915 dress advertisement. See also figs. 269, 293.

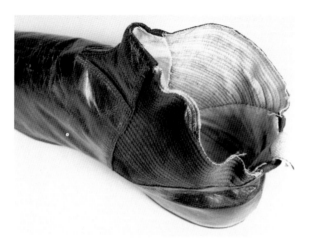

Fig. 281. Kid boot made with "shirred goods," ca. 1850–60. The faded and incomplete patent notice stamped on the inside reads ". . . AND EXCLUSIVE MANUFACTURER, [—]NDT ST. N.Y. GOODYEAR X SOLIS, . . . 44 - 48 - 49." The numbers refer to the years 1844 and 1849 when Goodyear received patents for vulcanizing rubber and making rubber fabrics, and 1848 for a patent received by Richards Solis on November 7 "for a mode of preparing the cloth for the rubber by stretching, also placing the rubber on the cloth obliquely." Catalog #4184. *Courtesy Lynn Museum.*

In some the vamp is leather while the top is of cloth, and in others a leather vamp merges with a leather heel fox, a technique to be more fully developed in the 1890s (fig. 278).

By the 1880s, side lacing was no longer an important fashion. *Demorest's* noticed in 1879 that "side-laced gaiters are always worn by a certain class of elderly ladies, who are conservative in all their ideas, and young ladies with very small feet affect this style of foot-dress for the promenade; yet there is no boot so universal a favorite as the buttoned, which has held, and continues to hold, so high a place in the favor of all ranks and degrees of society."[13] Only one side-lace boot was offered by Hirth, Krause and Wilhelm in 1890, and two by Montgomery Ward in 1895, the latter "made especially for those prejudiced against button shoes" (fig. 279). They appear once again in the fall of 1915 on the feet of some figures illustrated in *Ladies' Home Journal*, probably a French style that was never adopted in the United States (fig. 280) since no examples have been noted in the 1915 *Shoe Retailer*.

Boots with Elastic Adjustment

There are two main types of elastic boots. By far the most common is that which adjusts the boot by inserting a gusset of elasticized fabric called goring on each side. The other has one or two insertions of goring in the front, generally over the instep, below the regular laced or buttoned closing. Elastic-sided boots are most often made with a gypsy seam, much like side-lacing boots but with a roughly triangular gusset of elasticized fabric on each side of the ankle instead of a lace opening. The front side of the gusset is often straight while the back side is curved, the straight side continuing as a seam down to the sole at the waist. Occasionally the gusset is U-shaped, and then the seam is usually centered below it. These variations, however, do not help in dating.

Elastic-sided boots were first made in England in 1838, but they did not appear in America for nearly ten years. They were known here as Congress boots, and later as comfort shoes. *Godey's* was so delighted with the new style that a steel engraving and an entire column of text was devoted to it in August 1848 (see fig. 38).

Only about one year has elapsed since the Congress boot has been, to any considerable extent, introduced into the United States, and yet the demand has been so great that few have been able to obtain them. . . . The proprietor, believing the discovery to be valuable, has caused it to be patented, and this has limited the supply and prevented many fashionable shoemakers from adopting it [because they were unwilling to pay the license fee of six cents per pair]. . . . Shoemakers will eventually be induced to come into the manufacture of the graceful and comfortable Congress boot. It must be seen and worn to be admired and adopted. As a dress boot, it is the perfection of neatness. . . . They combine all the good qualities of a beautiful gaiter with none of the troubles and inconveniences. The elastic gore is an admirable and invaluable support to the ankle, making the boot fit snugly, and giving it a light, graceful and captivating appearance. . . .

The manufacture of the Congress boot is steadily progressing. The first experiments, we are told, failed, as the manufacture of elastic materials was not so perfect as at the present period. The difficulty was to get an India-rubber web so elastic that the boot would go on and off, and yet not so soft and yielding that it would [not] return to its original form. The exact elasticity required having been obtained, the boot is now believed to be the most perfect worn—certainly it is the most comfortable and economical.

Two kinds of elasticized fabric appear in the earliest surviving gored boots. One is a true elastic web in which rubber threads are incorporated into the weave. This "goring" is normally black on both sides, though it may have a slightly brownish cast (fig. 282), but for white boots it was woven with white silk and cotton so as to obscure the black rubber threads (fig. 287). The other, called "shirred goods," was made by cementing stretched-out rubber threads between two layers of fabric. The shirred goods used for shoes were made with black fabric facing outward, to blend with the black leather or serge of the upper, and an unbleached cotton toward the inside. When the cement dried and the rubber threads were permitted to relax, the fabric puckered up. In surviving examples it now looks a bit like seersucker (fig. 281). Shirred goods were not as elegant a solution to the problem of making elasticized fabric as the true elastic web, but it may have been easier than weaving in the early years when the rubber thread had to be cut by hand with shears and thus had a very uneven tensile strength. Better-quality vulcanized rubber thread could be imported from England in the 1850s and this is probably what was used in the earliest gored shoes having a true elastic weave, but such thread was not successfully made in the United States until 1863. Surviving shoes made with shirred goods all seem to date from the 1850s or very early 1860s, suggesting that once vulcanized thread was widely available, the elastic web was preferred.[14]

In October 1854 *Godey's* reported that gored boots were as popular as side lacing, and in 1860 it recom-

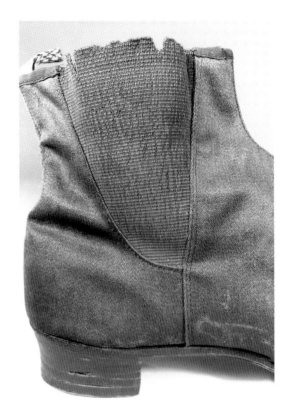

Fig. 282. Black serge Congress boot, ca. 1865–75, machine sewn, having the kind of goring in which the elastic threads are actually woven in. Catalog #3147. *Courtesy Lynn Museum.*

mended them for winter wear: "For walking shoes, there is nothing like the stout cloth boot, lined with canton flannel, and fitted to the ankle by an elastic gore. The soles are sensibly thick, the toes and heels comparing favorably with a gentleman's boots in that respect. No lady who can afford them should brave the pavement, in its present sloppy aspect, unless thus shod."[15] In December that same year *Godey's* mentions "congress boots with heels and soles a half inch thick, lined with cloth, Canton flannel, or flannel, and costing from $4.50 to $6.50" (quite expensive). The USMC collection at the Peabody Essex Museum is rich in examples of elastic-sided boots from the 1860s and 1870s. Many are made of black "stout cloth" with a black patent toe cap, and many have the thick soles suitable for walking (fig. 284). A few are trimmed with a black patent extension from the center front

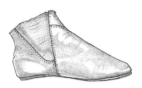

Fig. 283. Early side-gore boots had no heels and were quite low cut. This one of bronze kid with a turned sole ca. 1850–60.

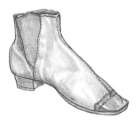

Fig. 284. By the 1860s, side-gore boots were more likely to have heels and patent toe cap. This boot of black serge with thick McKay-sewn sole is typical 1865–70.

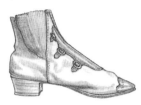

Fig. 285. The early 1870s saw attempts to make gored boots look stylish. This one has a decorative buckled extension to the center front seam, ca. 1865–75.

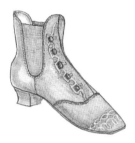

Fig. 286. The circular vamp was an alternative to the gypsy seam by the 1870s. White stitching, favored in 1865–75, here imitates a buttoned closure, 1876.

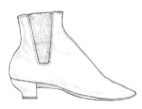

Fig. 287. Dressy white linen boot with white goring and knock-on heel, 1865–75, perhaps worn with the sheer white cotton dresses then fashionable.

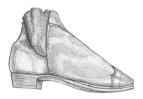

Fig. 288. Side-gore boots were also made in heavy utilitarian leathers like this black pebble-grain with scalloped tip and pegged sole, 1865–75.

seam that imitates a buckled closure (fig. 285). Those gored boots that are made of leather, like the leather side-lace boots of the same period, have a squarish piece inserted at the front top in place of the gypsy seam typical in serge boots (figs. 283, 288). In the 1860s and 1870s, elastic side gussets were still used in fairly dressy boots (figs. 286, 287), but they were increasingly associated with informal indoor shoes and with heavy everyday shoes of the type that often have pegged soles (fig. 288). By the 1880s, boots with elastic sides were no longer making any claim to a place among fashionable footwear, and references to them and examples from that decade are rare.

During the 1890s, shoemakers revived the elastic-sided boot by making it over the fashionable long-toed last and embellishing it with a fancy contrast leather tip that narrowed and extended up the entire front seam in a decorative band called a front stay. An early example of the new style was shown by Selz-Schwab of Chicago in the 1892–93 Columbian Exhibition, and the style seems to have become established in the next two years. The 1895 Montgomery Ward catalog notes for a similar boot that "this being the first season for [our offering] this very stylish Congress, we look for a large sale on same" (fig. 289). The updated version was given names such as "The Elite," the "Ladies' Up to Date Congress Shoe," or the "Juliet," the name most often associated with gored boots from the 1890s on. Boots of this type were made as late as 1907. Those made before 1900 often incorporated delicate cutouts in the front stay. After that date, front stays were less crisply designed and rarely had cutouts (fig. 291).

Later attempts to keep the elastic-sided boot in step with fashion were less successful. One such effort is illustrated in the January 1908 *Ladies' Home Journal*. The new version mimics a button boot with the whole foxing that was stylish at that time (fig. 292). Neat-appearing as it was, it seems not to have caught on. In 1915, a year in which all sorts of new ideas were tried, yet another effort was made to revive the Congress boot, this time christened the "Nancy Hanks" in the hope that it had become old-fashioned enough to be quaint and charming instead of merely dowdy (fig. 293).[16] But along with the other innovations of the midteens, this one was squelched by World War I, and by the time the spirit of experimentation returned in the 1920s, boots were dead.

Meanwhile, since the mid-1870s, more conventional versions of the gored boot had continued an inglorious existence as "comfort" shoes. These boots were made over broad-toed "common sense" lasts rather than whatever was currently fashionable, and as a rule were offered in wide widths only. Similar in pattern and ease to boudoir slippers, gored boots after 1900 sank ever deeper into the slough of slovenliness. In 1907 Sears reminded buyers that gored boots could be worn outdoors, but by then in all probability very few women still chose to wear them in public. The 1925 Charles Williams Store catalog describes such footwear as suitable for a woman "working around the house, or for comfort during her leisure hours."

These unfashionable gored boots appeared in two types. The earlier was very similar in pattern to the plain dressy gored boot of the pre-1875 period (compare fig. 287) and was advertised at least as late as 1908. It was made in both black serge and kid with a gypsy seam and low, stacked heel. It covered the ankle, and the goring extended all the way to the top edge. It had no decoration, but did have pulls at top front and back, unlike most other women's shoes. Often advertised as an "Old Ladies' Congress Gaiter," the style was apparently considered good for nothing better than accommodating swollen ankles, a task button boots were not well adapted for (fig. 290).

The second type of gored comfort shoe appeared by 1907 and continued until at least 1934. It was cut low enough to fall on the borderline between a boot and a shoe, and the goring itself did not usually reach the top of the leather front and back. Very often the gypsy seam was omitted, resulting in a smooth "seamless" vamp. This newer type was rarely if ever made in serge. The uppers were normally of kid or of cheap leather finished to imitate kid, and the heels were often of rubber. Many had a straight toe cap (fig. 236), and a few incorporated a debased version

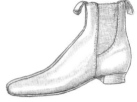

Fig. 289. Gored boots were updated 1892–1907 with a fancy front stay. Stays of the 1890s could have delicate cutouts. This example 1895. See fig. 520.

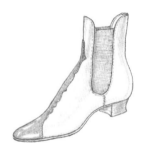

Fig. 290. Plain "Old Ladies' Congress" boot of black serge with gypsy seam and straight top, made from 1870s to 1908. This example 1902.

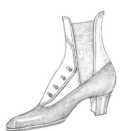

Fig. 291. Front stays used on Congress boots after 1900 did not have cutouts like those of the 1890s. This one 1907. Later ones were even duller. Compare fig. 240.

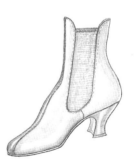

Fig. 292. In 1908 the gored boot was disguised to look like the more fashionable whole-foxed button boot. Compare fig. 267.

Fig. 293. Another attempt to update gored boots, this time with the stylish high Louis heel and a new name, "Nancy Hanks," 1915.

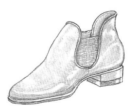

Fig. 294. "Restful easy Juliet," the frumpy shoe worn from 1907 to the 1930s. This example 1925. See also figs. 236, 240.

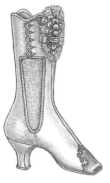

Fig. 295. Unusual combination of elastic gores below a buttoned flap lined with purple silk appears in this black kid boot, 1876.

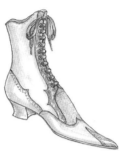

Fig. 296. The gored instep was introduced in the Rich Shoe Company's Julia Marlowe boot, patented 1896. This view advertised in Sears, 1897.

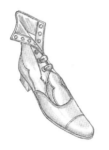

Fig. 297. This version of the gored instep was developed by Sears in 1902 to compete with the Julia Marlowe, which it no longer sold.

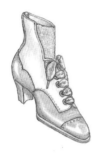

Fig. 298. Yet another short-lived variation appears in this boot with goring above an instep lacing. Offered by Sears, 1907.

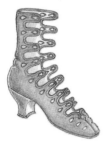

Fig. 299. The advantage of fastening the straps of a Grecian-style boot with ribbons is that it will adjust to the leg exactly. This one in black velvet, 1875–85.

of the front stay (fig. 240). Others are entirely plain (fig. 294). All make a strong claim to being the ugliest shoes illustrated in this book.

As side-gore boots were slipping irrevocably into dowdiness at the turn of the century, a new variation was introduced that centered the elastic goring on the instep at the bottom of the standard front lacing. Boots with elastic goring inserted below another fastening had been tried as early as 1876, when one is illustrated in *Harper's Bazar* (fig. 295). *Demorest's* appears to be describing a similar boot in 1879, when it mentions among other novelties that "walking boots of Indian goat are made to order, with silk elastic gores two inches deep set in each side at the ankle, and above this there are half a dozen buttons that close the boot in the usual manner."[17]

This early version does not seem to have been widely worn, but the one offered in the 1890s enjoyed a certain brief success. Front-lacing boots with an elastic insertion on the instep were patented by the Rich Shoe Company of Milwaukee on August 11, 1896, and marketed by 1897 under the name "Julia Marlowe" (fig. 296). The Julia Marlowe advertisements found in contemporary magazines explain that "The Special Feature of these shoes (Goring Instep) causes them to yield to every action of the foot, unlike any other style of shoes ever produced."[18]

A similar shoe was advertised in Sears by 1902, with the remark, "We formerly quoted the Julia Marlowe Lace Boot, with elastic instep, at $2.65, but the manufacturer refused to sell it to us longer unless we would charge our customers at least $3.00 for same [the price at which the maker was retailing it]. We refused to raise the price to our patrons, hence were compelled to build the shoe herewith illustrated. We have in this shoe combined all of the style usually found in the $4.00, $5.00 and $6.00 grades." The Sears boot apparently avoided patent infringement by dividing the goring into two sections separated by a strip of leather (fig. 297). A new variation was available from Sears by 1907 having the goring at the top of the boot and the lacing below it on the instep (fig. 298), but the idea of using front goring in boots seems to have been dropped about 1910 (see, however, the section in chapter 7 on gored shoes).

Boots with Straps or Ribbons across a Broad Front Opening

There is no one standard term for footwear that is as high as a boot in back but as open as a low-cut slipper in front, and that may fasten in a variety of ways. The most significant tradition identifies such boots with classical antiquity, and they are often referred to as Grecian or Roman sandals, or as being laced in the Greek style. Other writers use descriptive phrases such as "eight-strap sandals," but more fanciful terms appear as well. Fashion journals from the 1870s to the 1920s agree that the whole point of such footwear was to reveal the pretty colored silk stockings beneath.

In one version, the sides are fitted with lace holes through which a ribbon or silk lace is passed to cross over the opening (fig. 300). A second has a series of straps that button or buckle across the open front (fig. 301). In a third, the straps are short tabs, each bearing an eyelet through which a lace is run (figs. 299). Laced fastenings allow such boots to conform snugly to the ankle, while buttoned straps, being less easily adjusted, might sag on a thin leg. Therefore, in some boots the "straps" are really a series of cutouts, while the real closure is a side lacing (fig. 302).

French fashion plates around 1800 occasionally show shoes with extensions up the back of the ankle to keep the elaborate lacing in place (fig. 32). The idea was revived in the 1870s and continued as a fancy alternative to standard styles right through the 1920s. Laced versions appear in *Godey's* in 1870 and 1888, but for most of the 1870s and 1880s, the strapped style seems to have been preferred. The fashion for strapped boots reached its height between 1877 and 1883 (fig. 301). Boots in the Grecian style are rarely noted in the 1890s, but a black velvet "eight-strap sandal" trimmed with gold beads appears among the new styles in *The Shoe Retailer* for the fall of 1901 (fig. 303). A nine-strap version appears later in the decade. At a period when boots were increasingly limited to winter street wear, the usefulness of such dressy boots is questionable. But the answer is suggested by the Sears catalogs for 1907 and 1909, where a similar strapped boot is described as the "Stage Favorite, an exact duplicate of the sandal worn by

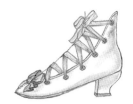

Fig. 300. Grecian boots laced over a broad opening are noted in *Godey's* in 1870 and 1888 but were presumably available 1870–90. This example, white kid, 1875–80.

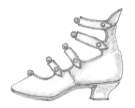

Fig. 301. The low Grecian boot with buttoned straps was particularly stylish 1877–83. This black kid boot has decorative black thread ball buttons center front.

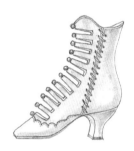

Fig. 302. As straps rarely fit well in high Grecian boots, they may be replaced by cutouts, the real adjustment being side lacing, a type stylish in 1874–83. This one 1877.

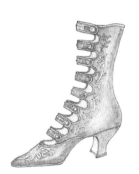

Fig. 303. When strap footwear in general returned to favor 1900–1905, eight- and nine-strap boots were offered with beading on the straps. This one 1901.

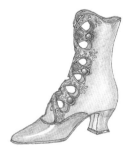

Fig. 304. This cross-strap Grecian boot, the Stage Favorite, probably designed before 1905, was still in the 1909 Sears Catalog.

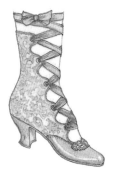

Fig. 305. Boots laced over a broad opening were revived 1914–17 as Tango Boots. Those with straps or cutouts became Roman Sandals. This one 1914.

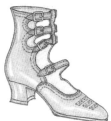

Fig. 306. This "four-buckle slipper" for 1922 apparently never caught on, but the buckles, stitching, and perforation are typical in the early 1920s. See fig. 146.

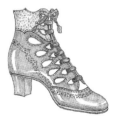

Fig. 307. The "Grecian Beauty Boot" offered by Sears in 1928 is really a higher version of the cutout oxford. See figs. 157, 207, 209.

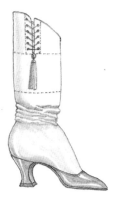

Fig. 308. Women began to wear solid leg boots for walking ca. 1915. This Russian boot has an ornamental lacing and tassel, 1915.

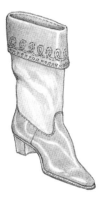

Fig. 309. Many 1920s Russian boots were made like riding boots but had a high Louis heel, but this one, Sears 1922, is gray suede and black patent stitched in red.

one of the leading prima donnas the past season. We thought it the most beautiful thing we had seen, so here it is at about one-third the cost of the theatrical boot makers, . . . a novelty for house, party or dancing." The Stage Favorite has beaded V-shaped straps that cross each other in front (fig. 304).

Every few years a new style of Grecian boot was tried, but none seems to have lasted very long. In 1914, the laced version reappeared as the "Tango Bootee" (fig. 305) while the strapped boot became the "Roman Sandal" with eight straps in 1914, and nine in 1917 when boots in general became higher. In 1921 the style reappeared with buckled straps (fig. 306), a taller variation of the ankle-strap shoes of that year (see fig. 146). The last revival noted is the "Grecian Beauty Boot" in Sears 1927 catalog. "Acclaimed at every Fashion Show in the United States, this latest Lace Shoe whim, recalling ancient days of glory, is decidedly modern and up to the minute. Supplies that snug fit liked so much in fall and winter while enhancing the charm of sheer fashionable hosiery through the 'Grecian sandal' cutouts" (fig. 307).

Solid Leg Boots

Boots without fastenings were a man's style for most of the nineteenth century. Women borrowed them first for riding (see chapter 5). The solid leg boot appeared for street wear in 1915, when it was illustrated in the February *Ladies' Home Journal* and called a "high Russian boot." This early version has a tassel hanging from a short side lacing that was probably ornamental rather than functional (fig. 308). Like other experimental styles of the mid-1910s, this one quickly disappeared, only to be revived in the early 1920s. Sears Roebuck sold a Russian boot in its 1922 catalog, and the fulsome description says, "If you were to walk down Fifth Avenue today you'd find the most fashionable women of the most fashionable city wearing the beautiful new Russian Boot. It's the 'last word' in footwear style, and the model we have selected is an unusually charming one" (fig. 309). Swann illustrates Russian boots of the 1920s in brown leather, black patent, and suede that look like contemporary riding boots except for the high Louis heel.[19]

CHAPTER NINE

Looking at the Bottom

Heels and Soles

Just as chapters 7 and 8 describe the uppers of shoes and boots, this chapter describes the bottoms. The first part deals with heels, first defining heel types as used in this book and in American shoe documents. Then, following a brief summary of the chronological changes in heel fashions, four detailed sections describe the variations found within each major heel type. The second part of the chapter deals with the shape of soles, of which the most conspicuous part is the toe. This material is organized into sections chronologically.

Looking at Heels

There are four major types of heels used on women's shoes between 1795 and 1930: Louis, knock-on, stacked, and spring (fig. 310). Both Louis and knock-on heels are normally made of wood[1] and covered with leather or fabric to match the upper. The difference between them is that in Louis heels the sole leather continues down the breast (forward face of the heel) while in knock-on heels it does not. The continuous sole typically appears in conjunction with the curved breast characteristic of Louis heels, but it can be used with a straight-breasted heel, and indeed it often is from the mid-1920s on. This latter type is sometimes called a Spanish Louis. The neck (back face) of a Louis heel traditionally forms a reverse curve to harmonize with the curved breast, but here too the curves are often straightened out from the 1920s on.

The knock-on heel, in contrast, is normally covered identically on all four sides, with the seam centered on the breast, although occasionally the breast is covered separately to mimic a continuous sole. The walking surface is provided with a sole leather top piece. Knock-on heels usually have a straight breast, and the neck may be either straight or curved. It is rare to find knock-on construction in very high heels—for those a Louis construction is preferred. While not in common use, the term "knock-on" is useful, because it implies that the heel is merely nailed on and because the type is so characteristic of the period 1860 to 1905 as to require some name. "Opera heel," the only contemporary term, is rarely used and not descriptive enough to be immediately understood.

Stacked heels are made of pieces of leather stacked one on top of another, each layer being called a lift. Stacked heels are naturally dark in color and are most often used on shoes with dark uppers. Shoes with white or light uppers are more likely to have wooden heels covered to match the upper so that the heel blends with the rest of the shoe. Stacked heels are used for most utilitarian footwear, and they are usually fairly low and straight in shape. But it is quite common to find a concave curve at the back, and a few were even cut to imitate the curves of a high Louis heel.

A spring heel consists of a single layer of leather (called a slip) inserted just above the sole at the back

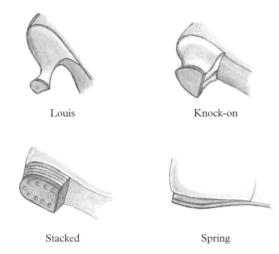

Louis   Knock-on

Stacked   Spring

Fig. 310. Four major heel constructions

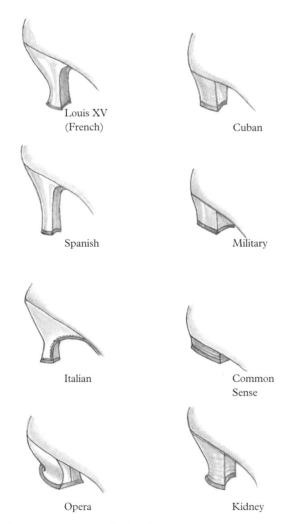

Louis XV
(French)   Cuban

Spanish   Military

Italian   Common
                         Sense

Opera   Kidney

Fig. 311. Eight common fashion shapes

of the shoe. When the edges are burnished, it may be difficult to see where sole leather ends and slip begins, but the stitching that attaches slip to sole (or the channel in which it is concealed) is often visible, running around the bottom of the sole near the edge.

A fifth kind of heel, called a wedge heel, extends forward to fill the space under the waist of the shoe (fig. 315). It is sometimes defined as being nailed to the outside of the sole rather than inserted between the sole and the heel seat like a spring heel, but this restriction is not observed in this book. Wedge heels are not a common type in the period 1795–1930. Those few that do appear tend to date 1790–1810 and develop from the partially wedged Louis heel called an Italian heel.

The definitions offered above are those used in this book, but readers cannot assume that other primary or secondary sources describing shoes will use terms in exactly the same way. American usage has generally differentiated heels in terms of their fashion shape, not by how they are attached to the shoe. For example, in American sources the term Louis tends to mean a high heel with curvy outlines, and not necessarily one made of wood with the sole continuing down the breast. Thus, the phrase "leather Louis" to refer to a curvy stacked heel is not a contradiction in terms, as it would be in British usage or in this book. The following definitions reflect American usage, primarily at the turn of the century, when the shoe industry was at its height (fig. 311).

Louis XV, or French: Any heel, usually of covered wood but sometimes of stacked leather, whose neck (back face) is shaped in a graceful reverse curve. This is the most characteristic shape for Louis heels (in the sense used in this book), since it harmonizes with the curve formed by the sole as it continues down the breast. By the early twentieth century, a low version of this heel was called a baby Louis, and a medium height a junior Louis.

Cuban: A term that came into common use about 1900 for a rather straight-sided heel. Unless it is modified, as in "Cuban wood" or "covered Cuban," the term implies a stacked heel. Depending on the period and the dressiness of the shoe, Cuban heels range from low and blocky to medium high and tapered at the bottom. It is not clearly distinguished from the military heel. In American usage, the covered wood version is felt to be related to the Spanish heel because both have straight sides, even though in Spanish heels the sole usually continues down the breast.

Spanish: A high, thin heel, normally of covered wood with straight, tapering sides and neck. In most cases the sole continues down the heel breast, even though it may lack the curved breast characteristically created by that construction. The term appeared by 1907 (but in that year the shape was similar to the kidney heel of 1914) and was in common use by 1923, first in the phrase "Spanish-Louis." Spanish heels are distinguished from Cuban heels first by their greater height and slenderness and second by being made of wood. By the mid-1920s, Spanish heels were so high and thin that they became known as spike heels.

Military: This term applies to a heel that is not consistently distinguished from a Cuban. In Swann's diagrams, the military heel has a concave curve to the neck, and can be fairly high. But in American periodical illustrations it has a moderately low, straight blocky shape, and when any distinction is made at all, the military heel is straighter than the Cuban. The term seems to imply a stacked heel unless expressly stated otherwise ("covered wood military"). By the 1920s, "military" replaced "Cuban" in referring to a straight-sided tapered heel of medium height.

Common Sense: A low, broad, stacked heel used for walking and sports shoes.

Opera: Term sometimes used around the turn of the century for a knock-on heel with straight breast and curved neck, presumably because it was used on the evening shoes known as opera slippers.

Kidney: A term used about 1913–14 to refer to a heel with a straight breast and curved neck, usually higher than the opera heel that preceded it. Previewing 1914 styles, the *Shoe Retailer* remarks that "kidney heels, properly speaking, are of leather, and this is the way most dealers want them. The wood kidney heel simply lightens up a shoe and is perhaps preferable for turns, while leather kidney heels will be used on welts."[2]

Italian: A slender Louis heel with a wedgelike extension that partially fills the hollow beneath the waist, a type very common during the 1780s and 1790s. The term was not in common use past the eighteenth century.

Heels are measured in eighths of an inch, so that an 8/8 heel is one inch high, a 17/8 heel is 2⅛ inches high, and so forth.

Chronological Overview

The Louis heel was standard in the eighteenth century. In the 1790s it became lower and lower until it was reduced to the merest wedge or replaced by a spring heel. Spring heels prevailed from 1800 to 1830, although low stacked heels with rounded sides were common in the 1820s. Entirely flat shoes, with no heel at all, appeared as early as 1812, became the norm during the 1830s, 1840s, and 1850s, and are found in evening slippers to the end of the 1860s.

Low heels, stacked or knock-on, slowly returned to fashion in the 1850s. Louis heels reappeared in the middle to late 1860s, when higher heels became fashionable. All three types continued in use right through the 1920s. Straight-sided stacked heels were preferred for walking and utilitarian footwear, while knock-on and Louis heels were used in dressier shoes. Among dressy shoes, Louis construction was preferred for higher heels and in higher-quality footwear.

Heels were in general higher in the 1870s than either before or afterward, but they rose again about 1900. About 1906 there was a strong reaction against curvy "French" shapes in favor of the straight-sided Cuban style. These had little competition until 1914, when Louis construction and curves returned together. From 1917 until about 1923, High, slender Louis heels were used for all higher-heeled footwear, including dress boots. Lower heels on more utilitarian boots and walking shoes, however, still had straight sides. In the mid-1920s, Spanish heels (straight-sided, high, and slender), became popular for dressy footwear. Lower, blockier heels of stacked leather or covered wood were chosen for afternoon wear and "dressy sports." For serious walking, however, women wore low, broad heels with a rubber top piece.

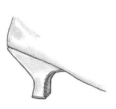

Fig. 312. Higher form of the wedged Louis known as an Italian heel, 1770–1800.

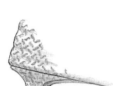

Fig. 313. Lower version of the Italian heel, 1785–1805.

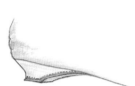

Fig. 314. Italian heel reduced to little more than its wedge-like extension, 1790–1810.

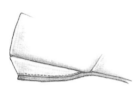

Fig. 315. Heel with full wedge under the arch, 1790–1810.

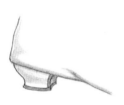

Fig. 316. Half-inch Louis heel without any wedge. Wedding slipper, 1801.

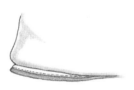

Fig. 317. Tiny covered heel stitched along the edge of the sole, 1795–1820. Closely related to spring heels (see fig. 326). This one 1797.

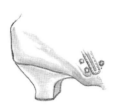

Fig. 318. The first Louis heels to return to use in the 1860s were not strongly curved. Some were higher than this one, 1865–70.

Louis Heels

All through the eighteenth century, women's shoes were made with Louis heels, some thick and blocklike, some slender, and ranging from 1½ to 4 inches in height. From about 1770 to the end of the century, the Italian heel (a Louis heel with a wedge-like extension beneath the arch) was worn, high at first, lower in the 1790s (figs. 312, 313).

During the 1790s, very low or even flat heels were gaining ground, but actual practice was not uniform. *Heideloff's* mentions entirely flat slippers as early as 1795, yet the heels actually illustrated are often rather high. Surviving wedding shoes also suggest an uneven rate of change. One pair dated 1797 has only a spring heel, but another from 1798 has heels over two inches high. Another of 1799 measures one inch, while one from 1801 is only half an inch (fig 316).

Nearly all these diminishing heels are variations of the Italian heel. In some lower versions, the wedged extension is so thick that the arch is reduced to nearly nothing (fig. 314), and indeed, true wedge heels were also made at the same time (fig. 315). The lowest examples are no thicker than a spring heel (fig. 317). But whether wedged or Italian, whether one inch thick or one-eighth inch thin, the slip or wedge or wooden heel is covered with upper material and in most cases a visible line of stitching passes through the covering directly next to the sole. In America, covered heels seem to have been replaced by spring or flat heels by 1810, but Swann notes later English examples,[3] and a thin covered heel appears on a boot brought from Italy in 1817.[4]

The Louis heel did not return to fashion again until the mid-1860s (fig. 318). Swann illustrates two French examples from circa 1864–65 and 1867,[5] and *Godey's* mentions "very high Louis XV heels" in January 1867. During the later nineteenth century, Louis heels could range from 1½ to 2½ inches in height (measured at the back), and more than one shape was in use at any one time (figs. 319–21). They were less likely to flare outward toward the top piece before 1880 than after 1880, and by the early 1900s the outward flare was nearly universal. There was a tendency toward higher heels in the 1870s and among high-style shoes at any time.

Louis-heeled shoes from this period appear less often in middle-class historical collections than they do in colections to which wealthy donors have given high-fashion clothing. Louis heels, being more difficult to make, made shoes more expensive, but they were preferred for very high heels because they were stronger than knock-ons. Wealthy, leisured women accepted the cost to obtain the better quality and the higher heel. Women who could not afford many shoes chose lower heels that were more generally useful, where the knock-on construction was not a disadvantage. The middle-class attitude toward Louis heels was primly expressed in the *Ladies' World* in 1899: "This is decidedly a season for frills and frivolity, therefore it is not surprising that the Louis XV heel has come in again and will be found on every sort of footwear from a walking boot to a dancing slipper. This heel seems inseparable from frills and furbelows, and has so little to recommend it in the way of common sense and healthfulness that it will be sure to be popular."[6]

Shoes with Louis heels, always with the outward flare at the bottom (fig. 322), and usually quite high, are frequently advertised from 1900 to 1905. The style suffered a serious eclipse from 1906 to 1913, however. In this period, most fashionable heels had straight sides and were stacked or knock-on, although dressy satin evening slippers continued to be made with high Louis heels. When Louis heels returned to fashion in 1914, they came in both the flared and unflared forms, the latter now given many new names, none of which stuck (fig. 323). The *Shoe Retailer* commented in 1913, "Wood heels have been in such demand for samples [for spring 1914] that heel makers have not been able to make deliveries on time. . . . There are many varieties of wood heels, . . . [and] top lifts for these heels are made in many shapes."[7] By 1917, the flared Louis, just as high and even more slender than it had been in 1905, predominated, and it appeared on dressy boots as well as shoes (fig. 324). But by 1923, the flared Louis had declined in favor of the straighter, unflared form. In the last half of the 1920s, slender straight-sided Louis heels 2½ inches or even higher were typical for dressy shoes (fig. 325) and were now known as spike heels.

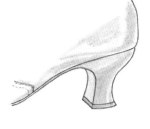

Fig. 319. High, slender Louis heels were common in the 1870s, although the outward flare toward the top piece was not universal.

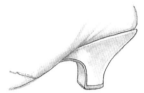

Fig. 320. High but thicker Louis sometimes used in the 1880s. This example does not flare outward at the bottom.

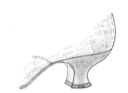

Fig. 321. Low Louis heel with the outward flare toward the top piece that became increasingly common after 1880.

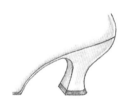

Fig. 322. High, flaring Louis heel was standard 1900–1905 and continued for evening slippers through 1913. This example 1904.

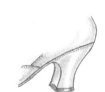

Fig. 323. A Louis heel only minimally flared at the top piece was in style 1914–16 and 1923–25 under various names. This example 1915.

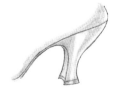

Fig. 324. Full Louis heel is slender, high, and flaring toward the top piece, 1916–23. Lower junior and baby Louis heels were also worn at this time.

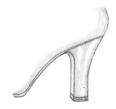

Fig. 325. Very high, thin, straight-sided Louis heels called spike heels came into wide use for dressy shoes 1925–30.

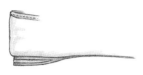

Fig. 326. The spring heel, a single lift inserted above the sole, is the most common "flat" heel in use 1800–1830.

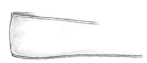

Fig. 327. Shoes truly without heels can date 1812–70. Before 1830, soles often show little curve when seen from the side. Compare fig. 328.

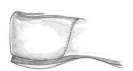

Fig. 328. Heelless shoe with gentle curvature in the sole almost universal after 1830. Compare the flat sole common before 1830 in fig. 327.

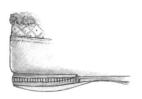

Fig. 329. Spring heels continued to appear in thicker-soled walking and winter shoes. This 1845–55 example has the slip obscured by wheeling.

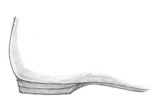

Fig. 330. Spring heels were considered children's wear when women wore high heels. In 1894 Montgomery Ward offered them again in women's sizes.

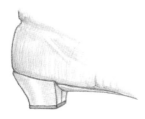

Fig. 331. Low knock-on heels appeared by 1855, of wood or leather covered to match a light upper. Low heels worn 1855–70 had a slightly concave neck.

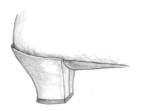

Fig. 332. From 1865 to 1880 knock-ons were often higher. Some still had the slightly concave neck.

Spring and "Flat" Heels

In the 1790s and early 1800s, the Louis heels of the eighteenth century became lower and lower until shoes appeared essentially flat. *Heideloff's Gallery of Fashion*, the great English series of fashion prints of the 1790s, mentions shoes "with flat heels" in 1795.[8] However, the "flat" shoes of this period are almost always made with a thin covered heel (fig. 317) or a spring heel, a single slip of leather inserted just above the sole (fig. 326). The slip may not be obvious, because the edges of sole and slip are often so carefully burnished that the two layers are indistinguishable and the sole merely appears thickened at the heel end. A check of the bottom of the sole, however, will usually show a horseshoe-shaped line of stitching running round the edge of the heel, or else a channel (slit) in which the stitching has been concealed. This stitching is what attaches the spring lift to the sole. The spring heel was mentioned by name in 1795 in *Heideloff's* ("purple Spanish leather spring heel slippers")[9] and continued in common use through the 1820s.

Spring heels were not particularly fashionable for women in the mid–nineteenth century, but they do appear on some thick-soled shoes (fig. 329). Later, when adult women were wearing higher heels, spring soles were routinely used on children's shoes. Montgomery Ward offered two styles of spring-heel button boots by 1894, noting that "in the past the largest size attainable in this style was No. 2. . . . Owing to the growing demand for a neat, stylish patent tip spring heel shoe, we have this made special, so as to meet the desired wants of many of our customers who are prejudiced against a heeled shoe" (fig. 330).

A truly heelless shoe appeared as early as 1812 (fig. 327) but was rather rare until after 1830. When heelless shoes did become usual, in the 1830s, 1840s, and 1850s, the soles were very thin and generally curved so as to contact the floor firmly only at the ball of the foot and the center of the heel (fig. 328). Heelless shoes were going out of fashion in the 1850s, but evening and wedding slippers continued to be made without heels to the end of the 1860s, and the type is more common in museum collections than they were in actual fact.

Knock-On Heels

Covered wooden knock-on heels are well represented in museums because they were routinely used on the light evening shoes saved as keepsakes from special occasions (fig. 334). But there is no evidence that they were worn in the early nineteenth century. The date Swann gives for their appearance is 1855,[10] and it is in that same year that *Godey's* first appears to refer to them, remarking that "white or light-colored satin boots, with light heels, are still seen in ballrooms."[11] Some early knock-ons were made of stacked leather rather than wood underneath the covering. Knock-on heels tended to be quite low and small in the 1850s and early 1860s (fig. 331), higher in the late 1860s and 1870s (figs. 332, 333), and lower again but somewhat heavier in the 1880s and 1890s (fig. 334). Two styles were offered in both heights, one fairly straight with a slightly concave neck, the other flaring outward toward the top piece to create a reverse "French" curve. From about 1890 to 1905, the latter style often had a slight ridge down the center back, echoing the point of the new shield-shaped top piece (fig. 334). Knock-on heels were never quite as chic as Louis heels, and they were usually somewhat lower.

When Louis heels suddenly went out of fashion in 1906, in favor of straight-sided, stacked leather heels, knock-ons also suffered a decline. They continued to be used on white wedding slippers and other dressy footwear where dark heels would be inappropriate but where straight lines were still desired (fig. 336). Covered wood heels of all types returned to fashion in 1914. While curvy Louis heels were used in the late teens for the dressiest boots and shoes, covered wood knock-on heels continued to be straight sided and were used as an alternative to stacked Cuban heels on oxfords and other walking shoes. As curvy shapes began to lose favor in the early 1920s and straight-sided styles took their place, covered wood knock-on heels were used on a broader variety of shoes. The lowest knock-ons were generally block-shaped (fig. 337), while the higher ones were tapered (fig. 338). For the highest "spike" heels that came in about 1926, Louis construction was preferred, but less extreme models were sometimes made as knock-ons (fig. 339).

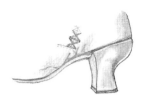

Fig. 333. Other high 1870s knock-ons had the curved neck associated with Louis heels, like this exhibition boot of 1876.

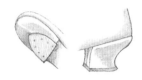

Fig. 334. Knock-ons commonly flared out toward the top piece and were fairly low 1880–1905. In the 1890s, the ridged neck and shield-shaped top piece were common.

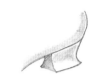

Fig. 335. Opera heel as illustrated in John Wanamaker's Catalog for 1901.

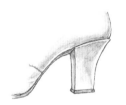

Fig. 336. Knock-ons acquired straight sides and some were fairly high from 1906 to 1913. But high-end evening shoes had Louis heels when height was wanted.

Fig. 337. Low and blocky knock-on heels for ordinary day wear were particularly common 1923–27.

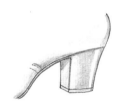

Fig. 338. Tapered knock-ons of medium height were widely worn throughout the 1920s and well into the 1930s.

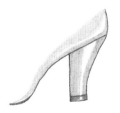

Fig. 339. Knock-on heels were occasionally quite high and slender in 1926–30, but a straight-sided Louis was usually preferred.

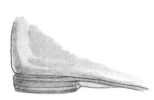

Fig. 340. Very low, stacked heels (only one or two lifts) appear occasionally on walking shoes and boots 1800–1820.

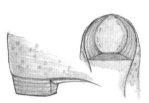

Fig. 341. A higher, rounded stacked heel is quite common on women's footwear 1824–30. This one 1824.

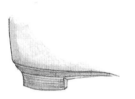

Fig. 342. Most shoes had no heels 1830–50, but this tiny heel was added to a dressy tan morocco tie shoe ca. 1835–45.

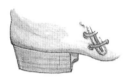

Fig. 343. Low, broad heel for ordinary wear was permanently established by 1860. This example 1852.

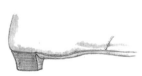

Fig. 344. Tiny stacked heels were often added to white slippers to update them in the later 1860s, sometimes with comical results. This example 1871.

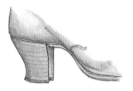

Fig. 345. Stacked heels, like others from the 1870s, could be very high. This one is on a dressy exhibition boot, 1876.

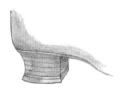

Fig. 346. Moderate stacked heels with concave necks were widely used 1870–1900. This example ca. 1885–92.

Stacked Heels

Stacked heels appear on some practical early-nineteenth-century footwear, including a pair of heavy calf slippers with pointed toes probably worn for everyday work (fig. 358), and on a pair of leather front-lace boots (fig. 340), both circa 1810. Both heels are quite low, only two or three lifts. Stacked heels are not common in dressy shoes until the mid-1820s, but judging from surviving dated examples, from about 1824 to 1830 they were nearly as common as spring heels and flats. These are typically three-quarters of an inch high, tapered, and rounded so that the top lift is nearly circular. They often appear with a domed waist (fig. 341).

Heels of any kind are uncommon among surviving shoes from the 1830s and 1840s, but the few exceptions have stacked heels about three-quarters of an inch high (fig. 342). In June 1846, *La Belle Assemblée*'s Paris correspondent reported, "There is also some talk of the revival of high heels; but this last report is, I think, unworthy of credit." By the early 1850s, however, heels were starting to appear again, first on boots. Heeled boots are illustrated in *Godey's* in October 1854. Frances French, who ran a hotel in Northampton, Massachusetts, mentioned heeled shoes as a novelty in November 1855, writing, "Mother has got on her high heeled shoes tonight. She has stretched herself on the lounge and joking all the while."[12] The earliest-noted documented heeled shoe from this period is a blue serge wedding boot of 1852 (fig. 343).

The stacked heels of the 1860s were still low, only one-half to one inch high, and some had a very small walking surface. Both stacked and knock-on heels were sometimes added to flat slippers and boots as a cheap way of bringing them up to date. In this early period, even when shoes came heeled from the manufacturer, they were still sometimes made over old lasts intended for flat shoes, and the result was awkward at best. If you put such a shoe on a table and press downward on the heel seat, the toe is quite likely to pop up into the air (fig. 344). Better-quality shoes and boots, of course, were made from the beginning on lasts designed with a bend to accommodate the heel. Fashionable heels in general became higher in the late 1860s and 1870s, and some of the boots made for the 1876 Centennial Exhibition have stacked heels two inches high with a curved neck (fig. 345).

While stacked leather heels had been used occasionally on dressy shoes in the 1860s, from 1870 to 1900 they were normally restricted to walking footwear. Most everyday boots had stacked heels (the Louis-heeled boots that commonly survive in museums were suitable only for dress wear or the carriage, and are not typical of the mass of footwear). Stacked heels were also used on the low summer walking shoes that became increasingly important from the mid-1870s on. Until 1900 these walking heels were of modest height, usually ¾ to 1¼ inches, with a broad walking surface and straight or concave sides (fig. 346).

From about 1901 to 1916, boots and shoes for dressy day wear, including Colonials and some oxfords, were made with what were at first called "spike heels," because compared to the stacked heels of the 1890s, they were somewhat higher and more tapered and had a smaller top piece. These could reach 2¼ inches in height, but 1¾ inches was closer to the norm. These classic Cuban heels generally had straight sides, but a few were concave at the neck (figs. 347, 348). From 1906 to 1913, tapered straight-sided, stacked leather heels in varying heights seem to have been used for nearly all footwear except the very dressiest light shoes (such as satin evening or wedding slippers), which called for a wooden heel covered to match the light upper. Utilitarian shoes, of course, continued to be made with lower, broader stacked heels (fig. 349).

Stacked heels declined as covered wood heels returned to favor in the mid-1910s, and by 1917 they were rarely used on dressy shoes. They now ranged in height from one inch, for utilitarian footwear, to 1¾ inches, for more stylish shoes and boots (fig. 350). A few boots were made with two-inch stacked heels cut to imitate the more stylish high Louis shape of 1917–23 (fig. 351). In the early 1920s, stacked heels were increasingly relegated to sports and utilitarian walking shoes (fig. 352), while the dressier oxfords and strapped shoes had covered wood heels. Many were equipped with rubber top pieces, a feature that had first appeared in the 1890s (fig. 353).

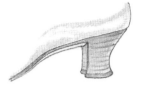

Fig. 347. Higher variant of the nineteenth-century concave heel, on a tan Colonial, ca. 1904. Compare fig. 346.

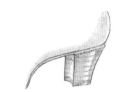

Fig. 348. Straight-sided, tapered stacked leather heels about 1¾ inches high were widely worn from 1901 into the 1930s. This example 1908.

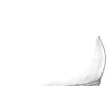

Fig. 349. Slightly lower and broader stacked heels were worn on less dressy footwear from 1900 into the 1930s. This example 1908.

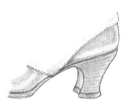

Fig. 350. The years 1914–16 saw experimentation in many aspects of shoe design. This stacked heel has the curved breast of a Louis but a straight neck.

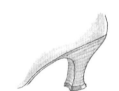

Fig. 351. When stacked heels imitated the more stylish Louis heels, 1917–21, they were called leather Louis heels.

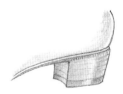

Fig. 352. Blocky military heels 1 to 1½ inches high were common on walking boots 1917–21 and continued in use on everyday shoes in the 1920s.

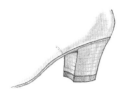

Fig. 353. Many heels were fitted with rubber top pieces in the 1920s. This example 1926.

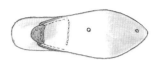

Fig. 354. 1770–90 buckle shoe: pointed toe, Louis heel, broad tread, waist wider than heel seat. See fig. 167.

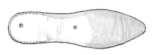

Fig. 355. 1797 wedding slipper: toe point slightly blunted, spring heel, sole shaped in gentle curves. See fig. 317.

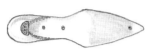

Fig. 356. 1799 wedding latchet-tie: pointed toe, narrow waist, low Louis heel. Tread forms an angle instead of a curve. See plate 1.

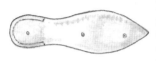

Fig. 357. 1800–1805 slipper: pointed toe not as long as often found. Note visible channel for stitching on the spring heel.

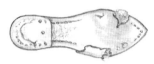

Fig. 358. 1800–1810 slipper: heavily worn and distorted everyday shoe with pointed toe, low stacked heel.

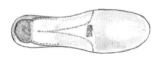

Fig. 359. 1805–10 sandal: new round toe, very low Italian heel, sole shaped in gentle curves. See figs. 35, 314.

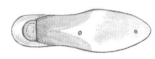

Fig. 360. 1805–10 sandal: oval toe, very low Italian heel, sole shaped in gentle curves. See fig. 443.

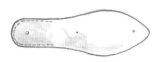

Fig. 361. 1805–10 strap shoe: narrow oval toe, unusual wedge heel. See figs. 130, 315.

Looking at Soles

Toe shape is a critical detail for dating shoes and the best way to see it is by looking at the sole. Other points to note are the contrast in width between waist and tread, how far back toward the heel the waist is placed, whether there are any decorative finishes, and whether the shoes are made as rights and lefts.

ca. 1700–ca. 1795: Shoes are straight, with oval or pointed toes. The waist is rarely narrower than the heel seat but instead gradually tapers from front to back (fig. 354).

ca. 1795–ca. 1805: Nearly all shoes have long, pointed toes, often sharply pointed, sometimes slightly rounded off (figs. 355–58). Most have a low heel in which the sole continues onto the heel breast. The tack marks from the last may be visible as little holes near the toe, at the waist, and in flat shoes, near the heel. Unlike earlier eighteenth-century shoes, the sole is now usually narrowest at the waist. The widest part of the sole, near the ball of the foot, may be cut as a gentle point rather than a curve (fig. 356).

ca. 1805–ca. 1828: In the first decade of the new century, heels became lower and lower until they seemed to disappear completely. However, most early-nineteenth-century shoes that at first glance appear heelless actually have spring heels, a single lift added above the sole. The stitching that attaches this lift—or the channel in which it is concealed—is visible on the bottom of the sole, running parallel to and near the edge (figs. 357, 363, 365). The spring heel continued in common use through the 1820s, and low stacked heels appeared by the mid-1820s (figs. 368, 369).

The pointed toe was no longer the dominant fashion after 1805, but pointed-toe shoes do exist that are said to have been worn in weddings in America in 1811[13] and in 1820. The 1820 date for a pointed toe is very late, but in this case the shoe also has a narrow waist placed far toward the back, a feature typical of the period 1815–30 (fig. 367). The waists of shoes 1805–15, by contrast, are often little if at all narrower than the heel end of the shoe (figs. 359–65).

French fashion plates, which at this period often show the shoes quite clearly, suggest that the transition from pointed- to round- or oval-toed shoes had taken place by 1804, and indeed, Empress Josephine's 1804 coronation slippers have oval toes. The *Lady's Magazine* for that year reports that "the ends of the shoes are still very round," but only a few months later says "the toes of ladies' shoes are no longer round, but almost pointed," as if no one style had become firmly established.[14] Documented examples with round toes include wedding shoes of 1812 and 1815 (figs. 364, 365). The very round toe and associated short vamp seem to have passed out of fashion about 1815.

The oval toe was worn at the same time as the rounder version, and it lasted longer, persisting at least through the 1820s and possibly as an alternative style through the 1830s. The earliest noted documented example is associated with a wedding of 1792,[15] but its very short vamp, more typical after 1804, suggests that at least the upper may have been altered. A more characteristic documented shoe was worn at a wedding in 1797, but it is so nearly pointed as barely to qualify as oval at all (fig. 355). Two others more clearly in the mainstream are both dated 1810 (fig. 363).[16] After 1815, the oval toe was the usual style, and many examples survive (figs. 366, 368, 369, 370).

No matter what the toe style, most shoes from the first two decades of the century are still undifferentiated for left and right feet. But in shoes circa 1824–30, right/left differentiation is fairly common (figs. 368, 370), along with stacked heels. Another feature of shoes from the late 1810s and 1820s is a very narrow waist, seen in documented examples of 1816, 1824, and 1828. In these shoes the narrowest part of the waist and the side seam tend to be placed somewhat farther back than at other periods (compare fig. 365 with fig. 369). Multiringed stamps were used in the 1820s to close and obscure the tack marks left from lasting, and in better shoes, one occasionally finds more elaborate sole finishes as well (fig. 369).

The use of wooden pegs to attach entire soles (as opposed to merely attaching heels or making repairs) was introduced in America by 1811,[17] and while pegged soles are rare in women's shoes before the 1840s, they are possible from the 1810s.

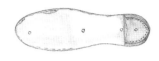

Fig. 362. 1805–15 front-lacing boot: round toe, low stacked heel, sole shaped in gentle curves. See figs. 246, 509.

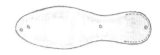

Fig. 363. 1810 wedding slipper: oval toe, spring heel, sole shaped in gentle curves. See fig. 442.

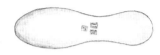

Fig. 364. 1812 wedding slipper: round toe, no heel, sole shaped in gentle curves. See figs. 421, 447.

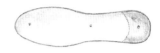

Fig. 365. 1815 wedding slipper: round toe, spring heel, sole shaped in gentle curves, heel end stained darker in typical design. See fig. 104.

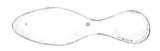

Fig. 366. 1816 slit-vamp shoe: oval toe now standard, spring heel; extremely narrow waist makes heel end look almost circular.

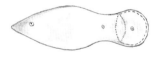

Fig. 367. 1820 wedding slipper: very late for a pointed toe, but has 1815–30 narrow waist and rounded heel end.

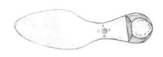

Fig. 368. 1824 evening slipper: oval toe, tapered stacked heel, very narrow waist, left/right. See figs. 341, 449.

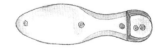

Fig. 369. ca. 1825 slit-vamp shoe: oval toe, tapered stacked heel, typical sole finish, and multiring stamps of the late 1820s. See fig. 188.

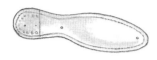

Fig. 370. 1828–30 side-lacing boot: oval toe and visible stitching channel. Left/right. See fig. 272.

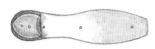

Fig. 371. 1830 wedding slipper: narrow square toe, small stacked heel, straights. See fig. 106.

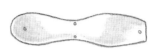

Fig. 372. 1831 wedding slipper: slightly broader square toe, no heel, waist placed more toward center. See fig. 448.

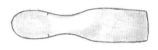

Fig. 373. 1835 wedding slipper: broad square toe typical until 1847, waist placed back of center.

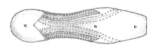

Fig. 374. 1839 side-lacing exhibition shoe: narrow square toe more typical of the early 1830s. Fancy sole finish fairly common in the 1830s.

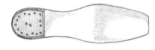

Fig. 375. 1835–45 slit-vamp shoe: square toe, rare stacked heel. See fig. 342.

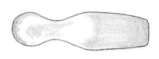

Fig. 376. 1846 slit-vamp wedding shoe: broad square tread contrasts with narrow waist and circular heel. See fig. 191.

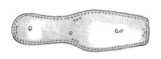

Fig. 377. 1840s utilitarian pegged slit-vamp shoe: broad toe with squared-off corners is most common sole shape ca. 1835–47. See fig. 190.

ca. 1828–ca. 1840: The next toe shape to appear in the nineteenth century is square—at first in a narrow version that looks as if a pointed toe has been chopped off near the end, and later in a broader form. Swann has found this toe on a man's shoe in an American painting of about 1819,[18] and it appears to be the type depicted in some French fashion plates even as early as 1813. The square toe appears with regularity in fashion plates by 1828. But in September 1830 the *Lady's Magazine* mentions that boots have square toes as if it were not yet taken for granted, and the only surviving documented American examples I have found with the narrow square toe are dated 1830, 1831, and 1839 (figs. 371, 372, 374). Judging from the few surviving examples, the narrow form of the square toe may never have been a very widespread style for women, or may have been quickly superseded by the broader type.

Documented shoes prove that the oval toe was worn at least until 1828, and there is some evidence to suggest that it persisted through the 1830s. But documented 1830s shoes are not common enough to provide any certainty. By the late 1830s, the trend had shifted to the broad and sharply square toe that was to be the standard style of the 1840s.

ca. 1835–ca. 1847: The broad form of the square toe appeared as early as 1835 (fig. 373), the sole being only slightly narrower at the toe than at the ball of the foot. The result is a sole where the forward part is almost rectangular in shape. The placement of the waist varies according to no very obvious rule during this period. Often, it is placed rather far back, so that the small narrow heel contrasts with the long broad tread (figs. 373, 376), but in many others, it is nearly centered.

Most shoes and boots were straights and were truly heelless in this period, having not even the single lift of the spring heel common before 1830. But though heelless, in one sense these turned shoes were less flat than before, because the soles nearly all curve upward slightly at the edges. The heel area in particular has a convex quality to the surface. This is easier to see from the side (see fig. 424). Pegged soles were increasingly available for utilitarian wear (figs. 62, 377).

ca. 1847–ca. 1870: The broad square toe, which usually had quite sharp corners in the preceding period, was now rounded off into a moderate shape that lasted thirty years. The soles of most surviving dress shoes from the 1850s and early 1860s are thin and extremely narrow—the tread is not much wider than the heel, and it is quite common to find that the soles of white satin dress slippers are only two inches across at the ball of the foot. These must be the "excruciating" French slippers mentioned by *Godey's* in 1850 as one of the sacrifices of a fashionable life[19] (fig. 378). Toward the end of the 1860s, walking boots were made somewhat broader across the sole, a trend that became more pronounced in the next decade.

After some twenty years of thin, flat soles, heels reappeared on some boots and shoes by the early 1850s—*Godey's* illustrated one in its October 1854 issue. However, heels are rare on documented surviving shoes until 1860, no doubt because flat soles were still the norm for the dressy shoes that tend to survive with histories. One surviving exception is a blue serge side-lacing boot associated with a wedding in 1852. This has a low, stacked heel, nicely tapered on the sides (fig. 380). Leather-covered wooden knock-on heels were also available, but heelless slippers continued to be made right through the 1860s.

Evening slippers continued to be made chiefly as straights, but the 1860s saw a slow drift toward making boots at least as rights and lefts. The right/left shoes of the 1860s are not as asymmetrical as those of the later nineteenth century. While the inner and outer curves are different, the sole as a whole still lies on a straight axis. Thus the outer edge is relatively straight from heel to toe, while the inner edge simply curves out farther at the ball of the foot (figs. 384, 385).

Shoes of the 1860s are more likely than those of the 1840s and 1850s to have a decorative finish on the sole. The simplest and most common of these is a darker, glossy finish forming a narrow border around the sole (figs. 382, 384). Documented examples of this practice date from 1854, 1862, and 1868.[20] Occasionally a wider band of dark finish will be added to the waist in order to make it look narrower, a practice even more common in the 1870s (fig. 383).

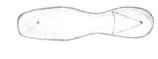

Fig. 378. 1852 side-lacing satin wedding boot: square toe with rounded-off corners; tread little broader than waist in dressy shoes 1847–67.

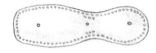

Fig. 379. 1850s utilitarian pegged slit-vamp shoe: similar to fig. 378 but broader overall. See fig. 62.

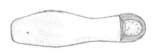

Fig. 380. 1852 side-lacing wedding boot: the small, tapered stacked heel was revived in the early 1850s, but left/right still unusual.

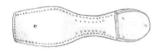

Fig. 381. 1860–75 utilitarian gored boot: heavy pegged sole with broad tread and broad, low stacked heel.

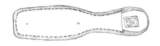

Fig. 382. 1860s everyday front-lace boot: McKay-stitched sole with visible stitches, stacked heel, and brown edge common in the 1860s.

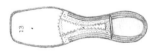

Fig. 383. 1865–75 everyday gored boot: broad tread, stacked heel, decorative finish at waist.

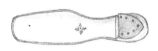

Fig. 384. 1860–65 dressy front-lace boot: narrow brown edge on sole, knock-on heel, left/right. See fig. 249.

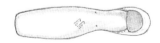

Fig. 385. 1865–70 side-lacing boot: Louis heel, left/right. See fig. 277.

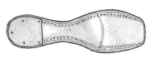

Fig. 386. 1870s Newport tie: double row of pegs on sole, narrow 1870s waist contrasts with broad tread, straight last.

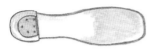

Fig. 387. 1873 wedding slipper: straight last a bit broader than on dressy shoes in the 1860s, knock-on heel. See fig. 480.

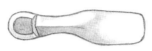

Fig. 388. 1876 side-lacing exhibition boot: knock-on heel, spade (ridged) shank, minimal left/right swing.

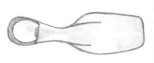

Fig. 389. 1876 side-lacing exhibition boot: common sole ornamentation, stacked heel, moderate left/right swing. See fig. 278.

Fig. 390. 1876 side-lacing exhibition boot: ornamented duck-bill sole shape, stacked heel, moderate left/right swing.

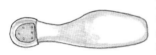

Fig. 391. 1877 buttoned boot: toe beginning to narrow slightly, knock-on heel, minimal left/right swing.

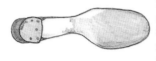

Fig. 392. 1877–80 French one-strap shoe: rounded toe, broad tread, Louis heel, moderate left/right swing. See fig. 475.

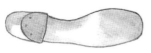

Fig. 393. 1877–85 button shoe: rounded toe, Louis heel, moderate left/right swing.

ca. 1870–ca. 1880: After the painfully narrow soles of the 1850s and early 1860s, somewhat broader ones began to appear after 1865, at least for utilitarian walking boots. But judging from contemporary remarks, the punishing narrow sole continued to be used in high-fashion footwear for some years yet (fig. 385). As late as 1875, the fashion editor of *Godey's* spoke as if broad soles were a recent innovation. "The boots worn by ladies at present are far more sensible than those lately in fashion. The design now is to give symmetrical shape and ease to the foot, rather than to cramp it into unnatural smallness. For this purpose, the best shoemakers now use French lasts, made precisely the shape of the foot, outlining the taper of the foot on top, and giving ample width of sole."[21] Two years later, the progress was confirmed. "There are but few changes in the styles of ladies' shoes. Each year brings into more general use comfortable broad shoes, that have full, wide soles, with extension edges. These prevent crowding, and leave the foot in its natural symmetrical proportions."[22]

The most stylish examples during this decade set off the wide forepart with a very narrow waist made to look even narrower by shiny finishes in elaborate designs and sometimes in two colors (figs. 389, 390). In well-made examples, the sole may be domed at the waist (fig. 388). The actual toe shape—a rounded-off square—did not really change, but the increased width makes it look boxier than the toes of the 1850s and 1860s. The toe became gradually more narrow and rounded at the very end of the 1870s. *Demorest's* mentions both narrow and broad toes being worn in 1879.[23]

By 1870, nearly all women's shoes had heels, Louis as well as the stacked and knock-on types, and some were quite high. The trend continued toward differentiating for left and right feet, though many dress slippers were still straights.

In the 1860s and 1870s, shoes and boots with pegged soles were made in enormous quantities for men, children, and to a lesser extent for women (fig. 386). Since pegging was normally used only for utilitarian footwear, pegged shoes were rarely preserved intentionally, but they do show up in quantity in the rubbish heaps of nineteenth-century archaeological sites.

ca. 1880–ca. 1895: Beginning in the very late 1870s, the broad, squarish toe gradually narrowed into a rounded shape and then into an oval that could be quite narrow by the mid-1890s (figs. 392–99). Right/left differentiation became the norm, although the shaping was not as asymmetrical as it could be later; and straight shoes continued to be made, especially in the dressier kinds of slippers. Heels were universal for adult women. The simpler kinds of sole decoration persisted (figs. 396, 399), but the age when shoes were as pretty on the bottom as on the top ended with the 1870s.

ca. 1893–ca. 1930: Shoes of this period can rarely be dated merely by looking at their soles. All have heels, generally higher than before, and nearly all are rights and lefts. The narrow waists contrast sharply with the broad sole at the ball of the foot. The right/left asymmetry, or "swing" in the last, tends to be more pronounced than before, but this waxes and wanes like any other fashion, tending to be less striking when toes are broad and vamps shorter. What makes identification most difficult is that more than one last was widely offered in each period from the mid-1890s on (fig. 409). As a rule, the narrower and more pointed lasts within any one period were used on the dressier shoes, and the broader toes on the sportier or more utilitarian shoes. Nevertheless, allowing for exceptions, the following generalizations often hold true.

In the early 1890s, toes were usually a moderate oval, but the trend was toward narrower and narrower styles. *Godey's* reported in 1894 that "although the French models are very graceful, English lasts are the most in vogue. All the French shoes have very pointed toes. . . . [Patent-leather slippers] must, of course, have a long, pointed toe"[24] (figs. 399, 400).

By the mid-1890s many shoes were made with a very shallow, narrow, and elongated toe ending in either a sharp point that was described by the 1897 Sears catalog as a "long, drawn-out needle toe" or a

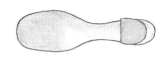

Fig. 394. 1881 wedding slipper: round toe, knock-on heel. Straight last still common for evening shoes. See also fig. 483.

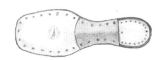

Fig. 395. 1880s utilitarian front-lacing boot: round toe, stacked heel, straight last, "standard screw" sole attachment. See fig. 253.

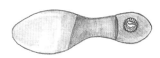

Fig. 396. 1885–92 button boot: oval toe, stacked heel, minimal left/right swing. See fig. 265.

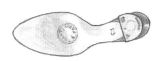

Fig. 397. 1885–90 French cross-bar shoe: oval toe, Louis heel, strong left/right swing.

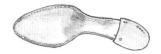

Fig. 398. 1890 button wedding boot: oval toe, stacked heel, pronounced left/right swing.

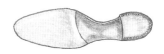

Fig. 399. 1893 front-lacing exhibition boot: oval toe, stacked heel, common sole finish, minimal left/right swing.

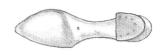

Fig. 400. 1896 silk T-strap: long pointed toe, knock-on heel, minimal left/right swing. See fig. 135.

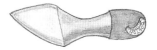

Fig. 401. 1898 oxford shoe: long pointed toe, stacked heel, moderate left/right swing.

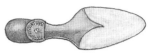

Fig. 402. 1901 dressy tie shoe: oval "coin" toe, Louis heel, minimal left/right swing.

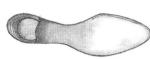

Fig. 403. 1904–5 Colonial: long oval toe, stacked heel, moderate left/right swing. See fig. 347.

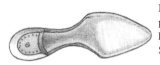

Fig. 404. 1908 one-eyelet tie: pointed oval toe, knock-on heel, strong left/right swing. See fig. 502.

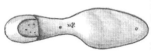

Fig. 405. 1911 wedding one-strap: shorter oval toe, high knock-on heel, minimal right/left swing.

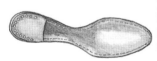

Fig. 406. 1911–14 button boot: rounded toe, stacked heel, moderate right/left swing.

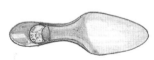

Fig. 407. 1915 advertisement for Cat's Paw rubber heels: longer oval toe, minimal right/left swing.

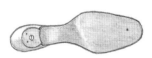

Fig. 408. 1916 front-lace boot: rounded toe, very high Louis heel, minimal right/left swing.

very narrow oval known as a coin toe, or a narrow square (figs. 41, 400, 401). Women who rejected such painful fashions could dress in dowdy shoes made over "common sense" lasts with a broad rounded toe and a low broad heel.

The pointed needle toe did not last more than a few years in the late 1890s, but the coin toe continued into the new century. Coin lasts were so called because they had round but very shallow toes. They varied in width and were described in terms of the coins they mirrored in size: dime toes were nearly pointed, toes the size of a quarter were somewhat less extreme, half-dollar toes approached a fashionable compromise with rationality. In general the toes of the period 1900–1905 were oval or rounded, and the forepart was slightly shorter than that of the 1890s (figs. 402, 403).

Beginning in 1905, some shoes began to be made with a shorter, deeper vamp and a narrower oval, very nearly pointed toe. This was a decided fashion by 1906 and continued through 1910 (fig. 404). The vamp or forepart continued to shorten at the end of the decade, and the short vamp effect was quite exaggerated in the years 1911 to 1913, especially as it often appeared in conjunction with a broader rounded toe that bulged upward at the very end, and a short stubby straight toe cap (figs. 405, 406).

From the extremely short-vamped, round-toed shoe of 1911–13, fashion moved to the opposite extreme, and, by the end of the decade, long vamps with extremely pointed toes were all the rage. The transitional years between the two styles were 1914 to 1916 (figs. 407–9). During 1914 especially, a great many different lasts were being offered. At one extreme, women in midwestern towns were still firmly loyal to the comfortable short, round stubby toe shape of the early teens, while the most advanced New York shoes already had vamps four inches long, a length not reached by the fashion mainstream until 1917[25] (fig. 410). At the same time, any one woman might own dressier shoes with relatively pointed toes and walking shoes with quite rounded ones.

The very long, pointed toe returned for nearly all footwear in 1916–17 (fig. 410) and continued very strong into the early 1920s. This was almost as extreme as the toes of the late 1890s, except that in the new version the vamp was not nearly so shallow. In the fall of 1921, Rochester shoemakers reported in connection with the new styles for spring 1922 that "lasts have undergone a remarkable change. The slender toes that sold a year ago, and which expanded slightly at the point in the spring, are now well rounded, some being broad enough to accommodate a silver half dollar, others an American quarter—and there is nothing that will not accommodate a dime. Last season many lasts were shortened and slightly rounded, while this season the last makers are in clover because of the decided change to roomy toes and square toes"[26] (fig. 411).

This interest in shorter vamps and broader toes, which was inspired by contemporary French styles, continued to be a factor in shoe styles throughout the 1920s, so that one finds a variety of lasts ranging from relatively narrow ovals to quite broad and square toes. The *Shoe Retailer* notes more than once that the American lasts tended to have longer vamps and narrower toes than their French prototypes, and these lasts are often described as "modified." "Manufacturers are shying away from the dollar toe or anything which is purely reflective of the French idea. American women do not like stubby foreparts, so the French lasts Americanized are fairly pointed at the end."[27] Nevertheless, there was a clear drift during the 1920s toward shorter vamps and stubbier toes, whether rounded or squarish (figs. 413–17).

With a broad choice in lasts, the narrow-toed styles tended to appear in the dressier shoes (and these are what usually survive), while the broader square-toed lasts were used for sportier shoes (fig. 417) and street oxfords. However, there were other distinctions as well. The *Shoe Retailer* says in 1926 that shoes with a short vamp and round toe were noticeably less popular in New England and the mid-Atlantic states than they were in the rest of the country.[28] One of the regional style charts published in 1928 notes that short vamps with square toes sold well on the cheaper shoes, but long vamps with narrower toes in the better-quality footwear.[29]

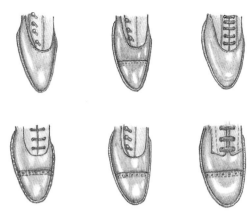

Fig. 409. 1915 boot lasts advertisement, G & R Shoe Company: (*top row, left to right*) Recede, Medium Recede, Narrow Stage (*bottom row, left to right*) English, Medium, Growing Girls.

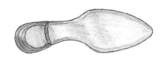

Fig. 410. 1918 advertisement for Neolin Soles: long pointed toe, high Louis heel, strong right/left swing in the last.

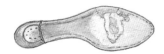

Fig. 414. 1931 oxford: oval toe, covered wood heel, well-worn sole, strong right/left swing.

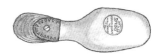

Fig. 411. 1922 cross-strap shoe: short-vamped round-toed French last became more important in the later 1920s. Moderate right/left swing.

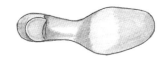

Fig. 415. 1928 cross-strap shoe: rounded toe, very high heel, strong right/left swing in the last.

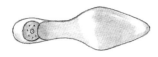

Fig. 412. 1923 wedding slipper: long pointed toe and high Louis heel a bit old-fashioned, minimal right/left swing.

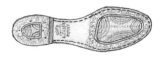

Fig. 416. 1928 advertisement for Plytex rubber sole: broad toe for sports, minimal right/left swing.

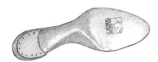

Fig. 413. 1923 button shoe: moderate oval toe, covered wood heel, strong right/left swing.

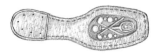

Fig. 417. 1933 sports shoe: square toe common on sports, cheaper shoes by late 1920s. Moderate right/left swing. Sports design pressed in rubber sole.

CHAPTER TEN

Variations in Lasts

While the upper pattern determines where the seams will come on a shoe, and whether it is a slipper, tie shoe, or boot, the wooden last over which a shoe is made is what gives it its distinctive three-dimensional shape, mass, and volume. The last is responsible for producing the characteristic profile of a shoe, the shape of the toe and its depth, and the angle of rise in the upper from the toe toward the instep. The shape of the last also governs the subtle curves of the sole. Sole leather, when it is first cut out, is quite flat. But when it is formed to the shape of the last and stitched to the upper, it acquires bends and curves, not only the bend upward toward any heel the shoe may have but also the upward curve at the toe and the slightly up-curved sides. The last is also what produces the differentiation in shape for right and left feet, while the upper pattern is sometimes identical for both.

Toe Profile and Instep

The single most conspicuous element in a shoe is the shape of the toe. The toe shape as seen from the bottom (pointed, oval, round, or square) is discussed in chapter 9, but the toe may also be distinctive from the side. The most common toe "profile" for women's shoes is called in the trade a recede toe, defined as one whose profile is comparatively narrow and pointed rather than blunt. The angle formed between

sole and upper in a recede toe is closer to forty-five degrees than the ninety-degree angle of a blunt toe.

The toe profile even of a recede toe, however, is affected by the way the sole and upper are sewn together. In welted and McKay-sewn shoes, the upper must first pass up and around the edge of the insole before receding back toward the instep. In turn shoes, because there is no insole, the upper and its lining merely fold back over a line of stitching. Thus, the most acute recede toe is possible in a turned shoe (figs. 418–19). Although the modern term may not yet have been in use, most nineteenth-century women's shoes through the 1870s had recede toes, simply because they were made of fabric or thin leather without any extra toe stiffening (figs. 421–24). Such soft-toed shoes crush easily and often emerge from decades of storage entirely flattened.

A shoe intended to retain a blunt shape generally incorporates a stiff lining called a toe box between the upper and the regular upper lining. It should be noted, however, that a similar stiffening effect can also be created by an external toe cap such as was added to women's utilitarian leather boots by the late 1860s (fig. 420). The toe box for ordinary shoes was generally made of leather or buckram (in protective boots it can be of steel), and an early reference to it for nineteenth-century women's dressy shoes appears in *Demorest's* for 1879: "Heels a little over one inch

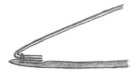

Fig. 418. Recede toe without boxing in a turned shoe: it is possible to form a very sharp angle at the toe end.

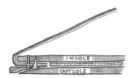

Fig. 419. Recede toe without boxing in a McKay shoe: the upper wraps around the insole edge before angling back (same effect occurs in welted shoes).

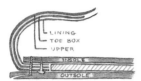

Fig. 420. Boxed toe: allows, if desired, a 90-degree angle with the sole, like a vertical wall at the toe end.

high, with boxed toes, both narrow and broad, are still the prevailing fashion for both ladies and children."[1] Toe boxes seem to have come into use in the mid-1870s in connection with the new trend toward more substantial footwear. A boot shown by Goodrich and Porter at the 1876 Centennial Exhibition incorporates the new toe box as a point of fashion, having a domed toe reminiscent of those worn by women in the late seventeenth century and by men into the eighteenth century (fig. 428).

The deep, blunt toe made possible by the toe box appeared more and more frequently from the early 1880s. A distinctive snub-nosed toe effect appeared even on dressy slippers in the early 1890s (figs. 42, 429). This extra depth made any shoe more comfortable and was particularly helpful when the vamp was rather short, as it was in the 1880s and very early 1890s. However, it took some time for the toe box to become universal, and silk evening slippers were sometimes made without it even after 1900.

In the late 1890s, the long, shallow "needle toe" became fashionable, and the toe box preserved the shape of the extreme end where it would not be filled by the foot (fig. 430). In reaction to such shallow toes, which lasted until about 1905, shoe fashions then began to swing toward deeper vamps. What was known in America as the high or full toe (and in England as a Boston or bulldog toe) began to develop in 1906 (fig. 432) and reached its extreme in the years 1911–13, when it formed a knobby bulge at the end of the shoe (fig. 433). Its most extreme form is most likely to appear on a short-vamped buttoned boot with a stubby straight toe cap (fig. 268). The dressy slippers made in the same period are not nearly as distinctive (figs. 93, 139). The high toe may be less fully represented in eastern museum collections, since it was apparently not as popular on the East Coast as elsewhere. The *Shoe Retailer* commented on several occasions that although "full round toes are to be the predominating features in lasts, especially for the Western trade, New York and vicinity still want medium narrow toes and do not seem to care for the high nob effects."[2]

The full toe was superseded in 1914 by a relatively deep recede toe stiffened by a toe box. This rational medium, however, lasted only a couple of years (fig. 269). By 1917, vamps became very long with pointed toes made over extremely shallow lasts, much like those of the late 1890s (fig. 434). Toes gained in depth about 1923, and moderate styles continued throughout the 1920s (figs. 150–58). At the same time, however, some short-vamped styles with square toes were quite blunt in outline (fig. 435).

Another style factor in the shape of the last is the treatment of the instep, since a high instep was considered an attractive feature. As early as 1823, the rationale given for slippers with shorter vamps was to "discover the beauty of the instep."[3] Skirts were too full and long from 1835 to 1865 for insteps to be of much importance, but with the shorter walking skirts of the late 1860s, they returned as an object of concern. In February 1871, *Godey's* noted that "the newest idea is to have the lacing begin at the foxing, and curve upward, giving ample room for a high instep," and a few months later it passed along the rumor "that false insteps and false eyelashes are among the late inventions."[4] Whether required by nature or artifice, many 1870s boots do have a higher instep than was typical in the 1860s. This was achieved simply by increasing the angle formed between sole and upper at the toe, from which the vamp rises inexorably to the thickened instep (fig. 426).

One of the effects of the long, shallow toe of the later 1890s was that it contrasted sharply with the instep rising behind it. In the most extreme examples, the vamp was made more shallow than seems possible over the ball of the foot, rising at the last moment in a dramatic hump over the instep (fig. 431). The abruptly humping instep continued to be a feature of fashionable boots into the early 1910s, and was used on men's shoes as well as women's. The best description of them is quoted by Swann from Max Beerbohm's *Zuleika Dobson* (1911): "so slim and long were they, of instep so nobly arched, that only with a pair of glazed ox-tongues on a breakfast table were they comparable."[5]

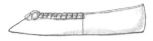

Fig. 421. The toes of most early-nineteenth-century shoes have no stiffening. As in this 1812 shoe, the soles are often quite flat.

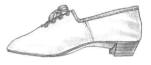

Fig. 422. In the 1820s the center of the sole was often thicker from the waist back, forming a domed waist when used with a stacked heel.

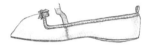

Fig. 423. Before 1840 many shoes had only a slightly curved sole, as in this 1837 slipper.

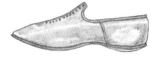

Fig. 424. Marked toe spring and greater curve in the sole were more common after 1840, as in this 1850s slit-vamp.

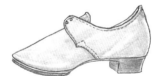

Fig. 425. Between 1865 and 1885 the marked toe-spring was more common in everyday footwear, as on this 1870s pegged Newport.

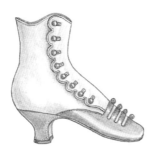

Fig. 426. Many high-style boots and shoes made between 1867 and 1881 barely touch the ground at the tip of the toe, emphasizing the high instep.

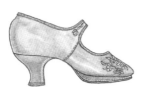

Fig. 427. The wedged sole of this French strap shoe (ca. 1877–80) permits both the high instep and firm contact with the ground.

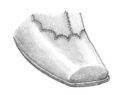

Fig. 428. Boxing made new toe shapes possible, such as the dome toe on this 1876 exhibition or the 1891 snub-nose toe in fig. 42.

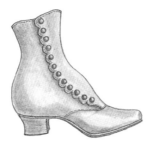

Fig. 429. The high toe spring returned to fashion 1882–93 while boxing added toe depth to many short-vamped walking boots. This one 1892.

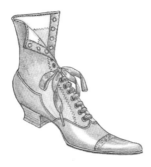

Fig. 430. The long needle-point toes of 1894–1900 would buckle when worn without boxing to support them. This one 1897.

Even in the 1920s, the high instep was being touted as an important attraction. A September 1928 advertisement in the *Ladies' Home Journal* for Arch Preserver Shoes, made by the Selby Shoe Company of Portsmouth, Ohio, warned readers, "You know, yourself, that the foot's chief claim to beauty is its perfectly curved instep. When you wear shoes that let the arch sag, the instep flattens, and the foot's aristocratic shapeliness is gone. This tragedy need not happen to you. It is forestalled forever by the famous arch bridge and other patented features in every Arch Preserver Shoe."

Toe Spring and Other Curves in the Sole

Just as the last determines the form and volume of the upper, most conspicuously the shape of the toe, it also governs the contours of the sole. "Toe spring" is the term for the upward curve of the sole at the toe end. A shoe that has no toe spring at all is said to have a "flat forepart." When high heels gave way to spring heels and then no heels in the 1790s and early 1800s, the soles of women's slippers were often truly flat, being made without even the gentlest echo of the natural curves of the foot. Tabitha Dana Leach's wedding slippers of 1812, for example, are impressive in their flatness and thinness and must have been uncomfortable to wear on anything but the smoothest floor or softest carpet[6] (fig. 421). Gradually, however, more shoes were made over lasts that rounded up slightly at the toe, arch, and sides, and these moderately contoured examples (figure 423 is typical) are found side by side with very flat soles all through the early nineteenth century.

The toe spring is usually moderate in women's footwear, but there are certain periods in which it is slightly more marked. Swann refers to *The Adventures of Tom Sawyer*, in which Mark Twain recalls the sharply turned-up toes of men's shoes in the 1840s.[7] Most women's shoes from that decade, certainly the dressy ones that tend to survive, fail to evince any extraordinary toe spring, perhaps because women did not spend their leisure hours with their toes against a wall like the young men of Twain's recollection. But the 1840s were a period when most women's shoes were still entirely heelless and not very comfortable for walking. An attempt was occasionally was made to compensate for this by shaping the sole more fully to the curves of the foot, bending it upward at the toe and the arch and cupping it around the heel. In some shoes, a fairly thick piece of sole leather was used that was then thinned out at the sides so that it did not appear so heavy, creating a domed effect on the sole. The shoe illustrated in figure 424 is rounded to fit around the heel of the foot, but the sole beneath the heel is still comparatively thick in the middle.

Toe spring was minimized in many stylish shoes during the 1870s. In fact, the point of greatest ground contact other than the heel was often the point of the toe. Instead of lying flat to the ground under the ball of the foot and then bending upward at the arch, the soles of chic 1870s shoes gradually angle up from the toe in a most implausible way. Seeing illustrations of such shoes, one would suppose that fashion artists had not yet learned how to draw high-heeled shoes, were it not that so many surviving shoes have the same feature (fig. 426). One exceptional French shoe of this period solves the problem by blocking up the sole at the ball so that the tread contacts the floor but the foot itself lies on a slope (fig. 427).

The awkward sole line of 1870s shoes passed out of fashion in the early 1880s for one in which the ball rests firmly on the ground and the toe rises slightly off it. Most shoes of the later nineteenth century display only moderate toe spring, but there were a few in which it was more pronounced in both the 1880s and 1890s (fig. 429).

Perhaps in reaction against the toe spring of the later nineteenth century, from about 1901 high-style shoes were made with a flat forepart; that is, without any toe spring at all. These shoes also tended to have a sharp break or corner where the flat tread turned upward toward the heel (fig. 431). The sharp break moderated about 1909 but the predilection for minimal toe spring seems to be a permanent feature of early twentieth-century shoes. Surviving shoes, it is true, do not always sit perfectly flat at the toe, but contemporary shoe illustrations are drawn as if they were supposed to.

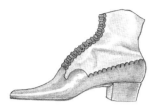

Fig. 431. Shallow but stiff flat foreparts were stylish from about 1900, as was the dramatic hump at the instep.

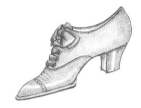

Fig. 432. Shoe designers tried out subtle new toe shapes supported by boxing 1906–16. This 1908 boot has the new deeper, narrower toe.

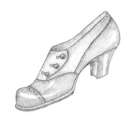

Fig. 433. Bulbous boxed toes peaked 1911–13, but slipper toes rarely bulged, though deeper and narrower than in 1900–1905. Compare figs. 91, 93, 139.

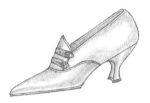

Fig. 434. In contrast to the high toes of the early teens, the long, pointed toes of 1917–21 were extremely shallow.

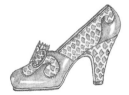

Fig. 435. From 1923 those shoes made with short vamps and square toes were more likely to have a blunt toe than were shoes with longer vamps.

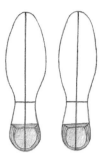

Fig. 436. Straight soles, not differentiated at all for right and left feet.

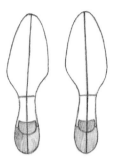

Fig. 437. Soles moderately differentiated for right and left feet, although the axis is still fairly straight.

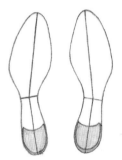

Fig. 438. Soles with strong swing (curve on the outside of the foot) and an axis that bends at the waist.

Right/Left Differentiation

Whether a shoe is shaped specifically for the right or left foot is a result of the shape of the last over which the shoe is made. Even when shoes are clearly lefts and rights, there are periods where the difference is more pronounced than at others (this is a matter of fashion just like anything else). Lasts that are more obviously altered for the different feet are said to have more swing, a term that refers to the outer curve of the sole (figs. 436–38). Another way to identify left/right differentiation is to determine whether an imaginary line drawn down the middle of the sole from the center back seam to the waist can continue toward the center of the toe without changing its direction at the waist. The greater the change of angle at the waist, the more swing is built into the shoe.

Shoes had been made as lefts and rights up through the sixteenth century, but in the seventeenth and eighteenth centuries most were made as "straights"; that is, the same shape for both feet. Men's shoes gradually began to be made in rights and lefts from the 1790s,[8] but among the dressier women's shoes that tend to survive, right/left differentiation is not common until the 1880s, and straight shoes for women were made well into the twentieth century. Nevertheless, women's shoes could be, and were, made in rights and lefts all through the period covered by this book. The invention of the pantograph and the development of a mechanized shoe industry in the 1860s may have played some role in making lefts/rights standard in the second half of the century, but they do not account for the fact that straight styling persisted longest among the dressiest shoes. Perhaps the symmetrical foot was considered an aesthetic advantage worth retaining for dressy footwear long after it had been rejected in everyday shoes because of the imperfect fit.

Left/right differentiation in nineteenth-century women's shoes first appeared in significant quantity in the 1820s, when there is a flurry of interest both in heels and rights/lefts. Shoes and boots of the 1830s–50s were rarely differentiated in the shapes of their soles. However, many evening slippers of this period were marked "droit" and "gauche" in the sock lining, so that one could, if desired, wear the same one always on the same foot—or else regularly alternate them. Shoes placed on alternate feet every day wore evenly instead of developing holes in one particular spot. "Ladies who are apt to run down shoes at the heel, would find gaiters that open in front, or the congress gaiters, to be more suitable for them. Such not being rights and lefts."[9] That is, even though their soles were cut straight, side-lacing boots were not so suitable for alternating because the lacing had to go on the inside of the ankle (otherwise it is extremely awkward to lace up). Right/left differentiation became very common in women's walking boots from the 1860s on, but dressy boots and evening slippers continued to be made as straights into the 1880s and even later, and since these are what survive in greatest quantity, museum collections show even less right/left differentiation than there really was. The issue was clearly not settled by 1879, or *Demorest's* would not have felt the need to write, "There used to be an old-fashioned notion about 'changing' the shoes to 'keep them straight.' Just take a good look at your feet, and you will observe that they are hollowed beneath the instep inside and the outer side of each foot touches the floor if you try to take a solid stand. There is then just as much reason in 'changing' gloves as in 'changing' shoes to keep them straight, and shoemakers realize the fact that intelligent customers want a shoe for each foot, a right shoe and a left shoe."[10]

From about 1904, lasts came into fashion that were more than usually unlike on the inner and outer sides, the inner side being nearly straight from the ball forward, and the outer one having a pronounced swing or curve (figs. 403, 404). This style grew in popularity toward 1906. In reporting on the new styles being offered for 1907, a Lynn shoe representative commented that "smart dressers will want some of the extreme shapes, but the most popular last will be straight with a little swing. Short foreparts will continue in vogue, but the pronounced swing will not be so much in evidence." But on the very same page a last maker warns that "shoe dealers should look very carefully when they are buying narrow toe shoes and get the swing in the last so there will be plenty of room for the feet."[11]

With the full, round toes that were especially popular in the Midwest in the early teens, a straighter last became more practical (figs. 406, 407). The *Shoe Retailer*, in previewing styles for spring 1912, noted that "the most pronounced effect in lasts is the improvement of the pump last with a tendency to straighter lines, wider bottoms and more wood over the toes. Retailers will gladly welcome the better fitting features which prevail the current season than in any previous period when extreme low cuts and shortened foreparts have predominated."[12]

CHAPTER ELEVEN

Materials and Decoration

As described in chapter 2, prevailing concepts of womanhood in the earlier nineteenth century encouraged women to choose very light, thin-soled shoes, while in the later nineteenth century they were allowed more substantial shoes and boots and, by 1900, even conspicuously mannish footwear. But the materials and ornamentation chosen for footwear depended not only on current social conditions but also on a complex interrelationship of aesthetics, utility, etiquette, and class. When skirts were short enough to show the foot, shoes and boots were often made of bright-colored materials, in more complex patterns, and with more ornamentation. When feet were hidden, footwear tended to be simpler. As a matter of both practicality and etiquette, shoes and boots for working and walking would typically be made in comparatively substantial leathers in neutral colors like black and tan. Special-occasion shoes, having to tolerate less wear, could be made of less practical materials like silk and in more conspicuous colors. The wealthy could afford shoes made in the same material as a particular dress, while less affluent folk would choose all-purpose colors like black or white, even in satin evening shoes. Class issues, however, did not always allot the most elaborate or colorful shoes to the wealthy. The poor materials used in cheap shoes were sometimes camouflaged by the use of bright dyes and overdecoration.

Since it was often the material rather than the pattern that made a shoe appropriate for one occasion rather than another, it is helpful to read chapter 4 on shoe etiquette along with this one. Because shoes and boots tended to be worn for differing occasions and because their cut required different kinds of ornamentation, this chapter is divided into two parts: the first describing typical materials, colors, and ornamentation in shoes, the second describing the same for boots. (See pages 250–56 and 263–65 for figures.)

Materials and Ornamentation in Shoes
ca. 1795–ca. 1815 (see figs. 439–47)

Among surviving shoes of this period, kid leather is about twice as common as silk or satin. Silks were usually either solid in color or striped. The rich floral brocades typical of mid-eighteenth-century shoes had gone out of fashion by the 1780s and even the tiny spotted silks of the 1780s were no longer typical after 1795. White shoes were worn, especially for the most formal occasions, but the period is memorable for its use of bright, clear colors: clear pink, lemon yellow, light blue, aqua blue, and occasionally bright red, purple, and pea green. The lighter-colored leathers were sometimes stamped with an all-over or border design in black, and there is at least one example of a darker color—purple—with the design in tan.[1] A pair at the Boston Museum of Fine Arts is of silvered leather.[2]

These bright shoes provided a splash of color that set off the many white dresses, and fashion plates usually show them with matching gloves, bonnet, or ribbon trims.

A few shoes have uppers made of two materials: kid and either silk or cotton. The Valentine Museum has a pair with white silk vamp and white kid quarters stamped with black,[3] but the more common pattern is an upper part of silk or cotton with a foxing of kid running round the lower edge of the shoe. The Boston Museum of Fine Arts has a pair of bright red morocco sandal shoes with uppers of tannish cotton, possibly nankeen, bound with red silk and tied with red ribbons.[4] A pair of light-blue kid slippers with brown cotton above survives at the Peabody Essex Museum.[5] In each case, one straight and one wavy row of chain-stitching is used to sew the leather onto the fabric, and this decorative stitching also forms a bowlike figure on the vamp. One example in this distinctive style is said to be a wedding shoe of 1797.[6]

Another shoe type found of this period has cutouts in a leather vamp. The cutouts are backed with satin, which may be embroidered with silver thread and sequins, and the edges are stitched down with chain stitching. Documented examples date 1801, 1810, and 1811.[7] Compare these with shoes dating 1855–80 that use a similar cutout technique but more elaborate patterns (figs. 467–71).

Simpler shoes were trimmed at the throat with a ribbon bow, a pinked leather or ribbon rosette, a fringed silk tassel sometimes secured by a tiny buckle, or silver thread and sequin embroidery. The *Lady's Magazine* for 1804 reports that "white shoes are worn, with a small branch or some kind of figure embroidered in silver."[8] Others were left quite plain. The use of a pleated length of ribbon to edge the throat persisted from the 1780s and 1790s and was also common in the next period.

In many of these early shoes, the side and back seams as well as the top edge are bound with silk tape about three-eighths of an inch wide in a harmonizing color. But in kid shoes, the side seams may be plain outside and reinforced on the inside with a strip of kid in some other fashionable shoe color. A white shoe may have pink reinforcements, a pink one may have blue, etcetera. The top edge may be bound with silk tape or have a leather binding that looks like the corded piping used in dresses.

1815–1830 (see figs. 448–53)

After 1815, the trend was away from bright colors. Among surviving shoes, grass green persists and one sees an occasional purple, but other colors tend toward the pastels: pale pink, light green, golden brown, light or aqua blue. Colors were now reserved almost entirely for day wear. Very gradually, gray, neutral shades of brown, and later black became more important in walking shoes. *La Belle Assemblée* reports that in Paris in August 1819, "grey shoes are universal; they are extremely convenient at this season of the year, either for the dusty suburbs, or for the well known poussière de Paris." Bronze shoes were mentioned as early as 1823,[9] but it is not clear whether the iridescent bronze produced by cochineal dye on leather was meant, or merely a greenish-brown color.

Shoes continued to be made of both kid and silk, but in the 1820s, silks woven with a small diaper pattern were used as often as plain satin. Soon after 1815, wool worsted also became very common. Worsted shoe fabrics are stout warp-faced twills with a smooth satinlike face or a small woven figure. They may have double warps and may show a different color on the back. They appear in black, white, shades of brown and tan, and in colors. Jean, a sturdy twilled or satin-weave cotton of the sort found in early nineteenth-century corsets, is mentioned as a shoe fabric in fashion periodicals by 1812,[10] and by 1820 we read of shoes made of "gros de Naples," a stout plain weave silk with a corded effect.[11]

A slipper at Old Sturbridge Village is made of blue and white ticking, the white stripes worked with overlapped cross-stitching in cream, brown, and green.[12] The Sturbridge example may date as early as 1815, but the technique was recommended as late as 1856 in *Every Lady Her Own Shoemaker*: "Quite a handsome shoe can be made of bed-ticking; when worked with worsted the material would hardly be known. Let the stripe run lengthwise, from the heel to the toe, and work the light stripe in cross-stitch, with two shades of worsted, that form a pleasing contrast, one over the other; say crimson and green; or rose color and brown; or straw color and purple. This is very good for gentlemen's slippers, and is very serviceable."[13] The Sturbridge slippers are in a woman's size and have a large blue silk bow on the vamp.

After 1815, shoes were much less elaborately ornamented. Stamped leather went out of fashion and cutouts were rare. Bows and rosettes at the throatline continued. In shoes of the early 1820s it is common to find two or three large bows nearly covering the long vamp (these bows are functional in tie shoes), but by the later 1820s, a relatively small round ribbon rosette is more usual. Another decoration characteristic of the period is a length of pleated ribbon edging the throatline. Silk tape is still used to bind the top edge, but it rarely covers the seams. Instead one finds a plain seam that in fabric uppers is reinforced with two rows of top stitching along the join.

1830–1850 (see figs. 454–57)

Shoes are less and less often described in fashion plates in this period, and to compound the problem, relatively few documented examples survive until the mid-1840s. There is enough evidence to be certain that full dress shoes were still usually made of white satin, but an increasing number of plates show black satin shoes with evening dress, though the use of black of itself was not apparently sufficient cause for remark in 1832: "The shoes are black satin, elegantly embroidered on the front of the foot, in colours to match the ribbons of the dress. All dress shoes are now embroidered"[14] (the word "all" should be taken with a grain of salt in this as in all other pronouncements about fashion). Once the skirts lengthened to obscure the foot in 1834, there was little point in lavishing much decoration on shoes (but see plate 5 for an exception). Most slippers have only a small silk bow at the throatline, and in the slippers imported from Viault/Esté/Thierry of Paris and London, the bow is minute, often being made of the same silk tape that binds the top edge. It should be noted that while these French shoes seem to have been made with only tiny bows, larger rosettes have very often been stitched over them by the retailer or the wearer.

The *Lady's Magazine* reported in October 1834 that "shoes and gaiters, or brodequins, as nearly the colour of the dress as possible, are more distingué than any others. Black shoes are, of course, always fashionable." Although fashion magazines throughout the century repeatedly refer to shoes matching the color or even the fabric of the dress, this must have been an expensive fashion that was indulged in only for rather special outfits. When the shoe remained invisible much of the time and neutral practical colors like black, gray, brown, and fawn were considered in perfectly good taste, most women must have considered it better sense and better economy to buy plain black shoes that could be worn with any dress.

Shoes continued to be made of silk, satin, and worsted, but fashionable shoes made entirely of leather became noticeably less common than they had been at the beginning of the century. The most important exceptions are the beige, fawn, and pumpkin-pie-colored kid and morocco slippers and low tie shoes that survive in some quantity, chiefly from the 1840s. These were fashionable enough to be worn with wedding day dresses. Black kid and morocco shoes also survive, but these were probably more or less everyday shoes, rather than high-fashion items. Other day shoes of the 1830s and 1840s have uppers of fancy serge (with diapering or sometimes even a minute plaid) foxed with kid, much like diminished boots (fig. 211).

ca. 1850–ca. 1870 (see figs. 458–68)

Slippers were made of worsted, kid, or morocco (for day), black satin (for dressy day or evening), and white satin (for the most formal of evening events). Bronze leather also became quite popular in this period. Bronze is a slightly iridescent or metallic-looking bronzy brown finish for kid or calf made from cochineal dye (the same cochineal, made from the bodies of a South American beetle, will dye fabric brilliant red). Boudoir slippers, always the most elaborate midcentury footwear, were made of embroidered velvet, Berlin work, or other fancywork, including straw—which characteristically was trimmed with pink or blue silk rosettes and pleated ribbons. By the 1860s, slippers were held on with a one-eighth-inch elastic band rather than narrow ribbon ties. Swann dates this change in England to the 1840s,[15] but I have not found it that early in the United States, perhaps because our rubber-thread industry was not as advanced.

The small bow at the throats of 1830s and 1840s slippers was replaced in the 1850s and 1860s by a more ostentatious bow or rosette. The earliest illustration I have found of the return of trimming on midcentury shoes is a fair-sized bow peeking beneath the skirt in a plate in *La Belle Assemblée* for October 1846. *Godey's* first mentions a small bow ornamenting the instep when reporting the new rounded square toe in May of 1849. Both bows and rosettes seem to have been used from the beginning of this fashion, and while they were usually placed at the instep, they were occasionally positioned farther down toward the toe. Lace mixed with the ribbon is mentioned by 1853, ribbons edged with a color by 1855, and rosettes ornamented with a steel buckle are illustrated in 1854 and reported as typical by 1860.[16] Among surviving shoes, documented wedding shoes of the early 1860s often have a rather broad oval bow or rosette. By the mid-1860s, the rosette is likely to be made of very thin and papery silk ribbon in a roughly circular shape with a little steel buckle in the middle. Another common form is a semi-spherical pompon-shaped rosette, of which a documented example survives from 1866.[17] By 1870, the rosette enlarged to become a long oval extending well above the throatline, and was often made of leather to match the upper; an alternative was to have a bow centered on each of two or three half-inch-wide elastic straps passing over the instep.

Two styles of ornament from the pre-1830 period were revived in the 1850s, both of them used primarily on the boudoir slippers worn with luxurious wrappers by leisured women in the morning at home. The first was a pleated ribbon at the throatline, now sometimes bordering the entire top edge. *Godey's* mentions this in February 1855, and it is seen into the early 1880s. The second was the pierced and embroidered vamp that had last been in fashion 1795–1815 and reappeared by 1854, perhaps earlier. Pierced vamps generally appear in bronze slippers backed with colored silk (usually rose or blue) beneath the cutouts. Each hole is edged with chain stitching to reinforce the leather edges and keep the satin inlay in place. In this period, the stitching borders the cutouts with decorative loops rather than the wavy pattern typical of the early 1800s, and the cutout designs suggest the strapwork elements typical of midcentury ornament. These shoes were often further embellished with pleated silk edging and elaborate rosettes incorporating lace and small buckles.

ca. 1870–ca. 1890 (see figs. 469–87)

Since boots rather than slippers were being worn for evening in the early 1870s, slippers were less often made in white satin than they had been in the 1850s and 1860s. Wedding shoes in the early 1870s were more often white kid with leather rosettes (figs. 465, 480). When boots went out of fashion for evening in the later 1870s and slippers returned to replace them, the slippers were once again more often made in the traditional evening fabrics, silk and satin, as well as kid. White and light colors continued in use, of course, but shoes made to match the richly colored silks of the late 1870s and 1880s were also fashionable, and it is not uncommon to find an elaborate afternoon or evening dress and its matching slippers preserved together (see plate 9). Glazed black and bronze kid were also common choices for slippers in the 1880s.

Low tie and strap shoes were most often made in black or bronze kid in the late 1870s and early 1880s, but black patent was mentioned more and more often through the decade of the 1880s, usually as a foxing with a black kid upper. Patent had been known and used for a hundred years and had appeared regularly in the foxings of women's boots. It was used occasionally for slippers as well (*Godey's* mentions patent slippers in February 1860), but it came into much wider use after 1880 for slippers, oxfords, and Molière shoes (which buckled or tied over a high flaring tongue). Wool/silk fabrics in black and colors continued in use for the tops of dressier boots and shoes. Tan kid is mentioned as a material for evening shoes in 1888, suggesting that at this early date tan was not yet clearly identified with informal day wear.[18] Alligator appears in women's oxfords in the *Jordan Marsh Almanac* printed for 1883 (fig. 40), and is mentioned along with seal leather in *Demorest's* "What to Wear" that same year. Alligator was used for women's tennis shoes in the 1880s (fig. 75), and *Godey's* lists crocodile skin among the materials used for stylish promenade wear in November 1888. But reptile leathers did not become of major importance in women's footwear until the 1920s.

From about 1877 to 1890, the vamp seam in some oxfords and boots was cut in a scalloped or waved pattern (figs. 194, 230). In the early 1880s, when this detail was most popular, dressy slippers sometimes had their top edges cut in scallops as well. Oxfords were provided with cordlike laces that very often had tasseled ends, but Molières tied with broad ribbons (figs. 174, 196).

In the 1870s, dark serge and leather footwear was often machine stitched with contrasting light thread (notably the toe caps), and the same light machine stitching was sometimes used to create simple linear embroidered loops and tendrils. More expensive shoes might be hand-embroidered with floral patterns in multicolored silk. Embroidery continued in occasional use right through the 1880s, usually in the form of a bouquet of flowers on the vamp. In addition to fancy stitching, shoes from the Centennial Exhibition of 1876 feature cutout vamps and quarters underlaid with gilded leather or colored satin.

By far the most common shoe ornament in the 1870–90 period was a complex bow or rosette. The distinctive oval rosettes of the early 1870s were so

long that the throat of the slipper was often extended into a tab to support them as they rested on the instep. Steel, mother-of-pearl, and jet buckles were often used in the center. Shoes of this type were known in America as Marie Antoinette slippers and were fashionable from 1869 to 1874.

Bows and rosettes changed their form from about 1875. Where before they had radiated loops in all directions from a central knot or buckle, now a simpler bow shape was typical—except that the bow had multiple loops, each one extending a little further than the one above it. These loops did not stick straight out to the side, but cradled the round throat of the slipper. Simple tiered bows of this type might have but two layers, but the more complex versions had as many as six. Tiered bows are most characteristic of the 1880s, but they were advertised in Sears as late as 1897.

Another silk shoe ornament of the 1880s seems to have developed from the pleated ribbon used to edge the throatline in the 1860s. In these shoes, a densely pleated ribbon as much as two inches wide was stitched to the throat, the stitching often covered with a bow. The loose edge of this ribbon, which lay on the instep, was turned back at two or three points and tacked down, creating a complex three-dimensional crumpled look (figs. 485, 486).

Both of these bowlike ornaments were often enriched with beading, cut steel on black shoes with black silk trim, and gold-color beads on bronze shoes with brown silk trim. The beads were sometimes merely dotted here and there on each tier of loops, but often the important edges were beaded to emphasize the folds and textures, creating an ornament in harmony with the complex draperies and fabric textures of the 1880s. In many shoes the space on the vamp below the bow was filled with still more beading.

1890–1910 (see figs. 488–91, 499–502)

During the two decades after 1890 several new materials became part of the standard repertoire in women's shoes. Chief among these was "tan" or "russet" leather. The word "tan" comes originally from the natural yellow-brown color of oak-tanned undyed leather, but the word came to mean any brown or tan color, whether the color was produced by the natural tanning process or by dyeing the leather afterward. Men had been wearing tan shoes for informal fashionable wear for some years before 1890, and even among women's shoes, tan had appeared from time to time. A pair of lovely tie shoes, ca. 1820, made of tan kid trimmed with blue silk ribbon survives at the Colonial Dames in Boston,[19] and tan kid is very common among the tie shoes and slippers of the 1840s (plates 3, 6). Utilitarian women's boots had also been made of natural undyed leather, often with a pebbled finish, in the 1860s and 1870s, but tan as a fashion color for women's shoes really came into its own after 1890.

Once the idea of tan rather than black shoes was accepted, variations in shade created in the dyeing or glazing process also came into fashion. This was encouraged by the development of chrome tanning after 1884. Chrome tanning took less time than the traditional oak tannage and was therefore less expensive, but it left the skins with a bluish gray tinge rather than yellow-tan. Thus it always had to be dyed to produce any shade of tan or brown. "Vici kid," a chrome-tanned kid available as early as 1893, was frequently advertised in the 1890s and early 1900s in a shade of dark brown called chocolate. Chocolate Vici kid was dark and glossy enough to look reasonably dressy, but it was not immediately settled when it was appropriate to wear the lighter natural tan. As a result, tan shoes waxed and waned in favor, to the consternation of shoe men, who could never be sure how many to produce or buy for the coming season. The *Shoe Retailer* mentions that the summer of 1904 saw a craze for tan shoes that caught many makers and dealers unprepared. In general, tan leathers in the 1890s and early 1900s were typically made up as summer oxfords intended for informal, outdoor use, but in 1908 tan pumps and Colonials came into fashion, and these were somewhat dressier.

Patent leather continued in frequent use in the 1890s for the toe caps, foxings, and lace stays of boots and tie shoes. It was now combined not only with black kid but also with tan and chocolate. Sometimes the entire vamp or even the entire shoe was of black patent, but this was more typical after 1900, when black patent became one of the most important leathers used. Patent finishes could be worked on any firm leather, and kid, calf, colt, and split sides were all used. The most frequently mentioned in the early 1900s was patent colt, the hides for which were imported from Russia, where colts were apparently slaughtered for meat and eaten much like veal.[20]

Heavier leathers such as oil grain, glove grain, and pebble grain (all split side leathers that did not take a very high finish), and calf were used far more often for men's footwear than women's in the nineteenth century. The standard leather for women's shoes had always been kid (but see fig. 62 and the section "Leather Shoes for Work and Country Wear" in chapter 4 for information about early-nineteenth-century shoes of calf and other heavier leather). Calf and split side leathers were occasionally used in later nineteenth-century heavy women's boots (which Montgomery Ward described as "Field and Farm Brands"), but the only low shoes that repeatedly appeared in such leathers in the 1890s catalogs were pebble-grain Newport ties and "grain slippers" for rough wear. One of the earliest of these heavier leathers to enter the fashion scene was "Russia," a calf leather originally made in Russia and characteristically a dark red color. One fashion commentator writing in 1894 felt that "Russia leather, with its deep reddish color, is the handsomest material for Bluchers and ties, and although expensive at first is the cheapest in the end."[21] Later the name was applied to chrome-tanned calf, and the leather could be dyed tan, brown, or black. Other calf leathers are mentioned after 1900, but more often in boots rather than shoes. The first type of calf commonly mentioned for low shoes was "gun metal," sometimes called "gun metal calf kid," suggesting that it imitated kid. It was finished dull or semi-bright and appears in advertisements by 1906. It was to find increasing use in the 1910s and 1920s.[22]

Other new materials that came into wide use in the late nineteenth century were canvas, suede, and felt. Like russet leather, canvas was considered suitable only for informal wear, and it appeared chiefly in summer oxfords (especially those intended for sports), usually in white but also in black and a shade of pumpkin brown. Tennis shoes advertised by Montgomery Ward in 1895 were even made of canvas check, unspecified in color but probably black and white (fig. 75). The same catalog listed gray linen oxfords with russet toe cap and lace stay.

Suede was important enough in the early 1890s to be suffering an eclipse by 1894: "Suede walking shoes are not so much worn this year, Russia and the various russet leathers taking their place."[23] Suede was made in soft shades of gray, green, cream, and beige and occasionally stronger colors such as rusty brown. Slippers, strap, and tie shoes were made of suede, and it was also used as a trimming or secondary contrasting leather. In the form of white buck it was used for summer shoes and boots. Reptile leathers continued in use but were not nearly as common as tan, canvas, or suede.

Felt boots and shoes were being advertised by 1889 by Daniel Green and Company under the name "Alfred Dolge's Felt Shoes and Slippers." They were a staple of the mail-order catalogs through the 1890s and early 1900s, in both high and low styles. The boot styles passed out of fashion, but the lower ones, which were essentially bedroom slippers, became a standard offering through the first half of the twentieth century. Nearly all were made without fastening, many in tabbed throat or nullifier styles. The soles could be of leather or felt, but leather seems to have been preferred. Felt slippers were routinely trimmed with fur or plush in the 1890s and 1900s, but with ribbon or with a contrasting felt collar in the 1910s and 1920s. Vamp embroidery was occasionally used in the early 1890s (fig. 52).

A sense of the range of materials available at the turn of the century is conveyed by an article in the *Shoe Retailer* about shoes being produced in Haverhill, Massachusetts, for the 1905 spring season. "The highest priced and most dependable leathers are to be found in the Haverhill lines as at present constituted. Patent colt, and patent kid, with patent split leather in the lower priced goods. Russia calf, colored kid, colored kangaroo in tans, and gun metal calf kid, mat kid, and kangaroo kid in the black goods indicates the wide range of materials, not to mention the many fancy leathers so largely used in this city. Colored shoes in goat and kid, other than tans, covert cloth and black and white canvas, and linen and basket cloth, as well as white kid, are all seen in the new lines."[24]

The characteristic embellishment for tie shoes in this period was the toe cap, usually pointed in the 1890s (fig. 176), straight after 1900 (fig. 178), and occasionally shield-shaped or winged from 1908 (fig. 68). The tip might be omitted in dressier oxfords. It was very often made of patent leather to contrast with the rest of the upper, and many shoes also had lace stays and foxing of patent to match. Contrasting collars (an extra band of material around the top edge) and perforations placed to imitate collars became particularly fashionable in 1908–9 and were used both on tie shoes and pumps (fig. 68). From 1904 it was common to make the entire vamp and sometimes the heel foxing of patent to contrast with a top or quarter of dull calf or suede (the latter more common from 1908). It was also in 1904 that oversized "porthole" eyelets came into widespread use. The laces for oxford shoes began to be made of flat silk in the 1890s rather than in the previous cord style. They gradually became broader still in the early 1900s, and by the end of the decade they appear to be a full inch and a half wide (figs. 197, 202).

Perforation was used on women's shoes by 1889 (fig. 196), and it remained an important style element throughout this period as a way of emphasizing the fashionable "mannish" quality in a shoe (figs. 68, 175, 178, 197–99). Toe caps, heel foxings, vamps and lace stays all might have perforated edges. The actual holes were usually round, combining larger and smaller sizes in some simple sequence, but about 1900 one sometimes sees them in star or diamond shapes as well (fig. 199). "Imitation tips" were created by perforating the vamp to suggest the shape of a toe cap but without incorporating the second layer of leather.

The Art Nouveau movement influenced shoe styles in a minor way in that there was a certain delight in elaborate curves. Vamps, foxings, and lace stays had been given scalloped or waved edges beginning in the 1880s and very typically in the 1890s (fig. 197), but patterns with short mechanical repeats such as these gave way about 1895 to patterns with longer, nonrepetitive curves (fig. 198). An extreme example is a shoe advertised in Sears in 1907 whose foxing is cut into a fanciful shape resembling a mermaid's tail (fig. 201). Some shoes were cut so that the side seam formed a much deeper curve than was typical in the earlier 1890s (figs. 180, 199).

Satin evening slippers in the early 1890s appeared in a variety of shades, notably ivory, pale yellow, gray, and pink, as well as black. The predilection for tiered and rumpled bows characteristic of the 1880s gradually died out in the early 1890s, and a narrow, neat, even prim, little flat silk bow took their place. The bow alone was sufficient for most white kid wedding shoes, but fashionable satin slippers were very often beaded on the vamp as well, a detail reported in 1894. "The toes of most evening slippers are embroidered in silk or beads to match the trimmings of the gown for which they are intended."[25] Unlike the beaded vamps of the earlier 1880s, which tended to employ beads of one type and color, whether cut steel, jet, or gold-colored, the early 1890s style of beading incorporates a variety of beads and sequins of various shapes and sizes, including some in pale colors, such as white, silver, and a touch of pink on a silver-gray slipper. Nonfunctional buckles and other small throat ornaments are mentioned with increasing frequency after 1890. They had appeared before, but usually within a rosette. Now they were used alone. "The fashionable slipper [of 1892] is made of black moire, the high heel being covered with the same material; a very small rhinestone buckle is the only decoration. These slippers will not increase the size of the

foot, as does velvet, and are not so warm, though it must be said that they have not the dressy appearance of satin."[26]

Plain opera slippers were not advertised as frequently as strap shoes ("sandals") from the early 1890s to 1908. In the 1890s, a single strap was most common, undecorated except for a large ribbon bow that may fasten the strap or conceal a buttoned fastening (fig. 134). The bow was often beaded on the knot, or was embellished with a paste buckle. Cross-straps were also available (fig. 133). In the early 1900s multiple straps and cutouts that imitated multi-strap shoes were more fashionable than single strap styles. These rarely had bows but they often had beading on the straps, white beading on white shoes, and black or steel beads on dark ones being common (figs. 138, 234). Both slippers and strap shoes were available in white and black kid and black patent as well as in satin, but bronze seems to have gone out of fashion soon after 1890 and did not return until about 1915.

1910–1930 (see figs. 492–98, 503–8)

The ever-quickening pace of change in shoe fashions after 1910 makes it difficult to give an unambiguous picture of style developments. The reality wasn't clear even for contemporary observers, and it certainly is not for us. To impose some order on the period, it seems best to discuss it in segments of three or four years each.

1910–1913: This was a period of mannish footwear and as a result calf leather was much used: dull calf, gun metal, Russia, and some tan and suede, as well as the staple black patent. White buck, white canvas, and white cravenette (a closely woven shoe fabric) are mentioned for the slippers and ties to be worn with white summer dresses. Satin continued for evening. Velvet is also mentioned, as is gold and silver brocade, although the latter did not reach its peak for some years yet.

Dresses in this period were short enough to expose the foot, and in the quest for a lighter-appearing foot, women began to wear slippers and Colonials on the street. In order to make these shoes stand up to harder use, those intended for walking were now often provided with welted soles rather than the turn sole traditional to slippers. From about this same time, the word "pump" came to be used for any slip-on shoe that was suitable for outdoor use (although usage was not yet consistent). Toe caps and perforations were also incorporated into pump and Colonial designs as a way of signaling that they were suitable for the street (fig. 96).

Shoe ornaments were very fashionable at this period and in 1912–13 were available separately so that the buyer could combine the pump and the ornament of her choice. The pumps and Colonials of 1910 generally had a modest leather or ribbon bow at the throat. By 1912, the bows on pumps were rather large and flat (no puckers) and the Colonials were fitted with large buckles, either covered to match the upper or made of cut or pressed steel, beads, silver, or bronze.

1914–1916: In the midteens, there was a swing toward lighter leathers, narrower toes, curvier heels, and more complex cutting in women's shoes, a trend that was interrupted by America's entry into World War I in 1917, but that bloomed again in 1921 after war-related limits on design were lifted. Black patent increased in use, but black kid vied with calf in popularity, and bronze enjoyed renewed importance. There was a new fashion for dark blue. Nineteen-fourteen and 1915 saw a fashion for two-tone shoes, usually a dark-colored vamp (generally black patent) with much lighter quarters, such as gray suede, white calf, putty cloth, or brocade (figs. 123, 204). The heels with these shoes might match either vamp or quarter. Two-tone shoes are less often illustrated in 1916 but they are noted, and one example reverses the earlier pattern and shows a light vamp and dark quarter. Gold and silver kid are mentioned again for evening, and satin continues to match the dress as before. Tan shoes seem to have gone out of fashion, and white was less important than in the early teens. The exception is in sports shoes, which were generally white canvas or buck with toe cap, foxings, or trim of tan, black, red, or green leather.

Perforation became less common in pumps and Colonials than in the early teens. The throat ornaments that had been so prominent in 1912 and 1913 were now smaller or absent entirely. In 1915 they were often round and no bigger than an ordinary button, made of cut steel for day and paste for evening (fig. 123). Paste jewels were also occasionally set into the heels of dressy evening shoes. A few Colonials still had buckles (more often rectangular than oval now), but more common still was an atrophied version of the Colonial with a peaked throat and no buckle at all (figs. 94, 97). One short-lived but distinct fashion of 1915–16 was for contrast piping or stitching on a black or dark shoe, a detail related to the interest in two-tone shoes. Strap shoes were another fad of these years that almost certainly would have developed further had it not been for the war. Two- or three-buttoned straps were the norm, but these were sometimes combined with cutouts to suggest even more (fig. 224). Multi-strap shoes were often embellished with steel beads on the vamp and straps (fig. 141). Beads were also commonly used on pumps.

1917–1920: When America entered the war in 1917, the trend toward elaborately strapped and cutout shoes made with contrasting leathers was interrupted, and there was an immediate reaction toward more utilitarian leathers, drab colors, and conservative styles. Thus while kid remained in use, more shoes were made of calf.

The increased showing of calf is due largely to the increased popularity of the tan shoe, which, in popular opinion, gives a greater opportunity for variety of tone and which, in the opinion of many dealers, is to be preferred for a strictly walking shoe. While the deeper shades of brown, tan, mahogany, cordovan and cherry red are popular, there is a decided tendency in the better grades toward a lighter shade of tan. Tan shoes were never brought out in a greater variety of shades than during the last few months and the retailer can find almost any color, shade or tone, from deep brown, that is difficult to distinguish from black, to nut brown, hazel and army khaki or chocolate, which latter is so well reproduced in kid stock.[27]

Besides this range of tans and browns, dark gray was also fashionable, but all these ranked behind black in sheer volume of sales. Two-tone shoes (fig. 124) were less common than solids, except in sports shoes, which were still made in white buck with contrasting vamp, foxing, and collar or lace stay of tan, blue, or other colored leather. White kid, linen, and canvas continued to be used for summer shoes. One notes an occasional pump or Colonial in black patent or suede, but far more common is satin (black or silver-gray) or kid (black, brown, or bronze, the brown being used for day wear, the bronze for evening). The *Shoe Retailer* mentions in 1917 that patent leather was being made in colors (light and dark tan, brown, gray, etcetera) but colored patent does not seem to have caught on.[28] One new material of interest was black celluloid, used to cover the wooden heels of black patent leather shoes from 1917 right through the 1920s. A detail often mentioned in the years 1917–19 is the insertion of an aluminum plate just above the top lift in Louis heels.

As would be expected during war time, ornamentation was subdued. Straps, which had made such a hopeful start in 1915–16, were cut off in their youth. "Pumps are shown with few decorations, except in the medium grades, where they are shown with small cut steel buckles or ornaments. A few ribbon bows, after the pattern of the old sailor tie, have been brought out, but in the better grades the plain pump is conceded to have the preference, and this without perforation and void of imitation tips, which are positively out of place in the pump pattern."[29] Perforation was by no means dead, however. It was still standard embellishment in most oxfords and continued to be used in many pumps despite the rejection of it in the "better grades" (fig. 117). "In the highest grade of oxfords perforations are small and inconspicuous. In the more popular-priced grades there are seen vamp perforations and quite fine perforated imitation tips, as well as foxings. Cheaper shoes have larger perforations, and, as usual, are over-decorated in this respect, toe punchings and perforations, wherever there is place for them, appearing in abundance."[30]

1921–1922: 1921 was a critical year in the development of shoe fashions because it marked the reintroduction of strapped shoes and black patent leather on a large scale. The report out of Rochester in September 1921 was that "patent leather is fast growing stronger in women's fine pumps. Patent last spring made a bid for popularity, and a kindly reception in some of the large cities paved the way for its greater popularity, so in the fall styles patent leather is stronger than for many years. It is generally believed that patent, satin and black suede or ooze will be the most wanted materials for evening footwear of the strictly dress variety."[31] Rochester shoe manufacturers catered to the middle class, but the same rage for patent seems to have prevailed among the makers of higher-grade shoes. "Patent leather is being bought extensively, and it can safely be said that about 65 to 70 per cent of the orders now going through Brooklyn factories call for patent leather. Twenty-five to 30 per cent of the styles are of black satin. These materials are good for several months, and to many it would not be surprising to see patent leather and black satin continue into the winter and spring."[32] At the other end of the scale, Sears notes in its 1922 catalog that "this is a 'patent leather' season." Black suede is usually listed as coming third after black patent and satin for dress shoes, with black kid and gun metal for less formal footwear. "Tans, from being the big style feature as a color, now occupy the position of the 'knockabout,' or sport shoe for ordinary wear, but with an intense black year ahead for dresses tan cannot be used as a dress shoe."[33] Rough weather, however, might bring out sensible brown welt shoes. White canvas straps were still appropriate for summer, and for sports white buck oxfords trimmed with contrasting patent or colored leather continued much as before. Otherwise, colored shoes were clearly in the minority.

This was not a strong period for shoe ornaments because pumps were so rarely worn—straps and ties carried the day (figs. 142–46, 182, 206). The trimmings used instead were stitching, perforation, and beading. Stitching appears most often as one to three parallel lines that follow the top edge, side seams, and straps, and can contrast in color with the upper. White stitching on black and orange stitching on tan were considered attractive. Perforations follow very much the same pattern as stitching, but they were also used to simulate straight tips, wing tips (including the elongated wing tip that suggests a moccasin-type vamp), and heel foxings or irregular arbitrary shapes on the quarter. Also making an appearance in 1921 were cutouts, sometimes left open, sometimes with contrasting underlay. These appear on vamp, quarter, or above the waist and are still fairly simple and regular in shape. Dressier strap shoes were decorated with beading (black satin with steel beads was mentioned as suitable for either evening or the street). The beading went around the top edge and along the strap rather than clustering on the vamp.

1923–1925: Black patent, satin, and suede continued to be the staple materials for a large proportion of mid-1920s footwear, but brown and beige shoes became more important than they had been at the beginning of the decade. Among shoes brought out for the spring 1924 season, "four general shades lead in the color class, ranging from the light beige down to the darker cinnamon color, with the big sale coming on the in-between colorings. In blacks, patent leads; satin is a good second, with black suede giving both patent and satin a hard race for position. Blacks are shown of all-over one material, but there are many pleasing combinations of two materials, as satin trimmed with patent; black ooze trimmed with patent, or vice versa. Then there are patent vamp shoes made with colored quarter and straps, but these are easily in the third place in the color scheme."[34] Like black shoes, brown footwear routinely combined two materials, one of them generally being suede. Some gray suede also appears, and Sears mentions "new light shades of satin footwear," such as blonde, in 1925. Reptile leathers began to appear, but they became more important in the next period.

Cutouts became more complex and strap patterns more inventive in the mid-1920s than they had been before (figs. 147–52). Where earlier there had been parallel straps or T-straps, shoes now displayed complex arrangements where it was hard to distinguish

straps from cutouts. The more complex shoes look almost as if they had been inspired by medieval Celtic ornamentation. One helpful detail in identifying the shoes of this period is that a second material tended to be used for the straps and to outline the cutouts, side seam, and top edge, where the earlier shoes merely edged the cutouts with stitching or perforations. While plain stitching and perforations did not completely disappear, and sometimes the trimming is made of the same material as the rest of the upper, the use of a second material is perhaps the most characteristic element in footwear of the mid- to late 1920s.

Multicolored brocades joined the standard gold and silver for evening. The *Shoe Retailer* mentions that in the fall of 1923, "the oats design is selling better than the rosebud pattern,"[35] suggesting that shoe brocades came in a limited number of standard patterns. Velvet combined with black patent or gold kid is mentioned from time to time, and black satin pumps were an acceptable, if conservative, choice for evening. Plain pumps could be dressed up with bright buckles or ornaments.

1926–1930: Black suede, satin, and especially patent continued as before to play a large role in women's shoes. Regional reports in the *Shoe Retailer* suggest that patent was the leading seller around the country in the fall of 1926, and in that same season the *Ladies' Home Journal* remarked that "not for many years past have black shoes made their appearance in such overwhelming numbers."[36] Light colors, including white and off-white shades with names like "parchment" and "sauterne," were worn in warm weather. White buck appliquéd with tan leather continued to be the standard while playing sports. But for most of the year, various shades of brown kid and suede, such as woodland brown and fawn, continued to follow black in popularity. In 1928 there was a fad for printed cloth shoes to match summer dresses.

The most important new additions to fashion were reptile leathers and their imitations. These materials added complexity of texture to shoe patterns that were already wildly complex, especially in the cheaper grades, where shoes reached depths of vulgarity that almost outstrip belief. "Never before has there been such a wide variety of material, style and color, or

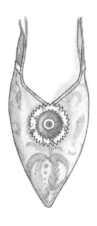 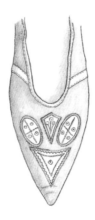 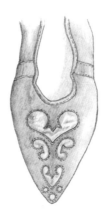 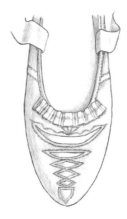 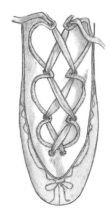

Fig. 439. 1795–1815 Bows and Rosettes Three flat leather disks, pink, green, and yellow, with sequin and bead, ca. 1800. Upper is much earlier silk.

Fig. 440. 1795–1815 Embroidered Cutout Pale-blue kid, white satin in cutouts embroidered with silver, 1801. Compare figs. 467–71.

Fig. 441. 1795–1815 Embroidered Cutout Black satin, the cut-outs backed with gray silk, 1811. Compare figs. 467–71.

Fig. 442. 1795–1815 Embroidered Cutout White kid, white satin behind cut-outs, throat edged with pleated ribbon, 1810. Compare figs. 467–71.

Fig. 443. 1795–1815 Contrast Materials Tan cotton (nankeen?) bound with red silk, red kid foxing with cream stitching in a bow design, 1805–10.

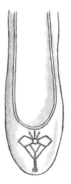 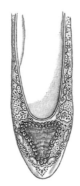 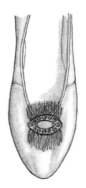 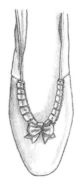 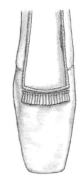

Fig. 444. 1795–1815 Embroidery Gold/silver sequin embroidery of this type appeared by the 1770s. White satin slipper 1805–15.

Fig. 445. 1795–1815 Embroidery Yellow kid slipper with black stamped pattern 1805–15. Sequins sewn on a buckram foundation stitched to vamp.

Fig. 446. 1795–1815 Buckle and Tassel Both knotted tassels and threads held in a buckle continued in use to ca. 1825. This one 1805–15.

Fig. 447. 1795–1815 Pleated Edging Pleated ribbon to edge a round throat up to the side seam was used from the 1780s. This shoe 1812.

Fig. 448. 1815–30 Pleated Edging Appears with a square throatline from 1815 to 1835 and again by 1858 (see fig. 467). This shoe 1831.

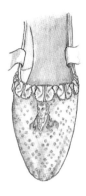
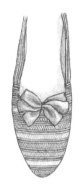
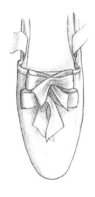
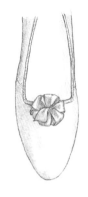
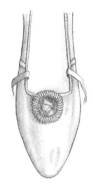

Fig. 449. 1815–30
Patterned Upper
Upper of silk with
tiny woven dots
typical in 1820s.
Picture of General
Lafayette on vamp,
1824.

Fig. 450. 1815–30
Patterned Upper
Cross-stitching on
white stripes of
ticking upper. ca.
1815. Single bow or
real tie can date
1800–1830.

Fig. 451. 1815–30
Bows and Rosettes
Some 1820s slit-vamp
shoes tie with two
separate bows, but
bows on this kid shoe
are not functional.

Fig. 452. 1815–30
Bows and Rosettes
Informal ribbon
rosette probably used
from at least 1800 to
1830. This shoe 1828.

Fig. 453. 1815–30
Bows and Rosettes
Carefully pleated
rosette used about
1810–35. This shoe
ca. 1825–30.

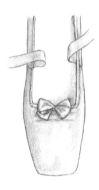
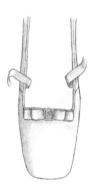
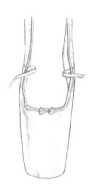
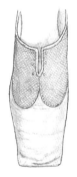
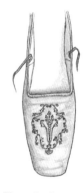

Fig. 454. 1830–50
Bows and Rosettes
Small, clearly
nonfunctional bow
probably had a long
period of use but
seems most common
1835–45.

Fig. 455. 1830–50
Bows and Rosettes
An exhibition shoe
with plain formal
bow and scroll-like
buckle, 1839.

Fig. 456. 1830–50
Bows and Rosettes
Typical minute bow
on 1840s and 1850s
slippers, often hidden
under a larger rosette
or bow after 1850.

Fig. 457. 1830–50
Patterned Upper
Slit-vamp shoe, with
patterned wool upper
and kid foxing, 1846.

Fig. 458. 1850–70
Gold Stamping
Black kid shoe,
design stamped in
gold on the vamp, ca.
1845–55.

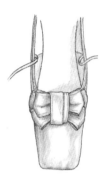
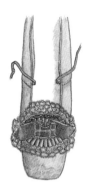
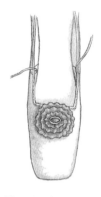
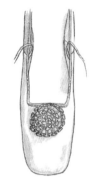
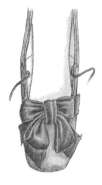

Fig. 459. 1850–70
Bows and Rosettes
Simple but fairly
large bow of silk
ribbon used 1846
through the 1860s.

Fig. 460. 1850–70
Bows and Rosettes
Lace and pleated
black silk ribbon
topped with black
velvet ribbon with a
white edge, 1855 to
1865.

Fig. 461. 1850–70
Bows and Rosettes
Spiral of pleated
ribbon with small
oval buckle, from
Godey's, 1861.

Fig. 462. 1850–70
Bows and Rosettes
Semi-spherical
pompon rosette of
crisp white silk
common in 1860s.

Fig. 463. 1850–70
Bows and Rosettes
Large multilooped
bows (this example is
black velvet) covered
most of the vamp by
the late 1860s.

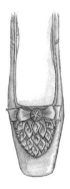
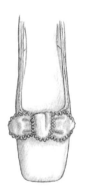
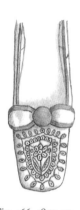
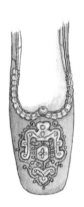
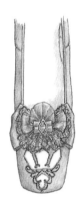

Fig. 464. 1850–70
Bows and Rosettes
Brown silk ribbon
pleated into leaflike
vandykes, similar to
one in *Godey's,* 1869.

Fig. 465. 1850–70
Bows and Rosettes
By 1869 and into the
1870s, bows and
rosettes were often
made of kid to match
the shoe. This exam-
ple 1871.

Fig. 466. 1850–70
Embroidery
White silk slipper
embroidered with
purple in looped
design. Purple
edging, ca. 1855–65.

Fig. 467. 1850–70
Embroidered Cutout
Chain-stitch edging
forms loops around
cutouts. Pleated
edging on bronze
shoe, 1855–65. See
figs. 440–42.

Fig. 468. 1850–70
Embroidered Cutout
Bronze kid, cutouts
in later style of 1865–
70 with larger rosette.
See figs. 440–42.

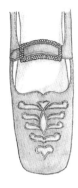

Fig. 469. 1870–90
Embroidered Cutout
Exhibition shoe, 1876,
strap with cut-steel
buckle, cutouts
backed with purple
silk.

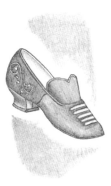

Fig. 470. 1870–90
Embroidered Cutout
Exhibition shoe,
1876, has cutouts
backed with gold kid.

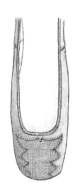

Fig. 471. 1870–90
Embroidered Cutout
Bronze shoe with
vamp cutout backed
with textured wool
fabric, ca. 1880.
Compare fig. 477.

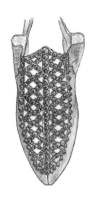

Fig. 472. 1870–90
Beaded Cutout
Gored shoe with
trellis-like open
cutouts outlined with
black "nail heads,"
ca. 1890.

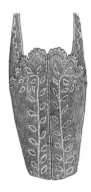

Fig. 473. 1870–90
Embroidery
Black kid shoe with
white machine stitch-
ing, goring under
high vamp, ca. 1875.

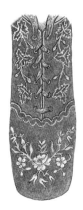

Fig. 474. 1870–90
Embroidery
Hand-embroidered in
several colors on
vamp, white vine leaf
design on quarters,
ca. 1875. French.

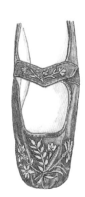

Fig. 475. 1870–90
Embroidery
Black satin with
multicolored hand
embroidery, ca.
1877–80. French.

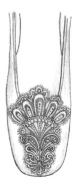

Fig. 476. 1870–90
Embroidery
White satin evening
slipper embroidered
in gold, shown in
Godey's and *Harper's
Bazar* in 1881.

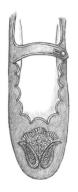

Fig. 477. 1870–90
Embroidery
Embroidered kid
slipper with scalloped
throatline, shown in
Harper's Bazar in
1882.

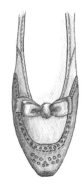

Fig. 478. 1870–90
Contrast Materials
Patent leather toe cap
on slipper shown in
Harper's Bazar in
1889.

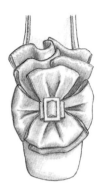 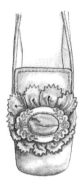 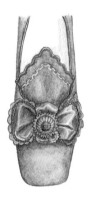 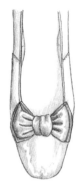 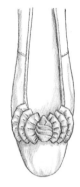

Fig. 479. 1870–90
Bows and Rosettes
Large oval rosettes
were stylish 1869–74.
This one of white
satin has a mother-
of-pearl buckle, 1871.

Fig. 480. 1870–90
Bows and Rosettes
Pinked edges are
typical on 1870s
leather bows and
rosettes. This, with
large silver buckle,
1873.

Fig. 481. 1870–90
Bows and Rosettes
Black kid shoe has
tongue stitched in
white. Kid bow
edged with braid, jet
button, 1870s.
Compare fig. 465.

Fig. 482. 1870–90
Bows and Rosettes
After 1875, bows
were smaller, with
layers that hugged
the round throatline.
This is from an 1880
wedding.

Fig. 483. 1870–90
Bows and Rosettes
Multitiered bows that
hugged the throat
were often enriched
with beading 1875–
95. This example
1881.

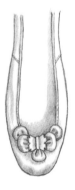 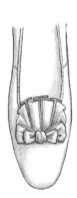 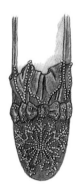 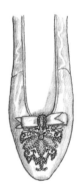 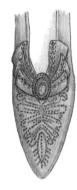

Fig. 484. 1870–90
Bows and Rosettes
This distinctive white
kid bow with "ears"
appears on wedding
shoes of 1885, 1887,
1891.

Fig. 485. 1870–90
Bows and Rosettes
A deep band of
pleated silk edges the
throat, with a bow
below, 1887.

Fig. 486. 1870–90
Bows and Rosettes
Silk pleated, as in fig.
485, is folded down
at three points,
forming a crumpled
effect, and then
beaded, 1880s.

Fig. 487. 1870–90
Bows and Rosettes
Satin slipper with the
beaded and sequined
vamp and neat
narrow bow that
came into style about
1890.

Fig. 488. 1890–1910
Bows and Rosettes
Late version of tiered
bow and beaded
vamp in a black satin
shoe of ca. 1895.

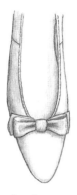

Fig. 489. 1890–1910
Bows and Rosettes
Prim satin bow in
sharp contrast to
previous crumpled
style, continues in use
1890 to early 1900s.

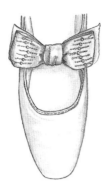

Fig. 490. 1890–1910
Bows and Rosettes
In strap shoes, the
bow was often on the
strap instead of the
vamp, 1890 to 1907,
and was often
beaded.

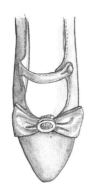

Fig. 491. 1890–1910
Bows and Rosettes
Simple, moderate-
size, soft leather or
ribbon bow is typical
1908–10.

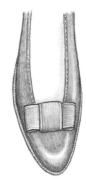

Fig. 492. 1910–30
Bows and Rosettes
Flat, unpuckered,
tailored bow is
common 1911–13 and
continues in use to
1920.

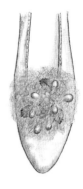

Fig. 493. 1910–30
Bows and Rosettes
A chiffon or tulle
rosette was used for
evening and wedding
shoes 1908–15 at
least. Wax buds on
this one, 1909.

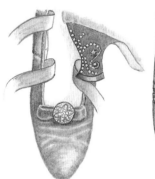

Fig. 494. 1910–30
Throat Ornament
Blue velvet tango
shoe has jeweled
heels, rhinestone
ornament, and ribbon
ties, ca. 1914.

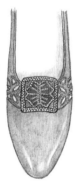

Fig. 495. 1910–30
Throat Ornament
Bucklelike throat
ornament conceals
goring for ease, 1928.

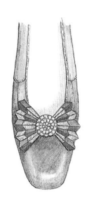

Fig. 496. 1910–30
Bows and Rosettes
Art Deco stylized
bow, 1928. Bows
were not very
common during most
of the 1920s.

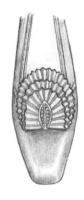

Fig. 497. 1910–30
Bows and Rosettes
Grosgrain ribbon
rosette has rhinestone
center. Art Deco
style, 1928.

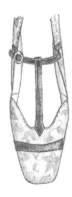

Fig. 498. 1910–30
Patterned Upper
Printed shoe fabrics
were a late 1920s fad.
This example is linen
with black patent
trim, 1928.

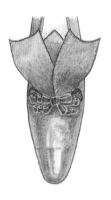

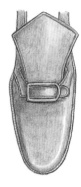

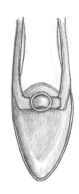

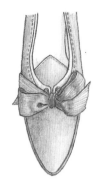

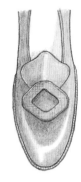

Fig. 499. 1900–1930
Colonials
Exhibition shoe, 1893,
with flaring three-part
tongue and small
velvet bow. Sears
1907 has similar shoe.

Fig. 500. 1900–1930
Colonials
Small functional D-
shaped buckle, 1902.
See fig. 177 for larger
1901 version.

Fig. 501. 1900–1930
Colonials
Very short tongue,
perforated collar
ending in straps
through a small oval
buckle, 1907–8.

Fig. 502. 1900–1930
Colonials
Tan suede, perfor-
ated, 1908. By 1915
string laces gradually
replaced the broad
ribbon ties of 1904–
10.

Fig. 503. 1900–1930
Colonials
The years 1911 and
1912 were the high
point of the fad for
Colonial shoes and
buckles.

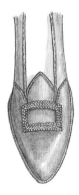

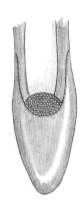

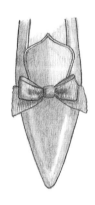

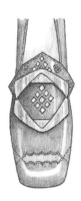

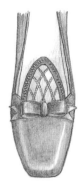

Fig. 504. 1900–1930
Colonials
"Colonial pumps"
had even smaller
tongues by 1913 and
were fitted with
purely ornamental
buckles.

Fig. 505. 1900–1930
Colonials
Beading at throat in
1915 is the ghost of
buckles past. See also
fig. 123.

Fig. 506. 1900–1930
Colonials
Large tongues were
stylish from 1917 to
1921, often with a
ribbon bow rather
than a buckle.

Fig. 507. 1900–1930
Colonials
Shoes with tongues
and buckles were rare
in the 1920s. This
example 1926. See
also fig. 126.

Fig. 508. 1900–1930
Colonials
Colonials returned
gradually in the late
1920s, but by 1930 a
perky bow was more
common.

such a universal use of inlays, bands, straps and other decorative touches. Dominating the various fabrics in point of quantity are the so-called reptile skin reproductions—alligator, lizard, snake, chameleon, baby leopard, shark and fish scales. Giving better service than the real skins and precluding the possibility of cracking, they are used on all kinds of shoes, with the exception only of those for evening wear."[37]

The complex styles of the mid-1920s continued to the end of the decade but there was a slow drift away from complicated straps and toward the use of one-strap and T-strap shoes. This was accompanied by a trend away from cutouts and toward the use of contrasting materials inlaid and appliquéd in capricious patterns that suggest the last distortions of a dying style. Instead of outlining the straps, cutouts, seam lines, toe caps, or counters, as had usually been the case before, the contrast material now began to be applied in arbitrary designs that did not relate to the structure of the shoe. These whimsical designs fall into two classes. The first consists of thin tendril-like strips of contrasting leather applied here and there on the shoe (figs. 101, 119, 158). The second arranges the two materials to cover approximately equal areas, making it unclear which is the main leather and which the trim (figs. 155, 156, 435). These stylistic changes appeared in novelty shoes but did not affect conservative shoes in simple strap or oxford styles.

Evening shoes were still made of silver, gold, and multicolored brocades as well as colored satins to match or set off the color of the dress. Large shoe ornaments with a distinctly Art Deco feel were sold in the late 1920s. Heels for evening shoes might be covered with black celluloid or silver and densely set with rhinestones, while gold-covered heels were studded with topaz.

Materials and Ornamentation in Boots
1790–1830

Boots from this period are rare, but surviving examples are made of a variety of materials, including silk, nankeen, kid, and a sturdy black leather that may be calf. (Refer to the illustrations in chapter 8 for more pictures of boots.) If so small a sample can suggest a

trend, then green was probably a common color. Jane Austen mentions half-boots made of nankeen foxed with black in her unfinished novel *The Watsons* (1804). The *Lady's Magazine* for November 1812 refers to crimson velvet back-lacing boots to match the mantle among the London fashions, and in February 1813 we hear of brown cloth ankle boots bound round the top and down the front to match the gloves.

After 1815, when boots became somewhat more common, the materials mentioned most often are morocco, kid, satin, and gros de Naples (a corded silk), with occasional references to jean and nankeen. Except for the nankeen, which was naturally a yellowish tan color, fashion magazines very often describe boots in colors to match the dress (blue seems to have been particularly popular), and in the more neutral shades of brown, gray, dark reddish-brown, and of course black. Contrasting tips (toe caps) are mentioned from time to time. White kid is described as suitable for carriage boots rather than walking. A spotted gros de Naples mentioned in 1828 probably refers to a monochrome woven spot rather than a contrasting colored one, but Swann illustrates an example of the late 1810s made of pale blue cloth printed with brown stars, along with two others of this period made of fawn silk and of yellow kid.[38] The chief decoration for these early front-lacing boots seems to have been rosettes at the throat (figs. 246, 509) or fringe placed round the top. Fringed boots appear in fashion plates all through the 1810s and 1820s and seem to have become particularly fashionable in the very late 1820s (figs. 247, 248, 271, 272, 510).

1830–1860

Some boots were still made to match the color of the dress, especially in the early 1830s, when the feet were visible beneath relatively short skirts. Very stylish boots might be embroidered above the toe cap, a detail that appears in some French fashion plates in the early 1830s (fig. 511). Occasionally one finds boot uppers in a wool fabric with a woven pattern, usually a minute plaid or spot (figs. 211, 273). But more and more often boots were made in a plain, dark-colored wool, generally black, brown, drab, or gray, woven with a satiny surface. The foxing normally contrasted with the upper in material if not always in color. For example, surviving boots of the 1840s appear in black wool with black morocco foxing, and in brown wool with brown or black morocco foxing (plate 6).

Hall's *History of Boots and Shoes,* reprinted as a series of articles in *Godey's* in both 1848 and 1853, says that "the leather best adapted for ladies' boots is morocco or goat-skin, which, when properly dressed, is sufficiently strong and durable. Kid being the skin of the young goat, is naturally finer and more delicate; the enamel or varnish leather, commonly called patent, is also very suitable, and being made of calfskin, is strong. For the little toe-caps and golashes [i.e., foxings] of ladies' Congress boots, it answers admirably, and as it requires no cleaning, always looks well. The upper part of the boot is constructed variously of morocco, prunella, cloth, silk or satin, according to the season."[39] Although Hall lists morocco as a possible boot-top material, presumably for winter, surviving boots made entirely of leather are rare until the very end of this period. Occasionally even the leather foxing was omitted, when the boot was of a dressy material like satin and was intended for indoor or carriage wear.

As in the 1840s, boots of the 1850s were likely to be made of black, brown, or gray serge with toe caps of black patent, or of black or brown kid or morocco. Linen was used for summer boots, and winter boots were sometimes made of quilted silk, or of wool cloth lined with flannel or fleece, both being foxed with leather. Occasionally boots are found that probably matched a dress.

1860–1890

By the 1860s boots of various types were worn for all kinds of occasions, from the farmyard to the ballroom, and therefore they were available in a range of materials. Evening boots in the 1860s were of white satin or kid, or of black or colored satin to match the dress. By the 1870s, although satin was still used for very elaborate examples, evening boots were most often of white kid with a buttoned closure, and white kid buttoned wedding boots are very common in museum collections. The boots of pink, blue, or even gilded kid that survive tend to appear in rather small sizes, suggesting that they may have been worn by young girls rather than grown women. *Godey's* does mention in February 1871 that "children wear pink or blue kid gaiters to match their evening dresses." Evening boots were unusual after 1885.

In the 1860s there was a growing tendency to wear colored boots during the day. "Now that the decree has gone forth in favor of short dresses, we must look to our boots. As harmony of color prevails to a great extent in dress, boots and shoes should also accord."[40] Boots from this decade that well-off women might have worn with matching carriage or visiting dresses survive in bright peacock blue, mint green, bronze, and other fashionable colors (plate 8). Ordinary walking boots continued to be made with cloth tops and leather foxing through the 1860s, but the standard everyday fabric was black serge rather than brown, and the foxing was more often than not black patent. The black patent was frequently used to strengthen the lace stay on front-lacing boots and it also trimmed the top edge (fig. 250).

The 1860s also saw a trend toward boots made with all-leather uppers. A pair of side-lace boots from the early 1860s, made entirely of bright red leather, survives at Northampton (plate 6), and an elegant pair in bronze leather made by Sulzer of Paris is preserved at the Colonial Dames (plate 8). Utilitarian front-lacing boots of the later 1860s at the Peabody Essex Museum are made of pebble-grained brown leather with black patent tips (fig. 241). Black kid foxed with patent is mentioned with increasing frequency in the early 1870s, and by the end of that decade *Demorest's* reported that "black kid, either French or Mat, is most used for the uppers of 'all leather' shoes, the foxings being of India straight or pebble goat."

Demorest's notes in the same column that "black cloth of the same quality and patterns as the heavy winter suitings and cloakings, is in great demand for the uppers of the fine grade of dress boots. Old English lasting or prunella, serge and satine of light quality are much used for single-soled boots for early fall wear; the linings are of white twill with kid insole, while for the heavier winter boots canton flannel is much used both for lining the uppers and as an insole for semi-invalids and people who suffer with cold feet."[41] In 1883, the situation was much the same. "French kid is the accepted material for the standard boot of the day; but a goodly number of cloth top kid foxed boots are worn by ladies who are not so unfortunate as to 'interfere' and take off the inner side of the ankles. Many ladies will wear holes the size of a dime through the cloth, before the foxings have lost their first gloss."[42]

Surviving walking boots of the 1870s and 1880s are likely to be made of plain black kid or calf, sometimes foxed with a leather of contrasting texture. *Godey's* reports in February 1871 that "all [shoemakers] agree in advising the plainest kid or pebbled leather boots, with very little, if any ornamental stitching, and with heels an inch and a quarter high. The white fan stitching bows and tassels on the boots and very high curved French heels are passée." But other evidence suggests that the desire for ladylike simplicity was by no means universal. Elaborate decoration was a high-style option from the mid-1860s to about 1884, and some of the boots illustrated in *Godey's* and *Harper's Bazar* are wildly elaborate, combining purple silk, black patent, white stitching, fancy cutouts, and ostentatious rosettes all in the same boot. Perhaps when most footwear was so predictable, only freaks were worth illustrating.

The interest in ornamented boots began in the early 1860s with the modest fashion for rosettes on the toe of dressy boots, echoing the rosettes on slippers (figs. 512, 513). *Godey's* mentions that "lasting boots [lasting is a glossy wool shoe fabric] are frequently trimmed with velvet rosettes" in September 1864. An 1863 white silk wedding boot has three lace rosettes down the front, each with a gilded butterfly in the middle, to match the dashing gilded heel[43] (fig. 46). Gilded heels are also mentioned in *Godey's* in November 1871. Rosettes on the vamp continued to appear on boots from time to time into the 1880s.

The shorter walking skirts of the mid-1860s and early 1870s, worn over hoops that swayed and tilted when the wearer moved, provided frequent opportunities to see a lady's ankles. Therefore boots were made a little higher, they were more colorful (purple seems to have been favored), and the decoration was placed not only on the vamp but also at the top, where it would be particularly alluring (plate 8). A dressy high front-lacing Polish boot was described in 1864 as being made of black leather bound with scarlet leather and trimmed with scarlet tassels.[44] Tassels were still the rage in January 1867 when *Godey's* reported:

One of the latest styles is of a bright cuir-colored leather buttoned up the sides, made with very high Louis XV heels, and finished with tassels. Some have very deep patent leather tips with kid uppers buttoned half way up the leg, and finished with loops of cord and two tassels. Others, again, have the uppers of cloth, lasting, or a checkered material, and are laced very high on the leg. Some are stitched with colored silk and trimmed with colored cords and tassels. For evening wear they are frequently of white lasting silk or satin with colored tips and heels.[45]

Tassels, like rosettes, were very fashionable at the tops of boots about 1869–73, and they also appeared in the early 1880s (fig. 518, plate 8). Another fashion of the same period was to trim the tops of winter walking boots with fur (fig. 514). Still other boots had a deep band of patent leather around the top that was further embellished with cutouts and embroidery, sometimes matching cutouts and embroidery on the vamp (fig. 515).

Perhaps the most characteristic ornament of this period was to use white thread for stitching dark materials, both for the functional seams and for ornament. The ornamental stitching often takes the form of loops or scallops bordering the edges of the toe caps, and in more elaborate examples, it may form a leaf and tendril pattern running along either side of the center front seam or lacing (fig. 516). In the most expensive and dressy boots, this embroidery might be done in colors and by hand (fig. 517). Fancy machine stitching was featured in the boots displayed at the 1876 Centennial Exhibition, and white stitching is mentioned in *Godey's* from the late 1860s right through the 1870s (figs. 252, 286, 518).

By 1885 the fad for elaborate boots seems to have run its course, and plain boots were worn with the more tailored dresses of the later 1880s. These had only the scalloped button fly and the potential contrast between the materials of the top and the foxing for decoration. As *Godey's* remarked in May 1885, "No fancy work, embroidery, stitching, beading, or even irrelevant fancy buttons are visible. The boot is ornamental only in its quality, which is of kid, the finest and softest." Of course, plain boots had been worn right along by plain people—it was only stylish belles who were rediscovering the merits of simplicity.

1890–1900

By the early 1890s, there was a modest turn back toward some decoration in boots. First, a peaked toe cap with perforated edges was added to the simple button boot. Then the heel foxing was cut into fancy shapes, or had scalloped or waved edges (figs. 431, 519). When front lacing was used, lace stays and trimming bands around the top edges were given scalloped and perforated edges, as were the stays covering the center front seams on gored boots (fig. 520). Lace stays and back stays of more substantial or hard-wearing leather served not only a decorative purpose but also to protect the upper from the constant friction of the skirts with their starched petticoats and stiff foundation materials.

The most frequently mentioned material in the early 1890s is Dongola kid, which was made in dull, satin, bright, and glazed finishes, but by the later 1890s Vici kid (the trademark name for chrome-tanned kid) had begun to live up to its name and conquer the vegetable-tanned competition. Leather boots of the later 1890s were generally black, but they were also made in the new tans and browns, specifically a dark brown called "chocolate," and more rarely in a dark wine red called "oxblood." Black patent was very widely used by the mid-1890s for the pointed toe caps and lace stays, and for the fancy heel foxing that came in a couple of years later.

With the new front-lacing styles, wool cloth tops came back into fashion. "Cloth top shoes are very stylish, more so in lace than button, as the former can be adjusted more easily than the latter."[46] These appeared in both black and brown to match the black and tan leather foxings, and they often had a small woven pattern (fig. 523, plate 10). Boots with uppers made entirely of serge or silk, however, were nearly nonexistent in the 1890s, except in the occasional Congress boot that was specifically advertised for "old ladies."

Felt, which was so widely advertised for bedroom slippers from the 1890s on, was also used to make warm but inexpensive winter boots, especially in the 1890s and early 1900s. Sears and Montgomery Ward advertised felt boots in button, front-lace, and elastic-sided styles. Some were made with felt soles and heels as well as uppers, but others had leather sole and heel, and sometimes a leather foxing, lace stay, or side patches at wear points (fig. 521). Fleece-lined, front-lace boots with felt tops but with leather vamps and quarters were advertised in Sears for both men and women as late as 1934. A boot dating from about 1890 made of black felt lined with scarlet wool and having a leather sole and heel is preserved at the Peabody Essex Museum.[47]

In the 1890s, only heavy-duty women's boots were made entirely of calf (if one does not count patent leather, which was often made of calf). Jordan Marsh, which catered to an urban clientele in the Boston area, listed a russet calf blucher boot with welted soles in its 1893 catalog as a "storm" boot, "especially adapted for winter wear." Montgomery Ward, which directed its catalog more toward country and small-town buyers, advertised calf boots as "Field and Farm Brands" in its 1895 catalog. These were made in both button and front-lace styles, and the front-lace versions came only with pegged soles.

Another leather used for women's sturdy and practical footwear in this period was oil grain. Oil grain was recommended for wet weather wear, since the oil-finished side leather would dry soft even after it had been wet. Another advantage was that its pebbled surface did not show the wear as immediately as a smooth-finished leather. Glove grain, a lighter split leather, could also be finished with oil to make it more waterproof.

One of the more interesting entries in the 1897 Sears catalog is for a "Ladies calf polish [high front-laced boot], made from the best all calf stock, half double soles and hand pegged. This is a strictly western custom made shoe, and there is nothing better for heavy wear at any price. . . . $1.70." This boot is plainer than most late 1890s front-lacing boots, lacking the long drawn out toe and contrasting fancy tip and lace stay characteristic of these years (fig. 522). It is not clear what makes this boot "western," but Sears could be catering to a specifically western regional taste. Another "western-made" closed-tab lace boot appears in the 1907 catalog as "A Beauty."

1900–1910

Beginning about 1900, when "mannish" styles with extension soles and masculine detailing became fashionable, heavier leathers became more acceptable for women's stylish walking boots. Dull mat calf was typically used for the tops of women's boots, while the vamps, foxing, and lace stays were of patent, itself by no means a soft or pliable leather. Chrome-tanned kid was also used for boot tops as a contrast to the shiny patent, and it replaced patent for the vamp when greater comfort and flexibility was desired. Box calf, glove calf, and gun metal were also frequently mentioned.

Patent, which had been used in the 1890s for toe caps and lace stays, became increasingly important through the early 1900s until by 1905 and 1906 nearly all the more dressy and expensive ($3-$4) boots advertised in Sears had the entire lower part made of patent leather (usually coltskin, when named at all). Dongola and chrome-tanned (Vici) kid were still widely used, but now more in the less expensive lines of shoes. Cloth tops were available in the early 1900s, but judging from advertisements and mail-order catalogs, they formed a rather small proportion of the boots made.

While tan leather was extremely popular for low shoes at this period, it was far less often used for boots, because boots were primarily a winter article while tan had come to be considered a summer color. This disapprobation of tan boots did not necessarily extend to the very dark shades of brown such as chocolate, but chocolate was not as common as it had been in the late 1890s. Sears advertised a chocolate

kid boot with black patent vamp and foxing in 1906, remarking "this is a very neat and tasty combination, the chocolate vici top being a nice relief from the regulation black." Suede appears only occasionally in descriptions of boots in this decade.

Aside from the contrast of bright and dull materials, boots were not often highly ornamented after 1900. Toe caps and top edges were generally straight, and even the traditionally scalloped edges of button flies were straightened out. Perforations were used to mark the toe cap and sometimes the edges of the foxing. The perforations varied in size, but around 1900 they tended to be large and sometimes cut in fancy shapes like diamonds or stars (fig. 524). Foxings were far less often cut in regular waved or scalloped shapes as they had sometimes been in the 1890s. More and more boots were "whole-foxed"; that is, they looked like a slipper with a boot-top above (fig. 525), although many were still made with separate vamp and heel foxing. The vamp usually curved gently down to the waist, but the heel fox came in a choice of shapes. Among the more common variations were a heel fox curved down to meet the vamp at the waist, angled down to meet the vamp at the waist, or extended forward to parallel the vamp seam and sometimes to merge with the lace stay (figs. 254, 256, 257). Congress boots usually had the front seam covered with a "front stay" that sprouted from the toe cap (fig. 291). Beginning about 1906, the mannish quality in some women's footwear was emphasized by creasing the vamp, a detail that continued in use until about 1915.

1910–1930

The period 1910 to 1921 falls into three periods: 1910–14, an era of mannish footwear; 1915–17, a brief period of experimentation; and 1918–21, a return to utilitarian footwear encouraged by World War I and the final decline of the boot. Patent vamps and foxing with dull-finished leather uppers continued as the most common style for dressier boots all through the teens, but more variety in material was admitted than had been seen in the first decade of the new century.

Dull-finished calf leathers were popular in the first

years of the decade. Gun-metal calf is frequently advertised and is mentioned specifically as being appropriate for wear with tailored suits. Tan was particularly fashionable for boots in 1911. White buck boots were much worn for summer at the beginning of the decade, thanks to the introduction in 1911 of an imitation white buck called "nubuck." Nubuck was preferred by manufacturers since real buck was so difficult to keep clean during the manufacturing process.

Boots in the early teens were not particularly decorative. They generally had straight perforated toe caps, and sometimes perforation marked the edge of the foxing, but otherwise most were quite plain. The variation in heel foxing typical in the previous decade faded from fashion as the simple and neat-appearing whole-foxed style became standard (fig. 268). Extension soles and creased vamps continued to appear in mannish walking boots.

Beginning in 1912, boots with black cloth tops came into fashion for use with a contrasting vamp and foxing, usually of black patent, sometimes of gun metal or black kid. The *Shoe Retailer* clearly associates the rise in cloth boots with the fashion for buttoned fastenings. The cloth-topped boot reached its peak in 1915, and declined thereafter, giving way to suede tops. Suede appeared in black, and in shades of gray, brown, and tan. It sometimes formed the entire boot but was more often used for the top of a boot with a darker vamp and foxing. The midteens also saw an increased interest in kid leather, since calf was expensive.

Between the fall of 1914 and spring of 1917, styles were slightly more variable and decorative than they had been earlier in the decade. One new pattern, the gypsy button boot, had a seam running from the tip of the toe straight up the center front. This was em-phasized by a contrast piping (often white on a black boot) or by a pointed toe cap that simply narrowed as it rose following the center seam, a detail borrowed from Congress boots (fig. 527). Some sports and walking boots had a "ball strap" applied across the vamp instead of or in addition to the toe cap (fig. 526).

The shortened skirts in the midteens encouraged the fashion for taller boots and by 1917, boots nine inches high above the heel were standard. Buttoned fastenings were not considered practical in the new height, and therefore most boots were now made to lace in front. The entry of the United States into World War I in 1917 caused a strong turn toward utilitarian styles and colors in the boots prepared for spring 1918. Nearly all were in the simpler whole-foxed pattern of the early teens. Calf made something of a comeback, thanks to the new interest in browns and tans. Many of the wartime and postwar boots were made of solid black or brown, but light gray and white were also available. Others were made with a dark leather vamp with a lighter top of gray, fawn, or white suede or cloth, but as boots sank out of fashion, to be retained only by conservative women, they were offered chiefly in utilitarian black and brown. Perforations appeared in the standard pattern, at toe cap and foxing and sometimes to mark the lace stay, but they were not universal.

A few boots were offered during the later 1920s, the most fashionable of which was the solid leg Russian boot (figs. 308, 309). Most twenties boots, however, were utilitarian wear for cold weather, made of kid, or occasionally calf leather, with a fleece or sheep's wool lining. These winter boots generally had low, broad heels made entirely of rubber or of leather with a rubber top lift (fig. 528).

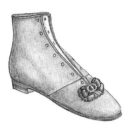

Fig. 509. 1790–1830
Bows and Rosettes
A bow or rosette at the base
of the front lacing is very
common in boots before
1830. This example 1805–15.

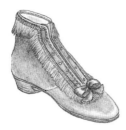

Fig. 510. 1790–1830
Fringe
Fringe, more often found
only around the top edge,
also borders the lace holes in
this 1820s boot.

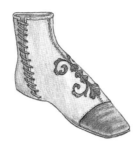

Fig. 511. 1830–60
Embroidery
Side-lacing boots with
embroidered insteps appear
in French fashion plates of
the early 1830s.

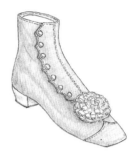

Fig. 512. 1860–90
Bows and Rosettes
The rosette on this silk
evening boot is similar to
those on slippers in the
1860s. This one 1866.

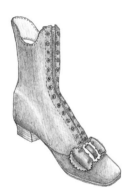

Fig. 513. 1860–90
Bows and Rosettes
This serge walking boot has
a bow and buckle typical of
the period 1865–75.

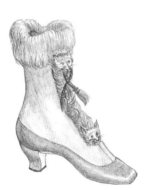

Fig. 514. 1860–90
Fur and Tassel
Fur trimming was stylish on
walking boots from 1869 to
1873, but compare the
carriage boots in figs. 83, 84.

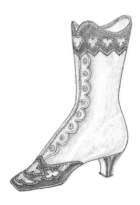

Fig. 515. 1860–90
White stitching
Cutouts stitched round the
edges are found only in the
most elaborate 1870s boots.
This example 1872.

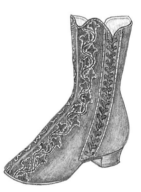

Fig. 516. 1860–90
Embroidery
White machine stitching was
widely used on dark uppers
from the late 1860s to the
early 1880s. This example
1876.

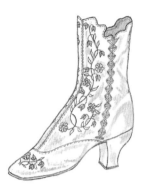
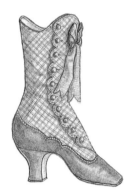
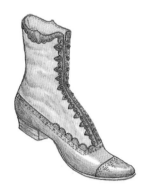
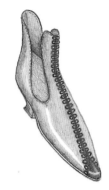

Fig. 517. 1860–90
Embroidery
More expensive and dressy boots were enriched with hand embroidery in the 1870s. This example 1876.

Fig. 518. 1860–90
Bows and Rosettes
Bows, rosettes, and tassels continued to ornament the top of boots into the early 1880s. This one 1882.

Fig. 519. 1890–1920
Elaborate Pattern
Exhibition boots from the 1890s were often decorated with scalloping and other fancy edges.

Fig. 520. 1890–1920
Elaborate Pattern
Gored boots were updated in the early 1890s by adding a scalloped front stay. This continued through the 1900s in a simpler version.

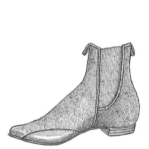
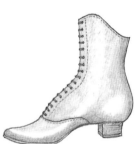
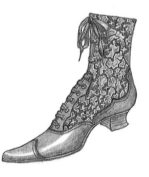
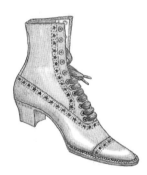

Fig. 521. 1890–1920
Felt Upper
Most felt boots were cut just like leather ones, but occasionally they had leather soles and reinforcements at wear points. This example 1897.

Fig. 522. 1890–1920
"Western" Boot
This simple front-lace boot with pegged half-double sole was described as a "strictly western custom made shoe . . . for heavy wear" in 1897.

Fig. 523. 1890–1920
Patterned Upper
Patterned silk and/or wool shoe fabrics called "vestings" were often combined with kid foxings and stays in the 1890s. This one 1900.

Fig. 524. 1890–1920
Perforations
Star- and diamond-shaped perforations are characteristic around 1900. See also fig. 199.

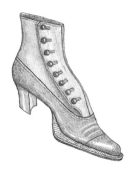

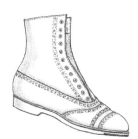

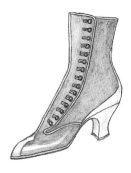

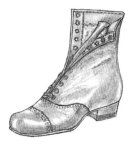

Fig. 525. 1890–1920
Creased Vamp
Creased vamps and
extension soles created a
mannish look in many boots
and shoes from 1906 to 1915.
This example 1907.

Fig. 526. 1890–1920
Elaborate Pattern
The "ball strap" (perforated
band across the vamp), used
in addition to a toe cap, was
a detail common in sports
shoes in the mid-1910s.

Fig. 527. 1890–1920
Contrast Materials
The gypsy pattern returned
to style in 1915–16,
emphasized by cording the
seam with a contrasting
color.

Fig. 528. 1920–40
Fleece Lining
The most common boot in
use after 1923 was a fleece-
lined, low-heeled, broad-
toed boot for utilitarian
cold-weather wear.

How Leather Is Made

Leather is the skin of any animal (usually a mammal) that has been chemically treated in such a way as to keep it from rotting. This chemical treatment is called tanning because it traditionally involves the action on the skin of tannin, a reddish, astringent substance found in many plants. The qualities of leather depend not only on what kind of animal skin is used but on the tanning and finishing processes applied to it.

The names given various kinds of leather can deceive the unwary reader of advertisements and fashion descriptions, because the name of a desirable but not very plentiful leather tends to become extended to include cowhide finished to look like the original. For example, there is a leather actually made from kangaroo skin, but kangaroo calf is simply calf finished to imitate kangaroo, and kangaroo sides refers to cowhide with some of the grain buffed off to make a leather suitable for work shoes. The tipoff is in the word "sides," which always denotes cowhide. Since cowhides are large and difficult to handle, they are normally divided in half lengthwise, each half being called a side. From this practice comes the term "side leather" for any leather made from cowhide (see the glossary for explanations of other leather terms). In the leather trade, the term "hide" is applied only to skins weighing over twenty-five pounds, that is, those taken from large animals—horses and full-grown cattle. The term "skin" is reserved for those weighing under twenty-five pounds, which may come from calves, goats, kids, sheep, etcetera. Lightweight cowhides between fifteen and twenty-five pounds are known as kips, and those under fifteen pounds are called calfskins.

The skin as it comes from the animal consists of three layers (epidermis, corium, and hypoderm), of which only the middle layer, the corium, or true skin, can be tanned. The upper side of the corium, or the leather made from it, is called the grain side, because of the fibrous pattern that is apparent on that side, while the underside is called the flesh side, because it is that side that connects with the muscles, blood vessels, and fat.

When leather is split into two or more thinner sheets, the layer bearing the grain is called the grain split; the bottom one, the flesh split. The grain split is stronger than the others and is the only one that can have a naturally smooth surface. Splitting requires a machine if all the splits are to be useful. While it was possible before the invention of the splitting machine to shave down leather to a more desirable thickness, the part pared off was no longer usable. Splitting is often done after tanning and before finishing, but it may be done at other stages as well.

Tanning is a very complicated process and subject to many variations, made either in order to produce a particular variety of leather or simply because the individual tanner prefers it so. In addition, there are changes in tanning practices from place to place and from time to time, so that it is quite impossible to provide a definitive description of tanning procedures in the context of a book on the history of clothing. However, the following simplified description is provided for those who wish to understand a little about the production of leather when they are trying to identify shoes or other leather accessories. The reader should remember that any of the following procedures may be carried out differently, and that a surprising number of them can be left out entirely and the resulting product will still be leather.

Perhaps the simplest kind of bark tanning involves digging a pit, putting a layer of oak or hemlock bark on the bottom, then a hide, then more bark, then a hide, and so forth, until the pit is full. Water may be added but does not have to be. A year later the pit is opened, and if the leather is not excessively thick it will be tanned through and may be subjected to finishing processes. This technique was used in colonial America by farmers to provide leather for their own personal use before commercial tanneries were widely established.

During the nineteenth and twentieth centuries, however, the process has been more or less as follows: When the tanner receives the hides or skins, they are dirty and bloody and may be salted and/or dried if they have been transported any distance. They must undergo a good deal of preparation before they are ready to be tanned. First, they are soaked to remove the dirt, blood, and salt, and to return dried skins to their natural condition of pliability. Then the outer and inner layers (epidermis and hypoderm) must be removed to expose the tannable corium. There are a number of ways to accomplish this, including soaking them in fermented plant material, damp smoking, and sweating (keeping the skins damp for several days). However, the most important process used was to soak the skins in a saturated solution of slaked lime for two or three days. All of these techniques rot the hair and epidermis, so that it can be scraped off manually in a process called "scudding." The remaining flesh, fat, and tissue on the underside is also scraped off. The alkaline lime must be washed off as much as possible, and the rest is neutralized by bating; that is, soaking the skins in a mild acid bath produced by mixing fermented manure in water. Then the bate has to be washed off before tanning proper can begin.

Tanning is done either with a vegetable tannin or in a chemical bath of chrome salts (the latter process in use only after 1884 and technically a species of tawing, since it uses mineral rather than vegetable substances), or for specialty leathers, with oils or with alum. Many plants contain tannin, and there are several that are used in leather making. The most important of these are oak bark, hemlock bark, sumac leaves, valonia (an acorn), and myrobalans (the immature fruit of a tropical tree), but a number of others are used in special applications or in combination with the above. The bark or other tanning material is ground small and then leached in water until nothing soluble can still be obtained. In the later nineteenth century, this "spent tan" was then used as the fuel for a special tan-burning furnace that produced steam to run the tannery machines.

The tanning itself may take anywhere from three months to a year, depending on how thick and heavy the leather is. It is done by soaking the hides in a solution of tanning extract in water. At first the solution is weak, but it is strengthened every day. The position of the hides in the vat is also changed daily, so that the tanning can take place evenly. This "handling" stage takes about six weeks. Then the hides are stacked in layers with tanning bark laid between each hide and allowed to rest for six weeks covered with an even stronger tanning solution. These processes may have to be repeated more than once before tanning is complete.

The chrome-tanning process is faster (taking a few days to six weeks, depending on the thickness of the leather) and has now largely superseded vegetable-tanning techniques. Skins are prepared for chrome tanning much as they are for vegetable tanning, since, of course, they are in just as much need of washing, unhairing, and scraping. When the preparation is complete, the skin is "pickled," that is, agitated in a bath in which salt and sulfuric acid are dissolved. The tanning is then done either in a "two-bath" or a "one-bath" process, the one-bath process being a refinement introduced in 1893. In the two-bath process, the skins are agitated in a bath of water to which salt, sodium bichromate (or potassium bichromate), and sulfuric acid are added. The sulfuric acid is necessary to allow the bichromate to penetrate the skin. When the solution is fully penetrated, the skins take on the yellow color of the bichromate. The second stage involves the addition of sodium thiosulfate, known to the photographer as "hypo." This chemical causes an insoluble chrome salt to precipitate between the fibers of the skin, resulting in chrome-tanned leather, a step that turns the skins blue; chrome-tanned leather retains its bluish-gray color unless it is bleached or dyed. The one-bath process differs only in that the final chrome salt desired is produced in advance and is milled into the skin in a single step, rather than being chemically formed within the skin from its separate components. The *Shoe and Leather Lexicon* notes in its entry on "Tanning" that "the process is very quick in comparison with bark tanning, and requires careful inspection in order to prevent burning of the leather by too rapid action of the acid. This effect is to be noted in the dry and papery surface sometimes seen in the chrome-tanned kid or goat skin."

There are two other tanning processes that should be mentioned here, which are used for special leathers. Tawing uses alum or a similar astringent mineral agent, produces a white leather, and is used chiefly for light, thin, supple leathers such as those for gloves. The skins are cleaned and prepared and then agitated in a vat containing alum, salt, flour, eggs, sometimes a little oil, and water. The skins may be tawed in as little as forty minutes.

Chamoising (or shamoying) involves impregnating the skin with fish oil. Again, the skin is prepared much as for other leathers, but in this process all but the very thinnest skins must have the surface grain scraped off. The oil is repeatedly rubbed on the skin and pounded in, and then allowed to oxidize in a heated room. The excess oil is washed out, and the result is a very soft, flexible, washable leather—not normally used for shoes, but sometimes for gloves. Any skin or hide may be chamoised, but it is done mostly on the flesh split of sheepskin. The name comes from the chamois, an alpine deer whose skin was prepared this way.

After tanning, the leather is too rough and stiff for use until it has undergone a number of finishing processes, which are traditionally the province of the currier rather than the tanner. These include smoothing the leather, shaving down the thicker spots to make it even, working in fats to make it soft and pliable, and giving it whatever surface finish is appropriate for its intended use.

Thick spots in the leather can be shaved off the flesh side, but further smoothing and equalizing can be accomplished by slicking; that is, stretching out the skin by rubbing it on the grain side while it is wet. This work also brings to the surface the bloom, a yellow deposit that covers vegetable-tanned leather when it comes from the tanning vats, so that it can be scraped off. A similar operation is performed on heavy sole leather to smooth and level it and to compress and solidify it. This equalizing process goes by a number of names, including striking out, pinning, stoning, and hammering on the lapstone.

The working in of fat may be limited to a light rubbing over with oil or may be an extensive milling in of fats, soaps, and greases known as fat-liquoring. Oil may be incorporated at more than one stage of the finishing—for instance, both before and after dyeing. The dyeing or coloring may be done either by dipping the entire skin into the coloring vat, in which case the dye can penetrate deeply into the skin from both sides, or simply by painting the surface.

Many leathers are given an artificial texture by a process called boarding (or sometimes graining), in which the grain side of the leather is folded against itself and the fold is rolled back and forth under pressure, resulting in many little parallel creases on the grain side. The rolling may be done again in the opposite direction to create a crosshatch texture, and again diagonally to produce a pebbled effect. Artificial surface textures can also be produced by running the leather between textured rollers under pressure.

If a shine is desired, the leather is glazed after it is colored by coating it with gelatin, shellac, or an albumen dressing. Then it may be burnished with a glass cylinder, a process that may be done repeatedly to create even shinier finishes. Patent leather is produced by a complex process involving painting the leather with successive coats of black varnish.

How Shoes Are Made

The following account of shoemaking is meant to serve merely as a basic introduction for the nonspecialist. The main steps in shoemaking are described only in the most general of terms, and many steps that are not done on all shoes, such as making eyelets and sewing on buttons, are not mentioned at all. In addition, the reader must remember that the way each step in the shoemaking process was carried out changed over time, and recent methods of using cement to attach sole to upper are not discussed here. The techniques of hand shoemaking naturally vary from those of the factory. Nevertheless, despite the many variations in practice, the shoemaking process can be broken down into four main steps: cutting, stitching, lasting, and bottoming.

Cutting is the process of cutting the upper from the hide, skin, or fabric. Upper pieces are likely to include vamp and quarters, and there may also be secondary pieces such as tongue, strap, lace stay, button fly, tip, foxing, etc. When the edges of the uppers are to be folded over before stitching, they are usually shaved thin or beveled on the flesh side (called "skiving") so that the fold is less bulky. Any decorative embroidery or perforations to be made in the upper must be done before the pieces are sewn together. The linings must also be cut from leather or fabric, and while they must fit with the uppers, the seams do not necessarily fall in exactly the same place. Stiff interlinings (toe box and counter) are prepared if desired.

Stitching is the process of sewing together the various parts of the upper. The lining is also sewn together, and the two attached to each other at the top of the shoe. This top edge may be finished by folding under either the lining or the upper leather, or by binding it with a strip of leather or fabric. Eighteenth- and early nineteenth-century women's shoes were often bound with a thin silk tape known as galloon, and this same galloon was sometimes laid over the side and center back seams as well.

Lasting is the process of shaping the uppers to the last, the last being a wooden form that imitates the shape of the shod foot, incorporating fashion details such as square or pointed toes. Each foot size requires a different last, and unless the shoes are to be straights, separate lasts are required for the right and left feet. Making straight shoes reduced the number of lasts needed by half. In the early days, this was an advantage to families making shoes at home or to traveling shoemakers who had to carry their lasts with them. Even when shoes were factory made, straights had the advantage of reducing the manufacturer's investment whenever new last styles were required (as when heels came into fashion, or when toes became narrower). When the variety of lasts available was small, doubtless many a foot suffered from ill-fitting shoes. On the other hand, when custom shoemaking was widely available, the good shoemaker could make a last to fit one's foot exactly, providing a luxury of fit available to very few people today.

When a shoe is lasted by hand, the last is either held in the lap or placed on a stand to hold it at working height, the sole upward, so that the shoe is worked upside down. The first step is to tack the insole, when there is one, to the top (that is, the sole) of the last. Then the upper is placed over the last. The lining is lasted first, the counter and toe box (if any) next, and then the upper. Pincers are used to pull the leather evenly around the last, working the leather and retacking as necessary, until the leather is smooth and wrinkle-free. Leather is easier to work when wet, so the upper is first mellowed by wetting it (the lighter and more flexible the leather, the less wetting is required). It also becomes more pliable as it is manipulated, so one can mold a piece of leather originally flat quite smoothly to the three-dimensional last by repeated stretching and tacking. When this process is complete, if tacks are to be used to attach sole to upper permanently, they are driven in against an iron-bottomed last, so that the points turn over, clinching them in place. If, however, the shoe is to be sewn together, the tacks are driven in only partway, so that they may be removed later. Lasting is a painstaking process that requires a good deal of judgment on the part of the shoemaker, lest wrinkles be formed in the upper or the leather be stretched so tightly that it will not flex when worn.

Bottoming is the process of attaching outsole and heel to the upper. Since about 1930, strong cements have often been used to bond sole and upper, but in the nineteenth century the most important construction types were welted shoes, turned shoes, pegged shoes, and stitched-down shoes.

Welted Shoes

Welting was the classic sewn technique used by hand shoemakers, and is the process used even today on the better class of men's shoes and women's sport shoes. It is a complex process that employs two rows of stitching. The first seam, called the inseam, connects the insole, the upper, and the welt. The welt is a narrow strip of leather about one inch wide laid around the edge of the sole so that part of it is hidden within the shoe and part of it sticks out beyond it and is visible on the outside of the shoe just above the sole. The second seam, the outseam, connects the visible part of the welt and the sole itself. The actual processes, however, are more complicated.

To sew the inseam, the insole must first be channeled. A channel is a slanting cut made in the bottom of the insole running around its entire edge (except where the heel is to be attached). This cut creates a "lip" that can be bent up toward the worker and that provides an accessible edge that can be sewn through. The upper is stretched over the last and fastened temporarily to the insole with lasting tacks. The tacks are not fully driven in and clinched as in pegged, nailed, or screwed shoes. Then the welt is laid around the edge of the sole and may be tacked in place. The inseam stitches pass through the lip in the insole, through the lining and upper, and through the inner edge of the welt. The tacks that are temporarily holding everything in place are removed one by one as the stitches are taken.

It would be possible to sew the outseam merely by stitching through the full thicknesses of both the welt and the outsole, but this would leave stitches exposed on the walking surface of the shoe that would eventually wear through with the friction of use and allow the outsole to come loose. To avoid this, a channel is cut into the edge of the outsole, creating a lip running around it entirely, much as was done with the insole. This lip is folded back, and the outseam is taken only through the welt and the partial thickness of the outsole lying between the channel and the welt. Then the lip is put back and cemented in place, protecting the stitches and ensuring the longer wear of the shoe. The outer edges of the outsole and welt are trimmed flush, so that when the shoe is completed, the welt looks as if it is part of the outsole.

Thus, welted shoes made with channeled insoles and outsoles show their stitching only on the welt around the outside of the shoe, but not on the inside of the shoe nor on the bottom of the sole. There are several advantages to a welted construction. Upper and sole are firmly held together, yet the shoe is reasonably flexible. Even without a sock lining, a welted shoe has a smooth surface next to the foot. There are no stitches to abrade the foot as in a McKay shoe. Nor are there stitches on the bottom of the sole to wear through with use. Welted shoes can be resoled easily without affecting the integrity of the original construction.

McKay-Sewn Shoes

Machinery capable of producing welted shoes was not perfected until 1877, with the appearance of the two Goodyear welting machines, one for inseaming and one for outseaming. Shoes were machine sewn, however, using a less complicated technique as early as 1860. Lyman R. Blake invented a machine to sew on the soles of shoes in 1858, but he sold the principal interest in it to Gordon McKay, who financed the construction of the first machines, worked with Blake

Methods for attaching the sole

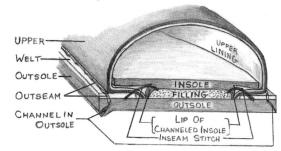

a. Welted shoe

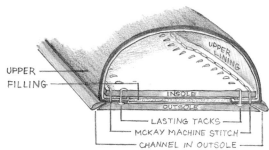

b. McKay-sewn shoe

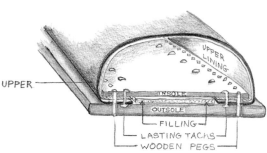

c. Pegged shoe

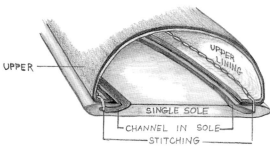

d. Turned shoe

to perfect them, and persuaded the Union Army to commission boots made by the new machine. Known as the McKay sole-sewing machine (in England as the Blake), it came into common use in the mid-1860s.

In the McKay-sewn shoe, the insole is permanently attached to the upper with clinched lasting tacks, and the last is then removed so that the sole can be sewn on by machine. This process uses no welt. The stitching goes straight through outsole, upper, and insole, except that the outsole is usually channeled to protect the stitching on the walking surface of the shoe. McKay-sewn shoes, therefore, are distinguished by the absence of any welt, and by the presence of both a seam and clinched lasting tacks on the foot side of the insole. Since these would make the shoe very uncomfortable to wear, a sock lining is placed over the insole. If this is lifted, the McKay stitching is visible.

Turned Shoes

There are two varieties of sewn shoes that do not incorporate insoles. The first is the turned shoe. In turned shoes, both upper and sole are put on the last inside out. The foot side of the sole (which is the side visible on the last) is channeled, creating a lip around its entire perimeter. The shoemaker bends the lip upward and stitches through it and the upper much as one would sew an ordinary seam in a dress, right sides together. Then the shoe is turned right side out (hence the name "turned shoe") and forced back over the last for shaping and drying. Then a sock lining is placed inside to cover the seam allowances. If the sock lining is lifted, you can see, not simply a row of stitching on the surface of the insole as in a McKay shoe, but the inner surface of the outsole with the seam allowances of the upper running round its edge.

This process can be used only for very light, flexible shoes with thin soles, and in practice it is limited chiefly to women's and children's shoes. Since women's and children's dress shoes make up by far the largest proportion of nineteenth-century shoes surviving today, the turned process is very fully represented in shoe collections. But actually turned shoes accounted for a minority of shoes produced, the majority being sturdier pegged, welted, or McKay-sewn shoes either for men or women.

Stitched-Down Shoes

An even simpler technique for sewing on soles is the stitched-down process. In this construction, the upper is turned toward the outside rather than under the last, and is then stitched directly to the outsole, requiring no insole. It was used in boots worn by soldiers during the Civil War.

Pegged and Screwed Shoes

Pegging, with its related processes of nailing and screwing, was used almost exclusively for hard-wearing shoes with heavy soles. In all shoes of this type, the lasting tacks were clinched against an iron-bottomed last to attach the upper to the insole. Then the outsole was attached to the insole and upper by driving through all three layers either a wooden peg, an iron or brass nail, or a screw. Any pegs that protruded up through the insole were planed off in the factory, but even retail shoe stores kept a peg cutter as standard equipment to shave off any recalcitrant ones that continued to annoy their customers. Pegged shoes are easily identified by the diamond-shaped peg ends that appear round the sole, sometimes in a double row. If the sock lining is lifted, both pegs and clinched lasting tacks should be visible inside on the insole.

Wooden pegs in shoes had long been used to build up and attach heels and to repair soles, but the use of pegs to attach sole to upper was a nineteenth-century innovation. The earliest American patent for making shoes and boots with wooden pegs was granted to Samuel Hitchcock and John Bement, of Homer, New York, on July 30, 1811.[1] Although a number of attempts were made to mechanize the pegging process (the Peabody Essex Museum has the first pair of pegged shoes made on a pegging machine invented in 1833 by Samuel Preston), pegged shoes were still often made by hand until 1859, when a successful pegging machine was run by power. By the middle of the nineteenth century, pegged shoes formed by far the greatest part of American shoe production, but the development of the McKay and Goodyear machines reduced the importance of pegged footwear until in 1910 it represented only two percent of shoes made. The earliest documented pegged shoe I have found may have been made as an exhibition shoe. It is a child's size, and the pegs in the sole are arranged to form on one shoe the motto "Remember your creator in the days of your youth" and on the other "E. B., A.D. 1816," with a border of overlapping scallops. E. B. was probably the maker, the father of donor Miss C. E. Blatchford.[2]

Using screws was tried about the same time nailing and pegging were developed, but the most important innovations in screwed shoes came with the invention of the screwing machine (1869, improved 1875). This employs not an ordinary screw with flat head and pointed tip, but a continuous length of heavy threaded wire, which the machine screws into the sole and cuts off flat when it has pierced all three layers. This results in a very strong bond, but makes the shoe difficult to repair later.

Littleway and Cement-Process Shoes

The following explanation of the Littleway and cement-process methods of attaching sole to upper has kindly been provided by Frederick A. Prahl, Jr. Mr. Prahl has fifty years of experience in shoemaking and shoe machinery development with first the United States Machinery Corporation and then the Compo Shoe Machinery Corporation, which introduced the cement process in the United States.

Up through the early 1930s, the majority of high-fashion, high-priced women's shoes were made by the turn, or turned, process because it produced the lightest, most flexible shoe. However, this process required more labor and skill, so it was limited to the higher-priced shoes such as I. Miller. The McKay process with lasting tacks clinched against the metal last bottom and a chain-stitched seam holding the insole, upper, and outsole together was limited to lower-priced shoes. In the early 1920s and through the early 1930s, two additional processes for women's shoes were introduced, which were the Littleway and the cement processes.

The Littleway was physically identical to the McKay process except that a staple lasting machine instead of a tack lasting machine was used for side lasting. The staple lasting machine created a staple from a reel of wire and drove the staple through the upper and lining but deflected the staple against an anvil so that the staple curled as it entered the insole and did not penetrate through the insole. The other feature of this process was that the horn sewing machine used to sew through the channeled outsole, the lining, the upper, and the insole was a lock-stitch machine. This machine had two threads, so that a lock was created in the outsole material making a more secure seam.

The cement process was introduced in Europe in the early twenties and was first practiced in this country by the Bresnahan Shoe Company in Lynn, Massachusetts. Originally the lasting procedure was the same as McKay or Littleway. After lasting, the bottom margin of the upper was roughed, using a rotary wire brush to remove the grain or top layer of the upper, and an adhesive was applied to the roughed margin. The outer sole was also roughed around its outer margin on the flesh side, and adhesive was applied to this margin. The original adhesive was pyroxylin or nitrocellulose, and required considerable time to dry. After the adhesive had dried on both bottom and sole, it was reactivated with solvent or a very light version of the cement on the sole, and the last with the upper, filler, and sole were placed in a press to hold the sole and shoe bottom together while the adhesive dried. Originally the machines had forty-eight stations on a belt, each having an inflated air bag that applied pressure on the outer sole against the shoe bottom while the adhesive dried. As the adhesive was developed to dry more rapidly, the number of stations were reduced to thirty-six, then to twenty-four, then to sixteen, and finally to eight. Different adhesives were later developed and used for both lasting and sole attaching. Nitrocellulose was replaced by heat-activated neoprene or vinyl cements that were activated by radiant heaters and only required a sole-attaching press with two stations, one for the right foot and one for the left.

The cement process is the major process worldwide for women's and a large percentage of men's shoes. The main reason is that the shoe remains on the last through all of the making operations except heel attaching.

Other Aspects of Bottoming

In shoes with insoles that have uppers of fairly heavy leather, a space is created between the insole and the outsole that must be filled if an uncomfortable depression is not to appear when the shoe is worn. This filling may be of leather, cork, or felt. It is also in this space that the thin metal or wooden shank may be inserted if the shoe requires reinforcement at the arch, as is particularly the case with high-heeled shoes.

After the sole has been attached, the edge is trimmed to the desired shape. This edge shape may be beveled, round, square, feather (a thin edge seen often in turned shoes), or "fudge." In this last type, a wheeled fudging tool is used to impress onto the welt a pattern of ridges that produces a decorative effect while covering the outseam stitches. Then the edge is "set"; that is, finished with polish applied by heavy rubbing. The bottom of the sole may be buffed with sandpaper to give it a smooth finished appearance.

Heels may be made either of wood or of layers of leather pegged (or, in the twentieth century, cemented) together. Wooden heels are usually covered with leather or fabric to match the upper. In either case, the heel is attached to the shoe either with nails clinched at the insole or with wooden pegs. The top piece, the tough piece of sole leather that provides the walking surface of the heel, is nailed or pegged on separately. Leather heels when attached are only roughly shaped, and they are trimmed to their final form afterward, when the breast is either squared off or hollowed into a curve. Then they are burnished to give them a smooth hard surface.

Before leaving the factory, a shoe was often subject to "treeing."

Treeing is done to give the boot or shoe the proper shape. In treeing a form is used that is just like the last [what we know as a shoe tree] and when the shoe is on this form any rubbing or cleaning that may be done to it does not damage the shape of the shoe, while it takes the dirt off and gives the treer a chance to put on a polish. A patent leather shoe or a colored shoe will get more or less dirt, cement, wax and other stuff on it in going through the factory, all of which must be taken off to bring the leather back to its original finish. In men's fine goods a calf shoe is about the only one now that has oil rubbed into it in treeing. This is the only fine shoe that has to be rubbed down hard with a rubstick. The stock is filled and made soft in treeing, which helps the calf upper.[3]

Rubber and
Elastic Webbing

Natural rubber is the coagulated liquid latex produced by a number of tropical trees and shrubs found around the world, but only in South and Central America did the indigenous peoples learn how to gather, cure, and shape it to produce a variety of useful articles. Europeans traveling in South America in the sixteenth century recorded that the native peoples made such things as rubber shoes, bottles, shields, breastplates, syringes, and playing balls, and there are later accounts of their making waterproof garments.[1]

Over two hundred years passed, however, before any European began to imagine rubber's potential usefulness. By the late eighteenth century, small quantities of rubber were imported to Europe from Brazil in the form of rubber bottles made by the Indians of the Amazon river valley. Cut up into small pieces, the rubber from these bottles was used for erasing or "rubbing out" pencil marks—which is where the common name "rubber" originated. In France, rubber is called "caoutchouc," a respelling of the Indian word "cahuchu" (weeping tree), and the French term was also used in English (pronounced "koochook") in the nineteenth century and even into the twentieth.

Both the elastic and the waterproof qualities of rubber interested early nineteenth-century inventors, but they were hampered by the fact that although rubber flows out of the tree in a liquid form, it soon solidifies and decomposes unless it is carefully dried. Therefore, it was available in Europe and North America only as a solid material already permanently shaped. This solid crude rubber came from the Amazon first in the form of bottles, and later as sixty- to eighty-pound balls, built up layer by layer, each layer painstakingly cured over smoky fires. To make these rubber bottles and balls into anything else meant either cutting smaller objects out of them (such as rubber erasers), or dissolving them so that they could be molded into something new.

The earliest objects made from rubber were things small enough to be cut out of one of the imported bottles. In 1820, Thomas Hancock opened a factory in London for making such small articles, including elastic inserts for the wrists of gloves, for waistcoat backs, trouser and gaiter straps, suspenders, garters, stockings, and stays, and for the straps of clogs and pattens to allow them to slip on without tying (before the use of rubber for such small elastic articles, a small wire spring or row of springs enclosed in leather was typically used). Hancock soon found that a large quantity of rubber scrap was accumulating, and he experimented with ways of putting this to use. He built a masticating machine intended to tear the scrap rubber to shreds, but discovered instead that it caused the scraps to amalgamate into a solid malleable mass. This could be pressed into a mold, producing a block that was more easily cut than the irregular bottles had been.

As of 1820, the best substances known to dissolve solid rubber were turpentine and ether. Ether worked fairly well, but was considered too expensive for common purposes. It was, however, used to produce rubber surgical tubing, known as "Grossart tubing" after its inventor. When rubber was dissolved in turpentine, it was left in a permanently gummy condition even more likely to melt when exposed to warmth than was the natural crude rubber. Then in 1823, Charles Macintosh of Glasgow discovered that naphtha, a cheap and until then useless by-product of the gas-lighting industry, would dissolve rubber and then evaporate, leaving it in its original condition. He spread the rubber and naphtha mixture on fabric, and then pressed two pieces of treated fabric together, rubber sides together. This safely enclosed the rubber, which was necessary because even when dissolved with naphtha, rubber would soften and get sticky in warm weather. In 1824 Macintosh began making waterproof fabrics. His name became a synonym for raincoats and the rubberized cloth from which they were made. Thomas Hancock found that he could produce a more concentrated rubber solution than Macintosh by using the new solvent with his masticated rubber, and eventually the firms of Hancock and Macintosh were combined. Thus, by 1825 in England, natural, unvulcanized rubber was being employed in clothing to a significant extent.

Rubber trade and manufacture started later in the United States and faced more serious trouble. The first American rubber manufacturing company was the Roxbury India Rubber Factory, begun in 1832 near Boston. Many others were incorporated soon after, most of them in the Boston area. The most important product made was shoes, but life preservers, coats, caps, suspenders, wagon covers, and carriage covers were also produced. All the American companies except the Roxbury Factory were using turpentine as a solvent, which made their products undesirably sticky. By 1836, the Roxbury company had a mill that transformed the crude rubber into a smooth sheet, and a calender that spread the rubber sheet onto the cloth without the use of any solvent at all, resulting in a better product.

This first boom in American rubber manufacturing occurred in the mid-1830s, only to collapse within a few years as Americans discovered the deficiencies of natural rubber. Macintoshes and other rubber articles had succeeded in England, where the climate was less extreme, but in the United States they fared less well. Even in New England, where rubber articles were first imported and manufactured, the summers were so hot that early rubber not only got sticky as it did in England, it melted and gave off a sickening smell. And the winters were so cold that the rubber got not merely firm, but iron-hard and so brittle it would crack. By the late 1830s, the American market for rubber collapsed, and even the Roxbury company went out of business.

In 1839, after five years of experimentation that are an epic in themselves, Charles Goodyear discovered that when rubber is heated with sulfur, its defects are cured. It does not melt or get sticky when warm or get brittle when cold, as natural rubber does. While all rubber gradually loses its original shape when repeatedly stretched, vulcanized rubber lasts longer than natural rubber and is also stronger. This critical discovery is the basis for the entire modern rubber industry, but Goodyear profited very little from it. Goodyear was so poor that he hadn't enough money to obtain a patent for his process until 1844. By that time the secret was out, and the patent rights in Great Britain went to Thomas Hancock the same year. One of Hancock's associates named the process vulcanization, by which it is known today. Between 1844 and 1850, a number of manufacturers received licenses to use the process legally, but many others pirated the discovery, and in spite of repeated lawsuits to protect his rights and those of his legitimate licensees, Goodyear was $200,000 in debt at his death in 1860.[2]

Many kinds of articles were made out of rubber from the time vulcanization made its use practical. In *America through Women's Eyes*, Mary Beard quotes Margaret Alsip Frink's *Original Journal of an Adventurous Trip to California in 1850*, in which the author describes the conveniences of the wagon in which the "adventurous trip" was made. "We had an India-rubber mattress that could be filled with either air or water, making a very comfortable bed. During the day we could empty the air out, so that it took up but little room. We also had a feather bed and feather pillows." These they used from the Missouri River all the way to California in 1850. The rubber mattress was laid on the wagon floor, which covered compartments full of provisions. "The wagon was lined with green cloth, to make it pleasant and soft for the eye, with three or four large pockets in each side to hold many little conveniences—looking glasses, combs, brushes and so on. Mr. Frink bought in Cincinnati a small sheet-iron cooking-stove, which was lashed on behind the wagon. To prepare for crossing the desert, we also had two India-rubber bottles holding five gallons each, for carrying water."[3]

Rubber shoes, though, were the most important rubber product made until the advent of rubber tires. In 1876, the National Rubber Company of Providence, Rhode Island, set up machinery at the Centennial Exhibition in Philadelphia in order to make rubber shoes on site, and the process was described in *Scientific American*:

Making rubber shoes, as demonstrated by the National Rubber Company of Providence, R.I., at the Centennial Exhibition in Philadelphia, 1876. *Scientific American,* October 21, 1876.

Fig. A

Fig. B

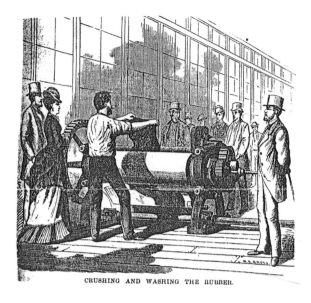

CRUSHING AND WASHING THE RUBBER.

Fig. C

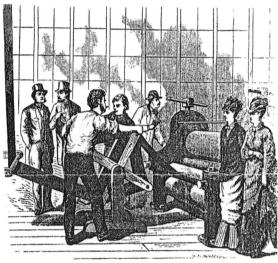

MAKING THE RUBBER INTO SHEETS.

Fig. D

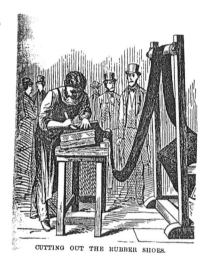

CUTTING OUT THE RUBBER SHOES.

Fig. E

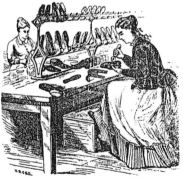

MAKING THE RUBBER SHOES.

Fig. F

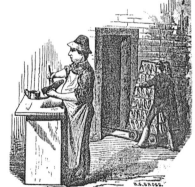

THE VULCANIZING OVEN.
VARNISHING THE SHOES.

A mass of raw rubber is represented in Fig. A. This, cut into suitable pieces by handknives almost as large as swords, is thrown between a pair of fluted cylinders, Fig. B, between which it is masticated and washed by streams of hot water, emerging in the mat-like form also represented in Fig. A. Next follows grinding, for from fifteen to twenty minutes between hot, smooth cylinders; and while the rubber is undergoing this process, the sulphur, tar, and other compounds to be mixed with it are added. The material now begins to form itself into a sheet; and after going through a pair of cylinders which stamp upon it the patterns of the shapes in which it is to be cut, besides ornamentation, etc., it is led to a reel, as shown in Fig. C. Meanwhile the black cloth, which is to form the backing, is led to the same reel, and as the latter is turned, alternate layers of rubber and cloth become wound about it. It remains now to consolidate the two materials, and this is done by passing the double sheet through heavy calender rollers under great pressure. From the sheets, thus prepared and of varying thickness, according to the parts which they are destined to form, the various portions of the shoe are cut (Fig. D), the workman following the stamped pattern with his curved knife. There are nine portions which go to make up the anatomy of the overshoe: the lining, the filling sole, the outsole, the insole, the forming strip up the heel, the strip around the shoe, the heel piece, the heel stuffing piece, and the junior or auxiliary heel piece; the respective uses of all these are sufficiently indicated by their names. As fast as they are cut out, they are passed to girls who sit beside a high table, perched on elevated stools. Running midway of the table are iron racks, and on pins thereon rest the lasts upon which the shoes are formed. The operation of putting the shoes together, which we illustrated in Fig. E, is by no means a difficult one, although it requires some skill. The lining and inside are attached to the last, and then the various pieces follow in succession, being secured in place by india rubber cement. Varnishing (Fig. F) is next in order, and then it might be supposed the shoe was complete—that is, to all appearances; but to feel the rubber is soon to be undeceived. It is soft and literally flabby; and although it has the shape of a shoe now, there is no reason to doubt but that, after a week's wear, the owner would find it half a dozen or so sizes too large, and more resembling a bag than a shoe. But here the vulcanizing process steps in to render the material hard and firm, yet elastic, and in a condition that, while the shoe may wear out, the shape will remain to the end. In Fig. F, in rear of the varnisher, a pyramidal iron carriage is shown, which a workman appears to be pushing into an open doorway. Across the framework of this carriage are tiers of bars, and on these bars are fastened the lasts with the varnished shoes upon them. When the carriage is filled it is pushed into the vulcanizing oven, a small brick chamber beneath which are large coils of steam pipes. The steam heat is gradually brought to about 270° Fah., causing, in about seven hours, the complete vulcanization or union of the rubber with the sulphur and other ingredients and leaving the shoes in fit condition for wear.[4]

Shoes dominated the rubber industry during the nineteenth century, but the other large category relevant to the history of clothing is the manufacture of elastic webbing, in which elastic threads are woven with other fibers into a stretchable fabric. In 1838 a precursor of true elastic webbing was made in England, a nonwoven elastic material made by stretching a sheet of rubber between two fabrics, using naphtha to make the layers adhere to one another. When the rubber was released it sprang back into shape, forming a wrinkled, stretchable fabric that was used for suspenders and elastic inserts for shoes (called gorings). This fabric did not breathe, of course, and was hot and binding. In 1839–40, Goodyear patented and began to manufacture "shirred goods," in which thin strips of stretched rubber were glued to fabric that was folded over to cover the rubber. Shirred goods were made throughout the 1840s and used for men's shirt ruffles, even though the product was not as durable as true elastic webbing, in which the elastic threads were actually woven in, not just glued. A version of shirred goods also seems to have been used in the earliest Congress boots (from the late 1840s through most of the 1850s). The Lynn Museum has a boot (fig. 281) in which the elastic threads were originally glued between two layers of fabric. This kind of goring is clearly identifiable because the outer layer of fabric is black and the inner one the tannish color of unbleached cotton. For another example using the same type, see the Peabody Essex Museum, United Shoe Machinery Corporation catalog #1808. There is in the Lynn shoe the faint remains of a stamped label, partly cut off when the goring was cut for use (as the bracketed hyphens indicate). It reads:

[-] AND EXCLUSIVE
[- MANU]FACTURER
[-]NDT ST. N.Y.
[- GOODYE]AR X SOLIS
[-] 44 - 48 - 49

The numbers 44, 48, and 49 refer to the years in which relevant patents were obtained. In 1844, Goodyear received patents both for vulcanized rubber and for a technique of making India-rubber fabrics, and in 1849 he received a patent for an improvement in rubber. The number "48" refers to the patent obtained on November 7, 1848, by Richard Solis, "for a mode of preparing the cloth for the rubber by stretching, also placing the rubber on the cloth obliquely."

According to Clifford Richmond, chronicler of the elastic web industry,[5] true weaving of elastic webs was first done in the United States by Hotchkiss and Prichard, Waterbury, Connecticut, in 1839, and in England at about the same time. This type is easily distinguished from the sandwiching technique used in shirred goods because it is a single layer of fabric with the elastic threads actually incorporated into the weave. The color is the same on both sides, normally black with a slightly brownish cast (fig. 282).

Early elastic webbing was made with natural rubber cut into strips with shears, resulting in an irregular thread of uneven tensile strength. Therefore, the early products were not very satisfactory. American companies made their own thread this way or else imported vulcanized thread from England (available circa 1850), since it was not successfully made in the United States until 1863. W. H. Richardson describes how cutting the threads was accomplished as of 1858.

A continuous strip may be cut from a bottle or any other curved mass of the India-rubber. The bottom of the bottle is cut off and is pressed into a round and tolerably flat form. The cake thus fashioned is fixed to the end of the horizontal shaft, or lathe-axis, and is made to revolve with great rapidity; and while so rotating, a circular knife, rotating at high speed, cuts through the substance, and advances steadily towards the centre of the disc; thereby separating the disc or cake into one continuous thread. This thread can be easily drawn out straightly and can even be separated into two or more finer threads, by drawing it through a hole where one or more sharp-cutting edges encounter it [the same principle was used to split straws for hat-making]. If a bottle or any other hollow piece of India rubber can be drawn over a cylinder of uniform diameter, it may be cut into a continuous thread by a modification of the same machine; the cylinder being made to revolve, a steel cutter is placed against it, and as the cylinder has a slow longitudinal motion given it, the gum is cut spirally from end to end—just on the same principle as a worm or thread is cut on a bit of iron by the screw-cutting machine. Machines of this kind were invented in France more than twenty years ago; but the machines used in our own country are of English invention and of later date.[6]

It seems likely that shirred goods were preferred as long as it was still difficult to produce elastic thread of even tensile strength. It must have been easier to glue the early irregular elastic thread between two layers of fabric than to actually weave them. It is only among the earlier styles of surviving Congress boots that shirred goods are found. Among the boots made in the styles of the mid-1860s, true elastic webbing with the rubber thread woven in is the type of goring employed.

Richmond reports that trademarks were used on rubber goring from the mid-1880s. The first was a shuttle design enclosing the words "Beatty and Taylor, Locked Rubber Patent" (1883–1884). The next important trademark appeared in 1884 or 1885, used by a Boston shoe goring company: a small heart enclosing the words "Hub Gore" and a date mark of the month it was made, stamped on the white back of the goring. The date mark was included because it was advertised to wear eighteen months after it was made, but apparently the date was not always easy to decipher. Hub Gore's chief competitor, Bridgeport Elastic Web Company, then adopted a trademark and the eighteen-month guarantee. In 1900, Hub Gore bought Bridgeport Elastic Web, but it is unclear whether Bridgeport retained its own name. In 1914, both companies with several others merged to form Everlastik, Inc., which still existed in 1946. "Double Arrows" was the trademark of John Buckley and Son, a firm that began in 1878. The trademark was used near the end of their existence, but no date is given.

Rubbers made in the United States in the nineteenth century were very often adulterated with other materials. Chalk, Paris white, Cornwall or porcelain clay, barytes, oxide zinc, white and red lead, ivory black, lamp black, black lead, and Spanish brown are the adulterants mentioned by W. H. Richardson in *The Boot and Shoe Manufacturer's Assistant and Guide* (1858). Some substances were added to change the rubber's color, and some actually improved the rubber, but others clearly did not. By the later nineteenth century adulteration seems to have been a great enough problem to discourage the buying of rubbers, and manufacturers countered by introducing more expensive rubbers of purer material. By the 1890s and early 1900s it was standard practice in many companies to carry two or three grades of rubbers called "firsts," "seconds," and "thirds." The *Shoe Retailer* listed the names of the trademarks used by rubber makers in 1901 to distinguish their various grades of goods (see chart):[7]

Name of Company	Firsts	Seconds
American Rubber Co.	American Rubber Co.	Para Rubber Shoe Co.
Apsley Rubber Co.	Apsley Rubber Co.	Hudson Rubber Co.
Banigan, Joseph, Rubber Co.	Banigan	Woonasquatucket
Beacon Falls Rubber Shoe Co.	Beacon Falls Rubber Shoe Co.	Granite Rubber Co.
Boston Rubber Shoe Co.	Boston Rubber Shoe Co.	Bay State
Bourn Rubber Co.	Providence Rubber Shoe Co.	Union Shoe Co.
Byfield Rubber Co.	Byfield Rubber Co.	Narragansett Rubber Co.
Candee, L., & Co.	L. Candee & Co. or Candee	Federals
Concord Rubber Co. (Mass.)	Concord Rubber Co.	Bunker Hill Rubber Co.
Goodyear's India Rubber Glove Mfg. Co.	Goodyear's India Rubber Glove Mfg. Co.	No seconds
Goodyear's Metallic Rubber Shoe Co.	Wales-Goodyear Shoe Co.	Connecticut Rubber Co.
Goodyear Rubber Co.	Special Brands: Crack Proof, Gold Seal, Snag Proof, Toboggan, Coasting, Newark Rubber Co.	Union India Rubber Co.
Grand Rapids Felt Boot Co.	Grand Rapids Felt Boot Co.	Wolverine Rubber Co.
Hood Rubber Co.	Hood Rubbers	Old Colony
Lambertville Rubber Co. (N.J.)	Stout's Patent Snag Proof	No seconds
Liberty Rubber Shoe Co.	2nds: Giant Rubber Co.	3rds: Atlantic Rubber Co.
Lycoming Rubber Co.	Lycoming Rubber Co.	Keystone Rubber Co.
Meyer Rubber Co.	Meyer Rubber Co.	No seconds
Milltown India Rubber Co.	Milltown India Rubber Co.	Crescent Rubber Shoe Co.
Mishawaka Woolen Mfg. Co.	Ball Band	Midland Rubber Co.
Model Rubber Co.	Model Rubber Co.	Fairmouth Rubber Co.
National India Rubber Co.	Tennis Shoes	
New Jersey Rubber Shoe Co.	No firsts	New Jersey Rubber Shoe Co.
Parker's Leather Soled	Made by Boston Rubber Shoe Co.	
Watkinson, Geo., & Co.	Geo. Watkinson & Co., Philadelphia	No seconds
Woonsocket Rubber Co.	Woonsocket Rubber Co.	Rhode Island Co.

Partial Listing of Shoe Manufacturers

As Compiled from Labels and Advertisements

The following list contains information from labels found in surviving shoes from the late eighteenth century to 1930, from advertisements culled from women's magazines between 1890 and 1930, and from a sample of issues of the *Shoe Retailer* between 1900 and 1928. Considering that the Philadelphia directory alone for a single year in the 1840s contains several pages of shoe manufacturers, jobbers, and retailers, it is obvious that this cannot be anything like a complete list of shoe manufacturers residing in the United States. It contains labels from shoes the author saw only when it was possible to note or photograph them. The advertisements come chiefly from the *Ladies' Home Journal* and the *Shoe Retailer*, although others were used when convenient. Because similar ads repeat from month to month in women's magazines, only the year and abbreviated periodical name are cited. Note that advertisements in the *Shoe Retailer* were directed at shoe retailers, not at the consumer, and therefore they often mention shoes' salability and counsel waiting to order shoes until retailers have seen the advertiser's samples. It is not always clear whether the prices listed were wholesale or retail, but if known, that fact is mentioned in the entry.

While the dates of advertisements and of surviving shoes suggest when certain makers were active, it is important not to assume that they existed only in the years for which advertisements were found. Many advertisements mention a history of twenty-five to fifty years, and some, like Daniel Green slippers and Red Cross Shoes, still exist today.

The following abbreviations explain such museum codes such as PEM USMC (Peabody Essex Museum, United Shoe Machinery Company Collection).

CD	National Society of the Colonial Dames
CHS	Connecticut Historical Society
CR	*Le Costume Royal*
DAR	Daughters of the American Revolution
DEL	*The Delineator*
DHS	Danvers Historical Society
FMH	Ferrar Mansur House, Weston Historical Society
GH	*Good Housekeeping Magazine*
HB	*Harper's Bazar*
HMG	*Hill's Milliners' Gazette*
HHS	Haverhill Historical Society
HN	Historic Northampton
HSW	*The Housewife*
LACMA	Los Angeles County Museum of Art
LHJ	*Ladies' Home Journal*
LM	Lynn Museum
LW	*The Ladies' World*
McC	*McCall's Magazine*
MFA	Museum of Fine Arts, Boston
NHMLAC	Natural History Museum of Los Angeles County
PEM	Peabody Essex Museum
PEM USMC	Peabody Essex Museum: United Shoe Machinery Corporation Shoe Collection
RIHS	Rhode Island Historical Society
SPNEA	Society for the Preservation of New England Antiquities
TSR	*Shoe Retailer*
USMC	United Shoe Machinery Corporation Shoe Collection
VHS	Vermont Historical Society
WHC	*Woman's Home Companion*

ABORN. C. H. Aborn & Co. Lynn, Mass.

1913: Illustrated a Colonial pump for 1914. TSR 9/20/13.

ADLER. B. Adler. New York City.

1921: Illustrated a strapped boot for 1922. TSR 9/17/21.

AIR MAIL SHOE CO. Sixth and Sycamore Streets, Cincinnati, Ohio.

Apparently a branch of the United States Shoe Company.

1927: "Air Mail Stock Shoes, a notable product and service of The United States Shoe Company, Cincinnati." Illustrated a rodeo boot at $6.25 and shoes from $4.25 to $5.35. TSR 12/17/27.

ALBERT. J. Albert & Son. Brooklyn, N.Y.

1921: Illustrated a fancy strap for 1922. TSR 9/17/21.

ALLEN SHOE CO. 31 Milk St., Boston, Mass.

1892: Boots $2.50 including postage. LHJ.

ALPINA. See HECHT.

AMERICAN HIDE & LEATHER CO. Boston, New York, Chicago, St. Louis, Cincinnati, Paris, and Northampton, England. The tanneries seem to have been located in Lowell, Chicago, Sheboygan, Ballston-Spa, and Curwensville.

1928: "Calf and side upper leather tanneries." "Special Willow Calf, the stylish women's shoe leather, beautiful and substantial with appearance and feel like kid." TSR 2/25/28.

AMERICAN LADY SHOE. See HAMILTON, BROWN SHOE CO.

ANTI-TENDER FOOT SHOE. See PETERSON, M. H.

APPLEBEE & NEUMAN, INC. 23–25 Greene St., New York City. Also Manila, Philippine Islands.

1917: "Fancy Shoe Buttons . . . pearl, ivory, pearlustre, inlays, etc." TSR 7/28/17.

ARCH PRESERVER SHOE. See SELBY SHOE CO.

ARCH REST. See DREW.

ARCHFIT. See KOLLOCK.

ARMSTRONG. D. Armstrong & Co. 115 Exchange St., Rochester, N.Y.

1901: "Manufacturers of Women's Boots and Low Shoes. Hand, Goodyear Welts and Turns. . . . The 'Dorcas,' $3.50, a Specialty." TSR 3/5/01, p. 98.

1902: Advertised Louis heel shoes. TSR 7/2/02.

1921: Illustrated a tie shoe for 1922. TSR 9/17/21.

1923: Illustrated a T-strap for 1924. TSR 9/15/23.

1928: Illustrated a one-strap. TSR 3/17/28.

ARNOLD. See NOVELTY KNITTING CO.

ARNOLD. M. N. Arnold Shoe Co. North Abington, Mass.

1921: Illustrated an oxford for 1922. TSR 9/17/21.

1923: Illustrated a one-strap for 1924. TSR 9/15/23.

ASHBY-CRAWFORD CO. Marlborough, Mass.

1916: Trot-Moc Back to Nature Shoes. Oxfords $4.00. Boots $4.50. "The genuine have the trade mark stamped all over the sole." Trademark: a vertical oval with an Indian holding a paddle [gun?] standing on a large ball with a shoe superimposed and "Trot-Moc" above the ball. LHJ.

AULT-WILLIAMSON SHOE CO. Auburn, Maine. Western and southern sales division in St. Louis.

1924: Constant Comfort Shoes. $2.50 to $6.00. LHJ.

1927: Constant Comfort Shoes. Trademark: an oval with words "Constant, AW, Comfort" and below the oval "Steel Arch Support." Constant Style Shoes. Trademark: an oval with words "Constant, AW, Style" and below the oval "Steel Arch Support." "Constant Comfort and Constant Style shoes are high-value Goodyear Turned shoes sold in volume at low price-range . . . $3 to $7.50 for all models, from boots to boudoir slippers." "Our factory [is] the largest in America devoted exclusively to women's 'turn' shoes." Goodyear Turned identification mark is an arrowhead pointing downward containing a large T below the smaller letters NO (the O is square and may be a D). LHJ.

BACHELLER & SPENCE. Lynn, Mass.

    1909: A sole shape containing the words "Bacheller & Spence, Lynn, Guaranteed old method Bark-tanned oak soles" may be a trademark. By this time much leather was chrome-tanned rather than bark-tanned. TSR 9/25/09.

BAKER. D. B. Baker, New York City. Probably a shoe ornament maker.

    1900: Illustrated slipper bows. TSR 4/1900.

BAKER. George W. Baker Shoe Co. Brooklyn, N.Y.

    1917: Illustrated a pump for 1918. TSR 9/22/17.

    1919: Illustrated a pump for 1920. TSR 9/20/19.

    1921: Illustrated a one-strap for 1922. TSR 9/17/21.

    1928: Illustrated a one-strap. TSR 3/17/28.

BALLOU. F. E. Ballou Co.

    1906–9: Front-lace boot with patent mark "Feb. 1906." RIHS 1969.11.23.

BARKE-GIBBON CO., INC. Philadelphia.

    1923: Illustrated a gore shoe for 1924. TSR 9/15/23.

BARTON, CLARA. See JOHNSON-BAIRD.

BATCHELDER & LINCOLN CO. 96 Federal St., Boston, Mass.

    1901: Advertised button and oxford models at $1.50. TSR 4/3/01.

BELL. Theodore Bell. Boston. Probably a retailer only.

    1835: Wedding slipper. Label: "Theodore Bell's Fashionable Boot and Shoe Store, Boston." MFA 21.265.

    1840–55: White satin slipper. Label: "Warranted Boots & Shoes, Particularly Made for Theodore H. Bell, 155 Washington Street, Boston, Opposite the Old South." Old South is a meeting house. PEM 123,052.

BELLAS-HESS. New York City. A general apparel mail-order house, not a shoe manufacturer.

    1915: White graduation pumps of canvas for $1.46 or "Nubuck leather" for $1.98. LHJ.

BELONGA & LEONARD. Lynn, Mass.

    1900: Illustrated a front-lacing boot at $1.60. TSR 7/1900.

BEMIS & WRIGHT. Lynn, Mass.

    1907: Advertised "FUTURE" shoes for women, "built to retail at $3.00, $3.50, and $4.00." Used a "Nail-less Cushion Heel Seat," covered by patents dated May 8, Nov. 13, and Dec. 11, 1906, and Jan. 22, 1907. "All nails and tacks are clinched below the Cushion. The thickness of the Cushion make it impossible for any nails or tacks to come in contact with the foot. This Cushion being resilient relieves all strain or jars while walking." TSR 9/28/07.

BLEECKER SHOE CO., INC. 138–40 Duane St., New York City. Offices in
Boston, Philadelphia, and Detroit.
1927: "Leap-Year Boots," price $4.50. TSR 12/31/1927.
BLISS & PERRY. Newburyport, Mass.
1928: Illustrated a cross-strap shoe. TSR 3/17/28.
BLUE RIBBON SHOEMAKERS, INC. St. Louis, Mo.
1928: Illustrated a T-strap. TSR 3/17/28.
BOARDMAN SHOE CO. 564 Atlantic Ave., Boston, Mass.
1913: Advertised boots. Trademark: a plain circle containing "The
Boardman Shoe, Trade Mark." TSR 9/20/1913.
BOND SHOE MAKERS. Cincinnati, Ohio.
1917: Mail order only, twenty-six styles offered, all for $3.00. "Regular
$4.00 and $4.50 shoes from our catalog, only $3.00." LHJ.
BOYD-WELSH SHOE CO. St. Louis, Mo.
1921: Illustrated a two-strap for 1922. TSR 9/17/21.
1928: Illustrated a one-strap. TSR 3/17/28.
BRADLEY CO. Haverhill, Mass. Boston Office, 183 Essex St..
1915: Trademark: "The Unity Shoe, Hand Turn" in a circle with the words
Style, Comfort, Quality in chain links below and some foliage above.
Apparently specialized in comfort shoes with low, broad, sensible rubber
heels, and cushion sock lining, some with a wide ankle. TSR 9/18/15.
BRADLEY-GOODRICH CO. Haverhill, Mass.
1876: Gilded kid slipper from Centennial Exposition. PEM USMC 2296
with others in this collection.
1928: Illustrated a one-strap. TSR 3/17/28.
BRAUER BROS. Shoe Co. St. Louis, Mo.
1928: Illustrated a pump. TSR 3/17/28.
BRESNAHAN SHOE CO. Boston, Mass.
1928: Illustrated a one-strap. TSR 3/17/28.
BRESNAHAN-MACLAUGHLIN SHOE CO. Lynn, Mass.
1919: Illustrated a one-eyelet tie for 1920. TSR 9/20/19.
BRIDGEPORT ELASTIC WEB CO. Bridgeport, Conn.
1901: Maker of Bridgeport Warranted Goring, used in elastic-sided shoes
and boots. TSR 3/12/01.
BRISTOLL & HALL. 82 Chapel St., New Haven, Conn.
1843–44: Listed in New Haven directory.
1844: Tan slit vamp shoe marked October 2, 1844. Label: "Bristoll & Hall
Makers, 82 Chapel St., New Haven, Ct." HN 66.645.
BROPHY BROS. SHOE CO. Lynn, Mass.
1900: Illustrated a front-lacing storm boot at $1.75. TSR 7/1900.
BROWN SHOE CO. St. Louis, Mo.
1909: White House Shoes for men, for women. Trademark: "Brown's Mark
Means Quality" around a rectangle with concave sides containing a ★5★.

This company also made "Buster Brown Shoes" for children. $2.50 for a woman's front-lace boot, $3.00 for a man's. Children's shoes ranged from $1.50 to $2.50. Advertisement in TSR 9/25/09.

    1911: Similar information. LHJ.

    1913: Illustrated a front-lace boot for 1914. TSR 9/20/13.

    1919: Illustrated a tongue pump for 1920. TSR 9/20/19.

    1926: Shoes from $3.85 to $5.35. TSR 12/4/26.

BUEK & CO. Philadelphia.

    1921: Illustrated a fancy side-gore shoe for 1922. TSR 9/17/21.

BUNN. Reuben Bunn. New York City.

    1801: Blue kid wedding slippers. Label: "Reuben Bunn, Ladies' Shoe Maker, No. 60, William Street, Formerly no. 39, Smith Street, Between Wall Street and Maiden-Lane." HN 1979.30.83.

BURRILL. I. Burrill. Lynn, Mass.

    1795–1805: White satin heeled slipper. Label: "Warranted Shoes made and sold by I. Burrill, In Lynn." SPNEA 1922.968.

BURROWS SHOE CO. Rochester, N.Y.

    1919: Illustrated a pump for 1920. TSR 9/20/19.

    1923: Illustrated a T-strap for 1924. TSR 9/15/23.

    1928: Illustrated a one-strap. TSR 3/17/28.

BURT. Edwin C. Burt.

    1917: Designed a front-lace boot. TSR 9/22/17.

BURT. E. W. Burt & Co. Lynn, Mass.

    1901: Advertised a "striking mannish Oxford." TSR 5/22/01.

BURT BROTHERS. New York City.

    1845–55: Black kid slipper, gilt-stamped on vamp. Label: "Burt Brothers, New York." HN 66.656.

CAMBRIDGE RUBBER CO. Cambridge, Mass.

    1926: "Raynboots" and "Cap'n Kidd Boots." Trademark: "caMco" with "Cambridge" and "Rubber Co." within the streamers depending from the enlarged M. TSR 10/15/27 cover.

    1927: Cap'n Kidd pull-on rubber boot. TSR 10/8/27, 11/26/27.

CAMCO. See CAMBRIDGE RUBBER CO.

CAMMEYER. 311 6th Avenue at 20th St., New York City.

    1914: Advertised a style book. LHJ.

    1916: Advertised a style book, "not only the popular and reliable styles, which we have been selling for over 50 years in our large New York store, but also the latest and most exclusive designs approved by fashion. . . . Fifty years experience in fitting by mail . . . over 92,000 customers each year buy this way." LW.

CANTILEVER SHOES. See MORSE & BURT CO.

CANTRELL. New York City.

    1863: Side-lace wedding boots with butterflies on three rosettes. Label:

"Cantrell, Maker, 813 Broadway Between 11 & 12 St. New York." HN 1979.30.86.

CAPITAL SLIPPERS. See WILEY-BICKFORD-SWEET CO.

CAPITAL SHOEMAKERS, INC. St. Louis, Mo.

    1923: Illustrated a strap shoe for 1924. TSR 9/15/23.

CAP'N KIDD BOOTS. See CAMBRIDGE RUBBER CO.

CARFAGNO SHOE CO. Rochester, N.Y.

    1919: Illustrated a plain pump for 1920. TSR 9/20/19.

    1921: Illustrated a one-strap for 1922. TSR 9/17/21.

CARLISLE SHOE CO. Carlisle, Pa. Offices in New York and Chicago.

    1903: Advertised boots and tie shoes for 1904. TSR 9/16/03.

    1915: Advertised a gypsy boot for $2.85. "Makers of women's shoes to retail at $3 to $5." TSR 9/18/15.

    1917: Advertised a "trench boot . . . with high khaki top made in imitation of a puttee, encircled with a strap which buckles at the top." Retail prices now range from $4.00 to $7.00. TSR 9/22/17.

CASH BUYERS UNION. First National Co-operative Society, 158 G Cash Buyers Building, Chicago.

    1904: "We Paralyze Competition. Co-operation does it. Send us a postal for our Big FREE 1904 Boot and Shoe Catalogue, fully describing all of these shoes and our full line of over 300 styles for Men, Women, and Children. . . . We can save you Big Money on your shoes and everything else you eat, wear or use." Women's shoes illustrated from $0.90 to $1.20, men's shoes illustrated from $1.20 to $1.95. McC.

CAT'S PAW. See FOSTER RUBBER CO.

CAUNT. Joseph Caunt & Co. Lynn, Mass.

    1900: Illustrated a strap shoe. TSR 7/1900.

    1904: Illustrated a latchet tie for 1905. TSR 9/28/04.

    1907: Illustrated a dressy tie for 1908. TSR 9/28/07.

CAUNT. Morris Caunt Shoe Co. Lynn, Mass.

    1904: Illustrated a tie shoe for 1905. TSR 9/28/04.

CHAMBERLAIN & SONS. Cheapside, London, England.

    1770: Blue silk wedding slipper of Mary Jones Colman. Label: "Chamberlain & Sons, Shoe Makers in Cheapside, London." SPNEA: 1966.43.

CHAMBERS. Box 607. [Part of ad missing.]

    1904: Eclectic Shoes. Advertises latest catalog (number 3), a "wide and long-established reputation for fine shoe-making," mentions twenty-seven styles and six widths and a price of $3.50. LHJ.

CHASE & COGSWELL. Haverhill, Mass. May be a retailer only.

    1815: White kid wedding slippers. Label "Chase & Cogswell's Variety Shoe Store, Main Street, Haverhill, Mass. Rips mended gratis." HHS 2821.

CHERRY. W. E. Cherry, Jr., & Co. Rochester, N.Y.

    1903: Advertised the "Rochester," a woman's front-lace boot wholesaling at $1.25. TSR 9/16/03.

CHICAGO SPECIALTY SHOE CO. Chicago, Ill.

    1921: Illustrated a two-strap for 1922. TSR 9/17/21.

CLEMENT CO. Apparently a retailer, possibly in Springfield, Mass.

    1922: Wedding shoe, colonial style. Label: "Made expressly for the Clement Co." HN 1981.40.2.

COHEN. 57 W. 19th St., New York City. Possibly the same as B. Cohen & Sons.

    1901: "The Only Makers of Felt and Warm Footwear," a statement that is probably not true unless they made the footwear marketed under the name Daniel Green. Romeos, 75c and up. TSR 4/3/01.

COHEN. B. Cohen & Sons. New York City.

    1900: Illustrated slippers, straps, ties. TSR 4/12/1900.

    1900: Illustrated four fur-lined "house shoes" [boudoir slippers]. TSR 7/1900.

    1901: Advertised dressy tie shoes. TSR 3/1901, 5/22/01.

COHEN AND FRANK. Brooklyn, N.Y.

    1904: Illustrated a front-lace boot for 1905. TSR 9/28/04.

COLT-CROMWELL CO., INC. 1239 Broadway, New York City. Est. 1899.

    1927: "It is the specialized line that gives distinction to the store. Imported English riding boots, aviator boots, field boots, jodhpurs, puttees, riding boot accessories." TSR 12/31/27.

COMFY. See GREEN.

CONSTANT COMFORT SHOES. See AULT-WILLIAMSON.

CONSTANT STYLE SHOES. See AULT-WILLIAMSON.

CONSUMERS' BOOT AND SHOE CO. Boston.

    1891: Boots $2.00 including postage. LHJ.

COON. W. B. Coon Co. 7 Canal St., Rochester, N.Y.

    1927: Wilbur Coon Shoes. "In all leathers and fabrics, for the unusual foot. Most models are priced $8 to $11." Trademark: "Stylish stout, Out Sizes, Trade Mark" in a rectangle with scallops on lower edge. Trademark: "Slender Foot, Arch Fitter, Trade Mark" in a rectangle with scallops on lower edge. LHJ.

CORNELL SHOE CO. 91 Adams St., Brooklyn, N.Y.

    1916: Shoe said to be the first one made by this company. PEM USMC 1491.

    1921: Illustrated a T-strap for 1922. TSR 9/17/21.

    1923: Illustrated a gore shoe for 1924. TSR 9/15/23.

CORONA KID CO. 95 South St., Boston, Mass.

    1902: Advertised Corona Colt ("It needs no polish, skirts do not deface it . . . for ladies' light footwear"). TSR 7/9/02.

COTTER SHOE CO. Lynn, Mass. Boston office at 183 Essex St..

    1909: Advertised low shoes, McKays retailing at $2.00–$2.50, and welts retailing at $2.50 and $3.00. TSR 9/25/09.

    1913: Illustrated a button boot for 1914. TSR 9/20/13.

COWARD. James S. Coward. 268–74 Greenwich St., near Warren St., New York City. Founded about 1880.

1903, 1904, 1908, 1909: The Coward Good Sense Shoe (characterized by a very broad noncramping toe). Made for men, women, and children. LHJ, DEL.

1914: The Coward Good Sense Shoe. "Coward Arch Support Shoe and Coward Extension Heel made by James S. Coward for over 34 years. For children, women and men. Send for catalogue. Mail orders filled. Sold nowhere else." LHJ.

CRAMER. John Cramer. Brooklyn, N.Y.

1919: Black Colonial slipper. PEM USMC 1521.

1919: Front-lace boot with plush top. PEM USMC 1522.

CRAWFORD SHOE MAKERS. 825 Broadway, New York City. Factories in New York City and Brockton, Mass.

1901: The Crawford Shoe. Sold through Crawford stores in New York, Brooklyn, Boston, Baltimore, Washington, and by "leading retailers everywhere." Boots $3.50 plus $0.25 postage. LHJ.

1903: Same. Philadelphia store now also listed. LHJ, DEL.

CREIGHTON. A. M. Creighton. Lynn, Mass.

1907: Illustrated a Colonial for 1908. TSR 9/28/07.

CREIGHTON. George A. Creighton & Son. Lynn, Mass.

1900: Illustrated a front-lace boot, "one of fifteen styles of the 'Try-Me' $1.50 Specialty for women." TSR 7/1900.

CROCKER. F. Crocker, Sole Owner. Washington, D.C.

1897: "Jenness Miller" Shoes. Boots: $5.00. LHJ.

1900: Sears sells a $2.65 boot called "Jenness from the fact that it is made over the famous Jenness Miller hygienic foot form last, which for comfort, fitting qualities, and stylish appearance excels anything on the market."

CROSS. John H. Cross. Lynn, Mass.

1907: Illustrated a pump for 1908. TSR 9/28/07.

1909: Illustrated latchet tie for 1910. TSR 9/25/09.

1921: Illustrated a strap shoe for 1922. Now listed as being in Haverhill rather than Lynn. TSR 9/17/21.

CURRIER. F. J. Currier & Co. Lynn, Mass.

1907: Button shoe illustrated for 1908. TSR 9/28/07.

CUSHING SHOE CO. Lynn, Mass.

1921: Illustrated a sporty shoe for 1922. TSR 9/17/21.

1923: Illustrated an oxford for 1924. TSR 9/15/23.

CUSHMAN AND HEBERT. Lynn, Mass.

1900: Illustrated a "popular priced kid oxford." TSR 7/1900.

CUSHMAN-HOLLIS CO. Auburn, Maine.

1928: Illustrated a sporty tie shoe. TSR 3/17/28.

CUTTING. See FLETCHER.

DALSIMER. S. Dalsimer & Sons. 1212 (later 1201) Market St., Philadelphia.

    1916: Nurses DeLyte Shoe. Boots $3.00 postpaid. Mentions thirty-sixth year, so presumably formed about 1880. LW.

    1917: Nurses DeLyte Shoe. Lace boots $3.50 postpaid, button boots $4.00. LHJ.

DAVIS. Edward Swain Davis. Lynn, Mass.

    1839: The Peabody Essex Museum has a group of shoes and boots exhibited by Davis "at the annual Fair of the Mass. Charitable Mechanics Association of New England, and for which he received a diploma." PEM USMC 1536–44.

DE FREEST & STOVER. 17 Second St., Waterford, N.Y.

    1905: "Slumber Slipper. Will keep the ankles warm. Worn in bed and out. Made of a handsome fleece-lined knit fabric; tops beautifully embroidered with silk. Dainty colorings. Two Pairs for 25c., Postpaid." DEL.

DEXTER SHOE MANUFACTURING CO. 122 Summer St. in 1891, 143 Federal St. from 1892, Boston, Mass. "Established 1880." Advertisements are small and cheap-looking.

    1891, 1892: Boots $1.50 postpaid. LHJ.

    1894: Boots $1.50. DEL.

    1899, 1901, 1904: Shoes and boots, $1.00 postpaid. LW, LHJ, McC.

DIAMOND. See UNITED FAST COLOR EYELET COMPANY.

DICK. Wm. H. Dick, Manufacturer. Dansville, N.Y.

    1891, 1900: Dick's Foot-Warmer Shoes (hand-woven, wool-lined seamless soft ankle-high boots). Ladies' sizes $1.25. LHJ.

DICKINSON. Joseph Dickinson. Lynn, Mass.

    1904: Illustrated a tie shoe for 1905. TSR 9/28/04.

DINGLEY-FOSS SHOE CO. Auburn, Maine.

    1928: Illustrated a tied strap. TSR 3/17/28.

DOLGEFELT. See GREEN.

DOLGE, ALFRED. See GREEN.

DODD. Dorothy Dodd Shoe Company. Boston.

    1902: Oxfords $2.50, boots $3.00. Advertising claims stylishness, fit, lightness, flexibility and arch support. LHJ.

    1908: Dorothy Dodd, *A Book of Authentic Shoe Fashions For Women of Taste, Autumn and Winter,* 1908. Logo is a shield with two Ds, straight sides facing each other. Contains twenty-five styles of boots, four of shoes.

    1917–20: Brown front-lace boot. HN 66.792.

    1928: See PLANT, which may have bought out Dorothy Dodd.

DODGE. Nathan D. Dodge Shoe Co. Newburyport, Mass. Offices in Boston, New York, Chicago, Kansas City, San Francisco, and Montgomery, Alabama.

    1917: Illustrated a pump for 1918. TSR 9/22/17.

    1921: Strap shoes from $5.00 to $7.00. TSR 9/17/21.

DODGE & BLISS. N. D. Dodge & Bliss Co. Newburyport, Mass.

    1901: Illustrated an eight-strap beaded boot. TSR 3/1901.

DOMO. See GOLO SLIPPER CO.

DR. A. REED CUSHION SHOES. See EBBERTS.

DR. EDISON CUSHION SHOE. See UTZ & DUNN.

DREW. The Irving Drew Co. Portsmouth, Ohio.

    1913: Illustrated a Colonial pump for 1914. TSR 9/20/13.

    1923: Illustrated a fancy strap shoe for 1924. TSR 9/15/23.

    1927: Drew Arch Rest shoes. Trademark on sole: a horizontal oval with
        pointed ends bearing words "Arch Rest, Drew, Portsmouth, O." Above
        oval: "Combination Last." Below oval: "Pat'd. [Nov?] 29 – 1921." LHJ.

    1928: Illustrated a one-strap. TSR 3/17/28.

DRIVER. S. Driver & Co. Salem, Mass.

    1816: White kid slit-vamp shoe. Label: "S. Driver & Co., Fashionable Boot
        and Shoe Store, No. 7 Old Paved Street, Salem. Rips mended gratis."
        PEM 135,384.

DRIVER. S. P. Driver & Bros. Lynn, Mass.

    1869: White kid wedding slippers worn by Addie Smith. Survive with
        original box. LM 5554.

DUANE SHOE CO. 143 Duane St., New York City.

    1928: "Women's specialties, latest styles at popular prices always in stock."
        Trademark: a circle with monogram in center (letters D, S, Co super-
        imposed) and "durability, style, comfort" in outer border. TSR 3/10/28.

DUCHAMP. Bordeaux, France.

    1780–1800: White silk slipper with silver vamp embroidery said to have
        belonged to Lady Pepperell. Label: "DuChamp, dit DuPuy, Maître
        Cordonnier pour femme, rue Pradel, près l'Archevêché à Bordeaux.
        [Duchamp, called Dupuy, master shoemaker for women, Pradel Street,
        near the archbishop's residence in Bordeaux." SPNEA 1966.253.

    1805–15: Pink dotted silk, embroidered vamp. Label: "Duchamp,
        Cordonnier, Rue L'Hôpital St. André No. 8 à Bordeaux." PEM 112,941.

DUGAN & HUDSON. Rochester, N.Y.

    1896: "Iron Clad Shoes" for children. LHJ.

    1917: Illustrated an oxford for 1918. TSR 9/22/17.

DUNN & McCARTHY. Auburn, N.Y.

    1919: Advertised boots. TSR 9/20/19.

DUPUY. See DUCHAMP.

DUTTENHOFER. Val Duttenhofer Son's Co. Cincinnati, Ohio.

    1904: Illustrated a dressy tie shoe for 1905. TSR 9/28/04.

    1919: Illustrated a pump for 1920. TSR 9/20/19.

    1923: Illustrated a strap shoe for 1924. TSR 9/15/23.

E.Z. CUSHION TURN. See KELLY.

E-Z WALK MFG. CO., INC. 62–70 W. 14th St., New York City.

1919: Made felt slippers called Foot-Pals. Trademark: a horizontal oval surrounded by scrollwork with the words "The E-Z Walk" above the oval, "Foot-Pals, trade mark" and a picture of a slipper in the oval, and "felt and novelty footwear" below the oval. TSR 9/20/19.

EASE ALL. See UTZ & DUNN CO.

EASTERN SHOE CO. 192 Broadway, Beverly, Mass.

1904: Whitcomb's Flexsole Shoes. Lace boot $3.00, button boot $3.25, oxford $2.50. "No tacks, no lining to wrinkle and hold moisture. No seams. Can be bent double." DEL.

1906: Whitcomb's Flexsole Shoes. Lace boot $3.00, button boot $3.25, oxford $2.00. LHJ.

EASTERN SHOE MFG. CO. 126–28 Summer St., Boston.

1907: Advertised calf-top boots at $1.60. TSR 9/28/07.

EBBERTS. John Ebberts Shoe Co. 213 Clinton St., Buffalo, N.Y.

1911: Dr. A. Reed Cushion Sole Shoes for Women. "The Lamb's Wool Cushion built into the shoe by our Patented process, assures perfect ease from the very start." LHJ.

1917: Illustrated a boot for 1918. TSR 9/22/18.

1917: Dr. A. Reed Cushion Shoes. Trademark stamped on sole: a circle with words "Dr. A. Reed Cushion Sole" above a rectangle with "John Ebberts Shoe Co. Makers." Men's styles were made by the J. P. Smith Shoe Co. of Chicago. LHJ.

1918: As before. LHJ.

1919: Illustrated a Colonial for 1920. TSR 9/20/19.

1928: Small ad for Dr. A. Reed Cushion Shoes for Women. TSR 3/10/28.

ECLECTIC. See CHAMBERS.

EDISON. See UTZ & DUNN.

EDUCATOR SHOE. See RICE & HUTCHINS.

ELKIN TURN SHOE CO. Philadelphia.

1921: Illustrated a multi-strap shoe for 1922. TSR 9/17/21.

1923: Illustrated a gored shoe for 1924. TSR 9/15/23.

ELLIS-EDDY CO. Haverhill, Mass.

1921: Illustrated an ankle-strap for 1922. TSR 9/17/21.

EMERSON SHOE COMPANY. Rockland, Mass.

1921: Two-strap shoes wholesaling at $6.00. TSR 9/17/21.

EMERY & MARSHALL CO. Haverhill, Mass.

1921: Illustrated strap shoes for 1922. TSR 9/17/21.

ENDICOTT-JOHNSON CORP. Endicott, N.Y. A very large company that handled every stage of the shoe business from leather production to retail stores.

1928: Illustrated a pump. TSR 3/17/28.

ESSEX RUBBER CO. Trenton, N.J., and other cities.

1928: "Plytex Soles and Heels . . . multiple layers of fabric overlapped and embedded in rubber." TSR 2/18/28.

ESTABROOK-ANDERSON SHOE CO. Nashua, N.H.

> 1900: "Said to have made 5,000 pairs [of tennis shoes] daily last year, and will probably make as many this year." TSR 5/1900.

ESTÉ, VIAULT-ESTÉ, VIAULT-ESTÉ/THIERRY & SONS. Paris, France.

Labels from the French maker Esté (later Viault-Esté) are the single most common type found in surviving shoes. They usually appear in plain black or white satin heelless slippers of about 1835–65 with a minute bow at the throat (sometimes obscured by a more elaborate rosette added later). The firm is first listed in Bottin's "Almanach du Commerce" in 1821, under "Bottiers," as "Esté, pour Dames, rue de la Paix 13." Viault seems to have bought or married into or inherited the business by 1838 or 1839. In the latter year, the firm is listed under Viault only, but from 1840, the name appears hyphenated as Viault-Esté. The labels in the shoes, however, may not have been changed to reflect the new name until at least 1849. In that year, the rue de la Paix was renumbered, and Viault-Esté's address changed from 13 to 17. Presumably the new address made revised labels desirable and the new design incorporated the Viault name as well as the new address. At any rate, no labels noted so far bear both the Viault name and the old address at No. 13.

The export side of the business seems to have expanded in the 1840s, judging from the great numbers of surviving shoes, and by 1852 or 1853, Viault-Esté had formed an association with Thierry & Sons in London. The Bottin directory entry for 1854, translated, reads, "Viault-Esté—[shoemaker] for ladies, licensed supplier to her Majesty the Empress. Admitted to the [Crystal Palace] Exhibition in London for the elegant cut of its court slippers and of its mules with quilted heels in the style of Louis XV, an article of taste and fantasy, choice fancy goods, shipments and exports for abroad. Honorable mention London 1851. Admitted to the exposition in New York (United States) 1853—Rue de la Paix 17."

Apparently exports fell into decline by the later 1860s, and may have been extinguished in 1870 by the Franco-Prussian war and the fall of the Second Empire. The number of Viault-Esté slippers manufactured with heels and thus clearly dating after 1865 that now survive in the United States is so small that one must assume they arrived as individual purchases abroad rather than mass imports. By the 1870s and 1880s, the firm's entries in Bottin are no longer embellished with bold typefaces or self-congratulatory descriptions. Sometime after 1880 and before 1885, Viault-Esté moved to rue de la Paix, 20, and it was probably shortly after this that the association with Thierry came to an end, since the Thierry name is cut off labels dating from the later 1880s. In 1890, the firm moved again, this time to Chauveau Lagarde, 18, and the company was still in business at that address in 1895.

See figure 5 for six common labels. Esté labels are found in most shoe collections. Examples of most styles can be studied at the Peabody Essex Museum.

EXCELSIOR.

>1877: Pink kid button boot bought for $15.00 at Rogers & Co. in Boston. Label (referring to V-shaped notch in button fly): "Excelsior Button Boot, patented August 25, 1868." PEM USMC 1342.

>1880s: Black boarded calf buttoned boot, stamped on sole: "Excelsior All Leather Boot, The Best Cheap Shoe Made." PEM USMC 1974.

EYRE. Fred. A. Eyre & Co. Brooklyn, N.Y.

>1923: Illustrated a high pump for 1924. TSR 9/15/23.

F. B. & C. KID. Appears to be the trademark of Amalgamated Leather Companies, Inc., New York City.

>1917–20: Advertised through "Fashion Publicity Company, Department L, New York City." In 1918, noted that tags were attached to the shoes as evidence of quality leather. LHJ.

FARGO. C. H. Fargo & Co. Chicago.

>1891: Boots $2.50. LHJ.

>1892: Boots $2.50 including postage. LHJ.

>1897: "Fargo's famous ball-bearing bicycle shoes" are advertised by name in the Sears catalog.

FARWELL, G. N. Farwell. Claremont, N.H.

>1846: Tan kid wedding slippers. Label: "Ladies' and Gentlemen's Boots and Shoes, Manufactured, warranted and sold wholesale and retail, by G. N. Farwell & Co., Claremont, N.H." HN 1976.137.2.

FAUST SHOE CO. Chicago.

>1921: Illustrated an oxford for 1922. TSR 9/17/21.

FENN. W. B. Fenn and Co. New Haven, Conn.

>1891: White suede beaded cross-strap wedding shoes. Label: "W. B. Fenn and Co., New Haven." CHS 1942.

FENTON. The John Fenton Shoe Mfg. Co. Columbus, Ohio.

>1921: Illustrated a one-strap for 1922. TSR 9/17/21.

FIRESTONE FOOTWEAR CO. Hudson, Mass.

>1927: A rain overshoe with tan jersey top and tan rubber sole. TSR 10/8/27.

FISCHER BUNION PROTECTOR. Fischer Mfg. Co. 380 Scott St., Milwaukee.

>1905: "The Fischer Bunion Protector enables one with bunions or enlarged joints to wear an unstretched shoe without inconvenience. The protector is a neat little soft-leather appliance that goes over the stocking, inside the same size shoe that one would wear with a bunion." $0.50. DEL.

FISHEL NESSLER CO. 184 Fifth Ave., New York City.

>1913: "Largest Manufacturers in the World of Fine Shoe Ornaments." Illustrates a set of five jeweled slides that attach to the sides of an ordinary slipper, through which a ribbon is laced, creating the effect of a tango-type sandal. TSR 9/20/13.

FISHER. A. Fisher & Son. Lynn, Mass.

1907: Illustrated a tan pump for 1908. TSR 9/28/07.

1909: Advertised new goods, including "the New Stage Last, a winner." TSR 9/25/09.

FLETCHER. John Fletcher & Sons. Acton, Mass.

1865–75: Pebbled calf front-lace boot with patent tip. Label: "Extra Quality Manufactured Expressly for Geo. W. Cutting & Son, Weston, Mass, by John Fletcher & Sons, Acton, Mass." PEM USMC 1981.

1865–75: Black serge gored boot with patent tip. Label: same as above. PEM USMC 2010.

FLEXSOLE SHOES. See EASTERN SHOE CO.

FOGG. Nathaniel Fogg, Exeter [N.H.?].

1775–85: White wool buckle shoes. Label: "Shoes, Made and sold by Nathaniel Fogg, Exeter." HHS 9362.

FOOT-FRIEND SHOES. See LAPE & ADLER COMPANY.

FOOTGLUV. See SULTANA MFG. CO.

FOOT-PALS. See E-Z WALK MFG. CO.

FOOT SAVER SHOES. See JULIAN & KOKENGE CO.

FORD. C. P. Ford & Co. Rochester, N.Y.

1921: Illustrated a sports oxford for 1922. TSR 9/17/21.

1928: Illustrated a pump. TSR 3/17/28.

FOSTER RUBBER CO.

1915: Cat's Paw rubber heels. Picture shows bottom of heel: "Cat's Paw, Non Slip," then two circles within an oval (for traction?), size number, "French heel, Foster Rubber Co." LHJ.

FOX. Chas. K. Fox. Haverhill, Mass.

1902: Made women's shoes using Corona colt leather. TSR 7/9/02.

1904: Button shoe illustrated for 1905. TSR 9/28/04.

1919: Illustrated a dress pump for 1920. TSR 9/20/19.

G & R SHOE COMPANY. Lynn, Mass.

1915: Advertised McKay-sewn boots over various lasts. Trademark: a shield bearing the overlapped letters G R, between the words "Lynn Made," all within a rectangle. TSR 9/18/15.

GAYTEES. See UNITED STATES RUBBER COMPANY.

GLOVE FITTERS. GLOVE FITTING. See AARON F. SMITH.

GLOYD. Arthur E. Gloyd. Lynn, Mass.

1900: Illustrated an oxford at $1.50. TSR 7/1900.

GOLLER SHOE CO. Lynn, Mass.

1909: Illustrated a button shoe. TSR 9/25/09.

GOLO SLIPPER CO. 129 Duane St., New York City.

1927: "Domo" trademark for their domestic slippers. TSR 12/10/27.

GOODRICH. B. F. Goodrich Rubber Co., Akron, Ohio. Est. 1870.

1927: Illustrated ankle-high zipper-front rubber overshoes. The boots themselves were called "Zippers." TSR 10/8/27, 12/31/27.

1928: "Goodrich Hi-Press Rubber Footwear." TSR 3/3/28.

GOODRICH. Hazen B. Goodrich. Haverhill, Mass.

1888: A black kid oxford tie said to have been made for a Vienna Exposition. Label: "Vienna Manufacture Warranted Hand Sewn First Quality." Label seems to contradict USMC attribution. PEM USMC 2268.

1888: A black kid slipper said to have been made for a Vienna Exposition. PEM USMC 2271.

1888: A black kid front-lace boot said to have been made for a Vienna Exposition. Label: "B. Strakosch & Sohn, Vienna." PEM USMC 2274.

1904: Illustrated a tie shoe for 1905. TSR 9/28/04.

1913: Advertisement suggests the firm specialized in turn shoes, especially pumps, and claimed "our spring [1912] showing has an intense artistic value," apparently reinforced by names such as "The Cubist Pump." TSR 9/20/13.

1915: Advertised pumps and strap shoes for 1916. TSR 9/18/15.

1917: Illustrated a tie shoe for 1918. TSR 9/22/17.

1922: Black kid pump, celluloid heel set with brilliants. PEM USMC 2285.

GOODRICH & PORTER. Haverhill, Mass.

1876: A group of shoes shown at the Philadelphia Exposition, including PEM USMC 2231, 2233, 2235, 2237, 2249, 2251, 2252, 2256, 2260, 2287, 2291, 2293, 2294, 2296, 2297, and 2300.

1893: One-strap for Columbian Exposition. PEM USMC 2187.

GOODYEAR INDIA RUBBER GLOVE MFG. CO. New York City.

1885–1900: Rubbers with knitted top added by owner. Label: "Goodyear's I.R.G. [picture of glove] Mfg. Co. New York." SPNEA 1933.1236.

1920–1930: Brown canvas tennis shoes. Label: "Goodyear's Glove M'f'g. Co. Naugatuck, CT, USA Keds" with tennis racket design molded into sole. See figure 76. LM 6842.

GOODYEAR TIRE AND RUBBER CO. Akron, Ohio.

1918: Neolin Soles. "Created by Science—to be what soles ought to be." LHJ.

GOODYEAR. See WALES GOODYEAR SHOE CO.

GRAYDON-PALMER CO. Market and Madison Streets, Chicago.

1899: Felt Juliet slippers, $1.45 plus $0.17 postage.

GREEN. Daniel Green Felt Shoe Company. Addresses all in New York City: 1889–90, 122 East 13th St.; 1898–1905, 119 West 23rd St.; 1912–20, various addresses on East 13th St.; by 1929, Dolgeville, N.Y.

1889: "The Alfred Dolge Felt Shoes and Slippers, Noiseless, Warm, Durable." Picture shows an old lady knitting, with caption, "Times Have Changed. 'Well, well; to think how, years ago, I put a slipper on to Tom, and yesterday he paid me up with interest by putting a pair on me. He says that he *felt* mine then, and it was warm enough for comfort; and now these are *felt* also, and, though likewise warm, are much more comfortable.'" DEL.

1890: "Alfred Dolge Felt Shoes and Slippers, Noiseless, Warm, Durable." Picture shows a wife and little girl coaxing a "pater familias" who says,

"There, there, do stop. I have heard of nothing but 'Alfred Dolge' and 'Felt Shoes' ever since those advertisements appeared in the papers. Go ahead and buy felt shoes for the whole family." HMG.

1892: "Alfred Dolge's Felt Slippers and Shoes." LHJ.

1898: "Dolge" pure wool felt slippers "especially designed for night wear, the bath room and the traveler made from ONE piece of DOLGE pure wool felt. Soft leather sole. Navy Blue and Scarlet: Ladies sizes, 85 cts." LHJ.

1900: "Dolgefelt" house shoes in black, brown, drab, red, and green, $2.00 including postage. "Dolgefelt" storm-proof inner sole in a kid street boot, $5.00. LHJ.

1901, 1902: "Dolgefelt" house shoes, low cut, $1.25; high-cut nullifer style, $1.50, delivered. LHJ.

1905: Nullifier style in black, red, brown, drab, green, blue, gray, and wine, $1.50. Low-cut "Comfy Slipper" in red, blue, brown, drab, $1.00. "Dolgefelt" no longer mentioned. DEL.

1912, 1914, 1915, 1916, 1920: Felt slippers continue, $1.25 to $2.00. Now ribbon-trimmed, and in more colors. Trademark "COMFY, Daniel Green" in a squarish scroll with words "Patented July 28, 1908." LHJ.

1929: Comfy slippers "priced from $2.50 to $6.50 and up to $15.00." Now made in satin, brocade, crepe de chine, and leather as well as felt. Trademark continues with squarish scroll, but with words: "Daniel Green, Comfy, Slippers, Patented Aug. 10, 1920." LHJ.

See also SIEGEL COOPER CO., a competitive distributor.

GREENOUGH. Probably Massachusetts, perhaps Salem, Lynn, or Boston.

1824: White silk slippers with picture of Lafayette printed on the vamp. Label partly illegible: "Warranted, Boots & Shoes, [-] sold wholesale and retail by [-] Greenough, [-] Middle Street, [-] M[ass?]." PEM USMC 1721.

GREILICH. William Greilich & Sons Inc. Brooklyn, N.Y.

1917: Designed and introduced a new spat style for 1918. TSR 9/22/17.

GRIFFIN-WHITE SHOE CO. Brooklyn or New York City.

1904: Illustrated dressy shoes for 1904 and 1905. TSR 9/21, 28/04.

1915: Illustrated a pump for 1916. TSR 9/18/15.

GRIPPER SHOE CO., INC. "Grippertown, Mass" (real address not identified).

1905–10: Brown leather open-tab front-lace boots. Label: "Modified Ground Gripper, Style No. 2, Made Only by Gripper Shoe Co., Inc, Grippertown, Mass." HN 66.790.

GROSSMAN. Julian Grossman, Inc. Brooklyn, N.Y.

1900: Illustrated an oxford. TSR 5/1900.

1913: Illustrated a three-strap tie for 1914. TSR 9/20/13.

1917: Illustrated two boots for 1918. TSR 9/22/17.

GROVER. J. J. Grover's Sons Co. Lynn, Mass. Specialized in comfortable shoes.

1893: Brown front-lace boot, slipper, and closed-tab tie, all with broad toes, exhibited at the Chicago World's Fair. Label: Grover Soft Shoes for Tender Feet, Trade Mark." PEM USMC 1290, no number, and 1298.

1921: Illustrated a tie shoe for 1922. TSR 9/17/21.

1923: Illustrated a three-strap for 1924. TSR 9/15/23.

GUPTILL. Hervey E. Guptill. Haverhill, Mass.

1900: Illustrated slipper, Colonial, and strap shoes. TSR 4 and 5/1900.

1902: "The name Guptill stands for the finest slippers. Offered in great variety in the Guptill line, Made in all materials and sewn on the Loop-lock Machine." Distributed in the southwest by Vinsonhaler Shoe Co., St. Louis. TSR 8/20/02.

1904: Advertised a carriage boot. TSR 9/21/04.

1915–20: A group of dressy shoes that may be associated with this company survives at the Danvers Historical Society. They all carry the trademark of a bare foot in a winged sandal surrounded by a sunburst.

HAGAN. H. E. Hagan. Boston.

1903: Illustrated a leather boudoir slipper. TSR 9/16/03.

HALLAHAN & SONS, INC. Philadelphia. Offices in New York and London.

1917: Front-lace boots, priced from $5.75 to $8.50, wholesale. "The designs are strictly new and . . . absolutely high grade in every detail." TSR 9/22/17.

1919: Illustrated a pump for 1920. TSR 9/20/19.

1923: Illustrated a one-strap for 1924. TSR 9/15/23.

HAMILTON, BROWN SHOE CO. St. Louis.

1897: "Own Make" Shoes. Boots, $2.50 including postage. LHJ.

1905, 1906: American Lady Shoes. $3.00 and $3.50. Style booklet called "Shoelight." Label: "American Lady" in script on the diagonal on the top facing. DEL.

1908: American Lady Shoes. Boots $3.00, $3.50, $4.00. "Largest makers of shoes in the world." LHJ.

1909: American Lady Shoes. $3.00, $3.50, $4.00. Trademark: Horizontal oval belt with words "Hamilton Brown Shoe Co." and in the center "Largest in the World." LHJ.

HANAN & SON. Bridge and Water Streets, Brooklyn, N.Y. Also a branch in Boston.

1906: Shoes, $5.00. "Write for our style book A 1, which tells you why unscoured sole leather used in ordinary shoes causes burning and aching feet,—we use only scoured sole leather—explains why you take a smaller size in a Hanan shoe."

1931: Imitation reptile skin open-tab ties. Label: "Made for Hanan & Son Retail Stores, Boston." SPNEA 1932.2301.

HARNEY BROS. Lynn, Mass.

1907: Illustrated a Colonial pump for 1908. TSR 9/28/07.

1909: Advertised the "Gypsy Button Oxford" for 1910. Retail prices of $3.00, $3.50, $4.00. TSR 9/25/09.

1911: Illustrated a colonial pump for 1912. TSR 9/16/11.

HARNEY. P. J. Harney Shoe Co. Lynn, Mass.

1909: Advertised low shoes retailing from $3.00 to $3.50. TSR 9/25/09.

1911: Advertised a Colonial pump for 1912. Goodyear welts, $2.10 and up; McKays, $1.75 and up. Trademark: a coat of arms with crowned lions on each side. Composite letter P and J in shield with "Harney" on diagonal. "Shoe Co., Trade Mark" on streamer below. TSR 9/16/11.

1913: Illustrated a baby doll pump for 1914. TSR 9/20/13.

1919: Illustrated a pump for 1920. TSR 9/20/19.

HARNEY, TRACY, CREHAN Co. Lynn, Mass.

1919: Illustrated a one-button shoe for 1920. TSR 9/20/19.

HARPER & KIRSCHTEN SHOE CO. Chicago.

1921: Illustrated a blucher oxford for 1922. TSR 9/17/21.

HARRIS SHOE [CO.?]. 59 Temple Place, Boston. Store in Boston and branches in Providence, R.I., and Buffalo, N.Y. Founded by 1874.

1899: The Harris Shoe. Boots $3.00 and $3.50. "Twenty-five years have been devoted to perfecting it. . . . The Harris Shoe is not machine sewed. Every pair is in a hand-sewed turn or welt, and every pair is made at our own factory. Genuine Harris Shoes can be bought only of us either by mail or at our stores. . . . 55 distinct styles." LW.

HARRISBURG BOOT AND SHOE MFG. CO., LTD. Harrisburg, Pa. By 1921 listed as the Harrisburg Shoe Mfg. Co. (boots were rarely worn by this date).

1902: Advertised shoes priced from $1.50 to $2.25. TSR 8/20/02.

1921: Oxfords wholesaling from $2.85 to $4.00. TSR 9/17/21.

1923: Mary Lee. Line under this name appears to be new: "Here are the first five—most shoe stores are selling them with my signature on their silk labels—if you can't find them readily, please write me personally. $5.00 and $6.00." Three strapped styles and two oxford ties. LHJ.

HAYDEN. Samuel H. Hayden. Haverhill, Mass.

1903: Illustrated gored shoes with cutouts. TSR 9/16/03.

HAYWARD RUBBER CO. Colchester, Conn.

1860–90: Remains of a rubber with a black knitted wool upper. Label: "Hayward Rubber Co., Colchester, Conn." SPNEA 1953.515.

HAYNES. Edward Haynes, Jr. Boston, Mass.

ca. 1845: Tan kid slipper with label "Warranted By Edw. Haynes, Jr. No. 219 Washington Street, Boston." PEM 112,452.

HECHT. F. Hecht & Co., Inc. 10 Spruce St., New York City.

1928: "Alpina reptile leathers are tanned, dyed and styled in Europe. They will not chip or peel, and are the most workable reptile leathers obtainable. Get the Hecht Sample Book! Shows hundreds of styles of novelty leathers." TSR 3/17/28.

HEER SHOE CO. Portsmouth, Ohio.

1902: Advertised women's shoes and boots from $1.50 to $2.50. TSR 9/24/02.

HEIM & TULL, INC. Brooklyn, N.Y.

1923: Illustrated a pump for 1924. TSR 9/15/23.

HELLSTERN. Paris, France.

1890. Pink silk slippers made to match a dress by Doucet. Label: "Brevet, Hellstern, Paris, Droit." CD 1961.32.

HELMING-MCKENZIE. Cincinnati, Ohio.

1909: Advertised a one-strap. Trademark: "The H+M Shoe," the words "the" and "shoe" resting in the curls of the H and M. $3.00, $3.50, $4.00. TSR 9/25/09.

HENNE. Wm. Henne & Co. 963–65 Kent Ave., Brooklyn, N.Y. Est. 1875. Trademark: a coat of arms with monogram, a large H with W above, & on the cross bar, and Co below. "Mark of reliability" on a streamer at bottom. 1911: Advertised colonial pumps. TSR 9/16/11.

1921: Illustrated a four-strap for 1922. TSR 9/17/21.

HIAWATHA. See SAWYER BOOT & SHOE CO.

HILLIARD & TABOR. Haverhill, Mass.

1917–20: Front-lace boot. PEM USMC 2078.

HIRTH, KRAUSE & WILHELM. 118 Canal St., Grand Rapids, Mich.

1890: "Manufacturers of Fine Custom Made Boot, Shoe and Gaiter Uppers." Catalog for 1890 was reprinted by the Early American Industries Association in June 1980. Shows a number of styles for men and a few for women. Catalog is shared with firm of Hirth & Krause, "Dealers in All Kinds of Leather & Findings," at the same address.

HOAG & WALDEN, MAKERS. Lynn, Mass. Boston Salesroom at 29 Lincoln St.

1901: "Ladies' Swell Shoes That Can Be Retailed at $2.00, $2.50, $3.00, $3.50. Modern Shapes Box-Stitched, Cross-stitched, Rope-Stitched, Etc. Extreme Edges made from Enamels, Patents, Velours, Box, Russia-Wax and Vici Leathers in Hand Welts, Goodyear and New McKay Process. Also Original Designs in Velvet Effects." TSR 4/3/01.

HOLDER. Joseph Holder. Bolton, Mass.

1828: White silk/cotton wedding slipper. Label: "Made and Warranted by Joseph Holder, Bolton, Mass." PEM 125,655.

HOLTERS CO. Cincinnati, Ohio.

1923: Illustrated an ankle-strap for 1924. TSR 9/15/23.

HOLTON. Lemuel Holton. 79 Court St. Boston.

1850–55: Black kid slipper. Label: "Lemuel Holton, 79 Court St., Corner Brattle St., Boston." CHS 1959-19-4.

HOMAN-HUGHES CO. Cincinnati, Ohio.

1919: Illustrated a one-eyelet tie for 1920. TSR 9/20/19.

1923: Illustrated a two-strap for 1924. TSR 9/15/23.

HON SING. Possibly Canton, China.

1795–1805: Blue satin latchet tie. CD 1948.50.

HOOD RUBBER CO. Boston.

1927: Illustrated a rubber-soled jersey overshoe. TSR 10/8/27.

HOOLEY. W. F. Hooley Shoe Co. Lynn, Mass.

1928: Illustrated a side-buckle shoe. TSR 3/17/28.

HOPKINS & ELLIS. Haverhill, Mass.

1921: "H & E" turn novelties, wholesaling at $5.25 to $7.00. TSR 9/17/21.

HOPPE & HEATH. 156 Minories. London, England.

1805–15: Yellow kid slipper with cutout vamp said to have been worn by Abigail Adams. Label: "Hoppe & Heath, Ladies' Shoe Makers, No. 156, Minories, London." PEM 112,450.

HORN MFG. CO. Brooklyn, N.Y.

1923: Illustrated a three-strap for 1924. TSR 9/15/23.

HOSE. Jonathan Hose & Son. London, England.

1758: Buckle shoe worn at a wedding in Newbury, Mass. Label partially illegible. LACMA M.89.144.1-2.

1750–65: Buckle shoe. Label: "Made by Jno. Hose & Son, At the Rose in Cheapside near Milk Street, London." CHS A341. Another example: DAR 3269.

Ca. 1772: Buckle shoe. LACMA 46.72.20.

HOSE. William Hose. London, England.

ca. 1750: Buckle shoe. DAR 2109.

HOWLAND. Bartlett Howland Co. Lynn, Mass.

1913: Illustrated a Colonial pump for 1914. TSR 9/20/13.

HOYT & ROWE. Lynn, Mass.

1900: Illustrated an oxford shoe at $1.00. TSR 7/1900.

HUB GORE MAKERS. Boston.

1910: "Hub Gore fabric" was the elastic fabric used in elastic-sided shoes and slippers. "Because it is guaranteed by the makers of Hub Gore it costs the manufacturer a trifle more. Because it is guaranteed for two years from date of stamp it is a protection to you and adds double the wear to the slippers. Look for the little "Heart" trade-mark on the inside of both panels." HSW.

HUNT-RANKIN LEATHER CO. 106 Beach St., Boston.

1927: Velvetta Suede. A non-crocking suede that won't rub off on hosiery. LHJ.

1928: Velvetta Suede and Velvetta Suede Dressing. LHJ.

HURRELL. Mrs. Hurrell. East 4th St., Cincinnati, Ohio.

1835–50: White kid slippers. Label: "Mrs. Hurrell, Maker., East 4th. St., Cincinnati." HN 66.646.

HURLEY SHOE CO. Rockland, Mass.

1923: Illustrated a T-strap for 1924. TSR 9/15/23.

INDEPENDENT SHOE MANUFACTURERS. St. Louis, Mo.

1928: Illustrated a one-strap. TSR 3/17/28.

INDIAN CURIO CO. Boise, Idaho.

1912: Indian moccasins "as worn by the Shoshone Indians" in "buck, squaw and papoose sizes." LHJ.

INTERNATIONAL SHOE CO. See PETERS SHOE CO.

IRON CLAD SHOES. See DUGAN & HUDSON.

J & K SHOES. See JULIAN & KOKENGE CO.

JACKSON. 54 Rathbone Place, Oxford St., London, England.

  1800–1805: White kid slippers. Label: "Jackson, Ladies' Shoe Manufacturer,
    54 Rathbone Place, Oxford Street, London." SPNEA 1936.823.

  1800–1805: Dotted kid slippers. Label: Same as above. RIHS 1983.14.5.

  1800–1810: Yellow kid slippers. Label: Same as above. CD 1952.532.

  1810: White kid wedding slippers. Label: Similar to above. HN 1976.137.1.

JAEGER HEALTH SHOE. See KELLY.

JANTZEN. H. Jantzen Co. New York City.

  1904: Illustrated a calf front-lace boot. TSR 9/21/04.

JEFFERSON IMPORT CO., INC. 47 West 34th St., New York City.

  1927: "New importations of fine French mules . . . for holiday selling."
    TSR 11/19/27.

JELLERSON-RAFTER CO. Norway, Maine.

  1928: Illustrated a cutout one-strap. TSR 3/17/28.

JENNESS MILLER. See CROCKER.

JOHANSEN BROS. SHOE CO. St. Louis.

  1921: Illustrated a three-strap for 1922. TSR 9/17/21.

  1928: Illustrated a T-strap. TSR 3/17/28.

JOHNSON. G & R Johnson. Norwich, Conn.

  1828: Beige serge wedding slippers. Label: "G & R Johnson, Norwich,
    Conn, Boot & Shoe Manufacturer, Rips Sewed Gratis." RIHS
    1980.86.16.

JOHNSON-BAIRD SHOE COMPANY. Fort Dodge, Iowa.

  1917: Illustrated buttoned boots. "A new and undeveloped field for every shoe
    merchant has been opened by the World Wide War. Women in every walk
    of life are performing duties which compel them to remain on their feet
    many hours. This has created an urgent, as well as immediate demand for
    shoes which give comfort and at the same time are not lacking in style.
    Clara Barton Shoes fill the specifications for this demand. . . . Reinforced
    by a built-in steel arch support, which scientifically distributes the weight of
    the wearer between the heel, arch and ball, eliminating foot fatigue so
    common with women constantly on their feet." TSR 7/28/17.

JOHNSON, STEPHENS & SHINKLE SHOE CO. St. Louis.

  1923: Illustrated a cross-strap for 1924. TSR 9/15/23.

  1928: Illustrated a one-strap. TSR 3/17/28.

JOLLY. Paris, France.

  1865–70: Bronze cutout slipper with rosette. Label: "Jolly 125." HN 66.659.

  1885–92: Black patent cross-strap shoe with rhinestone button. Label:
    "Jolly. Paris." SPNEA 1943.637.

JONES. V. K. & A. H. Jones Co. Lynn, Mass.

  1900: Illustrated a front-lace McKay boot for $1.50. TSR 7/1900.

JONES. Geo. R. Jones Co. Manchester, N.H. Also an office at 42 Lincoln St., Boston.

1915: "Bobby Boots . . . with Rubber-Krome Soles . . . a strong leather that is water-resisting, takes a clean edge and is pliable." Retails from $3.50 to $5.00. TSR 9/4/15.

JONES, PETERSON, NEWHALL Co. 48 & 50 Temple Place, Boston.

1903: Dressy tie shoe illustrated in TSR 9/16/03.

1908: Tan suede latchet tie. Label: "Jones, Peterson, Newhall Co., Makers, 48 & 50 Temple Pl., Boston." MFA 53.1067.

JOY, CLARK & NIER, INC. Rochester, N.Y.

1919: Illustrated a pump for 1920. TSR 9/20/19.

1923: Illustrated a cross-strap for 1924. TSR 9/15/23.

JULIA MARLOWE SHOES. See RICH SHOE CO.

JULIAN & KOKENGE Co. 424 E. Fourth St., Cincinnati, Ohio. Founded by 1899.

1900: Illustrated an oxford. TSR 12/1900.

1911: Trademark a triangle with the words The Heart/The Hand/The Mind along the three sides, and in the center the image of a wax stamp impressed with "The J&K Shoe for Women." "This stamp on any J&K pump or colonial insures a perfect fit. It is the great triangle of progress. . . . The J & K Shoe for young women. It fits the arch." Three new lasts were given the names "The Heart" (medium toe), "The Hand" (narrow toe), and "The Mind" ("growing girl last" with wide toe). TSR 9/16/11.

1915: Illustrated a button boot for 1916. TSR 9/18/15.

1917: Illustrated a sport pump for 1918. TSR 9/22/17.

1923: Illustrated a gore shoe for 1924. TSR 9/15/23.

1924: Foot Saver Shoes. Shows slightly differentiated styles for morning housework, afternoon shopping, afternoon tea, and evening dinner or theater, the latter a "more pronounced J. & K. style." "This program of shoe wearing will disperse wrinkles, headaches and bad nerves." The company "has been developing the Foot Saver principle of construction for over 25 years." J. & K. Shoes apparently a more stylish line than Foot Savers. LHJ.

1927: Foot Saver Shoes. Trademark: a circle with a bare foot and ankle. Above on a scroll "The Foot Saver." "Shoe" at the top of the circle. Below on a scroll "Controls the Arch," and in a bulge below the lower scroll, "J&K Co." LHJ.

1928: Foot Saver Shoes. Foot Saver shoes for men noted as being made by Commonwealth Shoe and Leather Co., Whitman, Mass. LHJ.

1928: Illustrated a cutout tie. TSR 3/17/28.

1930: Foot Saver Shoes. Men's Foot Savers now listed as also being made by the Slater Shoe Co., Ltd., Montreal, Canada. LHJ.

KAHLER. Park Square Building, Boston (according to USMC catalog card).

1923: Black buttoned shoe. Label: "Dr. Kahler Shoes, Famous Since 1858."
PEM USMC 2417.

KAHN, ALEXANDER & CO. 325–31 Lafayette St., New York City.
1911: Advertised shoe slides and buckles. TSR 9/16/11.

KEDS. See UNITED STATES RUBBER CO.

KEENE. Frank Keene Co. Lynn, Mass.
1900: Illustrated a front-lace boot at $2.10. TSR 7/1900.

KEITH. Geo. E. Keith Co. Campello (Brockton), Mass.
1896: Green silk T-strap, said to be made on order from A. H. Howe Co., and worn by Mrs. George R. Todd. PEM USMC 2351.
1900: "first engaged in business under the firm name of Green & Keith, on July 1, 1874. In 1880 we find him manufacturing shoes under his own name, which he continued up to 1896, when the George E. Keith Co. was incorporated. . . . The company produces more welt shoes than any other concern in the world. . . . The daily capacity is 7,000 pairs. . . . Besides the chief cities of the United States, they have branch offices in London, Melbourne, Cologne, Buenos Ayres and Santiago." TSR 9/1900, p. 24.
1912: Walk-Over Shoes. Button boot $5.00. LHJ.
1928: Illustrated "Walk-over's new tie effect." TSR 3/17/28.

KELLAM-GOLLER-LAND CO. Lynn, Mass.
1907: Illustrated a front-lace boot for 1908. TSR 9/28/07.

KELLY. John Kelly, Inc. Rochester, N.Y.
1904: Illustrated a tie shoe for 1905. TSR 9/28/04.
1909: Advertised a one-strap. "Specialties: Dr. Jaeger Health Shoe. E.Z. Cushion Turn. Lady Walker." TSR 9/25/09.
1911: Advertised buttoned boots at $2.50, $2.75, $2.85. TSR 9/16/11.
1915: Advertised in-stock boots from $2.35 to $2.85, and a pump for 1916. TSR 9/18/15.
1917: Illustrated a pump for 1918. TSR 9/22/17.
1919: Illustrated a pump for 1920. TSR 9/20/19.
1923: Illustrated a cross-strap for 1924. TSR 9/15/23.

KENWORTH SHOE CO. Cincinnati, Ohio.
1923: Illustrated a two-strap for 1924. TSR 9/15/23.

KEYSTONE SHOE MFG. CO. Kutztown, Pennsylvania. Branches in Philadelphia, Hartford, Chicago, and San Francisco.
1902: Advertised "Florodora Shoes" (button and front-lace boots) for $3.00. TSR 7/23/02.

KIELY. T. J. Kiely & Co. Lynn, Mass.
1909: "Kiely's Konquering Kid specialties at Prevailing Popular Prices." Women's and children's shoes. TSR 9/25/09.

KING. Mrs. A. R. King Corp. Lynn, Mass.
1911: Illustrated a misses pump with chiffon bow for 1912. TSR 9/16/11.

KINNICUTT. Thomas Kinnicutt. Possibly Rehoboth, Mass. Probably a retailer.

1795–1805: Light-blue kid latchet tie with pink tongue. Label: "Warranted and made by Wilber Mason for Thomas Kinnicutt. Rehoboth (Mass)." SPNEA 1918.934.

KOLLOCK. F. A. Kollock. Lynn, Mass.

1907: Advertised Archfit, a line of women's Juliets with steel shank and Pneumatic Cushion Rubber Heel. Also gymnasium shoes from $0.80 to $1.50, and "comfort shoes of every variety." TSR 9/28/07.

KOZY COMFORT SHOE MFG. CO. 1701 Richard St., Milwaukee, Wis.

1928: Advertised slippers in leathers, satins, woolskins, suedes. TSR 3/10/28.

KOZY SLIPPER CO. Lynn, Mass. Other offices at 214–16 Essex St., Boston, and 4 rue Martel, Paris, France.

1911: Illustrated a Congress shoe ($2.00) and a nullifer ($2.25). "Our new ideas include the Melville Hemped Sole Athletic Shoe, which will outwear three pairs of rubber soled sneakers, and is bound to revolutionize the cheap rubber sole shoe for men, women and children. It is the coolest and best shoe made for athletic purposes." They also made Kozy Travelling Slippers, Woodbury Foot Gluve, Kozy Flexible Welt— "Kozy Process," and Kozy Bath Slips and Novelties. TSR 9/16/11.

KRIPPENDORF-DITTMANN CO. Cincinnati, Ohio.

1928: Illustrated a one-strap. TSR 3/17/28.

KROHN FECCHEIMER & CO. Address in Cincinnati, Ohio, in 1905 at 820– 30 Sycamore St.; in 1908 and later at various addresses on Dandridge St. This company is a major advertiser in the *Ladies' Home Journal* from 1908 to 1923. Also noted in the *Shoe Retailer.*

1905: Red Cross Shoes. Oxfords $3.00. Boots $3.50. Trademark phrase: "It bends with the foot." Trademark is on the sole, a circle with "Krohn Fechheimer & Co—Cinti U.S.A—" around outer band, and "Red Cross Noiseless Shoe" in inner circle around a cross. DEL.

1908: Red Cross Shoes. Oxfords $3.50–$4.00. Boots $4.00–$5.00. LHJ.

1909: Red Cross Shoes. Sold direct and through dealers. Trademark phrase: "Bends with your foot." Trademark on sole as in 1905. LHJ.

1912: Red Cross Shoes. "There is none of the rubbing and burning that make stiff-soled shoes so unbearable in hot weather. The special Red Cross tanning process makes the sole so flexible that you can bend it almost double when new." LHJ.

1913: Red Cross Shoes. Prices as in 1908. LHJ.

1914: Red Cross Shoes, $4.00 to $6.00. LHJ.

1915–17, 1919–20: Red Cross Shoes continue as before.

1923: "Red Cross Shoes range in price from $7.50 to $10.00. There are some at $12.00. The Red Cross Arch-Tone Shoe, the special arch support model—"The Tonic for Tired Feet"—retails at $9.00 and $10.00." Also offers shoes for children and misses age four and up. LHJ.

KWIK GLIDE. See UNITED STATES RUBBER COMPANY, 1927.

LA FRANCE. See WILLIAMS, CLARK & CO.

LADY WALKER. See KELLY.

LAIRD, SCHOBER & CO. Philadelphia.

 1869: Founded as Laird & Mitchell, producing misses', children's, and infants' shoes.

 1872: Became Laird, Shober & Mitchell, and began making only high-quality shoes.

 1875–80: Boot open in front with silk laces. Partly illegible stamp on sole: "Laird Schober . . ." in a lobed design. CHS 1978.45.29.

 1870s: Three hand-sewn exhibition boots hold the current record for number of stitches per inch: 64, 64, and 50. LACMA, TR9025, gift Mrs. Charles D. Cline.

 1895: Became Laird, Schober & Co.

 1900: Won grand prize at Paris Exposition in 1900. The company was known for making its own lasts, for its highly skilled and highly paid workmen, and for its high-quality and very expensive product, which it exported all over the world. It made women's, misses', children's, and infants' footwear for street and house wear, fancy slippers, riding boots, "and other dainty specialties." Brief history of firm given in TSR 9/1900, pp. 25–26.

 1900: Advertised tie shoe and boot. TSR 3/5/1900.

 1901: Advertised a Colonial shoe. TSR 5/15/01.

 1913: Illustrated a Colonial pump for 1914. TSR 9/20/13.

 1915: Illustrated a pump for 1916. TSR 9/18/15.

 1917: Illustrated an oxford for 1918. TSR 9/22/17.

 1923: Illustrated a fancy strap for 1924. TSR 9/15/23.

 1928: Illustrated a one-strap. TSR 3/17/28.

LAMPE. W. H. Lampe Shoe Co. St. Louis.

 1928: Illustrated a pump. TSR 3/17/28.

LANE. Wm. Lane.

 1903: Illustrated two dressy shoes. TSR 9/16/03.

LANGLOIS. Washington, D.C.

 1897: Langlois Foot Form Boots, $3.00. LHJ.

LAPE & ADLER CO. Columbus, Ohio.

 1927: "Foot-Friend Shoes, Retail $8.50 to $10." TSR 12/31/27.

 1928: Illustrated a gored shoe. TSR 3/17/28.

LATTEMANN. John J. Lattemann Shoe Manufacturing Co. New York City.

 1900: Illustrated a button boot. TSR 3/1900.

 1903: Illustrated two-strap shoes. TSR 9/16/03.

 1904: Illustrated a fancy slipper. TSR 9/21/04.

 1904: Illustrated dressy tie and button shoes. "Since we first made shoes—and it's a long while—we have never been able to offer so much in daintiness. . . . The Lattemann line reflects the little peculiarities of style and nicety of workmanship which marks the distinctively 'New York' shoe. We're ready with samples, or a salesman, whenever you say so—

meanwhile we wish to say that wherever there are careful mothers—there should be shown 'The Lattemann Corset Shoe,' which is unique, in that it has a patent ankle-stiffening device which may be added to or totally removed, as is most needed." TSR 9/28/04.

1917: Illustrated pump and oxford for 1918. TSR 9/22/17.

LE SAL.

1945–50: Brown velvet pump. Label: "Pretties by Le Sal." HN 66.694.

LEACH SHOE CO. Rochester, N.Y.

1915: Advertised welt and turn boots from $2.15 to $2.75. TSR 9/18/15.

1917: Illustrated a pump for 1918. TSR 9/22/17.

1919: Illustrated a pump for 1920. TSR 9/20/19.

1921: Illustrated a one-strap for 1922. TSR 9/17/21.

1923: Illustrated an ankle-strap for 1924. TSR 9/15/23.

LEVIRS & SARGENT. Lynn, Mass.

1907: Advertised "'Prince Chap,' An Extreme Narrow Toe that makes retailers sit up straight and give orders. In Boots and oxfords. . . . To be retailed from $3.50 to $5.00, giving the dealer a splendid profit. This is only one of 175 styles for spring, representing The Longest Line of (exclusively) Goodyear Welts ever offered the shoe dealers of the United States." TSR 9/28/07, p. 45. Oxford is illustrated on p. 47.

1909: Illustrated a new one-strap for 1910 (retail $5.00). TSR 9/25/09.

1911: Illustrated a tie shoe for 1912. TSR 9/16/11.

1915: Illustrated a button boot for 1916. TSR 9/18/15.

LINDNER SHOE CO. Carlisle, Pa., with branches in New York City, Philadelphia, Washington, San Francisco, and Wilmington, N.C.

1900: Advertised a front-lace boot. TSR 5/1900.

1904: Advertised women's tie shoes and boots for 1905. TSR 9/14, 9/21, and 9/28/04.

1907: Advertised shoes and boots. TSR 9/28/07.

1911: Advertised button boot. TSR 9/16/11.

1913: Retail prices from $3.50 to $6.00. TSR 7/5/13.

1915: Retail prices from $4.00 to $6.00. TSR 9/18/15.

1919: Illustrated a dressy oxford for 1920. TSR 9/20/19.

LITTLE. A. E. Little & Co. 75 Blake St., Lynn, Mass. Trade Name "Sorosis" from 1898 to 1934.

1898: Sorosis, "the new shoe for women." Boots, $3.50. LHJ.

1906: Black buttoned boot. PEM USMC 2130.

1914–15: Oxblood (red) buttoned boot. PEM USMC 2917.

1915–16: Beaded bronze four-strap. PEM USMC 2152.

1915–16: Gray suede beaded four-strap shoe. Label: "Sorosis, Reg. U.S. Pat. Office." HN 66.691.

LITTLE, MAXWELL & CO.

1895: Buttoned boot said to have been made at the 1895 exhibit of the Goodyear Shoe Machinery Company to demonstrate the Goodyear welt system. PEM USMC 1472.

LOUNSBURY MATTHEWSON & CO. South Norwalk, Conn. Out of business in 1925.

> 1896–99: Black kid slipper. Label: "Lounsbury, Matthewson & Co." PEM USMC 992.

LUNN & SWEET SHOE CO. Auburn, Maine.

> 1919: Advertised shoes for 1920. TSR 9/20/19.

> 1923: Illustrated an oxford for 1924. TSR 9/15/23.

LYNCH SHOE CO. Lynn, Mass.

> 1921: Illustrated a three-strap for 1922. TSR 9/17/21.

LYNN SHOE CO. Boston.

> 1892: Boots $1.50, $2.00, $2.50, or $3.00. LHJ.

M & B. See MARSHALL & BALL.

MANDEL BROTHERS. Chicago. Almost certainly a retailer, not a maker.

> 1916: "By mail from one of Chicago's greatest stores—easier than 'going downtown for them'—you can get the new 'Hi-cut' shoes—with 9-inch tops" for $3.75 postpaid. Also offered free subscription of "Mandel's Magazine." LHJ.

MANHEIMER. Abe Manheimer & Co., Inc. Cook at Taylor, St. Louis, Mo. Maker of shoe ornaments.

> 1927: Jeweled heels (rhinestones on silver or black celluloid, or topaz on gold), clasp ornaments, and cut-steel buckles, "$1.00 to $20.00 per pair in steel or bronze." TSR 12/31/27.

> 1928: Throat ornaments for pumps and gores. TSR 1/21/28.

MANNING MEADOW-BROOK SHOES. See OUTING SHOE CO.

MANSFIELD. G. A. & E. A. Mansfield. Lynn, Mass.

> 1904: Illustrated a "Sixteen Threads Gore Buskin . . . a repetition of 'Ye Olden Days'" for 1905. TSR 9/28/04.

MANSS-OWENS CO. Cincinnati, Ohio.

> 1917: Illustrated a boot for 1918. TSR 9/22/17.

> 1919: Illustrated an oxford for 1920. TSR 9/20/19.

MANUFACTURER'S SHOE CO. 145 Main St., Jackson, Mich.

> 1896: Shoes, $3.00 hand-turned soles. Others $1.50–$2.50. LHJ.

> 1897: Boots, $3.50. LHJ.

MARSHALL & BALL. 807–13 Broad St., Newark, N.J.

> 1903: Shoes, $3.75 postpaid. "45 years manufacturing outfitters," suggesting it was founded about 1858. HB.

MARSHALL, MEADOWS & STEWART, INC. Auburn, N.Y.

> 1928: Illustrated a sporty tie shoe. TSR 3/17/28.

MASON. Wilber Mason. Probably Rehoboth, Mass.

> 1795–1800: Light-blue kid latchet tie with pink tongue. Label: "Warranted and made by Wilber Mason for Thomas Kinnicutt. Rehoboth (Mass)." SPNEA 1918.934.

MAYER. F. Mayer Shoe Co. Milwaukee, Wis.

> 1928: Illustrated a T-strap. TSR 3/17/28.

MAYNARD SHOE CO. Claremont, N.H.

   1900: described as a "large manufacturer" of tennis shoes. TSR 5/1900.

MAURELLI. Erasmo Maurelli. Florence and Rome, Italy.

   1875–80: Black satin buttoned boot embroidered on vamp. Label translates:
   "Erasmo Maurelli, supplier to Her Majesty the Queen of Italy; successor
   to Mr. Antinucci. Great assortment of shoes of all kinds. Rome: Via due
   Macelli 101. Florence: Borgo Ognissanti 2. On parle français. English
   Spoken. SPNEA 1935.1.

McELROY-SLOANE SHOE CO. St. Louis.

   1917: Illustrated a boot for 1918. TSR 9/22/17.

   1919: Illustrated a pump for 1920. TSR 9/20/19.

MCKAY SEWING MACHINE CO. This company made the first machine
   capable of sewing soles to uppers. Shoemakers using the McKay machine
   were required to buy license stamps and affix one to each pair of shoes
   made. This license is a postage-stamp–sized label bearing a handwritten
   number and "McKay Sew. Mach. Co. License Stamp. Patd. Aug. 14, 1860"
   in an oval that surrounds the representation of the partial bottom of a shoe.

   1860–70: Serge front-lace boot with license stamp. PEM USMC 2005.

   1860–70: Serge gored boot with imitation buckle front and license stamp.
   Retail price was $2.75. PEM USMC 2016.

   1860–70: Gored boot with license stamp. LM 3147.

   1880–90: Girl's buttoned boot with license stamp. PEM USMC 1548.

MELVILLE HEMPED SOLE ATHLETIC SHOE. See KOZY SLIPPER CO.

MENIHAN CO. Rochester, N.Y.

   1921: Illustrated a three-strap for 1922. TSR 9/17/21.

MENZIES SHOE CO. Fond du Lac, Wis.

   1926: "Jiffy Boot for hunting, fishing, camping, touring and hiking" having
   a "hookless fastener," known today as a zipper. Cover TSR 9/25/26.

MIDDLETON. C. Middleton. 279 Broadway, New York City.

   1846: White satin wedding slippers. Label: "C. Middleton, Maker, 279
   Broadway, New-York." VHS 59.19.3.

MILLER. J. B. Miller & Co. 387 Canal St., New York City. Probably a retailer.

   1835 (possibly later): White kid wedding slipper. Label: "J. B. Miller & Co.,
   Ladies' French Shoe Store, 387 Canal St., N. Y." CHS 1960.24.5.

   1855–70: Bronze slipper with cutouts and large rosette. Label: Same as
   above. PEM 123,789.

MILLER. Sam Miller. 5 Cornhill, London, England.

   1799: Dark blue-green kid latchet tie wedding shoe. Label: "Sam Miller,
   Boot and Shoe Maker, No. 5, Cornhill, London." HN 66.635.

MILLER RUBBER CO. New York City and Akron, Ohio.

   1927: Rubber "Shuglov" rain boot. TSR 10/8 and 12/3/27.

MILLER SHOE MFG. CO. Cincinnati, Ohio.

   1915: Illustrated a Congress boot for 1916. TSR 9/18/15.

MILLER. I Miller, Inc. Brooklyn, N.Y.

   1921: Strapped shoes, wholesale prices from $7.00 to $8.50. TSR 9/17/21.

1923: Illustrated a one-strap for 1924. TSR 9/15/23.

MINOR. P. W. Minor & Sons, Inc. Batavia, N.Y.

1923: Illustrated a cross-strap for 1924. TSR 9/15/23.

1927: Shoes from $4.65 to $6.50. "Treadeasys, Style Welts, Littleways." TSR 12/31/27.

MITCHELL Mfg. Co. Portsmouth, Ohio.

1913: Advertised the "'Latestyle' (two in one) shoe lace, . . . the re-enforced combination flat and tubular oxford lace in black, white, grey or tan, retails 10 cents per pair." These were tubular toward the middle of the length, where the lace would pass through the eyelets, but flat and broad toward the ends, the part that would form the bow. TSR 9/20/13.

MONGUIGNON. 356 rue St. Honoré, Paris, France.

ca. 1890. Label: "Monguignon. de Suc^r L. Perchellet. Rue St. Honoré 356. Paris." PEM 127,397 or 8.

MOORE SHOE CO. St. Louis.

1928: Illustrated a T-strap. TSR 3/17/28.

MOORE-SHAFER SHOE MANUFACTURING CO. 200 Main St., Brockport, N.Y.

1900: Illustrated a boot, $3.50. Trademark: "The Ultra, Fit for a Queen" around a monogram M over S. LHJ, TSR 5/1900.

1904: Advertised "the Ultra Shoe for Women. It's comfortable. . . . Our patent cushion insole protects the feet from dampness and cold in Winter and heat in Summer. . . . A catalog illustrating fifty or more styles for home or street wear furnished free by your dealer or by us." TSR 9/14/04.

1915: Advertised in-stock boots from $2.35 to $3.15, and a pump for 1916. TSR 9/18/15.

1917: Illustrated an oxford for 1918. TSR 9/22/17.

1919: Illustrated an oxford for 1920. TSR 9/20/19.

1921: Illustrated a walking oxford, Ultra Shoes, $5.20. TSR 9/17/21.

MORLEY BUTTON CO. 20 Boylston St., Boston.

1911: Advertised Milo Buttons for shoes. TSR 9/16/11.

MORNING STAR SHOE CO., Lynn, Mass.

1900: Misses' front-lace boot, $1.15. TSR 7/1900.

MORSE & BURT CO. 6 Carlton Ave., and later 410–24 Willoughby Ave., Brooklyn, N.Y.

1924: Cantilever Shoes. "The distinctive feature of the Cantilever Shoe gives the foot extra support on the inner and weaker side and yet the sole is flexible from toe to heel." LHJ.

1926: Cantilever Shoes. "The heel of the Cantilever is slightly higher on the inner side to induce the wearer to toe straight ahead and swing the weight of the body to the outer and stronger side of the foot. The Cantilever heel encourages correct posture and is never too high to destroy Nature's balance." LHJ.

1928: Name of company now Cantilever Corporation. TSR 3/10/1928.

MORTON. Joseph Morton. 39 Marlboro St., Boston. Retailer.

    1823–28: Pale-blue kid slit vamp. Label: "Joseph Morton's Fashionable Variety Shoe Store, No. 39, Marlboro' Street, Boston." PEM 104,997.

MOSELEY. T. E. Moseley & Co. Temple Place, Boston. Retailers.

    1871: Pink silk wedding slipper said to have been purchased from T. E. Mosely & Co., "well-known dealers in high grade shoes in Boston for many years." PEM USMC 2131.

MURPHY & SAVAL CO. Chicago.

    1926: Fancy welt-type McKay pumps to retail $8.50 to $10. "America's Fastest Growing Factory." TSR 12/18/26.

    1928: Illustrated a strap shoe. TSR 3/17/28.

MURRAY SHOE CO. Lynn, Mass.

    1915: Illustrated a button boot for 1916. TSR 9/18/15.

NAHM BROTHERS, Philadelphia.

    1880s: Girl's pebble goat buttoned boot. McKay stamp. PEM USMC 1548.

    1895–1900: Dressy buttoned boot. PEM USMC 1568.

    1895–1900: Child's front-lace boot. PEM USMC 1569.

NARROW FABRIC CO. Reading, Pa.

    1919: "Makers of the famous Nufashond fabric tip shoe laces." Trademark: "Nufashond Porpoisette Shoe Lace" within a whale shape. TSR 9/20/19.

NATIONAL SHOE MFG. CO. Medinah Bldg., Chicago.

    1897: Woman's buttoned low shoe, $2.00, "is one of 1,000 styles of footwear shown in our catalogue . . . men's bunion shoes a specialty." LHJ.

NEOLIN SOLES. See GOODYEAR.

NETHERSOLE SHOES. See ROCK ISLAND SHOE CO.

NEWELL. James Newell. Middle St., Boston.

    1785–1800: Blue and white satin slippers embroidered on vamp. Label: "Women's Shoes & Slippers, of all Sorts made & sold By James Newell, Middle-Street, Boston." PEM 128,306.

NEWTON. J. R. Newton & Co. Philadelphia.

    1901: Advertised a latchet tie. TSR 5/5/01.

NICHOLSON. George E. Nicholson & Co. Lynn, Mass.

    1900: Illustrated a misses' front-lace boot at $1.20. TSR 7/1900.

NOVELTY KNITTING CO. 312 Broadway, Albany, N.Y.

    1901: "Arnold" knitted bedroom or bed slippers for $0.15. LHJ.

NOVELTY SHOE CO. Chicago, Ill.

    1921: Illustrated a sporty shoe for 1922. TSR 9/17/21.

NUFASHOND. See NARROW FABRIC CO.

NURSE'S DELYTE. See DALSIMER.

O'CONNOR & GOLDBERG. Chicago.

    1913: Originators of the Bulgarian Sandal. See article. TSR 9/20/13, pp. 35, 41.

O'DONNELL SHOE MFG. CO. St. Paul, Minn.

1919: Illustrated a two-strap pump for 1920. TSR 9/20/19.

OLDHAM. John Oldham. 5 Arran Quay, Dublin, Ireland.

1770–85: White satin buckle shoe with embroidered vamp. Label: "John Oldham, Ladies' Shoe Maker, No. 5 Arran Quay, Dublin." FMH 118.

OLYMPIC FOOTWEAR CO. 183 Essex St., Boston.

1914: Ped-Speed Shoes "are made of chrome-tanned brown mocha calf uppers with Juniper soles, or soft white buck uppers with white Ivory soles. Goodyear welts—sewn throughout, full counter support for heel. Soles are waterproof—wetting won't harm or stiffen them. All sizes and widths for all ages." Trademark: "Ped-Speed" in a pair of outspread wings. LHJ.

ONE PROFIT SHOE CO. 238 Monroe St., Chicago.

1897: Boots, $3.00, including postage. LHJ.

ORIENTAL SLIPPER MFG. CO. 101 Reade St., New York City.

1915: Hand-turned satin slippers, $1.15 with Cuban heel, $1.25 with Louis heel. TSR 9/18/15.

O'SULLIVAN RUBBER CO. Lowell, Mass.

1901: O'Sullivan's Comfort Heels, $0.35 pair plus attaching price. "The lives of ladies lengthened by this rubber blessing. The springy step of youth brought back to the aged, and muscle-weary women may again realize the joy of buoyancy." LHJ.

1905: "Don't [sic] it stand to reason that the heel of new rubber is essential? That it sheaths your walk through life with comfort, because they carry out what nature intended? . . . There is only one kind of heels made of new rubber, 'O'Sullivan's.'" $0.35 a pair or $0.50 attached. GH.

1912: "The pounding leather heel is as unsatisfactory compared with the resilient heel of new, live rubber, as a motorcar without tires compared to a smooth-riding completely equipped machine of the latest model." CR.

OUTING SHOE CO. 530 Atlantic Ave., Boston.

1923: Manning "Meadow-Brook" Shoes. Features white canvas shoes, leather soles, and rubber heels, all with buttoned straps. LHJ.

OWN MAKE SHOES. See HAMILTON, BROWN SHOE CO.

PARIS. N. A. Paris. 91–101 Ingraham St., Brooklyn, N.Y.

1927: "Paris of Brooklyn, producer of ultra-fashionable McKays." TSR 12/31/27.

PARSONS. James Parsons & Co. Brooklyn, N.Y.

1904: Illustrated a front-lace boot on "a new last for women" for 1905. TSR 9/28/04.

PCRH CO. See PNEUMATIC CUSHION RUBBER HEEL CO.

PEABODY, Ellery. 213 Washington St., Boston. Probably primarily a retailer.

1860s: White kid slipper. Label: "Ellery Peabody. 213 Washington St., Boston" with pictures of two front-lace boots and one shoe. PEM 124,400.

PECK SHOE CO. Worcester, Mass.

1928: "with insoles that will sta-smooth." TSR 3/10/28.

PED-SPEED SHOES. See OLYMPIC FOOTWEAR CO.

PEDIGO-WEBER SHOE CO. St. Louis.

    1928: Illustrated a one-strap. TSR 3/17/28.

PERKINS. Warren Perkins. Reading, Mass.

    1812: White kid wedding slippers. One shoe has label reading "Shoes, Particularly made for retailing, By Warren Perkins, Reading, Rips Mended gratis." The other shoe has VOSE retailer's label. DHS 60.70.1.

PERCHELLET. L. Perchellet. Paris, France. French maker of high-quality shoes.

    1877–80: Black satin one-strap with embroidered vamp. Label: "Perchellet. 26 Rue Louis Le Grand, au coin de la rue du 4 Septembre. L. Perchellet. Breveté S. G. D. [C or G.] Fab^t des Chaussure à Ressorts pour Hommes et pour dames. Paris." SPNEA 1920.61.

PERRY, DAME & CO. 150 East 32nd St., New York City. A general mail-order house, not a shoe manufacturer.

    1917: Advertised catalog and featured a boot for $3.98. LHJ.

    1918: Advertised "wearing apparel—quality shoes for women and children" and featured an oxford for $3.98. LHJ.

PETERS SHOE CO. St. Louis. A branch of International Shoe Co.

    1921: One-strap shoes at $4.60 and $4.75. Trademark: a diamond enclosing "Peters Shoe Co's DiamonD Brand, St. Louis." TSR 9/17/21.

PETERSON. M. H. Peterson & Co. 154 Fifth Ave., Chicago.

    1904: "<u>Your</u> Shoes Hurt? . . . Peterson's Anti-Tender Foot Shoes for Men and Women . . . never fail to give relief for bunions, corns and callouses." Trademark: a circle with "Peterson's, The Natural Foot Cover" running round the outer band, and "Anti-Tender Foot Shoe" in the center with a picture of a boot. McC.

PHELAN. James Phelan & Sons. Lynn, Mass.

    1900: Illustrated a front-lace boot at $1.60. TSR 7/1900.

PHILIPSON-LOCKWOOD, INC. Long Island City, N.Y.

    1928: Illustrated a T-strap. TSR 3/17/28.

PILGRIM SHOE CO. Danvers, Mass.

    1904: Illustrated a front-lace boot for 1905. TSR 9/28/04.

PINCUS & TOBIAS, INC. Brooklyn, N.Y.

    1915: Illustrated a button boot for 1916. TSR 9/18/15.

PINGREE CO. Detroit, Mich.

    1915: Illustrated a pump for 1916. TSR 9/18/15.

PLANT. Thomas G. Plant Co. 110 (later 107, later 2) Bickford St., Boston. Branch "in-stock" departments in New York City and Chicago. "Sold in 2500 Cities and Towns. Only one dealer in a town."

    1900, 1901: Queen Quality Shoes. Boots $3.00, Oxfords $2.50, plus $0.25 postage. LHJ.

    1912: Queen Quality Shoes and boots from $3.50 to $5.00. LHJ.

    1913: Same as 1912, with "a few unusual styles at $5.50 and $6.00." LHJ. Also advertised in TSR 9/20/13.

1919: Queen Quality Shoes. "World's largest factory making women's shoes exclusively." LHJ.

1927: "Hi-Toppers," boots with cuffs that can be worn up or down. Trademark: "Queen Quality" in oval of laurel leaves with crown at the top. TSR 12/10/27.

1928: Illustrated a strapped "Dorothy Dodd pattern." TSR 3/17/28.

PLASTIC SHOES. See THAYER, MCNEIL.

PLYTEX. See ESSEX RUBBER CO.

PNEUMATIC CUSHION RUBBER HEEL CO. 19 Lincoln St., Boston.

1905: "The most comfortable shoes for women's wear are juliets, oxfords and old ladies' balmorals with 'pneumatic cushion rubber heels' attached." DEL.

1907: Trademark: PCRH CO, PAT MAY 11, 1897 in a circle. TSR 9/28/07.

1910: Same trademark. HSW.

QUEEN QUALITY. See THOMAS G. PLANT CO.

R-G SHOE. Also R & G SHOE CO. See RICKARD-GREGORY.

RADCLIFFE SHOE CO. 179 Lincoln Street, Boston.

1901: Radcliffe Shoes. Boots, $2.50. LHJ.

1902, 1903, 1904: Same price, heavy advertising. LHJ, DEL.

1909: Advertised boots wholesaling at $2.20 and $3.25 in TSR 9/25/09.

RAMIREZ. Probably California.

Date uncertain: Blue satin slipper in early-nineteenth-century style. Sole stamp: "Ramirez" in a tilted cursive. NHM-LAC A.3580–1300.

RAMSFELDER-ERLICK CO. Cincinnati, Ohio.

1913: Advertised boots. Trademarks: "It Stands Supreme." "Restshu" with "for women with tender foot" in a streamer below. "The Best Flexible Sole Shoe in the World." TSR 9/20/13.

RAUH. S. Rauh & Co. 310–18 Sixth Ave., New York City.

1886–95: Bathing shoes, marked on sole "Rauh's Standard Indestructible Cork Sole, Trade Mark, Pat. August 17th, 1886." NHM-LAC A.10030–82.

1927: "Standard Rau-Craft Slippers, Best for Rest." TSR 12/17/27.

RAYNBOOT. See CAMBRIDGE RUBBER CO.

REA. Pelatiah Rea. Boston. Probably primarily a retailer.

1805–15: Turquoise kid slipper. Label: "Pelatiah Rea's Variety Shoe Store, No. 2, North-West corner of the Old State-House, Boston. Rips mended gratis." CD 1970.65.

RED CROSS SHOES. See KROHN, FECHHEIMER & CO.

REED, DR. See EBBERTS.

REED. E. P. Reed & Co. Rochester, N.Y. Branches in New York and Chicago.

1909: Advertised boots at $2.50. TSR 9/25/09.

1915: Advertised boots from $2.60 to $3.10. TSR 9/18/15.

1928: Illustrated a strapped shoe. TSR 3/17/28.

REGAL SHOE CO., INC. 703 Summer St., Boston. Factory in East Whitman, Mass. Mail-order branches at factory and in San Francisco and London.

   1904: Shoes $3.75 postpaid. "Regal styles are exact reproductions of those Pinet originals." "M. Pinet in Paris [is] the famous custom boot-maker whose designs set the fashions in feminine footgear." "We are now satisfying over 300,000 well-satisfied mail order customers." "Exclusive Regal Women's Stores in Boston, New York and Philadelphia. Sixty-two Regal Men's Stores in all the principal cities from San Francisco to London." Partial list of addresses given. DEL, LHJ.

   1905: Shoes $3.75 postpaid. Special custom bench-made $4.00. "They are the only shoes in the world made in Quarter Sizes." DEL.

   1906: Shoes $3.50–$4.00. "The largest retail shoe business in the world." LHJ.

RESTSHU. See RAMSFELDER-ERLICK.

RICE & HUTCHINS, INC. 137 High St., Boston. Factory may have been in Marlboro, Mass.

   1903: Tan front-lace boot. PEM USMC 2320.

   1915: Broad-toed Educator Shoes. "Prices $1.35 to $5.50. But EDUCATOR must be branded on the sole or it isn't the genuine orthopaedically correct Educator shape." LHJ.

   1922: Cross-strap shoe. Label: "The Vera, Made in America by Rice and Hutchins, Boston, [illegible]." PEM USMC 2344.

RICE-O'NEILL SHOE CO. St. Louis.

   1928: Illustrated a one-strap. TSR 3/17/28.

RICH SHOE CO. Milwaukee, Wis.

   1897: Sears advertised "Rich's Patent Julia Marlowe Lace Boot. . . . Elastic Goring Over the Instep." $2.85 per pair. Trademark stamp on sole: "Rich's Julia Marlowe Lace Boot Pat'd Aug. 11–96." The patent apparently refers to the elastic on the instep.

   1899: "Rich's Patent Julia Marlowe Shoes." Boots $3.00. Oxfords $2.00. Hand turning, add $0.50. Hand welting, add $1.00. Fancy vesting top, add $ 0.25 (oxfords) or $0.35 (boots). LW.

   1901: Advertised Julia Marlowe Lace Oxford, Pat. Oct 23rd, 1900. Basic oxford price now $2.25. "Unprincipled Counterfeiters in the shoe business are trying to imitate them and deceive the public. Therefore, when buying, see that the name "Julia Marlowe" is on every sole." TSR 4/3/01. Also LHJ.

   1903: Boots as before. Oxfords $2.00–$2.75. DEL.

   1908: Boots as before. Turned shoe elastic instep $2.75. Welted two-eyelet $3.50. LHJ.

   1911: Advertised shoes and boots for 1912, no elastic in evidence but Julia Marlowe name still used. TSR 9/16 and 9/30/11.

   1913: Illustrated a button boot for 1914. TSR 9/20/13.

RICHARDSON. Wm. Richardson Co. Hornellsville, N.Y.

   1900: Illustrated a front-lace boot. TSR 12/1900.

1901: Advertised a woman's balmoral boot with star-shaped perforations and extension sole. TSR 3/1901.

RICKARD SHOE CO. See RICKARD-GREGORY SHOE COMPANY.

RICKARD-GREGORY SHOE CO. Lynn, Mass. Salesroom at 72 Lincoln St., Boston. In 1911, the name given is The R & G Shoe Co., Geo. Gregory Pres. & Gen. Mgr.; in 1914, it is The Rickard Shoe Co., Lynn; in 1923, it is the Rickard Shoe Co. of Haverhill.

1907: Illustrated boots and shoes as the "R-G" Shoe, retailing at $3.00, $3.50, and $4.00. TSR 9/28/07.

1909: Illustrated a low tie, and a selection of shoe buckles and bows for 1910. TSR 9/25/09.

1911: Advertised button boots retailing at $3.00, $3.50, $4.00 for 1911, and pumps for 1912. Trademark: a rectangle with R & G diagonally from upper left to lower right, with "The" in the upper right corner, and "Shoe" in the lower left corner. TSR 9/16/11.

1913: Illustrated a button boot for 1914. TSR 9/20/13.

1923: Illustrated a cross-strap for 1924. TSR 9/15/23.

RILEY SHOE MFG. CO. Columbus, Ohio.

1913: Advertised button boots, pumps, and Colonials. Welts and turns at $2.10 to $2.50. Same lasts and patterns in McKays at $1.75 to $2.10. TSR 9/20/13.

1928: Illustrated a T-strap. TSR 3/17/28.

ROCHESTER SHOE MANUFACTURING CO. Probably Rochester, N.Y.

1918–22: Slipper with high Louis heel. Label: "Rochester Shoe Mfg. Co." PEM USMC 968.

ROCK ISLAND SHOE CO. 402 Third Ave., Rock Island, Ill.

1901, 1902: Nethersole shoes. Boots, $2.50. postpaid. LHJ.

RUBY KID.

1928: Ruby Glazed Kid used in shoes. TSR 1/21/28.

RUEPING. Fred Rueping Leather Co. Fond du Lac, Wis. Branches in major American cities, Paris, Frankfurt, and Northampton, England.

1928: Kin Kin, fine elk tannage, colors and black. Shoe illustrated is made "from Kin Kin Veal Sides Smoked with Kiltie Tongue. Gristle sole and heel." TSR 2/25/28.

RYAN. Wm. Ryan. Philadelphia.

1845: White kid wedding shoes. Label: "Wm. Ryan, Maker, No. 18 N. 4th St, Phila." HN 66.643.

1845–60: White kid slit vamp shoe. Label: "Wm. Ryan & Co., Makers, No. 16 S. 4th St., Phila." PEM 127,755.

SACHS SHOE MFG. CO. Cincinnati, Ohio.

1923: Illustrated a fancy strap shoe for 1924. TSR 9/15/23.

SAIFER. Dave Saifer Shoe Co. Chicago. See also TOBER-SAIFER.

1921: Illustrated a three-strap for 1922. TSR 9/17/21.

SARGENT. Don D. Sargent Shoe Co. Salem, Mass.

1917: Illustrated an oxford for 1918. TSR 9/22/17.

SARGENT SHOE CO. Lynn, Mass.

1921: Illustrated a tie shoe for 1922. TSR 9/17/21.

SAWYER BOOT & SHOE CO. Bangor, Maine.

1911: Advertised Hiawatha Indian moccasins. Trademark: "Hiawatha" in script with "trade mark" in the streaming tail of the H. TSR 9/23/11.

SCHEIFFELE SHOE MFG. CO. Cincinnati, Ohio.

1911: Advertised a misses' one-strap for 1912. TSR 9/30/11.

SCHMIDT. Carl E. Schmidt & Co. Detroit, Mich.

1909: Advertised calf leathers for 1910. "Specify these most popular tan calfskin shades: Hazel Brown, Color R, Color C B. . . . You can always be sure of the genuine by our indelibly stenciled mark on every inch of the back of every Calfskin we tan." TSR 9/25/09.

SEARS ROEBUCK & CO. Chicago.

1894: Boots, $2.00 to $4.25 (at least).

1897: Boots, $1.00 to $3.50. Shoes: $0.60 for serge buskin slippers to $1.98 for satin slippers. Carpet slippers $0.24, leather-soled, fur-trimmed felt slippers $1.15.

1900: Boots, $1.50 for felt to $2.65 for "Jenness" last.

1901: A factory was apparently built to allow Sears to make many of its own shoes. The 1902 catalog included a picture of Sears' "new 20th century shoe plant," saying, "Our factory was taxed to its fullest capacity last season, and to the increased demand for home made shoes we have added more new machinery, thus placing us in a position to make the very best at the lowest prices. One order of 35,000 pairs is now being made for the United States Government, thus demonstrating the high quality of the goods produced."

1902: Boots, $0.85 for serge Congress to $2.95 for extra high welted calf. Shoes, $0.95 to $1.95. House slippers $0.24 to $1.05.

1906: Boots, $1.25 to $3.50. Shoes, $0.85 to $2.50. House slippers $0.75 to $1.39.

1908: Boots, $0.97 to $1.58. Shoes, $0.92 to $1.68.

1909: Boots, $1.05 to $2.23. Shoes, $1.19 to $2.25.

1927: Boots, most fleece-lined, $1.89 to $3.98. Shoes: $1.88 to $4.95. Bedroom slippers $0.49 to $1.79.

SEAVIEW. Not clear whether this is a company or a style name. Possibly located in Maine.

1920–25: Red satin, rubber-soled, front-lace bathing boots. Label: "Seaview Bathing, Made in USA." HN 1976.121.

1920–25: Same as above, but green satin. DHS 91.34.319.

SELBY SHOE CO. 133 7th St. (later 432 7th St. and later still 764 7th St.), Portsmouth, Ohio. Founded by 1880.

1911: Illustrated a Colonial for 1912. TSR 9/30/11.

1913: Illustrated a Colonial for 1914. TSR 9/20/13.

1915: Illustrated a front-lace boot for 1916. TSR 9/18/15.

1919: Illustrated a Colonial pump for 1920. TSR 9/20/19.

1921: Illustrated an oxford for 1922. TSR 9/17/21.

1923: Arch Preserver Shoes, "makers of women's fine shoes for more than forty years!" "Unlike the ordinary shoe arch construction which sags under the weight of the body and quickly lets the foot become strained and uncomfortable, the Arch Preserver Shoe has a special concealed built-in arch-bridge that supports the foot arch perfectly no matter how high the stylish heel of the shoe raises the foot arch from the ground." LHJ.

1926: Arch Preserver Shoes. Trademark on sole lining: a pedestal with curved words "Arch, Preserver, Shoe" inside. Above pedestal, a circle divided in half vertically with A/P on left and the sole of a foot on right. Below pedestal, "Keeps the foot well." LHJ.

1928: Arch Preserver Shoes ("For men and boys by only E. T. Wright & Co., Inc., Rockland, Mass."). "You know, yourself, that the foot's chief claim to beauty is its perfectly curved instep. When you wear shoes that let the arch sag, then the instep flattens, and the foot's aristocratic shapeliness is gone. This tragedy need not happen to you. It is forestalled forever by the famous arch bridge and other patented features in every Arch Preserver Shoe." LHJ.

SELZ-SCHWAB CO. Chicago.

1893: Boots and shoes exhibited at Chicago World's Fair. PEM USMC 2457, 2470, 2478, 2483, 2487. Men's shoes from this company also survive in the USMC collection.

SHERWOOD SHOE CO. Rochester, N.Y.

1917: Illustrated an oxford for 1918. TSR 9/22/17.

1928: Illustrated a T-strap. TSR 3/17/28.

SHILLABER E-Z GLOVE SHOE. See AARON F. SMITH CO.

SHOE SPECIALTY MFG. CO. St. Louis.

1919: Illustrated a one-eyelet tie for 1920. TSR 9/20/19.

SIEGEL COOPER CO. Sixth Ave. at 18th and 19th Streets, New York City. A general apparel mail-order house, not a shoe manufacturer.

1905: Advertises "Comfy Slippers" for $0.90, and fur-bound red, black or brown felt "Juliettes" for $0.98, "though we know that the maker of these shoes sells them direct to some of his customers for $1.50." Presumably Daniel Green Felt Shoe Co. is the maker referred to, since the Juliettes appear identical to those made and advertised by Green for $1.50 in the same year, and the Comfy Slipper to Green's $1.00 comfy. DEL.

SLATER & MORRILL, INC. South Braintree, Mass.

1915: Illustrated a white buck front-lace boot for 1916. TSR 9/18/15.

SLUMBER SLIPPER. See DE FREEST & STOVER.

SMALTZ GOODWIN CO. Philadelphia.

1913: Illustrated a Colonial pump for 1914. TSR 9/20/13.

1915: Illustrated a pump for 1916. TSR 9/18/15.

1919: Illustrated a pump for 1920. TSR 9/20/19.

1921: Illustrated a two-strap for 1922. TSR 9/17/21.

1923: Illustrated a one-strap for 1924. TSR 9/15/23.

SMITH. Aaron F. Smith Co. Lynn, Mass. Est. 1864.

   1909: Advertised Goodyear welt boots at $2.25. TSR 9/25/09.

   1911: Advertised oxfords at $2.15, boots at $2.25. Carried a line called
      "Glove Fitters" or "Glove Fitting Welts," and also the "Shillaber E-Z
      Glove Shoe." TSR 9/16/11.

SMITH. J. P. Smith Shoe Co. Chicago.

   1928: Illustrated a two-eyelet tie. TSR 3/17/28.

SMITH. Wm. Sumner Smith. 325 Monroe St., Chicago.

   1928: Small ad for $1.00 shoes. TSR 3/10/28.

SMITH & SISLEY. 188 Chatham St., New York City.

   1840–45: Tan morocco and serge slit-vamp shoes. Label (much worn):
      "Smith & Sisley, Makers, 188 Chatham St., N.Y." CHS 1970.

SOROSIS. See A. E. LITTLE & CO.

STANDARD BOOT AND SHOE LASTING CO.

   1885–90: Black buttoned boot with royalty stamp on sole: "Standard Boot
      and Shoe Lasting Co., License Stamp, [stamped number], Pat. Aug. 11,
      '85, Reiss[ued] Sep. 1, '85, Lasted, Without Tacks." PEM USMC 2418.

STANDARD KID MFG. CO. 207 South St., Boston.

   1919: Advertised "Vode [glazed] Kid, a leather which lasts in footwear, is
      made only from fine imported kid skins, dyed thru and thru. . . . Just now
      all womankind is fascinated with Vode Kid in Field Mouse. This shade is
      being featured in the smart shops, where you will also find shoes of Vode
      Kid in other popular colors—Havana Brown, Gray, Tan, Blue and
      Black." Trademark: a goat standing on a shield bearing words "Standard,
      Kid, guaranteed selections, Standard Kid Mfg. Co., Boston." LHJ.

STANDARD SCREW.

   1885–90: Front-lace boot stamped on sole: "Registered Trademark—
      Standard [picture of screw] Fastened." PEM USMC 1733.

STARNER-COPELAND CO. Columbus, Ohio.

   1904: Advertised front-lace boots. "True Merit Shoes Retail for $2.00,"
      $1.50 wholesale. TSR 9/21/04.

STETSON SHOE CO. South Weymouth, Mass.

   1928: Illustrated a summer oxford. TSR 3/17/28.

STONE. K. M. Stone Importing Co. 12-14-16 East 22nd St., New York City.

   1919: Advertised boudoir slippers from $8.50 to $12.50 per dozen. If these
      were imported (as company name implies), the materials suggest an
      origin in the Far East. Also illustrated a Colonial pump. TSR 9/20/19.

   1921: Illustrated a strap shoe for 1922. TSR 9/17/21.

STROOTMAN. John Strootman Shoe Co. Buffalo, N.Y.

   1913: Advertised low shoes for 1914. TSR 9/20/13.

   1917: Illustrated an oxford for 1918. TSR 9/22/17.

SULLIVAN. Edward E. Sullivan. Haverhill, Mass.

   1921: Bench-made turns for $5.00 "for retailers who cater to the worth-
      while trade." TSR 9/17/21.

SULLIVAN. P. Sullivan & Co. Cincinnati, Ohio.

1917: Illustrated shoes for 1918. TSR 9/22/17.

1919: Illustrated a pump for 1920. TSR 9/20/18.

1923: Illustrated a gore shoe for 1924. TSR 9/15/23.

SULTANA MFG. CO. 317 Findlay St., Cincinnati, Ohio.

1915: "Footgluv" boudoir slippers that folded into their own case, costing $8.00 to $24.00 per dozen. TSR 9/18/15.

SULZER. Alexandre Sulzer. 7 rue du 29 Juillet, Paris, France.

1865–70: Bronze buttoned boot with tassel. Label: "Fournisseur de S. M. la Reine de Saxe, Alexandre Sulzer, Cordonnier, pour Dames, Rue du 29 Juillet, 7, Paris." CD 1955.1.

SWEET. Alfred J. Sweet. Division of United States Shoe Co. Auburn, Maine. See also LUNN & SWEET.

1928: Illustrated a one-strap. TSR 3/17/28.

SYRACUSE SHOE MFG. CO. Syracuse, N.Y.

1909: Advertised a Colonial pump. TSR 9/25/09.

TAPPAN SHOE CO. Coldwater, Mich.

1911: Advertised a pump for 1912. TSR 9/30/11.

TAS CO. (TAS may be an acronym).

1917–20: Front-lace boot. Label: "The TAS Co." HN 1976.121.3.

TAYLOR. L. W. Taylor. 78 Railroad Ave., Brockton, Mass.

1915: Kid, suede, and canvas boudoir slippers from $3.60 to $5.00 per dozen, $0.50 more with quilted sock lining. Also felt slippers in all colors. TSR 9/18/15.

TESSIER & BOWDOIN CO. Haverhill, Mass.

1923: Illustrated a T-strap for 1924. TSR 9/15/23.

THAYER, MCNEIL CO. 12 West St., Boston.

1914–16: Brown cloth buttoned boot foxed with black patent. Label: "Thayer McNeil Co., Boston." SPNEA 1990.51.

1916, 1917: Plastic Shoes, for men, women, children. Lace, button, high- and low-cut ("plastic" meaning "flexible," not the modern synthetic material). Sold by mail only or at Boston salesroom. Claims to relieve foot troubles by proper shoe construction. "New England's leading shoe house." LHJ.

1924–30: White canvas strap shoe with black patent trim. CD 1956.138.

THAYER, MCNEIL & HODGKINS. Boston. Address in 1884, 22 Temple Place; by 1900, 47 Temple Place.

1885–90: White silk button boot. PEM 129,782.

ca. 1895: Black satin beaded slipper. Label: "Thayer, McNeil & Hodgkins, 47 Temple Place, Boston." HN 66.683.

1906–9: White kid latchet-tie shoes. Label: "Thayer, McNeil & Hodgkins, 47 Temple Place, Boston." HN 66.685.

1915–16: Steel-beaded gray suede multi-strap shoe. Label: "Thayer, McNeil & Hodgkins, Boston." CD 1956.134.

THIERRY. See ESTÉ.

THOMSON-CROOKER SHOE CO. Roxbury Crossing (later 18 Station St.), Boston. Factory at Lynn, Mass.

1909: Advertised boots at $1.50 and $2.10 ($3.00 retail). Label: monogram on top facing appears to be H.W. superimposed on a large C, with a smaller "s co." fitted inside the C. TSR 9/25/09.

1913: Advertised boots from $2.10 to $2.85.

1921: Advertised strap and tie shoes from $3.75 to $5.50 wholesale. TSR 9/17/21.

1923: Advertised strap shoes from $4.15 to $4.75. TSR 9/15/23.

TILT. J. E. Tilt Shoe Co. Chicago.

1921: Illustrated an oxford for 1922. TSR 9/17/21.

TOBER-SAIFER SHOE CO. 1312 Washington Ave., St. Louis. See also SAIFER.

1923: Advertised strapped shoes from $4.50 to $5.75. TSR 9/15/23.

TRAVERS CO. Cincinnati, Ohio.

1919: Illustrated a side-gore shoe for 1920. TSR 9/20/19.

TROT-MOC. See ASHBY-CRAWFORD CO.

TROY. Seymour Troy & Co., Inc. Brooklyn, N.Y.

1923: Illustrated a cutout pump for 1924. TSR 9/15/23.

TRUE MERIT SHOES. See STARNER-COPELAND CO.

TUTTLE. Henry Tuttle & Co. 259 and 261 Washington St., Boston. Probably primarily a retailer.

1868: White satin wedding shoes. Label: "Henry H. Tuttle & Co., French & American Shoe Store, 259 & 261 Washington St., Boston. Warranted." HN 66.662.

1875–95: Black velvet and fur carriage boots. Label: "Henry H. Tuttle & Co. Boston." HN 66.793.

1900–1905: Cream kid sandal slipper. Label: "Henry H. Tuttle & Co. Boston." CD 1989.22.

1917–20: Silver evening slippers. Label: "The H. H. Tuttle Co. Boston." CD 1947.1.

TWEEDIE BOOT TOP CO. St. Louis. By 1923 the name was changed to the Tweedie Footwear Corp., since spats (boot tops) were no longer worn; by 1928 "General Offices and Factory—Jefferson City, Missouri."

1920, 1921: "Tweedies, BooTop, Trade Mark" on spats. LHJ.

1921: "How am I to fit 'spats' over the new strap effects?" The ad recommends trying the new Tweedie Swing Button pattern of spats. TSR 9/17/21.

1923: Illustrated a cross-strap for 1924. TSR 9/15/23.

1928: Advertisement. TSR 1/28/28.

ULTRA SHOE. See MOORE-SHAFER.

UNITED FAST COLOR EYELET CO. 205 Lincoln St., Boston.
  1900: Thomas Plant (Queen Quality shoes) mentions using "fast color eyelets." LW, LHJ.
  1902: Dorothy Dodd mentions using "fast color eyelets." LHJ.
  1905: Hamilton, Brown Shoe Company (American Lady Shoes) mentions using "fast color eyelets." DEL.
  1928: Makers of Diamond Brand Visible Fast Color Eyelets. Diamond Trade Mark. TSR 1/28/28.
UNITED LACE AND BRAID MFG. CO. Providence, R.I.
  1909: Advertised shoe laces "made in all colors, pure silk and mercerized silk" with "beaded tip." TSR 9/25/09.
UNITED STATES RUBBER CO. New York City.
  1900:Information about this company in TSR 5/1900, p.34, includes:
  1893: Began making tennis shoes. "Two styles were only produced at first . . . the Defender and Champion, first and second grades. The Defender, the highest quality, . . . is of white, black or brown duck. It has a corrugated rubber sole, with several raised bars across and a double heel. The jobbers' net price to dealers [in 1900] is 65 cents for men's oxfords and 80 cents for bals. The second grade, known as "Champion," has a wide sale, for the price is very moderate. Dealers pay this year [1900] 45 cents for men's oxfords and 60 cents for bals. . . . These are the popular 'sneaks.'"
  1893–96: Probably introduced the dressy all-white canvas yachting shoe.
  1897: Introduced a lighter-weight gymnasium shoe.
  1898: Introduced a bathing shoe.
  1900: The company produced about 7,200 pairs daily. Introduced the "vacation shoe," with canvas top and heavy red rubber sole.
  1917: Advertisement for rubber overshoes. "Pressure Process rubber footwear has 'life' and 'spring.'" Trademark: a circle with "US Rubber System" in center surrounded by "United States Rubber Company and Associated Companies." TSR 9/22/17.
  1917: Introduced Keds. "A new shoe—a new name—a new attractiveness in style—a new comfort in coolness and graceful flexibility—a new economy worth while. These are reasons why you, too, will appreciate the charm of this big new American shoe family called Keds. Keds have cool tops of the firmest and finest of canvas. The soles are made of rubber, full of grace and spring. Keds prove a necessity to the well-dressed woman who values perfect ease in all of her outdoor games and sports. They are so comfortable out-doors that she also wears them for housework, shopping and leisure dress-up hours. Three price levels: National Keds (from $1.50 up), Campfire Keds ($1.23–$2.00), Champion Keds ($1.00–$1.50)." LHJ.
  1927: Rain overshoes with jersey top and rubber sole known as "Gaytees," fastening either with a concealed snap or a "kwik glide fastener" (a zipper). TSR 10/29/27.

UNITED STATES SHOE CO. See AIR MAIL SHOE COMPANY. See also
  SWEET.
UPHAM BROS. SHOE CO. Stoughton, Mass.
  1919: Illustrated an oxford for 1920. TSR 9/20/19.
UTZ AND DUNN CO. 50 (later 88) Canal St., Rochester, N.Y. Offices at
  200 Fifth Ave., New York City, and also in Denver and Los Angeles.
  1900: Illustrated a front-lace boot. TSR 5/1900.
  1902: Advertised oxfords for $1.60, $1.85, $2.25. "Terms: 4 Per Cent. off
    30 Days. 'Discount Pays the Freight.' . . . Remember this—We guarantee
    that no cut-off vamps or two-piece counters go into any of our shoes."
    TSR 7/16/02.
  1904: Illustrated a fancy two-strap for 1905. TSR 9/28/04.
  1909: Advertised dressy shoes. TSR 9/25/09.
  1911: Dr. Edison Cushion Shoe. Boots, $4.00.
  1912: Dr. Edison Cushion Shoe. Boots $4.00, 4.50. Oxfords $3.40, 4.00. LHJ.
  1915: Dr. Edison Cushion Shoe. Boots $4.50. LHJ.
  1915: Advertised button boots from $2.25 to $3.25 (presumably wholesale
    prices), claimed fifty styles in stock. Illustrated a two-strap for 1916. TSR
    9/18/15.
  1917: Illustrated shoes for 1918. TSR 9/22/17.
  1917: Dr. Edison Cushion Shoe. "An insole of live wool felt excludes all
    cold and dampness, removes pressure from sensitive joints and nerves,
    and yet does not sacrifice one stylish line." LHJ.
  1919: Ease-All Shoes. "The shoe of invisible comfort and visible style." LHJ.
  1920: Ease-All Shoes. LHJ.
  1923: Ease-All Shoes. Trademark: "Ease All" on a banner with curled
    pointed ends, with a diagonal band bearing words "Utz & Dunn Co."
    across the middle. LHJ.

VELVETTA SUEDE. See HUNT-RANKIN.
VIAULT-ESTÉ. See ESTÉ.
VINSONHALER SHOE CO. St. Louis.
  1902: Mentioned as a southwestern distributor for Hervey E. Guptill, a
    Haverhill slipper manufacturer. TSR 8/20/02.
VODE. See STANDARD KID.
VOSE. Josiah Vose's Shoe Store, 32 Newbury St., Boston. Probably primarily
  a retailer.
  1812: White kid wedding shoe. Label: "Warranted Shoes Made in particular
    for Josiah Vose's Shoe Store No. 32, Newbury Street, corner of West
    Street—Boston (Rips mended gratis)." The other shoe has a Perkins
    label. DHS 60.70.1.

W. B. C./W. B. COON CO. See COON.
WALES GOODYEAR SHOE CO. Probably Connecticut.

1885–95: Rubbers, with knitted tops added by owner. Label: "Wales Goodyear Shoe Co. Trade Mark. [size:] 5F." SPNEA 1946.339.

WALK-OVER SHOES. See KEITH.

WANAMAKER STORE. New York City. A retailer, not a maker.

1903: Wanamaker-Reliable Shoes for Women. $3.00 plus $0.25 postage. Line consists of thirty-two different styles of women's boots. "If you have other needs in shoes for men, women, and children, send for our Shoe Catalogue No. 15, telling all about the largest retail shoe stock in the land. John Wanamaker. New York." HB.

WATSON SHOE CO. Lynn, Mass.

1911: Illustrated a button shoe for 1912. TSR 9/16/11.

1913: Advertised new styles for 1914 at $3.50 and $4.00. Trademark of "The Triangle Line": a triangle with a boot in the center and "Watson Shoe Company" around the sides. TSR 9/20/13.

1915: Illustrated a button boot for 1916. TSR 9/18/15.

1919: Illustrated a pump for 1920. TSR 9/20/19.

1921: Illustrated an oxford for 1922. TSR 9/17/21.

1923: Illustrated a fancy strap for 1924. TSR 9/15/23.

WEBER LEATHER CO. West Lynn, Mass.

1904: Advertised Lorraine leather, made in black and colors. "Shoes made with Lorraine cost no more than ordinary kid," in TSR 9/21/04.

WELCH & LANDREGAN. Lynn, Mass.

1907: Illustrated a welt boot on cover, and buttoned shoe inside. TSR 9/28/07.

1909: Advertised Goodyear Welt Boots, $1.90. $2.00, $2.25. Goodyear welt oxfords, $1.60 to $2.00, McKay-sewn boots and oxfords, $1.50 and $1.60. Also illustrated a two-strap retailing at $3.00 for 1910. TSR 9/25/09.

WELCH, MOSS & FEEHAN CO. Haverhill, Mass.

1923: Illustrated a cross-strap for 1924. TSR 9/15/23.

WELCOME SHOE CO. Lynn, Mass.

1896: Women's boots $2.00–$3.00. Misses $1.50. Children's $1.00. LHJ.

WHITCHER. Frank W. Whitcher Co. Boston or Chicago. Made Velvet Rubber Heels.

1911: Trademark: an oval with VEL within one side and VET within the other. "Made in whole and half heels, made with and without friction plug." TSR 9/16/11.

WHITCOMB'S "FLEXSOLE" SHOES. See EASTERN SHOE CO.

WHITE HOUSE SHOES. See BROWN SHOE CO.

WHITMAN. M. J. Whitman Co. Rochester, N.Y.

1904: Illustrated a tie shoe for 1905. TSR 9/28/04.

WHITMAN & KEITH CO. Brockton, Mass.

1917: Illustrated a boot for 1918. TSR 9/22/17.

1919: Illustrated a sports oxford for 1920. TSR 9/20/19.

WICHERT. Little information. Apparently New York City.

1917: Illustrated a boot. TSR 9/22/17.

WILEY-BICKFORD-SWEET CO. Worcester, Mass., and Hartford, Conn.

    1924: Capitol Slippers. Trademark: the word "Capitol" in back-slanting cursive style over a representation of the capitol dome and clouds. LHJ.

WILLIAMS, CLARK & CO. 362 Washington St., Lynn, Mass.

    1904: LaFrance $3.00 Shoe for Women. "If your dealer don't [*sic*] have them send us your size and $3.00. We will send a pair prepaid and guarantee satisfaction. An interesting novelette, 'A Bunch of Roses,' sent free on request." DEL.

    1905: LaFrance $3.00 Shoe for Women. Style booklet "One Day." "Write for catalog and novelette `Her Photograph.'" DEL.

    1908: LaFrance Shoes. Trademark stamped on lining appears to have "LaFrance" diagonally in a shield flanked by lions and topped by a crown or fleur-de-lis. LHJ.

    1909: LaFrance Shoes, $3.00-$4.00. LHJ.

    1923: Illustrated a strap shoe for 1924. TSR 9/15/23.

WILLIAMS, HOYT & CO. Rochester, N.Y.

    1919: Illustrated a pump for 1920. TSR 9/20/19.

WILLIAMS-KNEELAND CO. South Braintree, Mass.

    1917: Illustrated oxfords for 1918. TSR 9/22/17.

WILSON. Charles E. Wilson. Lynn, Mass.

    1907: Colonial illustrated for 1908. TSR 9/28/07.

    1913: Illustrated a four-strap for 1914. TSR 9/20/13.

WISE, SHAW & FEDER CO. Cincinnati, Ohio.

    1919: Illustrated a pump for 1920. TSR 9/20/19.

WITHERELL. E. A. & M. C. Witherell Co. Haverhill, Mass.

    1923: Illustrated a strap shoe for 1924. TSR 9/15/23.

WOODBURY FOOT GLUVE. See KOZY SLIPPER CO.

WOODRUFF. Samuel Woodruff. Branford, Conn.

    1810: Blue kid wedding slippers said to have been made by the groom, Samuel Woodruff, for his bride, Betsy Harrison. CHS 1983-80-1.

YPSILANTI INDIAN SHOE CO. 349 Cross St., Ypsilanti, Mich.

    1912: Yipsi Silent House Shoes, genuine buckskin, handsewn. Trademark: YPSI in a horizontal diamond within a black rectangle. LHJ.

ZIEGLER BROS. Philadelphia.

    1904: Illustrated tie shoes for 1905. TSR 9/28/04.

    1915: Illustrated a gypsy pump for 1916. TSR 9/18/15.

Glossary

While in the early nineteenth century, American shoemakers still depended on British works about the craft of shoemaking, by the mid–nineteenth century, the American industry had begun to develop independently. As Americans invented new machines and methods, their technical terminology also began, perhaps inevitably, to diverge from its British roots. By 1910, the American and British shoe manufacturers were in many cases using different words for the same things, or using the same words to mean slightly different things, or using words that no longer meant the same thing they had a century ago. Because that state of affairs is confusing to readers today, this glossary attempts to distinguish between American and British usage, and also to indicate the way some words changed their meanings over time. Most of the American definitions given here are closely adapted from the *Shoe and Leather Lexicon.* This was first published in 1912 and went through several successive editions. I have relied chiefly on the editions of 1916 and, to a lesser extent, 1947. The less comprehensive glossaries in the *Shoe and Leather Encyclopedia* of 1911 were also consulted. For British terms I have relied on Thornton and Swann's *Glossary of Shoe Terms,* as well as the glossary in Swann's history, *Shoes.* Where all these failed, I have extrapolated definitions by noting how terms were used in contemporary documents.

Adelaide. Nineteenth-century British term for a side-lacing boot, named after the queen consort of King William IV, during whose reign (1830–37) they came into fashion.

Adjustment. A term applied generally to the fastening of a shoe or boot, whether button, buckle, or lace, etc., by which it is adjusted to the foot; or more specifically, to the degree of play available in the fastening. The lace is the most flexible of all adjustments; the buckled strap has less adaptability. Buttons are adjustable by resetting.

Alaska. An overshoe with a rubber sole, cloth upper, and fleece lining made higher in front and back than on the sides, thus covering the shoe but not the ankle and requiring no fastening. American term.

Ankle. The joint connecting the foot with the lower leg; or more loosely, the slender part of the lower leg. Any footwear that covers those anklebones that bulge slightly at each side of the foot is, in this book, considered a boot. When footwear leaves these bones uncovered, it is considered a shoe.

Arch. The part of the foot underneath the instep on the inner side in which the bones form a bridge between the heel and the ball. Also, by extension, the corresponding part of the shoe or last.

Arctic. An overshoe with rubber sole, thick cloth upper, and fleece lining, cut higher than an alaska, enough to cover the ankle, and fastening with one or more buckles. American term.

Backpart. The back half of the shoe, including both upper and bottom.

Back seam. Seam joining parts of the upper (generally the quarters) at the back of the shoe.

Backstay. In American usage, a strip of leather covering and strengthening the back seam of a shoe. The British equivalent is "back-strap" or "back-strip."

Bal. Short for balmoral.

Ball. The fleshy part of the bottom of the foot directly behind the toes, especially the roughly ball-shaped area behind the big toe. When a last is measured, the "ball measurement" is a girth measurement taken around the last at the ball of the foot (below the girth measurements taken at the instep and waist).

Balmoral. American lexicons define a balmoral merely as a medium-height front-lacing boot different in pattern from a blucher. A closed-tab pattern is clearly implied. British usage specifies a closed-tab, front-lacing boot in which the vamp continues round to the back seam, forming a golosh. The buttoned equivalent is known as a button balmoral. Like the balmoral petticoat, this was named after Balmoral Castle in Scotland, which Queen Victoria rebuilt for her own use in 1853–55.

Bar shoe. British usage for a strapped shoe, usually cut like a slipper with one or more straps added over the instep.

Basil. Heavy bark-tanned sheepskin used for linings or insoles.

Beaded. (1) Decorated with glass, steel, or jet beads, usually sewn to the vamp.

(2) Having the edges of the upper leather skived thin and folded in, instead of being left raw.

(3) Thornton and Swann define "bead" as "a strip of material inserted in upper seams for reinforcement."

Bellows tongue. A broad tongue used in an open-tab shoe or boot, that, rather than hanging free like an ordinary tongue, is stitched to the upper along each side of the front opening. When the boot is fastened, the tongue folds down flat; but when unfastened, the tongue can spread out so the foot can be put in or out. It is designed to keep out snow or wet, and among women's footwear it is most often found in rubber overshoes.

Binding. (1) The silk or leather strip that is laid over the top edge of a shoe and sometimes the upper seams, roughly synonymous with "galloon." The term is not in the twentieth-century American lexicons.

(2) The process of sewing the galloon or binding around the top edge of the shoe. In the early nineteenth century, when the galloon was also used to join vamp and quarters at side and back seams, the term binding could be synonymous with "stitching," but modern usage distinguishes "stitching," which means joining the various parts of the upper, from "binding," now limited to adding the binding around the top edge. "The uppers were sent out to women and children to be stitched together and bound. 'Hannah binding shoes' might have been found in almost every home in the shoe towns in eastern Massachusetts"[1] (see fig. 8).

Blind eyelet. An eyelet concealed on the inner side of the lace stay, the lace hole being left raw on the outer side.

Blucher. An open-tab shoe or boot; that is, one in which the quarters extend forward over the throat of the circular vamp but are not stitched down where they meet at the center front to lace over the tongue. Named for a general of the Prussian army during the Napoleonic Wars. In Britain, "blucher" is generally limited to boots, while "Gibson" (as in "Gibson girl") is used for women's open-tab shoes and "derby" for men's. Early-twentieth-century American sources, however, tend to call all tie shoes oxfords if they have three or more lace holes. They may use the word "blucher" in descriptions of open-tab ties, or they may name them "blucher oxfords," which in Britain would be a contradiction in terms, since oxfords there are by definition closed tab. The term "Gibson" was known in the United States but was not in common use. In the attempt to introduce a gender distinction, one unfortunate Montgomery Ward catalog called a woman's open-tab tie a "blucherette oxford,"[2] which is a vulgarity on both sides of the ocean.

Boarded. Leather finished with a lined surface faintly indented or stamped. See appendix A, "How Leather Is Made."

Boot. In this book, British usage is followed, defining boots as encasing at least the ankle and sometimes part of the leg. American usage has been less consistent, sometimes limiting it to a man's solid leg boot or heavy laced hunting boot, while the term shoe covered most high-cut footwear with some sort of fastening. More recently, it has also been used to refer to a high-cut overshoe. See **Shoe.**

Bootee. (1) According to the *Shoe and Leather Lexicon,* a boot with a short leg, sometimes made with elastic goring over the ankle, and sometimes made with a front lacing. It is a term more often associated with men's footwear than women's. Once men were wearing their boots under long trousers rather than knee breeches, boots that were only ankle-high were easier to fasten and less bulky than full-length designs, yet they looked similar when in use.

(2) An infant's knitted boot made high enough to come above the ankle but not as high as the knee.

Botte. French for "boot." Defined as a very thick walking boot in Myers (1892).[3]

Bottines. French for "ankle boot." In English fashion magazines, the term "bottines" is noted most commonly after 1830, when the term "half-boot" fell out of use. It is possible that by the end of the century, English speakers associated bottines with cloth-topped rather than all-leather boots. Myers, writing in 1892, says it was "applied chiefly to house boots."[4]

Bottom. All those parts that comprise the underside of the shoe, such as insole, outsole, welt, heel, etc.

Bottom finish. The final polishing, painting, buffing, or other processes applied to the bottom of a completed shoe. The British use "fiddle finish" to refer to soles with shaded waists.

Boudoir slipper. An easy-fitting slipper, often elaborately trimmed, worn indoors with a dressing gown or informal morning dress. The rough modern equivalent is the bedroom slipper. Also known as a toilet slipper.

Box calf. According to the *Shoe and Leather Lexicon,* a proprietary name for calf leather finished with the grain side boarded or stamped with irregular rectangularly crossed lines.

Box toe. The toe of a shoe having a stiff interlining called a toe box or boxing intended to preserve the toe shape. "When a shoe has a box toe it is often called a hard toe, and so it is, but a genuine hard toe is flexible enough to spring back in shape if pressed out of place. It is because of this quality that a sole leather box has always been popular."[5] See **Boxing.**

Boxing. The stiff reinforcement placed between vamp and lining at the toe of the shoe to preserve its shape, or in work shoes to protect the toes from injury. Leather, composition, zinc, wire net, drilling stiffened with shellac, etc., have all been used for this purpose.

Steel is used in safety-toe shoes. See **Box toe.** Equivalent terms are "toe box" (American usage) and "toe puff" (British usage). Boxing seems to have been the term used in the early twentieth century.

Breast. The forward surface of the heel (the back surface is called the neck).

Brodequin. French term for "ankle boot." Sometimes adopted in British and American fashion descriptions in the early nineteenth century.

Brogan. A heavy pegged or nailed ankle-high work shoe, normally open tab. These were mass-produced in New England, and many were exported south and to the West Indies for use by slaves.

Brogue. A heavy oxford trimmed with perforations, stitching, and pinking, and typically having a winged toe cap ("wing tip").

Bronze. Leather, usually kid or calf, finished with cochineal, a dye made from the dried and crushed bodies of the cochineal beetle, which, although it dyes cloth red, gives a bronzelike, metallic semi-iridescence to leather. The true cochineal is delicate and tends to rub off when wet, and therefore it was eventually imitated with less fragile aniline dyes.

Buckskin. Tanned or tawed skin of a male deer, or when used loosely, other leathers suede-finished in white or light shades. In the early twentieth century, "buck" usually meant suede-finished cowhide.

Buskin. The word buskin originally referred to a boot worn by actors in Greek tragedy and was later loosely used to refer to half-boots, as when the 1916 *Shoe and Leather Lexicon* defines buskin as "a peculiar antique type of laced or gored half-leg boot, seldom used." The definitions most relevant to women's footwear in the period of this book, however, are the following:

(1) References in *Godey's* indicate that in the mid-nineteenth-century buskins were understood to be tie shoes, and the fact that they were routinely recommended for walking implies that they had welted rather than turned soles, but it is not clear whether they were open tab or slit-vamp. "For the street, we have buskins, ties, Jeffersons, and Jenny Linds, all made of kid or morocco. We would recommend the first and last for country wear. . . . 'Jenny Linds' are high buskins, laced from the toe to the top of the instep, in such a way that the white stocking shows beneath, with a very pretty peasant-like effect."[6] This

suggests some variation of a slit-vamp shoe in which the slit was too wide to close when laced up (see fig. 66 for a later example of this type). However, a reference in 1872 clearly describes an open-tab style. "For country wear is the garden shoe, a low buskin, tied over the instep like the brogans worn by gentlemen. This is similar to the Newport tie of last summer. It is made of kid or morocco."[7] Brogans are usually open tab, and Newport ties definitely are.

(2) Later twentieth-century editions of the *Shoe and Leather Lexicon* define buskin as a "woman's low cut house shoe of either cloth or leather, having small, triangular-shaped goring on top of front at instep." The shoes listed as "buskin slippers" in mail-order catalogs from the 1890s to about 1910 were probably of this type, although the elastic gusset is not specifically mentioned. The *Shoe Retailer,* however, illustrated an identical shoe in 1904, identifying it as a "Sixteen Threads Gore Buskin . . . a repetition of 'Ye Olden Days,'"[8] and a similar shoe survives in the Peabody Essex Museum (see fig. 235).

Button fly. In American usage, the doubled strip of leather in the front of a button shoe that carries the buttonholes. The British equivalent is "button piece."

Calfskin. Untanned cattle skin weighing under fifteen pounds. See **Kip** and **Side leather.**

Cameleons. Swann reports finding a description in the *Englishwoman's Domestic Magazine* for 1867 of "cameleon" slippers, bronze slippers with "open lace appliqué. Satin is inserted under in a kind of pocket. . . . Satin of various shades is sold with these shoes ready to fit in, so with your blue dress your shoes are blue, and so on." Swann found no surviving shoes with removable colored inserts and considered it "a last desperate fling at the end of a style."[9] Bronze slippers with satin inlay edged with chain stitching that fixes the satin in place, however, are quite common ca. 1850–70 (see plate 13).

Cap. Alternative term for toe cap (British) or tip (American), and used in both countries.

Carriage boot. An overshoe, usually of fabric, often fur trimmed, worn over ordinary shoes or especially over dancing slippers for warmth en route to a winter party (see figs. 82–84). Or, sometimes merely a boot too dressy to be suitable for walking, such as the "carriage boot of kid and quilted satin" depicted in *Godey's* in December 1877.

Chameleon. See **Cameleon.**

Channel. A slanting cut made around the edge of a sole or insole where concealed stitching is to be done. The stitches pass through only the thickness of leather remaining below the base of this cut or groove, the lip of which is then cemented down to conceal the stitches and protect them from wear. (See diagrams in appendix B, "How Shoes Are Made.")

Chaussure. French for "footwear," or "a pair of shoes"; used to create an elegant tone in fashion writing.

Chrome sole. Strong, light sole leather made from the full thickness of cowhide, chrome tanned. It is slippery and porous and has a rough edge. Sometimes stuffed with grease to make it waterproof. Used chiefly in outing and athletic shoes.

Circular vamp. See **Vamp.**

Clog. In the most general sense, any footwear made of wood or with a wooden sole.

(1) The most common American type, which was worn in the first half of the nineteenth century before vulcanized rubbers were widely available, is a wooden-soled sandal-like overshoe. It may have a strap over the instep, and an abbreviated upper much like a toe cap and counter, and/or a leather-covered spring around the heel. Sometimes the sole is hinged at the ball of the foot. "Pattens" are a subcategory of clogs having a wooden sole raised on an iron ring (see fig. 78 and plate 16).

(2) A second type of clog has a complete leather upper with a wooden sole (see fig. 80). Wooden-soled shoes of this kind were rarely worn in the United States except by comedians and "clog dancers," or where there was a particular practical need, as in slippery workplaces like laundries, dairies, and breweries. They were, however, quite commonly worn as everyday footwear in the north of England well into the twentieth century, and some of these English clogs were brought back to the United States as souvenirs. To reduce wear on the wood, the sole was often edged round heel and toe with a grooved iron strip rather like a horseshoe (see fig. 79).

(3) "Clog" is also the term normally used for a partial overshoe in which the sole is not wood but

thick leather (although a block of wood may fill the space under the arch). The most common version of this is a dressy eighteenth-century clog having merely a leather sole fitted to receive the high-heeled shoe and a strap covered with silk brocade to harmonize with the shoe worn with it (see plate 1 and fig. 81).

Closed tab. A useful British term for the upper pattern of a laced shoe or boot whose eyelet tabs are stitched down to (or under) the vamp (in contrast to "open tab"). Oxford shoes and balmoral boots are both closed-tab styles. Also called "closed front." American lexicons occasionally use the term "straight lace" as a rough equivalent. See **Open tab.**

Closing. British term for sewing together the uppers. The equivalent American term is "stitching."

Collar. A narrow strip of leather stitched around the outside of the top edge of a shoe. Modern athletic shoes may have padded collars, but in the period 1795–1930 the collar in women's shoes was ordinarily decorative and usually contrasted in material, color, or texture with the rest of the shoe upper. (See figs. 55, 96.)

Colonial. A late-nineteenth/early-twentieth-century American name for a woman's shoe with a buckle (only sometimes functional) and a high, flaring tongue, meant to suggest mid-eighteenth-century styles. At some periods the tongue is smaller, and occasionally the term is used for a tongued shoe with a bow instead of a buckle. The British equivalent is the Cromwell.

Congress. American term for a boot or shoe having a gusset of elasticized fabric called goring set into each side of the upper to allow the foot to be slipped in without other fastening. (See figs. 281–94.)

Construction. A term more often used in British than in American sources for the method by which upper and bottom are joined together. See appendix B, "How Shoes Are Made."

Continuous sole. A sole that continues down the breast of a wooden heel and sometimes under the heel as well, replacing a separate top piece. The continuous sole with or without separate top piece is the diagnostic feature of a Louis heel. A descriptive term used by Thornton and Swann.

Cordovan. Originally a fine, expensive, close, waterproof leather made from the butt of horsehide, later imitated in calf and side leather finished on the flesh side. Named after Cordova, the city in Spain where it was first made.

Counter. In American usage, the stiffening placed inside the quarter (or between it and a quarter lining) that keeps the back part of the shoe from caving in. In British usage this stiff lining is called the stiffener, and the word "counter" is reserved for a similarly shaped and located piece applied to the outside of the shoe. This outside counter is roughly equivalent to "heel foxing" in American usage. See **Foxing.**

Court shoe. British term for a pump.

Cravenette. According to the *Shoe and Leather Lexicon,* a proprietary name applied to a closely woven cloth used for shoe uppers in the early twentieth century.

Cromwell. See **Colonial.**

Croquet sandal. Late-nineteenth-century term for a rubber overshoe cut lower than a storm rubber.

Cuban heel. See **Heel.**

Cutouts. Holes cut into the uppers, usually on the vamp and normally for decoration. Cutouts are often backed with a contrasting material that is held in place by a row of stitching (often chain stitch or buttonhole stitch) running around the edges of the cutout.

Domed sole. Defined by Swann as a "sole rounded up at the sides."

Dongola. Heavy, plump goatskin with a semi-bright finish, tanned with a combination of vegetable and mineral acids. Named after a region in the Sudan where it originated. The terms "Dongola," "kid," and "morocco" are sometimes loosely used interchangeably.

Enamel. Leather with a shiny finish on the grain side as distinguished from patent leather, which is usually finished on the flesh side or on the surface of a split leather.

Extension sole. A sole that extends farther than usual beyond the upper, an occasional feature of women's shoes when made in masculine styles from the 1870s on.

Eyelet. The reinforcement (usually a ring of metal or, later, plastic) inserted in the holes through which the shoe laces are threaded. The term is also used for the reinforced hole itself. Plain, unreinforced holes are called lace holes, and those reinforced only with stitching are called "worked eyelets" (or in British usage, "stitched lace holes"). Lace holes in which the reinforcement is visible only on the inside are called "blind eyelets."

Eyelet tab. British term for that part of the quarter that extends over the instep and bears the eyelets or lace holes. Latchets are straplike eyelet tabs with only one or two pairs of lace holes.

Facing. The diagrams printed as an appendix in Swann's *Shoes* use this term to describe a strip of leather or other material applied to either the inside or outside front of a lacing shoe to strengthen and reinforce the part bearing the eyelets or lace holes. Thornton and Swann's *Glossary of Shoe Terms*, however, defines the facing as "the front part of the quarters carrying the eyelets/lace holes" (although they more often use the term "eyelet tab" when referring to this part of the shoe), while the term "facing stay" is used for the reinforcement. The American term for the extra reinforcing strip is "lace stay."

Findings. As defined by the *Oxford English Dictionary*, it refers chiefly to a shoemaker's tools, but the *Shoe and Leather Lexicon* defines it as nearly every material used in making, trimming, or caring for shoes except the actual leather. The examples listed apply to the shoe store and include among other things shoe laces, polishes, shoe trees, rubber heels, shoe horns, and fancy buckles.

Flesh side. The underside of leather or skin that originally attached to the muscles, fat, etc. Suede leathers have the flesh side outward.

Foothold. A low rubber overshoe with an opening in the back half of the sole for the heel of the shoe to pass through; so the backpart consists of little more than a strap.

Forepart. Roughly the front half of the shoe, including both upper and bottom.

Foxing. In American usage, a piece of leather forming or covering the lower part of the quarter of a shoe, similar to an outside counter. What British writers call the "counter" or "outside counter" Americans call "heel foxing." The term was loosely used to mean the vamp as well, especially in the nineteenth century. Thus foxing was the term used for the leather pieces forming both the heel and the toe of mid-nineteenth-century cloth gaiter boots. "Slipper-foxed" or "whole-foxed" were equivalent to the more modern American term "whole vamp" or to the British term "golosh." A boot that is slipper-foxed has a vamp continuing around to the back seam, so that the vamp alone takes a shape similar to a slip-on shoe. The part of the boot above the slipper foxing is often made of a contrasting material to suggest the appearance of a gaiter encasing the foot above a low shoe.

French calf. Wax-finished calf leather of firm quality and high grade. The 1916 edition of the *Shoe and Leather Lexicon* remarks that "our importations of both French calf and French kid have fallen off very largely since the great improvements in American tanning, as this country is the exporter of leather to a much greater extent than it is imported. In recent years, our exports have been five times the amount of our imports."

French heel. See **Heel.**

Gaiter. (1) A covering for the ankle and top of the foot, worn over a separate shoe or boot. Gaiters are usually made of cloth, fastened with buttons and kept in place by either a buckled strap or an elastic band beneath the shank of the shoe. Also called spats (an abbreviation for "spatterdashes"). Gaiters extending to the knee or thigh were called leggings and were advertised throughout the late nineteenth and early twentieth centuries. See figure 89.

(2) Also commonly used from about 1840 for side-lacing or elastic-sided fabric boots that when foxed at toe and heel looked rather like gaiters worn over shoes (see fig. 60). In order to distinguish between true gaiters and gaiter boots, the separate article was sometimes called an "over-gaiter."

(3) As side-lacing boots retreated into the past, the term "gaiter" began to be understood as referring to an elastic-sided boot.

(4) A term in use from the 1890s through the 1920s for a winter overshoe with rubber bottom, cloth top, and fleece lining, usually calf-high and fastening with buttons, buckles, or, by the late 1920s, with a zipper.

Galloon. In the general sense, according to an 1882 definition, galloon is a metallic lace or braid or a narrow ribbon used to trim furniture or clothing.[10] In the context of this volume, it refers to the narrow, thin, flat silk tape used to bind the seams and top edges of shoes up through the early nineteenth century. "Bind the top [of the shoe] and around the slit with galloon to match the shade of the outer material. The galloon should be merely placed over the edge and stitched once around; as the edge of it is not raw, it is not necessary to turn it in at all."[11] See **Binding.**

Ghillie. A British term defined in Thornton and Swann as "a shoe of Scottish origin in which the lace passes crisscross through loops in the front of the quarters instead of through eyelets." Rarely used in America.

Gibson. A British term occasionally used in America for a woman's shoe (as opposed to a boot) in the blucher pattern. Named after the Gibson girl, it became fashionable in the late 1890s. The most used American equivalent is "blucher oxford." See **Blucher.**

Glazed kid. Tanned goatskin with the blacking or coloring pounded in to make the skin smooth and glossy; the usual way of finishing goatskin for shoes.

Glove grain. Light, soft-finished split leather for women's and children's shoes. Used for cheaper grades of shoes.

Golosh. (1) An overshoe (in this sense usually used in the plural, "goloshes"). According to the 1916 edition of the *Shoe and Leather Lexicon*, "an English term not often used in this country, meaning a rubber overshoe." The American spelling is usually "galoshes."

(2) In British usage, a whole vamp; that is, one that extends along each side of a shoe or boot to meet at the back seam. A closed-tab boot made with a golosh is called a "balmoral." Sometimes spelled "galosh." The American equivalent is "whole fox." See **Foxing.**

Goodyear welt. A shoe made by the Goodyear welting machines (patented 1877), one of which did inseams, the other outseams, thus stitching soles to uppers in a way similar to hand-welted shoes. See **Welt** and appendix B, "How Shoes Are Made."

Gored. (1) A gored shoe is a slip-on shoe cut high enough to require an insertion of elastic goring on the side or instep to allow it to slide on and off. By substituting goring for a laced fastening, a lighter, dressier, and more decorative effect can be created in a higher-cut shoe. (See figs. 227–40.)

(2) A term used in dressmaking, meaning roughly triangular or wedge-shaped. When a length of material used in a skirt is narrower at the top than at the bottom, it is said to be gored. When skirt panels are not gored, the entire fullness of the skirt must somehow be gathered or pleated into the waistband. Goring the skirt panels maintains the same circumference at the bottom of the skirt but creates less bulk at the waist and hip.

Goring. A fabric woven with elastic thread and used in the stretchy gussets in an elastic-sided (Congress) shoe or boot. Named from the triangular or wedge (i.e., gored) shape of the inserted gusset. The type of goring that became standard had the elastic thread woven in. Some early gorings produced about 1850 were made with stretched elastic threads glued between two layers of fabric. When the tension was released, the fabric crinkled. This elastic material was known as "shirred goods."

Grain side. The outer side of leather or skin that originally bore the hair or fur. The grain side is smoother than the flesh side and, except in suede, it is usually the side that shows. Each animal species has a characteristic texture that helps identify the leather made from it, although these grain textures can also be imitated artificially.

Grecian. (1) British term defined in Thornton and Swann as "a low-heeled or heel-less slipper, plain front, cut away at the sides and with no fastening." This is usually a man's style of bedroom slipper.

(2) In the phrase "Grecian sandal," a term occasionally used in American sources about 1921 for a woman's strapped pump, especially one with several straps or complex cutouts. See the section on boots with straps or ribbons across a broad front opening in chapter 8.

Guêtres. French term for "gaiters."

Gun metal. A proprietary name for a fine grade of chrome-tanned calfskin finished dull or semi-bright.

Gutta-percha. Like rubber, gutta-percha is made from a tree resin, but the resulting product, while somewhat flexible, is not elastic like rubber. A thin strip of it can bear a considerable weight. It does not stick to other materials as rubber does. It softens when warmed, can be drawn into fibers, rolled into sheets, or molded. When soft, it takes fine impressions and retains them when hard. It is not affected by water but degenerates in the presence of oxygen and light. While its nonclothing uses are most important, it has been used for buttons and overshoes. The 1886 edition of the *Encyclopedia Britannica* remarks that "a very considerable trade exists in boots and shoes with outer soles of gutta-percha in place of leather, the headquarters of that trade being in Glasgow."

Gypsy. An upper pattern having a seam running straight down the center front of the shoe from top edge to toe, creating a "split vamp" or "gypsy vamp," the seam itself being called a "gypsy seam." A late-nineteenth-/early-twentieth-century American term, and one particularly common in 1915–16, when this cut was very fashionable.

Half-boot. A boot cut high enough to cover the ankle, but not extending all the way to the knee. The term came into use by the end of the eighteenth century and was the standard term for women's ankle-high front-lacing boots in fashion plate descriptions from 1800 to 1830. When side-lacing boots made to imitate gaiters came into fashion about 1830, the term "half-boot" gradually fell out of use, being replaced by the French terms "bottines" and "brodequins." By the later 1830s, when skirts were long enough to cover the feet, fashion plates rarely mentioned footwear at all. When references to boots began to reappear in the 1850s, they were referred to simply as boots, or sometimes as gaiter boots.

Heel. A leather or wooden addition to the sole that raises the heel of the foot higher than the toe. Heels are measured in eighths of an inch, so that an 8/8 heel is 1 inch high, a 17/8 heel is 2⅛ inches high, etc. The terminology for heels is not consistently applied in contemporary documents. American lexicons do not clearly distinguish heels in terms of how they are made, only by their fashion shapes, but it is necessary in this book to distinguish both. There are five basic categories of heel, based on how they are made:

Stacked: Made of one or more layers of leather, each called a lift, which are stacked one on top of the other, pasted, sewn, nailed, and/or pegged together, trimmed to a uniform shape, and nailed to the bottom of the sole. The lift that touches the ground, a thick piece of sole leather, is called a top lift or top piece.

Louis heel: Made of a block of wood, usually covered to match the upper, except that the sole of the shoe continues down the forward face (breast) of the heel, and sometimes also forms the top piece. In American usage, this word designates a shape. (See *French heel.*)

Knock-on heel: Made of a block of wood, usually covered on all sides to match the upper, and nailed on to the shoe. The walking surface is then finished with a thick piece of sole leather called a top piece. A knock-on heel is rarely very high. When a very high covered heel is wanted, a Louis construction is preferred because it is sturdier. Louis heels were also more time-consuming to make and therefore more expensive. Thus, Louis heels tend to appear on better-quality footwear, while the knock-on heel was used for cheaper shoes. The term "knock-on" is not in common use, but it does describe the way the heel is made, and the type is so characteristic of the period 1860–1905 as to require some name. One source, John Wanamaker's *Catalog for Spring and Summer 1901,* seems to call knock-on heels "opera heels," presumably from their frequent use in "opera slippers."

Spring heel: A single lift called a slip inserted between the sole and the heel seat.

Wedge: A heel that extends forward to fill the space under the waist of the shoe. It is sometimes defined as being nailed to the outside of the sole rather than inserted between the sole and the heel seat like a spring heel but this restriction is not observed in this book.

Stacked construction tends to be used when lower heels are wanted on dark shoes. Light-colored and dressy shoes generally get covered wooden heels so that the heel will not contrast with the upper (but occasionally in the 1850s and 1960s, stacked leather heels were covered to match light-colored uppers). When a very high heel is wanted, a Louis construction tends to be preferred, and if the shape is to be quite high and slender, it may have to be reinforced with a spike. The habitual conjunction of certain constructions with certain shapes in heels has led to a good deal of confusion in their names and the following will not cover every reference. The more common names by which the shapes of heels are known are:

Louis, or French: A heel whose neck (back face) is shaped in a graceful reverse curve. This is the most characteristic shape for Louis heels, since it harmonizes with the curve formed by the sole as it continues down the breast of a Louis heel. This conjunction is so persistent that the terms "French" and "Louis" have become nearly interchangeable, and in American usage this shape is called a Louis or Louis XV ("the baby," or "junior Louis," is a shorter version). The same shape, however, is occasionally imitated in stacked heels. It is also common in knock-on heels, though in this form the breast is normally straight.

Opera: The knock-on heel with straight breast and curved neck is sometimes referred to as an opera heel in late-nineteenth-/early-twentieth-century sources. The same heel may also be called a Louis.

Kidney: A term used about 1913–14 to refer to a heel with a straight breast and curved neck, usually higher than the opera heel that had preceded it. Previewing 1914 styles, the *Shoe Retailer* remarks that "kidney heels, properly speaking, are of leather, and this is the way most dealers want them. The wood kidney heel simply lightens up a shoe and is perhaps preferable for turns, while leather kidney heels will be used on welts."[12]

Cuban: A term that came into common use about 1900 for a rather straight-sided heel. Unless it is modified, as in "Cuban wood" or "covered Cuban," the term seems to imply a stacked heel and as stacked heels are most often relatively low and blocky, "Cuban" tended to be associated with lower and more blocky shapes, while "Spanish" was used for the higher and more slender straight-sided heels made of covered wood. Also compare the "military heel."

Spanish: A rather high, thin Louis heel with straight, tapering sides and neck. The term appears by 1907 but commonly from 1923, at first sometimes as "Spanish-Louis." The British seem to distinguish it chiefly by its being narrower than a Cuban heel (having a smaller top piece). The American lexicons distinguish it chiefly by its being made of covered wood, but still in the Cuban shape.

Italian: A Louis heel with a wedgelike extension that partially fills the hollow beneath the waist; very common in the 1780s and 1790s.

Military: This term applies to a heel that is not consistently distinguished from a Cuban. In Swann's diagrams, the military heel has a concave curve to the neck and can be fairly high. But in American periodical illustrations they have a moderately low, straight blocky shape, and when any distinction is made at all, the military heel is straighter than the Cuban. The term seems to imply a stacked heel unless expressly stated otherwise ("covered wood military").

Common sense: A very low stacked heel used for walking and sports shoes.

Heel seat. The area of the sole to which the heel is attached.

Inlay. A contrasting piece of leather or fabric inserted under a cutout in a shoe upper and stitched in place for ornamental effect.

Insole. See **Sole** and appendix B, "How Shoes Are Made."

Instep. The top of the foot not including the toes or the ankle, and by extension the corresponding part of the shoe or last. When a last is measured, the instep measurement is a girth measurement taken around the last at the highest (thickest) part of the instep (above the girth measurements taken at the ball and the waist).

Jenny Lind. A Swedish opera singer who toured the United States in 1850–52 to great acclaim. Many fashionable articles were named after her, including a buskin.

Juliet. See **Nullifier.**

Kid. Shoe leather made from the skins of mature goats. Leather made from young goats is too delicate for shoes but is used for gloves.

Kidney heel. See **Heel.**

Kip. Leather made from a lightweight cowhide weighing fifteen to twenty-five pounds when untanned ("green"). See appendix A, "How Leather Is Made."

Lace hole. Unreinforced hole in the shoe through which the shoe lace is threaded. See **Eyelet.**

Lace hook. A metal hook that for convenience's sake may replace the eyelets in the upper part of a laced boot. Lace hooks are most familiar today in ice skates. They were also used in women's bicycle boots in the late 1890s.

Lace stay. A strip of leather applied to either the inside or outside of the eyelet tabs to strengthen and reinforce the eyelets or lace holes. The British term is "facing" or "facing stay."

Last. The wooden form or mold over which a shoe is constructed and that gives the shoe its shape. It imitates the shape of the shod foot, incorporating such fashion details as square or pointed toes. Some lasts have an iron bottom against which the lasting tacks are clinched in certain shoe constructions.

Latchets. A useful British term for the straps formed by extending the quarters over the instep in a shoe. If the latchets overlap, a buckle is used to fasten them. If they stop just short of meeting, they bear one or two pairs of lace holes and are tied together. The latter style of shoe is often called a latchet tie. (See plate 1, figs. 162, 171–75.)

Leg. British term for the part of a boot upper encasing the ankle and leg above the vamp and quarter. The American equivalent is "top."

Leg boot. American term for a boot that extends some distance above the ankle without lacing or buttoning. Sometimes, for the sake of clarity, the phrase "solid leg boot" is used in this book to emphasize the lack of any opening or fastening.

Legging. A covering for the leg, extending from the ankle to the knee, held in place by straps or lacing. See **Puttees.**

Lift. One of the separate pieces of sole leather used in making a stacked leather heel, the one that touches the ground being called the top lift or top piece.

Louis heel. See **Heel.**

Mat kid. Thin calfskin with a dull mat surface, frequently used in uppers as a contrast to brighter leathers or patent leather.

McKay-sewn. See appendix B, "How Shoes Are Made."

Military heel. See **Heel.**

Moccasin. A soft-soled shoe traditionally made by shaping a single piece of hide, skin, or leather round the foot, stitching it up the center of the top and up the back, and sometimes tying it on by means of a thong run around the topline. Another version is made with an additional U-shaped piece called an apron inserted over the top of the foot. During the nineteenth century, moccasins were worn as casual house shoes. They were made of velvet as well as leather, and were typically decorated on the apron and around the top edge with brightly colored beadwork or embroidery, sometimes on a ground of scarlet wool. Moccasins were among the tourist items sold by Native Americans, but they were also often made at home. Shoes whose uppers imitate moccasins but that have a separate sole are now also called by this name.

Molière. A woman's open-tab shoe that buckles or ties over a prominent tongue. The Molière, intended to suggest seventeenth- or eighteenth-century styles, was usually made of dressy materials and with a relatively high heel. The name, current in the 1870s and 1880s, was replaced in England by "Cromwell" and in the United States by "Colonial" when the type was revived about 1900.

Morocco. Originally a sumac-tanned goatskin made in Morocco, finished in black or bright colors, most characteristically in red. It is clear in color, elastic, soft, and firm, with a fine grain. Eventually the term was expanded either to refer to any goatskin used for shoes, or for any thin leather made to imitate the grain and finish of the original morocco.

Mule. A slipper made with an upper consisting of a forepart only. Since it has no quarters, it exposes the heel of the foot. Mules were particularly fashionable in the 1870s.

Nankeen. Originally a cotton from Nanking in China that has a natural tannish-yellow color. From the mid–eighteenth century, however, it was imitated in the West by dyeing ordinary cotton yellow. It was used in the very early nineteenth century for women's boot uppers and for gaiters worn over shoes.

Neck. The back face of the heel (the forward face is called the breast).

Newport. A woman's low-heeled, open-tab shoe, usually two-eyelet, roughly equivalent to a man's brogan or blucher. This basic pattern is a recurring one, but it appears under this name from about 1871 to 1907. Newports are pictured in Sears, and the exact equivalent survives in the USMC collection (see figs. 172, 179).

Nubuck. A proprietary name for a white or cream-colored buck leather.

Nullifier. A shoe with high vamp and quarter, dropping low at the side and having a U-shaped goring inserted; made loose fitting and appropriate for house wear. The term is most common ca. 1890–1910. A nearly identical type that sometimes omitted the goring was the "Juliet" (the man's version was, naturally, a "Romeo"). The British term is "Cambridge." (See figs. 51, 52.)

Oak sole. The best bark-tanned sole leather.

Oil grain. Heavy, bark-tanned side leather finished with oil and with a pebbled surface on the grain side; for heavy work shoes.

Ooze. Originally a proprietary name for velvet- or suede-finished calfskin and loosely equivalent to suede.

Open tab. Useful British term for a pattern of shoe or boot upper where the eyelet tabs (that is, the extended quarters) are left unattached to the vamp at the center front. Also called "open front." Americans are likely to use the term "blucher" for this type. Compare **Closed tab**. (See figs. 162–64.)

Opera heel. See **Heel**.

Opera slipper. A dress slipper for women, having a turned sole and covered wood heel, usually with a curved neck. The upper is normally made of satin or other fine fabric or kid (commonly ornamented with beading, embroidery, rosettes, etc.) in a whole-vamp or circular-vamp pattern. Also a particular cut of house slipper for men.

Outsole. See **Sole**, and appendix B, "How Shoes Are Made."

Oxford. In American usage, any low-cut shoe, whether an open tab or closed tab, that adjusts with laces, buttons, or straps, but preferably with three or more lace holes. British usage is limited to a front-lacing shoe with the quarters (the part bearing the lace holes) fully stitched under the vamp; that is, a closed-tab shoe. (See figs. 40, 164, 194–210.)

Patent leather. Leather with an extremely glossy black finish, created by painting the flesh side with a black syrupy varnish, drying or pumicing between coats, and alternating further coats of varnish, oil, etc., with periods of oven drying and sun drying, according to a complicated formula that varied from producer to producer. According to Swann, patent leather for shoes developed in England in the 1790s, probably from the older practice of japanning leather, and appeared in the United States in Newark, N.J., in 1822.[13]

Patten. A type of clog having a wooden sole raised on an iron ring. See **Clog**.

Pattern. The metal or cardboard sheets that served as guides by which to cut the various parts of the uppers. These were made in graded sizes to fit a particular shaped last. By extension, the word was also used to refer to basic classes of cut, such as slipper, closed or open tab (balmoral or blucher), etc. "There are two principal points in the style of a shoe. Pattern is one and the last is the other. . . . In some seasons the principal differences are in the toes and other variations in the last. In other seasons the style changes seem to involve more changes in the pattern."[14]

Pebbled goat. Tanned goatskin with a pebbled surface on the grain side created by passing the leather between heavy rollers.

Pegged. Footwear in which the sole is attached to the upper by means of wooden pegs. Pegging was introduced about 1811 and was common in the United States for heavy cheap shoes and men's boots, especially from the 1820s through the 1870s.

Plimsoll. British term for a rubber-soled canvas shoe used for boating and the seaside. It was named after Samuel Plimsoll, a British reformer concerned with the welfare of seamen, who was instrumental in passing the Merchant Shipping Act of 1876. One provision of this act was the "Plimsoll line," which is painted on British ships to mark the point beyond which they would be too heavily loaded. Plimsoll himself had nothing to do with the shoe. The name was a marketing idea of the Liverpool Rubber Co. and was registered in 1885.[15]

Polish. American term for a front-lacing closed-tab boot measuring at least five inches from heel seat to top, a pattern said to have originated in Poland. Balmoral boots are also closed tab, but distinguished in

American usage by being lower. See **Balmoral,** whose British meaning was slightly different.

Prunella. A specially woven wool serge used frequently for uppers of women's and children's shoes in the nineteenth century.

Pump. A low-cut slip-on shoe made without adjustable fastening, essentially equivalent to a slipper. In older references the single sole was mentioned as characteristic, but this was no longer true by the early twentieth century. In fact, the word first came into common use to describe women's slippers when they began to be worn on the street and were therefore often made with welted soles and a heel (about 1906). "Pump," however, was not consistently used to differentiate slippers with welted soles from those with turned soles, but instead became the term of choice for any slipper not confined to the boudoir. The British equivalent is "court shoe."

Puttees. Knee-high leggings formed from a spirally wrapped strip of wool or leather, not typically worn by women, except occasionally in the early twentieth century for riding.

Quarters. The two side sections in the backpart of the shoe, each connecting to the vamp at the side seam and to each other at the back seam. In tie and button shoes, the quarters meet over the instep and bear the lace holes or buttons.

Recede toe. Toes of shoes or lasts that seen from the side are relatively shallow, the vamp being drawn down so sharply toward the sole at the toe that its profile is comparatively narrow and pointed rather than blunt in outline.

Rubber. (1) An elastic, waterproof material produced from the sap of a tree from the Amazon River valley.

(2) An overshoe made from rubber.

See appendix C, "Rubber and Elastic Webbing," and chapter 6 on protective footwear.

Russet. Tan-colored—and by extension bark-tanned—leather in its natural, undyed state. Sometimes incorrectly used to mean "Russia."

Russia. Originally calfskin tanned with willow bark and dressed with birch oil, which gave it a characteristic pleasant odor. A very watertight, strong, and insect-repellent leather. Heavier grades in black or tan were used for shoes. Lighter ones were dyed with Brazil wood to produce a distinctive deep red used in bookbinding.

Sandal. In the narrowest sense a sandal consists only of a sole held on to the foot by straps, but by extension the term often refers to any low-cut shoe in which the straps or ties are conspicuous or in which there is profuse slashing or cutting-out in the vamp. Thus, in the early nineteenth century the ubiquitous low-cut evening slippers with ribbon ties that crossed and tied round the ankles were sometimes referred to as sandal slippers: "Sandal slippers are worn in the morning by the pedestrian fashionables" (1802), and "black satin slippers tied 'en sandales'" (1829).[16] In the 1830s, "sandal" came to mean the ribbon ties themselves. In the late nineteenth and early twentieth centuries, "sandal" commonly meant an ordinary strapped pump or slipper.

Satin calf. Not calf but the grain split of cowhide, dressed with oil and smooth-finished.

Serge. A thick and firm twill-woven wool fabric specially designed for use in shoe uppers. "Since the advent of short dresses, shoe dealers are surfeited with complaints of cloth uppers splitting or rubbing to pieces in a short time. This is due in a great measure to starched skirts, but . . . if cloth tops of a closely woven pattern are selected there will be less cause for dissatisfaction" (1879).[17]

Shank. A strip of metal used to stiffen the sole of a shoe between the heel and the ball, especially useful when the shoe has a heel. Loosely used in American sources to mean the corresponding part of the sole.

Sheepskin. A leather used mostly for linings, since it is not strong enough for uppers, tending to scuff and tear.

Shirred goods. See **Goring.**

Shoe. Loosely used, any kind of footwear. In this book, a shoe is defined as footwear that encases only the foot, not including the anklebone. The distinction between boots and shoes, however, has not always been straightforward. Sometimes, especially in American usage, "boot" has meant chiefly strong and heavy working footwear or a solid leg boot, while the term "shoe" has extended to cover any street or formal footwear no matter how high it is, as long as it has some sort of fastening such as laces or buttons. In the shoe trade and in older British usage, "shoe" may mean specifically an oxford shoe as opposed to a pump, slipper, or sandal.

Side leather. Tanned cowhide that may be split to whatever thickness its intended use requires. See appendix A, "How Leather Is Made."

Side seam. The seam connecting the vamp to the quarters. This may be straight, dogleg, or curved. In many kinds of shoes, the side seams meet and join over the vamp. One or both side seams may be absent, resulting in a "three-quarter vamp" or "whole vamp" upper.

Skive. The shoe-trade term for shaving or paring thin. For example, leather uppers may be pared thin at the edges to make them less bulky where they are turned under before stitching.

Slipper. Although today "slipper" has come almost exclusively to mean bedroom slippers, this book follows common nineteenth- and early-twentieth-century American usage in using "slipper" to mean a slip-on shoe that has no fastening built into the cut but that is supposed to stay on by means of the snug fit. Because it has to slip on, the slipper must have a flexible sole (usually of turn construction), a fairly low-cut upper, and must be made of cloth or lightweight leather. Since snugness and slip-onableness are frequently at odds, one often finds ribbon ties or elastic bands attached to footwear that is otherwise a slipper in cut, and the word "slipper" is extended to refer to these as long as the basic slipper pattern is not altered. This has its precedents from at least April 1802, when the *Lady's Magazine* reports that in Paris "almost all slippers have coloured ribbons which cross upon the leg" (see fig. 32).

Americans were likely to use the term slipper for strapped shoes as well, as in "two-strap slipper," and by the early twentieth century the term was considered broad enough to include Colonials, which fasten with a buckled strap over a tongue, and even one- or two-eyelet ties as well. This departure from logic is not followed in this book, except when quoting directly from original sources.

Slippers were standard wear for dancing and formal occasions and for indoor daytime wear as well. From time to time in the nineteenth century, they supplanted boots or tie shoes for light walking, and they were frequently worn on the street by the early twentieth century, at which time they became known as pumps and could be made with welted as well as turned soles. (See **Pump.**) Mid-nineteenth-century newspaper advertisements often use the word "slips" for slippers.

Slips. Used in mid-nineteenth-century American newspaper advertisements to refer to slip-on shoes (slippers), often occurring in the phrase "slips and ties." The modern equivalent is "slip-ons," a term still used by shoe retailers.

Slit-vamp. A fairly high-cut tie shoe commonly worn by women and children ca. 1800–1860 and available in two styles. One version is cut like a slipper; that is, the quarters end at the side seams rather than meeting over the instep. The vamp is very long and in order to get the shoe on, the vamp is slit down some distance from the top edge. The slit is bordered with one or more pairs of lace holes but there is rarely any tongue. Shoes originally intended as slippers were sometimes slit in this way if the wearer found them too tight. The second version does have quarters that extend over the instep and bear the lace holes, but this degree of opening being insufficient, it continues as a slit in the vamp. (See figs. 186–88, 192, 193.) If the slit is part of a seam that extends all the way to the tip of the toe, the pattern is called a "gypsy" or "split-vamp."

Sneaker. American term for a rubber-soled canvas tie shoe. According to *The Household* in 1893, "Tennis shoes with rubber soles . . . the kind known among boys as 'sneakers' are inexpensive and desirable [for mountain-climbing] if made with a ventilated inside sole of leather."[18] The *Shoe Retailer* reported seven years later that

the second grade [of tennis shoes sold by the United States Rubber Company], known as "Champion," has a wide sale, for the price is very moderate. Dealers pay this year 45 cents for men's oxfords and 60 cents for bals. . . . These are the popular "sneaks" that have been widely advertised by this euphonious name by hundreds of dealers from Maine to California. Thousands of young people virtually "live in them" all summer.

Since 1893 the increase in the demand for tennis shoes has been continuous. They are inexpensive and can be worn with comfort to the feet. A great many of the sales are to boys, who do all varieties of "stunts" in them, from riding a wheel to playing ball. Their sale is by no means confined to boys however.[19]

Snuffed. "Snuffed" leathers have had defects in the grain rubbed off ("snuffed off") against an abrasive wheel. They are sponged with black dye and finished dull.

Sock lining. The lining on which the foot rests inside the shoe.

Soft toe. A shoe that has no boxing to stiffen the toe. Also soft tip.

Sole. The main piece or pieces forming the bottom of any footwear. Many shoes, including welted, McKay-sewn, and pegged shoes are made with an insole as well the outsole that is visible on the bottom, and some heavy shoes have a midsole as well. Turn shoes have only a single sole, the outsole. A half-sole is one that extends only from toe to waist. When used without qualification, "sole" usually means the outsole.

Spanish heel. See **Heel.**

Spats. Short for spatterdashes, a British term for cloth gaiters. See **Gaiters.**

Split-vamp. See **Gypsy** and compare **Slit-vamp.**

Spring heel. See **Heel.**

Stiffener. British term for "counter."

Stitching. American term for sewing together the various parts of the uppers. The British equivalent is "closing." Compare **Binding.**

Storm boot. An extra-high-cut women's boot coming well above the ankle, made of heavy leather and intended to meet bad weather conditions.

Storm rubber. Rubbers covering the entire foot and shoe and cut with a tonguelike tab on the instep.

Straights. Shoes not differentiated for right and left feet, but symmetrical in shape.

Suede. Originally kid but frequently calf leather whose flesh side is buffed to raise a velvety nap and that is used with the flesh side out. The buffing is sometimes done on the grain side, but losing the grain weakens the leather.

Swing. The curvature of the outer edge of the sole of a shoe. The degree of swing is one element that differentiates shoes made on a straight last from those made as rights and lefts. See chapter 10.

Tab. (1) British term for an extension from the throatline of a low shoe suggesting or imitating a tongue. American usage does not distinguish between the functional tongue in a tie shoe and the tongue-shaped tab added for decorative purposes. What the British would call a "tab court," Americans would call a "tongue pump."

(2) British term for that part of the quarters that extends over the instep in a lacing shoe and bears the lace holes or eyelets, usually called the eyelet tab. See **Closed tab** and **Open tab.**

Tag. The reinforcement around the end of a lace that stiffens it enough to allow one to push it through the lace holes.

Tan. (1) To treat an animal skin so as to keep it from rotting. See appendix A, "How Leather Is Made."

(2) A tawny, yellowish brown, the natural color of unfinished oak-tanned leather. The *Shoe and Leather Lexicon* notes that since mineral tanning (chrome tanning) does not naturally leave the leather with this yellow-brown color, but rather bluish-gray, the tan color is achieved in most twentieth-century shoes by dyeing.

Throat. The center back section of the vamp at the lower part of the instep, a common location for decoration.

Throatline. The front edge of the opening of a shoe when this edge passes through the throat area as it often does in a slipper or pump. The throatline may be round, square, peaked, tabbed, etc.

Tip. An older American term for "toe cap." A "diamond tip" has a long pointed shape; a "wing tip" spreads back along the sides of the vamp.

Toe. In a foot, one of the five terminal digits. In a shoe, the extreme forward end, often described in terms of its shape as seen from the bottom: pointed, round, oval, square, etc.

Toe box. See **Box toe** and **Boxing.**

Toe cap. An extra piece (often of contrasting material) added over the vamp at the toe. Toe caps may be straight, peaked, or winged. "Toe cap" is correct in both British and American usage. The older American term is "tip," preserved in the phrase "wing tip."

Toe puff. See **Boxing.** According to Jonathan Walford of the Bata Shoe Museum Foundation, toe puff can also refer to the wad of cotton batting or crumpled rags that is sometimes found filling out the pointed toes of eighteenth-century footwear and occasionally in shoes as late as 1910.

Toe spring. The distance between the surface on which the shoe rests and the toe end of the shoe. A shoe with little or no toe spring is said to have a flat forepart.

Toilet slippers. A common nineteenth-century term for loose slippers for wear indoors. Also boudoir slippers.

Tongue. In a laced or buckled shoe, an extension of the vamp or a separate piece sewn on to the vamp at the throat. It lies under the lace holes or latchets, filling the opening and protecting the foot from the pressure of the laces or buckles.

Top. American term for the parts of a boot or shoe above the vamp. In boots, the top generally includes those parts covering the ankle and leg. The rough British equivalent is "leg."

Top edge. The upper edge of the shoe, where the foot is put in. Sometimes called the topline. In slippers, where the top edge cuts through the throat area, the top edge may be called the throatline.

Top facing. A binding or lining sewed round the inside top of the boot upper on which the name of the maker or dealer is often stamped or woven.

Top lift. See **Top piece.**

Top piece. The British term for the thick layer of sole leather applied to the heel where it contacts the ground. Very occasionally in Louis heels, the top piece will be an extension of the sole. In American usage, often known as a "top lift," but this is more appropriate for stacked heels than those of covered wood.

Tread. In American usage, the part of the sole (not including the heel) that contacts the ground, in British usage only the widest part thereof.

Turned shoe. A shoe with a single sole that is sewn to the upper right sides together and then turned right side out. Turned shoes must be made of thin, flexible materials, and are therefore generally recommended only for indoor use or very light walking. See appendix B, "How Shoes Are Made."

Upper. All parts of the shoe covering the top of the foot, including vamp, quarters, linings, etc., in contrast to the bottom, which includes the heel and sole and their component parts.

Vamp. That part of a shoe upper that attaches to the sole and covers at least the front part of the foot. When this piece stops at the side seams, it is called a circular vamp. When it extends from an inner side seam to the back seam, it is called a three-quarter vamp. When it extends around the whole shoe to the back seam, it is called a whole vamp, or in British usage a golosh. In American usage, an upper with three-quarter vamp was sometimes referred to as "three-quarter foxed," and a whole vamp as "whole-foxed" or "slipper-foxed." A vamp that is divided in two parts by a seam from throat to toe is called a "split-vamp" or "gypsy vamp," the seam being called a "gypsy seam."

Vesting. A patterned fabric, usually of silk and wool with the figure brought out in the silk, used for the tops of boots and high shoes. "You will observe that we have a kid back stay and a kid lace stay both of which come just high enough to protect the vesting top from coming in contact with the skirts."[20]

Vici. A trade name used by Robert Foerderer (who perfected the development of chrome-tanned leather) for his chrome-tanned glazed kid. The name was extended to refer to all such leather, not just that produced by Foerderer.

Waist. The narrow part of the sole under the arch of the foot. When a last is measured, the "waist measurement" is a girth measurement taken around the last above the ball but below the instep measurement. It is called the waist because its girth is normally smaller than the girth at either the instep above it or the ball below it.

Wax calf. Heavy calfskin with a wax finish, among the earliest and best methods of finishing calfskin.

Wedge heel. See **Heel.**

Wellington. British term originally applied to a man's knee-high riding boot with a curved top edge, but now used for a rubber boot.

Welted shoe. A shoe with both an insole and an outsole in which two seams are used to attach them to the upper. The inseam stitches the upper to the insole and to the welt, which is an extra flat strip of leather laid around the edge of the sole. The outseam stitches the welt to the outsole. See appendix B, "How Shoes Are Made."

Notes

1. Rice, in Depew, *One Hundred Years of American Commerce*, 567.

2. *Montgomery Ward Catalog*, no. 57, Spring and Summer 1895, 509, 511.

3. Myers, *Home Dressmaking*, 312.

4. Ibid.

5. *Shoe Retailer*, September 25, 1909, 65.

6. *Godey's Lady's Book*, August 1851, 128.

7. Ibid., August 1872, 198.

8. *Shoe Retailer*, September 28, 1904, 81.

9. Swann, *Shoes*, 48–49.

10. Caulfield and Saward, *Dictionary of Needlework*, entry under Galloon.

11. *Every Lady Her Own Shoemaker*, 11–12.

12. *Shoe Retailer*, September 20, 1913, 31.

13. Swann, *Shoes*, 42, 56.

14. The *Shoe and Leather Lexicon*, entry for "patterns," 45.

15. Swann, *Shoes*, 42, 56.

16. *Lady's Magazine*, January 1802. *La Belle Assembleé*, August 1829.

17. *Demorest's*, Autumn/Winter, 1879/1880, 32.

18. *The Household*, August 1893, 265.

19. *Shoe Retailer*, May 1900, 34.

20. *Sears Catalog for 1900*, 488.

Notes

Introduction

1. *Shoe Retailer*, September 17, 1921, 88, and September 15, 1923, 54.

2. Swann, *Shoes*, 63.

3. *Shoe Retailer*, September 20, 1919, 85.

4. Swann, *Shoes*, 65.

5. For more information about the shoe collection in the Peabody Essex Museum, including a history of the United Shoe Machinery Corporation collection, see Paula Richter's essay "Following the Footprints of the Past: The Shoe Collection of the Essex Institute," 115–37.

6. The fashion illustrations entitled "Costume Parisien" appeared first in the French periodical *Journal des Dames et des Modes* (1797–1839). The series of plates was also sold separately, and these ancillary editions appear to have been published in various languages with alternate numbering systems, colorings, labels, and varying selections of images. For this reason, references to *Costume Parisien* will note the library where the plate was found under the cited number (in most cases, the set housed in the Textile Department at the Museum of Fine Arts, Boston). Readers should be warned that these plate numbers will not necessarily match those in other surviving sets of plates having the title *Costume Parisien*.

For example, the Los Angeles County Museum of Art (LACMA) has a set of what appears to be the original French periodicals with articles and captions in French and the years written in standard form. There are occasional plates showing English fashions and others showing only half-length figures. In contrast, the set at the Boston Museum of Fine Arts contains the plates bound alone without articles or extended captions. These have headings and labels in French and dates in the Revolutionary style until it returns to standard practice in 1806. No English plates are included, and some of the plates that are only half-figures in the LACMA periodical appear in Boston's set as full figures. Sometimes a plate has been turned (presumably redrawn) and the numbers of similar plates are unrelated.

1. Makers and Marketers: A Brief Look at the American Shoe Industry

1. Hazard, quoting the *Palladium* of February 6, 1827, in *The Organization of the Boot and Shoe Industry in Massachusetts before 1875*, 29.

2. William Rice, "The Boot and Shoe Trade," in Depew, *One Hundred Years of American Commerce*, 567.

3. Hazard, *Boot and Shoe Industry*, 29.

4. Ibid., 62.

5. Ibid., 61.

6. Ibid., 51.

7. Richardson, *The Boot and Shoe Manufacturer's Assistant and Guide*, 14–16.

8. Hazard, *Boot and Shoe Industry*, 13–14.

9. This advertisement, cut from an unknown newspaper, is preserved in the ephemera relating to the shoe industry at the Lynn Museum.

10. Danvers Historical Society, catalog #60.7.1.

11. Haverhill Historical Society, catalog #2821.

12. Jackson shoes can be seen at Historic Northampton (1810 wedding shoes of Sarah Poole Brewer, catalog #1976.137.1), the Colonial Dames (catalog #1952.532), and the Society for the Preservation of New England Antiquities (catalog #1936.823).

13. Colonial Dames, catalog #1948.50.

14. Hazard, *Boot and Shoe Industry*, 63 (footnote), 79.

15. Peabody Essex Museum, catalog #123,335.

16. Natural History Museum, Los Angeles County, catalog #A3580-193.

17. Connecticut Historical Society, catalog #1960-24-5.

18. Historic Northampton, catalog #66.662.

19. Richardson, *The Boot and Shoe Manufacturer's Assistant and Guide*, xviii, xix.

20. Swann, *Shoes*, 39.

21. Rice, in Depew, *One Hundred Years of Commerce*, 567.

22. *Every Lady Her Own Shoemaker*, iv–v.

23. Swann, *Shoes*, 38.

24. Historic Northampton, catalog #66.646.

25. Hazard, *Boot and Shoe Industry*, 74.

26. Ibid., 94.

27. Ibid., 76.

28. Ibid., 77–78.

29. Ibid., 94.

30. Johnson, *Sketches of Lynn*, 341.

31. Hazard, *Boot and Shoe Industry*, 78–79.

32. Saguto, "The Wooden Shoe Peg," 8–9, quoting Bishop, *A History of American Manufactures*, vol. 2, 509, and vol. 1, 464.

33. Peabody Essex Museum, USMC catalog #2005 and #2016.

34. Rice, in Depew, *One Hundred Years of American Commerce*, 568.

35. Richardson, *The Boot and Shoe Manufacturer's Assistant and Guide*, 14–15.

36. Rice, in Depew, *One Hundred Years of American Commerce*, 568.

37. Banks, *First-Person America*, 15.

38. Society for the Preservation of New England Antiquities, catalog #1920.61.

39. *Shoe Retailer*, October 1900, 54–55.

40. Swann, *Shoes*, 51.

41. Swann, "Prize Work."

42. Entry on "Patterns," *Shoe and Leather Lexicon*, 44–45.

43. Hazard, *Boot and Shoe Industry*, 51.

44. Sterling Last Corporation, *Highlights of American Shoemaking*, 34.

45. *Shoe Retailer*, September 24, 1909, 50–51.

46. Ibid., September 17, 1921, 88.

47. Ibid., September 20, 1913, 31.

48. Ibid., September 25, 1909, 45.

49. Ibid., September 16, 1911, 50.

50. Ibid., 43.

51. Ibid., September 25, 1909, 45.

52. Ibid., September 17, 1921, 90.

53. Ibid., September 15, 1923, 63.

54. Ibid., February 25, 1928, 30–31.

55. Ibid., January 20, 1923, 63.

56. Ibid., September 15, 1923, 46.

57. Ibid., January 20, 1923, 64.

58. Ibid., September 25, 1909, 59–62.

59. Ibid., September 20, 1919, 71.

60. Petsche, *The Steamboat Bertrand*, 60–62.

61. Society for the Preservation of New England Antiquities, catalog #1966.42.

62. Natural History Museum, Los Angeles County, catalog #A3580-1300.

63. Calderón de la Barca, *Life in Mexico*, 194.

64. Ibid., 133.

65. Ibid., 198.

66. Ibid., 200–201.

67. Ibid., 91.

68. *Shoe Retailer*, September 16, 1903, 168.

69. Ibid., September 25, 1909, 45.

70. Ibid., September 16, 1911, 50.

71. Ibid., September 20, 1913, 28.

72. Ibid., September 20, 1919, 77.

73. *Ladies' Home Journal*, March 1924.

2. Stepping Out or Staying In? Women's Shoes and Female Stereotypes

1. Peabody Essex Museum, catalog #127,626.

2. Trollope, *Domestic Manners*, 300.

3. Mrs. A. M. F. Annan, "The Cheap Dress," *Godey's Lady's Book*, September 1845, 88–89.

4. Sarah Josepha Hale, "Editors' Table," *Godey's Lady's Book*, July 1844, 45–46. The book Mrs. Hale reviewed, L. Aimé-Martin's *The Education of Mothers*, was translated from the French and published by Lea & Blanchard of Philadelphia.

5. Woloch, *Women and the American Experience*, 17.

6. Bremer, *Letters*, 290.

7. Park Benjamin, "The True Rights of Woman," *Godey's Lady's Book*, June 1844, 273–74.

8. Ibid. 271–74, passim.

9. *Demorest's*, Spring/Summer 1883, 71.

10. Benjamin, "True Rights of Woman," 274.

11. Hale, "Fashions of Dress and their Influence," *Godey's Lady's Book*, April 1865, 370.

12. Dickens, *American Notes*, 81.

13. "Chit-Chat upon Watering-Place Fashions," *Godey's Lady's Book*, July 1850, 62.

14. Mary A. Livermore, *The Story of My Life*, 81.

15. George Sand, *The Story of My Life*, 203–4.

16. *Harpers New Monthly Magazine*, April 1856, 714.

17. *Every Lady Her Own Shoemaker*, 32.

18. Ibid., 8.

19. Benjamin, "True Rights of Women," 273.

20. Flint, "Travellers in America," 289.

21. Ibid., 291.

22. Ibid., 286.

23. Trollope, *Domestic Manners*, 300, in an editorial note quoting the Cincinnati *Mirror and Ladies' Parterre*, August 18, 1832.

24. Farrar, *The Young Lady's Friend*, 98.

25. Trollope, *Domestic Manners*, 300, 413, 423.

26. Bremer, *Letters*, 244–45. This was recorded in a letter dated November 7, 1850.

27. Austen, *Mansfield Park*, 73.

28. Warner, "Public and Private," 49–50. The material referred to is preserved in the Mount Holyoke College Archives, South Hadley, Mass.

29. *Demorest's*, Spring/Summer 1883, 41.

30. Slocum, Jr., *Lawn Tennis in Our Own Country*, 90.

31. Bernice V. Rogers, "The Rev. Abiel—Convert," *Household*, November 1896.

32. "The Athletic Age," *Godey's Lady's Book*, August 1884, 204.

33. *Godey's Lady's Book*, February 1874, 198.

34. Ibid., February 1885, 227.

35. *Demorest's*, Spring/Summer 1883, 16.

36. *Ladies' World*, December 1899, 27.

37. Ibid., January 1899.

38. *Shoe Retailer*, September 16, 1911, 42.

39. *McCall's Magazine*, July 1904, 790.

40. "My Ideal Sweetheart, by 'Bob' the Gibson Man," *Ladies' World*, December 1913, 8.

41. For an interesting glimpse of contemporary attitudes toward women's roles, see the series of articles by Edith Rickert, "What Has the College Done for Girls?" Parts 1–4 in *Ladies' Home Journal*, January, February, March, April, 1912. The acceptance of physical exercise, the swing toward domestic science, and the tendency to limit women's range of activity are all described in this series.

42. Dudley A. Sargent, M.D., "Are Athletics Making Girls Masculine? A Practical Answer to a Question Every Girl Asks," *Ladies' Home Journal*, March 1912, 11.

43. *Godey's Lady's Book*, March 1881, 268.

44. Duffey, *Our Behavior*, 24–26.

45. *Demorest's*, Spring/Summer 1883, 16.

46. Duffey, *Our Behavior*, 250.

47. *Demorest's*, Spring/Summer 1883, 16.

48. Hartley, *The Ladies' Book of Etiquette* (1873), 25.

49. *Demorest's*, Autumn/Winter 1879/1880, 32.

50. *Godey's Lady's Book*, November 1862, 516.

51. *Ladies' Home Journal*, August 1892.

52. Ibid., July 1896.

53. Stratton-Porter, *A Girl of the Limberlost*, 22.

54. Ibid., 35, 37.

55. *Woman's Magazine*, November 1904.

56. *Shoe Retailer*, September 20, 1913, 34.

57. *Ladies' Home Journal*, January 1908.

58. *Godey's Lady's Book*, September 1857, 216.

59. Claudia Brush Kidwell, "Making Choices: The Real and Pictorial Dresses of Margaret Marston Philipse Ogilvie (1728–1807)," in *The 44th Washington Antiques Show* catalog (1999), 87.

60. *Ladies' Home Journal*, January 1908.

61. Ibid., May 1928.

62. Linda Wells, "Ups and Downs," *New York Times Magazine*, October 1989, 68.

63. Swann, *Shoes*, 30. Quoted from "Receipt for Modern Dress," 1753.

64. The advertisement can be seen on page 20 of "Fashions of the Times," Part 2 of *New York Times Magazine*, February 25, 1990.

3. A Chronological Overview of Shoe Fashions

1. *Every Lady Her Own Shoemaker*, v.

2. *Costume Parisien*, 1809, #1013 in the series owned by the Museum of Fine Arts, Boston. The plate may also be seen in Monique Levi-Strauss's *The Cashmere Shawl* (New York: Harry N. Abrams, Inc., 1988), 37.

3. Advertisement placed by R. Sacket on February 12, 1840, in a Northampton, Mass., newspaper (name not preserved), found in the clipping files at Historic Northampton.

4. *Every Lady Her Own Shoemaker*, 37.

5. Swann, *Shoes*, 42.

6. *Every Lady Her Own Shoemaker*, 38.

7. *Godey's Lady's Book*, June 1877, 558.

8. Ibid., September 1880, 300.

9. Ibid., January 1867, 107.

10. Ibid., February 1885, 227.

11. *Shoe Retailer*, September 17, 1921, 82.

4. The Correct Dress of the Foot

1. *Godey's Lady's Book*, June 1881, 567.

2. *Ackermann's*, January 1810.

3. *Godey's Lady's Book*, January 1851, 71.

4. Ibid., November 1855, 478–79.

5. White kid 1884 wedding boots of Clara Bailey Lowe of Montpelier. Vermont Historical Society, catalog #71.11.2.

6. *Godey's Lady's Book*, February 1873, 198.

7. Society for the Preservation of New England Antiquities, catalog #B3146.

8. *Godey's Lady's Book*, February 1874, 198.

9. *Demorest's*, Spring/Summer 1883, 17.

10. *Ladies' Home Journal*, February 1892, in a brief answer to "Belle."

11. *Godey's Lady's Book*, July 1894, 120–21.

12. *Ladies' World*, April 1899.

13. *Shoe Retailer*, September 18, 1915, 54, advertisement by the Oriental Slipper Mfg. Co. of New York City. Satin slippers with high Cuban heels were made in "black, white, red, pink, light blue, nile, yellow, lavender, Royal blue, Emerald green and gold," at $1.15 a pair. With a half Louis heel only black, white, pink, and blue were available, and the cost was $1.25.

14. *Ladies' Home Journal*, January 1920.

15. Ibid., June 1913.

16. *Shoe Retailer*, September 20, 1913, 32.

17. *Godey's Lady's Book*, May 1857, 479.

18. Ibid., July 1857, 196.

19. Ibid., February 1853, 190.

20. Ibid., April 1859, 382.

21. Ibid., January 1854.

22. *Ladies' Home Journal*, January 1892.

23. Historic Northampton, catalog #66.799.

24. *Godey's Lady's Book*, April 1856, 383.

25. Ibid., January 1889, 88–89.

26. *Peterson's Magazine*, December 1878.

27. *Ladies' Home Journal*, December 1901.

28. *Petit Courrier des Dames*, plate #679, November 1829. This plate is copied in the English periodical *La Belle Assemblée* in December 1829.

29. Ibid., plate #945, January 1833.

30. Peabody Essex Museum, catalog #122,803.

31. Brown and Brown, *Diaries*, 38.

32. Historic Northampton, catalog #66.796, worn by Dr. Samuel Shaw (1790–1870) of Plainfield, Mass. A similar pair of moccasins is catalog #66.795.

33. *Godey's Lady's Book*, December 1854, 485.

34. Ibid., November 1862, 516.

35. Ibid., July 1858, 96.

36. Ibid., April 1873, fig. 18, caption p. 388.

37. *Demorest's*, Spring/Summer 1883, 17.

38. *Ladies' Home Journal*, October 1892.

39. Ibid.

40. *Ladies' Home Journal*, September 1891. The Society for the Preservation of New England Antiquities has a pair of mustard-yellow kid mules with turned-up toes in the Turkish style said to have been bought in Paris in 1890. They are edged with a thick cord but have no beading (catalog #1933.1142). Another pair of mules bought at the same time are of beaded gray satin (catalog #1933.1141).

41. *Harper's Bazar*, December 26, 1891, 1025.

42. *Ladies' Home Journal*, January 1919.

43. *Godey's Lady's Book*, February 1862, 210.

44. Ibid., August 1872, 198.

45. Ibid., April 1875, 390.

46. Ibid., September 1880, 300.

47. *Every Lady Her Own Shoemaker*, 7.

48. *Godey's Lady's Book*, July 1857, 96.

49. *Ackermann's*, August 1815.

50. Trollope, *Domestic Manners*, 300. See chapter 2 in this volume, "Stepping Out or Staying In."

51. *Godey's Lady's Book*, August 1848, 119.

52. Ibid., May 1849. A very similar remark appears in *Godey's*, July 1848, 60.

53. *Godey's Lady's Book*, November 1855, 478–479.

54. Ibid., September 1845, 88.

55. *Maine Farmer and Journal of the Arts*, vol. 1, no. 50, December 28, 1833, 399. A copy of this advertisement was kindly provided by Paige Savery.

56. Ibid.

57. *Barre Gazette*, November 11, 1839. This advertisement is transcribed in the files at Old Sturbridge Village and was kindly shown to me by Curator Jessica Nicoll.

58. *Hampshire Gazette*, February 1840. This advertisement is preserved in the files at Historic Northampton.

59. *Godey's Lady's Book*, September 1849, 228.

60. Ibid., August 1851, 128.

61. *Massachusetts Spy*, April 16, 1834, advertisement for the Worcester Boot and Shoe Store. This advertisement is transcribed in the files at Old Sturbridge Village and was kindly shown to me by Curator Jessica Nicoll.

62. *Hartford Times*, advertisement for the Brimfield Boot and Shoe Store, No. 46 State Street, at the "sign of the BIG BOOT" first placed in the newspaper on November 11, 1840.

63. *Etiquette for Ladies*, 63.

64. Saguto, "The Wooden Shoe Peg," 9, quoting Bishop, *A History of American Manufactures from 1608–1860*, vol. 1, 464.

65. Peabody Essex Museum, USMC Catalog #593 and #1959. See also Lynn Museum, catalog #3207.

66. Rawick Sup. Series II, vol. 4: 1126–27. Quoted in Starke, "U.S. Slave Narratives: Accounts of What They Wore" in *African American Dress and Adornment*, 72.

67. Rawick Sup. Series II, vol. 2: 40. Quoted in Starke, "U.S. Slave Narratives: Accounts of What They Wore" in *African American Dress and Adornment*, 72.

68. "Letter Second" by "Susan," *Lowell Offering*, IV (June 1844), 169–72. Reprinted in Bode, *American Life in the 1840s*.

69. Old Stone House Museum, catalog #C.1392. Identification courtesy June Swann, who suggests that the heel may originally have been two inches high. The heel is a type for which she has documentary evidence dating 1819 and 1829.

70. *Godey's Lady's Book*, August 1848, 119.

71. Ibid., September 1864, 276.

72. Swann, *Shoes*, color plate 4b.

73. *Demorest's*, Autumn/Winter 1879/1880, 32.

74. *Godey's Lady's Book*, September 1880, 300.

75. *Demorest's*, Spring/Summer 1883, 16.

76. *Godey's Lady's Book*, February 1874, 198.

77. *Demorest's*, Autumn/Winter 1879/1880, 32.

78. *Godey's Lady's Book*, October 1877, 357.

79. See the illustration "The Quarrel" of a country couple in a barn in *Peterson's*, April 1863, and the illustration "Summer" of a family working on the harvest in *Godey's Lady's Book*, July 1880. In both cases, the women are wearing heavy front-lace boots.

80. *Godey's Lady's Book*, August 1872, 198.

81. Ibid., May 1875, 485.

82. Ibid., June 1877, 558.

83. Peabody Essex Museum, USMC catalog #1714 and #1724.

84. *Demorest's*, Spring/Summer 1883, 16–17.

85. Ibid., 30.

86. *Godey's Lady's Book*, July 1894, 120–21.

87. *Ladies' Home Journal*, August 1892.

88. Ibid., July 1896.

89. Ibid., April 1908.

90. Ibid., June 1913.

91. Ibid., June 1909.

92. Swann, *Shoes*, 41.

93. *Godey's Lady's Book*, July 1894, 120.

94. *Ladies' Home Journal*, December 1913.

95. Ibid., July 1896.

96. *Woman's Magazine*, May 1906.

97. *Ladies' Home Journal*, July 1917.

98. Ibid., June 1913.

99. *Shoe Retailer*, September 15, 1923, 48.

100. Ibid., October 2, 1926, 44–46.

101. *Ladies' Home Journal*, March 1917.

102. Historic Northampton, catalog #1976.121.2.

103. *Ladies' Home Journal*, September 1925.

104. Trollope, *Domestic Manners*, 300.

5. Shoes Adapted for Sports

1. Cunnington and Mansfield, *English Costume for Sports*, 99; Swann, *Shoes*, 21.

2. Swann, *Shoes*, 30.

3. *Costume Parisien*, An 9 (1800/1801), #303 in the series owned by the Museum of Fine Arts, Boston.

4. Ibid., An 12 (1803/1804), #518 in the series owned by the Museum of Fine Arts, Boston.

5. Calderón de la Barca, *Life in Mexico*, 230.

6. *Costume Parisien*, 1806, #740 in the series owned by the Museum of Fine Arts, Boston; *Ladies' Magazine*, October 1806.

7. *La Belle Assemblée*, June 1817.

8. *Ackermann's*, 1818. Reprinted (no month given) in *Ackermann's Costume Plates*, ed. Stella Blum (New York: Dover, 1978).

9. *La Belle Assemblée*, November 1829.

10. *Godey's Lady's Book*, August 1848, 108.

11. *La Belle Assemblée*, October 1848.

12. Gallery of English Costume, *Costume for Sport*, plate 6a.

13. *Godey's Lady's Book*, July 1851, 64.

14. Ibid., March 1861, 288.

15. Duffey, *Our Behavior*, 271.

16. *Demorest's*, Autumn/Winter 1879/1880, 32.

17. *Harper's Bazar*, April 14, 1888, 245.

18. *Ladies' Home Journal*, July 1915.

19. Ibid., September 1927.

20. Kidwell, *Women's Bathing and Swimming Costume*, 17.

21. *Godey's Lady's Book*, July 1874, 83.

22. *Peterson's*, June 1878.

23. Swann, *Shoes*, 56.

24. *Godey's*, July 1881, figs. 20, 21; *Delineator*, July 1884.

25. Duffey, *Our Behavior*, 284.

26. Peabody Essex Museum, catalog #131,162.2.

27. Connecticut Historical Society, catalog #1959-72-20.

28. *Ladies' Home Journal*, June 1918.

29. Colonial Dames, catalog #1957.81.

30. Historic Northampton, catalog #1976.121.1.

31. Kansas City Museum, catalog #67.43.

32. Kidwell, *Women's Bathing and Swimming Costume*, 28.

33. *Ladies' Home Journal*, July 1915.

34. Connecticut Historical Society, catalog #1983-45-1; Peabody Essex Museum, catalog #135,574; Old Stone House Museum, catalog #C.1396.

35. *Shoe Retailer*, March 19, 1901, 18. The buyer worked for the department store of Frederick Loeser & Co. of Brooklyn.

36. *Demorest's*, Spring/Summer 1883, 41.

37. *Ladies' Home Journal*, August 1892.

38. *Good Housekeeping*, July 1902.

39. *Ladies' Home Journal*, July 1900.

40. Ibid., July 1915.

41. Ibid., July 1917.

42. *Shoe Retailer*, September 20, 1919, 83–84.

43. *Ladies' Home Journal*, April 1926.

44. Ibid., October 1926.

45. Ibid., June 1928.

46. Ibid., October 1928.

47. Ibid., September 1929.

6. Shoes Adapted for Protection

1. Jane Austen, *Persuasion*, 135.

2. Simcoe, *Diary*, 33.

3. See Vigeon, *Clogs or Wooden Soled Shoes*, for a discussion of wooden-soled shoes in England.

4. *Shoe Retailer*, July 1900, 45.

5. *Montgomery Ward Catalog #57* for 1895, 519.

6. Banks, *First-Person America*, 58.

7. Information from the files at Old Sturbridge Village kindly provided by Curator Jessica Nicoll.

8. Winslow, *Diary*, 8.

9. Bowne, *A Girl's Life*, 92.

10. Ibid., 95.

11. Ibid., 96.

12. Laura Ingalls Wilder, *These Happy Golden Years*, 69.

13. Simcoe, *Diary*, 39.

14. Ibid., 40.

15. Society for the Preservation of New England Antiquities, catalog #1937.1079

16. Swann, *Shoes,* 33.

17. *Barre Gazette,* November 11, 1839, advertisement placed by Moses Mandell of the Barre Shoe Store. A transcription of this advertisement in the Old Sturbridge Village files was provided kindness of Curator Jessica Nicoll.

18. Letter from Elizabeth Russell of York (Toronto) to a friend in England, November 1797. Information from the files at the Bata Shoe Museum Foundation, kindly provided by Jonathan Walford.

19. Society for the Preservation of New England Antiquities, catalog #1923.102.

20. Wolf and Wolf, *Rubber,* 33. The early history of rubber is given in a number of sources, and the details vary slightly from account to account. See Wolf and Wolf, *Rubber,* for the most detailed description of the early history of the industry, and Richmond, *The History and Romance of Elastic Webbing,* for information about elasticized fabrics. W. H. Richardson describes the development of the rubber and gutta-percha industries up to 1858 in his *Boot and Shoe Manufacturer's Assistant and Guide,* and a brief introduction is given in the *Scientific American,* vol. 35, 262–63, which also describes how rubber shoes were made in 1876.

21. Wolf and Wolf, *Rubber,* 295.

22. Ibid., 34.

23. Ibid.

24. "Rubber Shoe Making at the Centennial," *Scientific American,* October 21, 1876, 262. The rubber-covered boots at the Peabody Essex Museum are catalog #112,865 and #113,169.

25. Wolf and Wolf, *Rubber,* 296–98.

26. Ibid., 302.

27. *Godey's Lady's Book,* February 1847.

28. "Letter Third," by "Susan," in the *Lowell Offering,* IV, August 1844, 237–40. Reprinted in Bode, *American Life in the 1840s,* 35–40.

29. *Every Lady Her Own Shoemaker,* 32.

30. *Godey's Lady's Book,* January 1853.

31. Connecticut Historical Society, catalog #1960-37-14G.

32. *Demorest's,* Autumn/Winter 1879/1880, 33.

33. Stratton-Porter, *Girl of the Limberlost,* 63.

34. *Demorest's,* Spring/Summer 1883, 17.

35. Swann, *Shoes,* 42.

36. *Shoe Retailer,* October 8, 1927, 41.

37. Society for the Preservation of New England Antiquities, catalog #1933.1236, #1946.339, and #1953.515.

38. *Godey's Lady's Book,* November 1862.

39. *Peterson's,* March 1863.

40. Historic Northampton, catalog #01.425 and #01.426.

41. *Ladies' Home Journal,* June 1892.

42. *Shoe Retailer,* September 22, 1917, 55.

7. Upper Patterns in Shoes

1. But what may be an even earlier example appears in *Harper's Bazar,* May 25, 1889, 384.

2. *Godey's Lady's Book,* February 1874, 198.

3. Ibid., September 1880, 300.

4. *Shoe Retailer,* September 16, 1911, 46.

5. Ibid., September 20, 1913, 28.

6. Ibid., September 20, 1919, 77.

7. Ibid., September 15, 1923, 68.

8. Ibid., December 3, 1927, 36; February 4, 1928, 34.

9. Ibid., September 30, 1911, 34, 38.

10. *Lady's Magazine,* April 1802.

11. *La Belle Assemblée,* August 1829.

12. *Shoe Retailer,* September 28, 1904, 97; Peabody Essex Museum, USMC catalog #2351.

13. Ibid., September 17, 1921, 71.

14. Ibid., September 15, 1923, 65.

15. Ibid., September 17, 1921, 71.

16. For more information on buckles, see Hughes, *Georgian Shoe Buckles,* and Swann, *Shoe Buckles.*

17. Historic Northampton, catalog #66.635.

18. For more information on this subject, see Swann, "Shoes Concealed in Buildings."

19. *Godey's Lady's Book,* August 1872, 198.

20. *Costume Parisien,* 1806, #730 in the series owned by the Museum of Fine Arts, Boston. The shoes are yellow and shown with walking dress. Other plates show similar shoes but less clearly.

21. Peabody Essex Museum, catalog #135,384. Label: "S. Driver 3d & Co. Fashionable Boot and Shoe Store, No. 7, Old Paved Street, Salem. Rips mended gratis."

22. Swann, *Shoes,* 41, fig. 35-5.

23. *Shoe Retailer,* September 22, 1917, 43, 46.

24. *Godey's Lady's Book,* June 1877, 558.

25. *Shoe Retailer,* September 20, 1913, 29.

26. Peabody Essex Museum, catalog #137,689.

8. Upper Patterns in Boots

1. Swann, *Shoes,* 30.

2. *Ackermann's,* April 1809. *Costume Parisien,* 1809, #982 in the series owned by the Museum of Fine Arts, Boston.

3. For three more examples of early front-lacing boots, see Swann, *Shoes,* 38.

4. *Shoe Retailer,* September 22, 1917, 48.

5. *La Belle Assemblée,* September 1828.

6. *Every Lady Her Own Shoemaker,* 37.

7. Society for the Preservation of New England Antiquities, catalog #1936.203.

8. Society for the Preservation of New England Antiquities, catalog #1930.255.

9. *Costume Parisien*, 1822, #2072 in the series owned by the Museum of Fine Arts, Boston.

10. *La Belle Assemblée*, November 1828. The first picture noted is in the same periodical in March 1828.

11. Trollope, *Domestic Manners*, 300. See chapter 2 in this volume for more discussion of this topic.

12. *Godey's Lady's Book*, April 1875, 390.

13. *Demorest's*, Autumn/Winter 1879/1880, 32.

14. See Richmond, *The History and Romance of Elastic Webbing*, a not very organized history of the industry apparently compiled by reviewing the old records of one Easthampton, Mass., company.

15. *Godey's Lady's Book*, February 1860, 192.

16. Nancy Hanks, mother of Abraham Lincoln, was a popular icon of virtuous motherhood. However, she died in 1818, thirty years before the introduction of gored footwear.

17. *Demorest's*, Autumn/Winter 1879/1880, p.75.

18. For example, the *Ladies' World*, May 1899, 11. Advertisements also noted in *Ladies' Home Journal* and *Shoe Retailer*.

19. Swann, *Shoes*, 62, 68.

9. Looking at the Bottom: Heels and Soles

1. Some of the earliest knock-on heels in the 1850s and 1860s appear to have been made of stacked leather rather than wood, and then covered to match the upper. Unless the covering is deteriorated enough to show the bare heel block, it is not obvious which are made of which material.

2. *Shoe Retailer*, September 20, 1913, 31.

3. Swann, *Shoes*, 38, fig. 33.

4. Museum of Fine Arts, Boston, catalog #1988.1160.

5. Swann, *Shoes*, 46, fig. 40c, and plate 4c.

6. *Ladies' World*, September 1899, 13.

7. *Shoe Retailer*, September 20, 1913, 31, describing advance styles for spring 1914.

8. *Heideloff's Gallery of Fashion*, April 1795, fig. 47.

9. Ibid., June 1795, fig. 44.

10. Swann, *Shoes*, 48.

11. *Godey's Lady's Book*, November 1855, 478–79.

12. Frances French to her parents Mary and Nathaniel Abbott, November 4, 1855, Northampton, Mass. Historic Northampton, French family papers, #1-456.

13. Wedding shoe of Frances Mary Eldredge Lyman of Brooklyn, Conn., June 26, 1811. Rhode Island Historical Society, catalog #1928.8.1.

14. *Lady's Magazine*, May and August 1804.

15. Wedding shoe of Mary Little Pearson, Newbury, Mass., 1792. The shoe has her maiden initials embroidered in silver on the vamp, but the short vamp is more typical after 1804.

Possibly the throatline was cut down or the shoe entirely remade, using the original embroidery. Peabody Essex Museum, catalog #126,347.

16. The other example not illustrated in fig. 363 is the light blue kid wedding shoe of Betsy Harrison, Branford, Conn., 1810, said to have been made by the groom, Samuel Woodruff. Connecticut Historical Society, catalog #1983-80-1.

17. Saguto, "The Wooden Shoe Peg," 8.

18. Swann, *Shoes*, 34.

19. *Godey's Lady's Book*, July 1850, 62.

20. (1) *Godey's Lady's Book*, October 1854, 363.
   (2) White kid wedding shoe of Jennie Kimball Brook, April 10, 1862. Haverhill Historical Society, catalog #9534.
   (3) White satin wedding shoe of Bertha Olmsted Niles, June 5, 1862. Connecticut Historical Society, catalog #1974-24-2.
   (4) White satin wedding shoe of Mrs. Theodore Topping, 1868. Historic Northampton, catalog #66.662. See figs. 6, 39.

21. *Godey's Lady's Book*, April 1875, 390.

22. Ibid., June 1877, 558.

23. *Demorest's*, Fall 1879, 32.

24. *Godey's Lady's Book*, July 1894, 120–21.

25. *Shoe Retailer*, September 20, 1913, 28.

26. Ibid., September 17, 1921, 79.

27. Ibid., 88.

28. Ibid., December 11, 1926, 28.

29. Ibid., February 4, 1928, 34.

10. Variations in Lasts

1. *Demorest's*, Fall 1879, 32.

2. *Shoe Retailer*, September 16, 1911, 50.

3. *La Belle Assemblée*, March 1823.

4. *Godey's Lady's Book*, February 1871, 206, and June 1871, 584.

5. Swann, *Shoes*, 51. Beerbohm, *Zuleika Dobson*. New York: Modern Library Edition, 31.

6. Danvers Historical Society, catalog #60.7.1.

7. Swann, *Shoes*, 42.

8. Ibid., 32.

9. *Every Lady Her Own Shoemaker*, 31–32.

10. *Demorest's*, Autumn/Winter 1879/1880, 33.

11. *Shoe Retailer*, September 28, 1907, 45.

12. Ibid., September 30, 1911, 31–34.

11. Materials and Decoration

1. Colonial Dames, catalog #1952.7.

2. Museum of Fine Arts, Boston, catalog #49.1021. Slippers of silvered kid, ca. 1805–15. It is also possible that the

metallic coating was gilding (the tarnish and wear makes it difficult to identify), but if the slippers were gold, one would expect the binding to be yellow rather than white.

3. Valentine Museum, catalog #60.160.2.

4. Museum of Fine Arts, Boston, catalog #51.346. A very similar sandal survives at the Society for the Preservation of New England Antiquities, catalog #1940.435.

5. Peabody Essex Museum, catalog #121,772.

6. Bedford Historical Society, Prudence Dean wedding shoe, 1797, catalog #C-24.

7. Documented shoes with cutouts at Historic Northampton include wedding shoes of 1801 (catalog #1979.30.83) and of 1810 (catalog #1976.137.1). The Rhode Island Historical Society has wedding shoes with cutouts dated 1811 (catalog #1928.8.1). These three shoes are illustrated in figs. 440, 441, and 442.

8. *Lady's Magazine*, February 1804.

9. *La Belle Assemblée*, November 1823.

10. The Peabody Essex Museum has a ca. 1805–10 slipper of brown cotton edged all around with light blue kid, in which the cotton fabric may be jean (catalog #121,772).

11. See Montgomery, *Textiles in America*, entries on "Everlasting" (235–36), "Gros de Naples" (250–52), "Jean" (271), and "Prunella" (328–29).

12. Old Sturbridge Village, catalog #26.25.78.

13. *Every Lady Her Own Shoemaker*, 28–29.

14. *Lady's Magazine*, June 1832.

15. Swann, *Shoes*, 41.

16. *Godey's Lady's Book*, July 1853, 96; August 1854, 190–92; October 1855, 359; February 1860, 192.

17. Haverhill Historical Society, catalog #5429.

18. *Godey's Lady's Book*, November 1888.

19. Colonial Dames, catalog #1952.105.

20. *Shoe and Leather Lexicon*, entry on "Coltskin," 15–16.

21. *Godey's Lady's Book*, July 1894, 120.

22. Descriptions of leathers are adapted from those given in *Shoe and Leather Lexicon*.

23. *Godey's Lady's Book*, July 1894, 120.

24. *Shoe Retailer*, September 28, 1904, 63.

25. *Godey's Lady's Book*, July 1894, 121.

26. *Ladies' Home Journal*, September 1892.

27. *Shoe Retailer*, September 22, 1917, 46.

28. Ibid.

29. Ibid.

30. Ibid.

31. *Shoe Retailer*, September 17, 1921, 82.

32. Ibid., 78.

33. Ibid., 71.

34. *Shoe Retailer*, September 15, 1923, 49.

35. Ibid., September 25, 1923, 62.

36. Ibid., October 2, 1926, 44–47, and *Ladies' Home Journal*, October 1926.

37. *Ladies' Home Journal*, April 1926, "The Fashions of Our Head and Heels Make or Mar Our Costume."

38. Swann, *Shoes*, 38, fig. 33.

39. *Godey's Lady's Book*, March 1853, 161.

40. Ibid., January 1867, 107.

41. *Demorest's*, Autumn/Winter 1879/1880, 32.

42. Ibid., Spring/Summer 1883, 16.

43. Historic Northampton, catalog #1979.30.86.

44. *Frank Leslie's Lady's Magazine*, May 1864.

45. *Godey's Lady's Book*, January 1867, 107.

46. *Montgomery Ward Catalog*, no. 57 for Spring and Summer, 1895, 509, in the description of a boot called "The Charmer."

47. Peabody Essex Museum, catalog #137,676.

Appendix B: How Shoes Are Made

1. Saguto, "The Wooden Shoe Peg," 8.

2. Peabody Essex Museum, USMC catalog #1384.

3. *Shoe Retailer*, September 25, 1909, 65.

Appendix C: Rubber and Elastic Webbing

1. Wolf and Wolf, *Rubber*, 15–29 passim. As stated in note 20, chapter 6 above, the early history of rubber is given in a number of sources, and the details vary slightly from account to account. The Wolfs provide the most detailed description, and theirs is the source most relied on here.

2. Ibid., 287–308, passim, for an account of the early nineteenth-century industry in England and the United States.

3. Beard, *America through Women's Eyes*, 118.

4. "Rubber Overshoe Making," 262–63.

5. Clifford Richmond, author of *The History and Romance of Elastic Webbing*, worked in the industry and drew on the limited company records available to him in producing his book.

6. Richardson, *Boot and Shoe Manufacturer's Assistant and Guide*, 58. Richardson describes the development of the rubber and gutta-percha industries up to 1858.

7. *Shoe Retailer*, March 12, 1901, 19.

Bibliography

Allen, Frederick James. *The Shoe Industry.* Boston: Vocation Bureau of Boston, 1916.

Annan, Mrs. A. M. F. "The Cheap Dress: A Passage in Mrs. Allanby's Experience." *Godey's Lady's Book* 31 (September 1845): 86–91.

"The Athletic Age." *Godey's Lady's Book* 109 (August 1884): 204.

Austen, Jane. *Mansfield Park.* 1814. Edited by R. W. Chapman. London: Oxford University Press, 1934.

Austen, Jane. *Persuasion.* 1818. Edited by R. W. Chapman. London: Oxford University Press, 1934.

Banks, Ann, ed. *First-Person America.* New York: Alfred A. Knopf, 1980. [Life-history narratives produced by the Federal Writers' Project during the 1930s.]

Beard, Mary. *America through Women's Eyes.* New York: Macmillan, 1933.

Benjamin, Park. "The True Rights of Woman." *Godey's Lady's Book* 28 (June 1844): 271–74.

Bishop, J. Leander. *A History of American Manufactures from 1608–1860.* 3 vols. 1868. Reprint. New York: Johnson Reprint Corporation, 1968.

"Bob," the Gibson man [pseud.]. "My Ideal Sweetheart." *Ladies' World,* December 1913, 8.

Bode, Carl, ed. *American Life in the 1840s.* Documents in American Civilization Series. Garden City, N.Y.: Doubleday & Co./Anchor Books, 1967.

The Boot and Shoe Industry in Northampton. Reprinted from "Life in Old Northampton" (pp. 40–53). Northampton, England: Northamptonshire Libraries, 1975.

Bowne, Eliza Southgate. *A Girl's Life Eighty Years Ago: Selections from the Letters of Eliza Southgate Bowne.* Introduction by Clarence Cook. New York: Charles Scribner's Sons, 1887. Reprint. Williamstown, Mass.: Corner House, 1980.

Bremer, Fredrika. *America of the Fifties: Letters of Fredrika Bremer.* Selected and edited by Adolph B. Benson. New York: American-Scandinavian Foundation, 1924.

Brown, Sally, and Pamela Brown. *The Diaries of Sally and Pamela Brown, 1832–1838, Plymouth Notch, Vermont.* Edited by Blanche Brown Bryant and Gertrude Elaine Baker. Printed with *The Diary of Hyde Leslie.* 1887. 2d ed. Springfield, Vt.: William L. Bryant Foundation, 1979.

Buck, Anne M. *Victorian Costume and Costume Accessories.* Rev. ed. Carlton, Bedford, England: Ruth Bean, 1984.

Butterworth, Jeffrey. "Simply Stupendous: A Century of Exposition Shoes, 1839–1939." *Essex Institute Historical Collections* 127 (April 1991): 138–60.

Calderón de la Barca, Frances. *Life in Mexico: The Letters of Fanny Calderon de la Barca.* With new material from the author's private journals. Edited and annotated by Howard T. Fisher and Marion Hall Fisher. New York: Doubleday & Co., 1966.

Caulfield, S. F. A., and Blanche Saward. *The Dictionary of Needlework: An Encyclopedia of Artistic, Plain and Fancy Needlework.* London: A. W. Cowan, 1882. Reprinted as *Encyclopedia of Victorian Needlework.* New York: Dover, 1972.

"Chit-Chat upon Watering-Place Fashions." *Godey's Lady's Book* 41 (July 1850): 62.

Colazzo, Charles, Jr. *The Foot and Shoe, A Bibliography.* Toronto: Bata Shoe Museum Foundation, 1988.

Cunnington, Phillis, and Alan Mansfield. *English Costume for Sports and Outdoor Recreation from the Sixteenth to the Nineteenth Centuries.* London: Adam & Charles Black, 1969.

Dawley, Alan. *Class and Community: The Industrial Revolution in Lynn.* Cambridge: Harvard University Press, 1976.

Depew, Chauncey M., L.L.D. *One Hundred Years of American Commerce, 1795–1895.* New York: D. O. Haynes & Co., 1895.

Derwin, Luke. "Woman's Influence." *Peterson's Magazine,* November 1849, 171–73.

Dickens, Charles. *American Notes and Pictures from Italy.* 1842. London: Oxford University Press, 1957.

Duffey, Mrs. E. B. *Our Behavior: A Manual of Etiquette and Dress of the Best American Society.* Philadelphia: J. M. Stoddart & Co., 1876.

Etiquette for Ladies: With Hints on the Preservation, Improvement and Display of Female Beauty. Philadelphia: Carey, Lea & Blanchard, 1838.

Every Lady Her Own Shoemaker: or, A Complete Self-Instructor in the Art of Making Gaiters and Shoes. By a Lady. 1856. Reprint, with introduction by Carolyn R. Shine. Davenport, Iowa: Amazon Drygoods, 1989.

Faler, Paul G. *Mechanics and Manufacturers in the Early Industrial Revolution: Lynn, Massachusetts, 1780–1800.* Albany: State University of New York Press, 1981.

Farrar, Mrs. John. *The Young Lady's Friend.* Rev. ed. New York: Samuel & William Wood, 1849.

"Fashions and Manners." *McCall's Magazine* (July 1904): 790.

Flint, Timothy. "Travellers in America." *The Knickerbocker, or New York Monthly Magazine* 2 (October 1833): 283–302.

French family papers. Historic Northampton, Mass.

Gallery of English Costume. *Costume for Sport.* Picture Book No. 8. Edited by Anne Buck. Manchester, England: Art Galleries Committee of the Corporation of Manchester, 1963.

[Hale, Sarah Josepha.] "Editor's Table: Fashions of Dress and Their Influence." *Godey's Lady's Book* 70 (April 1865).

[———.] "Editor's Table." Review of *The Education of Mothers* by L. Aimé-Martin. *Godey's Lady's Book* 29 (July 1844): 45–46.

Hartley, Florence. *The Ladies' Book of Etiquette.* Boston: Lee & Shepard, 1873.

Hazard, Blanche. *The Organization of the Boot and Shoe Industry in Massachusetts before 1875.* Reprint. New York: Augustus M. Kelly, 1969.

Hide and Leather and Shoes Encyclopedia of the Shoe and Leather Industry. Chicago: Hide and Leather Publishing Co. 1941.

Hughes, Bernard, and Therle Hughes. *Georgian Shoe Buckles: Illustrated by the Lady Maufe Collection of Shoe Buckles at Kenwood.* London: Greater London Council, 1972.

Johnson, David N. *Sketches of Lynn or the Changes of Fifty Years.* Lynn, Mass.: 1880.

Kidwell, Claudia. "Making Choices: The Real and Pictorial Dresses of Margaret Marston Philipse Ogilvie (1728–1807)." In *The 44th Washington Antiques Show* catalog, 1999. 86–93.

———. *Women's Bathing and Swimming Costume in the United States.* Washington, D.C.: Smithsonian Institution Press, 1968.

Leno, John Bedford. *The Art of Boot and Shoemaking: A Practical Handbook Including Measurement, Last-Fitting, Cutting-Out, Closing, and Making, with a Description of the Most Approved Machinery Employed.* London: Crosby Lockwood and Co., 1885.

Livermore, Mary A. *The Story of My Life.* Hartford, Conn: A. D. Worthington & Co., 1899.

Melder, Keith. *Life and Times in Shoe City: The Shoe Workers of Lynn.* Salem, Mass.: Essex Institute, 1979.

Montgomery, Florence M. *Textiles in America, 1650–1870.* New York: W. W. Norton, 1984.

Myers, Annie E. *Home Dressmaking, A Complete Guide to Household Sewing.* Chicago: Charles H. Sergel & Co., 1892.

Petsche, Jerome E. *The Steamboat Bertrand: History, Excavation, and Architecture.* Washington, D.C.: National Park Service, 1974.

Rees, John F. *The Art and Mystery of a Cordwainer: or, An Essay on the Principles and Practice of Boot and Shoe-Making with Illustrative Copper-Plates.* London: Gale, Curtis, and Fenner, 1813.

Rexford, Nancy. "The Speaking Shoe." *Essex Institute Historical Collections* 127 (April 1991): 161–84.

Richardson, W. H., Jr. *The Boot and Shoe Manufacturer's Assistant and Guide, Containing a Brief History of the Trade, History of India-Rubber and Gutta-Percha and Their Application to the Manufacture of Boots and Shoes, etc.* Boston: Higgins, Bradley & Dayton, 1858.

Richmond, Clifford A. *The History and Romance of Elastic Webbing.* Easthampton, Mass.: Easthampton News Company, 1946.

Richter, Paula. "Following the Footprints of the Past: The Shoe Collection of the Essex Institute." *Essex Institute Historical Collections* 127 (April 1991): 115–37.

Rickert, Edith. "What Has the College Done for Girls?" Parts 1–4. *Ladies' Home Journal,* January–April 1912.

Rogers, Bernice V. "The Rev. Abiel—Convert." *The Household,* November 1896.

"Rubber Overshoe Making at the Centennial." *Scientific American* 35 (October 21, 1876): 262–63.

Saguto, D. A. "The Wooden Shoe Peg and Pegged Construction in Footwear—Their Historical Origins." *Chronicle of Early American Industry* 37 (March 1984): 5–10.

Salaman, R. A. *Dictionary of Leather-Working Tools, c. 1700–1950 and the Tools of Allied Trades.* London: George Allen & Unwin, 1986.

Sand, George. *The Story of My Life.* Translated and adapted by Dan Hofstadter. New York: Harper & Row, 1979.

Sargent, Dudley A. "Are Athletics Making Girls Masculine? A Practical Answer to a Question Every Girl Asks." *Ladies' Home Journal,* March 1912.

Shoe and Leather Encyclopedia: A Book of Practical and Expert Testimony by Successful Merchants. St. Louis: Shoe and Leather Gazette, 1911.

Shoe and Leather Lexicon: An Illustrated Glossary of Trade and Technical Terms Relating to Shoes, also Leather and Other Shoe Materials, and Allied Commodities, with Especial Reference to the Production, Distribution and Retail Merchandising of the Finished Article. 3d rev. ed. Boston: Boot and Shoe Recorder Publishing Co., 1916. 14th rev. ed. New York: The Shoe and Leather Lexicon, 1947.

"Shoe Shopping—The Congress Boot." *Godey's Lady's Book* 37 (August 1848): 119–20.

Sigourney, Mrs. L. H., et al. *The Young Lady's Offering: or, Gems of Prose and Poetry.* Boston: Phillips, Sampson & Co., 1851.

Simcoe, Elizabeth. *Mrs. Simcoe's Diary.* Edited by Mary Quayle Innis. Toronto: MacMillan of Canada, 1965.

Slocum, H. W., Jr. *Lawn Tennis in Our Own Country.* New York: A. G. Spalding Bros., 1890.

Starke, Barbara M., Lillian O. Holloman, and Barbara K. Nordquist. *African American Dress and Adornment: A Cultural Perspective.* Dubuque, Iowa: Kendall/Hunt, 1990.

Sterling Last Corporation. *Historical Highlights of American Lastmaking and American Shoemaking.* In commemoration of the fiftieth anniversary of Sterling Last Corporation, 1932–82. N.p., 1982.

Stratton-Porter, Gene. *A Girl of the Limberlost.* 1909. Reprint, with afterword by Joan Aiken. New York: NAL Penguin Inc./Signet Classics, 1988.

Swann, June. "Prize Work." *The Crispin Courier* [Newsletter of the Honourable Cordwainers' Company] 5 (August 1989): 4.

———. *A History of Shoe Fashions.* Northampton, England: Northampton Borough Council Museums and Art Gallery, 1975.

———. *Shoe Buckles.* Northampton, England: Northampton Borough Council Museums and Art Gallery, 1981.

———. *Shoemaking.* Shire Album #155. Aylesbury, Bucks, England: Shire Publications Ltd., 1986.

———. *Shoes.* Costume Accessories Series. Edited by Aileen Ribeiro. London: Batsford, 1982.

———. "Shoes Concealed in Buildings." *Northampton Museum Journal* 6 (1969).

Thornton, J. H., and J. M. Swann. *A Glossary of Shoe Terms.* 4th ed. Northampton, England: Central Museum, 1986.

Timbs, John. *Stories of Inventors and Discoveries.* New York: Harper and Bros., 1860.

Trollope, Frances. *Domestic Manners of the Americans.* 1832. With a history of Mrs. Trollope's adventures in America. Edited by Donald Smalley. New York: Alfred A. Knopf, 1949. New York: Random House/Vintage Books, n.d.

Vigeon, Evelyn. *Clogs or Wooden Soled Shoes.* Reprinted from the *Journal of the Costume Society* (1977).

Warner, Patricia Campbell. "Public and Private: Men's Influence on Women's Dress for Sport and Physical Education." *Dress* 14 (1988): 48–55.

Wells, Linda. "Ups and Downs." *New York Times Magazine,* October 8, 1989, 68.

Wilder, Laura Ingalls. *These Happy Golden Years.* New York: Harper & Row, 1943.

Winslow, Anna Green. *Diary of Anna Green Winslow, a Boston School Girl of 1771.* Edited by Alice Morse Earle. 1894. Reprint. Williamstown, Mass.: Corner House Publishers, 1974.

Wolf, Howard, and Ralph Wolf. *Rubber.* New York: Covici, Friede, 1936.

Woloch, Nancy. *Women and the American Experience.* New York: Alfred A. Knopf, 1984.

Credits for Part II Illustrations

Fig. 90. Generic illustration of typical slipper 1830–50.

Fig. 91. *Shoe Retailer*, April 3, 1901, p. 22. "A design by Newman, 'The Shoeman,' of Boston."

Fig. 92. *Ladies' Home Journal*, March 1908. Advertisement for Red Cross Shoes. Model No. 98, "Priscilla pump, patent colt, gun metal or tan, $3.50."

Fig. 93. *B. Altman Catalog* 103, Spring/Summer, 1911, p. 106. Item #2371, "Gray or black suede beaded slippers . . . $5.00."

Fig. 94. *Ladies' Home Journal*, March 1915. Red Cross Shoe. "Model No. 385. The 'Gladys' Colonial. Very chic, yet delightfully simple. In either fawn or grey dreadnought quarter, patent vamp."

Fig. 95. *Bellas Hess Catalog*, Spring 1918, p. 242. "#20x411 Handsome custom dress pump made of very fine brilliant black patent leather. A stylish shoe for dancing or general dress wear. It has high leather Louis Cuban heels, fitted with aluminum heel plate, which prevents the heel from wearing down. It fits snugly at sides and well up under arch. Has light weight flexible dress soles and is finished with fancy perforations, as pictured. Black only. . . . $3.49."

Fig. 96. *Ladies' Home Journal*, April 1912. Advertisement for Red Cross Shoes. Model No. 259.

Fig. 97. *Shoe Retailer*, September 18, 1915, p. 29. "Mat kid gypsy pump, light welt, vamp with front seam from toe to tongue with four rows of white stitching and perforations, 16/8 straight breasted louis leather heel. Shown by Ziegler Bros., Philadelphia [for Spring and Summer 1916]."

Fig. 98. *Shoe Retailer*, September 22, 1917, p. 62. "Metropolitan Footwear Fashion Glimpses [for Spring 1918]. . . . Bristol pump in brown kid and suede; orange fitted, point foxed. An artistic creation by George W. Baker."

Fig. 99. *Shoe Retailer*, September 20, 1919, p. 86. "Women's Spring and Summer Styles [1920]. . . . The Aeroplane sport pump, white eve cloth, high tongue and wing throat of patent leather, 18/8 celluloid covered louis heel with plate. Lunn & Sweet Shoe Co., Auburn, Me." On page 53, the same style is listed at $7.00.

Fig. 100. *Shoe Retailer*, January 28, 1928, p. 33. "A clever combination of tan kid and genuine watersnake by Sak's Herald Square."

Fig. 101. *Ladies' Home Journal*, August 1930, p. 64. Advertisement for Foot Saver Shoes, made by Julian and Kokenge Co., Cincinnati, Ohio.

Fig. 102. Connecticut Historical Society, #1960-57-2A. White kid slipper with pointed toe and spring heel, ca. 1795–1805. Needle holes on vamp (not included in illustration) show placement of original trimming.

Fig. 103. Peabody Essex Museum, #103,126. White kid slipper with round toe and spring heel, ca. 1805–15.

Fig. 104. Haverhill Historical Society, #2821. White kid slipper with round toe, spring heel, and ruche at throatline, worn by Mrs. Thomas Newcomb at her wedding on January 17, 1815. Label: "Chase & Cogswell Variety Shoe Store, Main Street, Haverhill, Mass. Rips mended gratis."

Fig. 105. Peabody Essex Museum #118,057. Green wool serge slipper with oval toe and spring heel, ca. 1815–30.

Fig. 106. Connecticut Historical Society, #1972-63-2. White satin slipper with narrow square toe and low stacked heel, worn by Almira Barnes Fletcher at her wedding, May 5, 1830.

Fig. 107. Historic Northampton #66.644. White silk slipper with square toe worn by Susan L. B. Munroe, age sixteen, at her first ball, 1837.

Fig. 108. Historic Northampton, #66.656. Black kid slipper with rounded square toe, ca. 1845–55. Stamped gilt design on vamp is illustrated in fig. 458. Label: "Burt Brothers, New York."

Fig. 109. Danvers Historical Society, #45.5.3. White kid slipper with rounded square toe and knock-on heel, worn by Emily P. Abbott at her wedding in 1869.

Fig. 110. Connecticut Historical Society, #1974-114-2. White kid slipper with oval toe and knock-on heel, worn by Alta Harriett Farr Bigelow at her wedding in Connecticut, June 10, 1885.

Fig. 111. Peabody Essex Museum, #127,398. White satin slipper with oval toe, beaded vamp, and Louis heel, ca. 1890. Label: "Monguignon, Suc^r de L. Perchellet, rue St. Honoré 356, Paris."

Fig. 112. Peabody Essex Museum, USMC #690. Black kid slipper with long pointed toe and low stacked heel, ca. 1898.

Fig. 113. *Sears Roebuck Catalog*, 1902. "Women's Patent Leather Sandals, $0.95. . . . Made with patent leather vamp, kid quarter, high heel and with bow strap."

Fig. 114. *The Ladies' Home Journal*, June 1909. Advertisement for the American Lady Shoe (made by Hamilton, Brown Shoe Co. of St. Louis and Boston).

Fig. 115. *Shoe Retailer*, September 16, 1911, p. 58. Advertisement by Julian and Kokenge Co., Cincinnati, for three new lasts for spring 1912. "The Heart: Medium wide toe that carries a 12/8, 13/8, or 14/8 heel."

Fig. 116. Historic Northampton, #66.692. Bronze kid slipper with oval toe, high Louis heel, and gold beads on vamp, ca.1914–16. Label: The Clements Co., Springfield, Mass."

Fig. 117. *Bellas Hess and Co.* catalog, Spring, 1918, p. 242. "Dress Pump of fine soft, dull kid . . . built on the latest fashionable last . . . Has high leather Louis Cuban heels, fitted with aluminum plate above top lift of heel, which prevents the heel from wearing down and another piece of leather can easily be set on when the heel wears down to the plate. Shoe has plain pointed vamp and is trimmed with perforated foxings. Has light weight soles. This pump fits snugly and will hug the arch of foot. Black only. . . . $3.49."

Fig. 118. Peabody Essex Museum, USMC #2285. Black kid slipper with oval toe, celluloid-covered heel, and covered buckle, made over a Stage last by Hazen B. Goodrich of Haverhill, Mass., in 1922.

Fig. 119. *Ladies' Home Journal*, May 1926. Advertisement for the Arch Preserver Shoe, made by the Selby Shoe Co. of Portsmouth, Ohio. Style name: "The Barrie."

Fig. 120. *Sears Roebuck Catalog*, 1930, p. 226. Reprinted in Blum, *Everyday Fashions of the Thirties*, p. 17. "4-Inch Heels! Savoy Last. Black brocaded satin or patent leather for these regally correct D'Orsay bow pumps on perfectly poised 4-inch covered spike heels with short vamp on Ritz 'fashion' last." Model numbers: 15D2214–17.

Fig. 121. Connecticut Historical Society #1958-2-1-6. White satin slipper with pointed toe, tabbed throat, and Louis heel worn by Catherine Wadsworth Terry at her wedding in Hartford, Conn., on March 14, 1798.

Fig. 122. Historic Northampton #66.670. White kid slipper with tabbed throat, oval rosette, and knock-on heel, ca. 1869–74.

Fig. 123. *Ladies' Home Journal*, April 1915. Advertisement for Red Cross Shoes. "Model No. 396. The 'Corinne.'"

Fig. 124. *Shoe Retailer*, September 20, 1919, p. 74. "Women's Spring and Summer Styles [for 1920]: Gypsy tongue pump, patent vamp, mat kid quarter over, narrow toe last, four-inch vamp, 17/8 covered louis wood heel, combination mat and patent gypsy tongue, turn sole. Joy, Clark & Nier, Inc., Rochester."

Fig. 125. *Shoe Retailer*, September 15, 1923, p. 53. Styles for spring 1924. "Gore pump of black suede with patent trim, slashed front, the buckle concealing the goring; round toe, two inch Spanish heel. Barke-Gibbon Co., Inc., Philadelphia."

Fig. 126. *Shoe Retailer*, December 31, 1927, p. 80. Advertisement by P. W. Minor and Son, Inc., Batavia, N.Y., for shoes in stock in January and February 1928. "The Amy, style no. 802, light welt, honey alligator, price $5.25."

Fig. 127. *Costume Parisien*, An 12 (1803/4), #514 in the series at the Boston Museum of Fine Arts.

Fig. 128. Metropolitan Museum of Art, Costume Institute, #60.22.23. Purplish-pink kid shoe with oval toe and three pairs of tabs for silk tape lacing, ca. 1804–10. The thickness and attachment of the sole suggests that this shoe was worn for walking.

Fig. 129. *Costume Parisien*, 1807, #806 in the series owned by the Boston Museum of Fine Arts.

Fig. 130. Lynn Museum #2978. Black kid shoe with oval toe, wedged heel, and single strap tied low on the instep, ca 1805–10.

Fig. 131. *Harper's Bazar*, March 4, 1876, p. 149. Reprinted in Blum, *Victorian Fashions and Costumes from Harper's Bazar*, p. 108. Black kid shoe with kid-covered high heel. Straps are bound with black silk ribbon and have buttonholes in both ends. Black silk ribbon bow. "For evening toilettes the bands and buttons should be made of material to match the color of the dress."

Fig. 132. Historic Northampton, #66.677. Black kid three-strap slipper with oval toe, knock-on heel, and black beads on vamp, ca. 1885–90.

Fig. 133. Connecticut Historical Society, #1942. White

suede cross-strap shoe with oval toe, knock-on heel, and beading on the straps, worn by Ellie Munger Lines Chapin at her wedding on March 24, 1891. Label: "W.B. Fenn and Co., New Haven."

Fig. 134. *Montgomery Ward Catalog*, 1895, p. 512. "Ladies kid strap sandal slipper . . . very popular for house or dance wear." The identical shoe is advertised in the *Sears Roebuck Catalog* for 1897 and nearly identical ones in the *Sears Roebuck Catalogs* for 1902 and 1907.

Fig. 135. Peabody Essex Museum, USMC #2351. Light-green figured-silk T-strap shoe with pointed toe and knock-on heel, made by the Geo. E. Keith Co. of Boston on order from A. H. Howe Co. of Boston, and worn by Mrs. George R. Todd in 1896. See also fig. 400.

Fig. 136. *Shoe Retailer*, April 3, 1901, p. 22. Black patent shoe with Louis heel, four eyelets, and velvet tie, "a design by B. Cohen & Sons, of New York."

Fig. 137. *Shoe Retailer*, September 24, 1902, p. 102. Advertisement by The Heer Shoe Co., Portsmouth, Ohio. "Fine chrome kid, Queen Sandal, imitation turn sole, style 623. $1.50."

Fig. 138. *Shoe Retailer*, September 16, 1903, p. 135. "New Styles Designed for House and Evening Wear. . . Tan castor beaded three-strap sandal" made by the John J. Lattemann Shoe Manufacturing Co. for the spring 1904 season.

Fig. 139. *Ladies' Home Journal*, June 1909. Advertisement for the American Lady Shoe, made by the Hamilton, Brown Shoe Co. of St. Louis and Boston. "This ankle strap pump is one of this season's newest creations, —the Hebe last. Made in two leathers No. 6241, patent leather with turned sole, and No. 6242 in the swell new Suedes—London smoke, black and tan, with light welt sole."

Fig. 140. *Shoe Retailer*, September 25, 1909, p. 64. Advertisement by John Kelly, Inc., Rochester, N.Y., for spring 1910.

Fig. 141. *Shoe Retailer*, September 18, 1915, p. 36. Advertisement by Hazen B. Goodrich and Co., Haverhill, Mass., for spring 1916.

Fig. 142. *Shoe Retailer*, September 17, 1921, p. 12. Advertisement by I. Miller, Inc., Brooklyn, N.Y., for "beautiful shoes in stock." This model, called "The Pandora," is offered for $8.00 in black kid or patent with a high Louis or baby Louis heel, and in tan calf with welted sole and baby Louis heel.

Fig. 143. *Shoe Retailer*, September 17, 1921, p. 41. Advertisement by the Emerson Shoe Company, Rockland, Mass., for two-strap shoes currently in stock. "No. 1587, Wollaston, $5.75 Black diamond kid, 15/8 Cuban heel."

Fig. 144. *Shoe Retailer*, September 17, 1921, p. 77. "Women's Advance Styles [for spring 1922]: Patent two buckle sandal, new French toe, cutout vamp, square edge turn, 15/8

Spanish-Louis covered heel. Shown by Smaltz-Goodwin Co., Philadelphia."

Fig. 145. *Shoe Retailer*, September 17, 1921, p. 72. "Women's Advance Styles [for spring 1922]: A new two buckle and strap patent leather pump, showing new cut-out side effect, modified round toe French last, Cuban-Louis covered heel, square edge turn sole. Shown by J. Albert & Son, Brooklyn."

Fig. 146. *Shoe Retailer*, September 17, 1921, p. 73. "Women's Advance Styles [for spring 1922]: Combination sandal and ankle strap pump, all patent leather, junior Louis covered heel, new medium round toe last, square edge, turn sole. Shown by Ellis-Eddy Co., Haverhill."

Fig. 147. *Shoe Retailer*, September 15, 1923, p. 52. "Black brocade cross-strap turn with black ooze straps and trimming. Black suede covered Louis heel. [Style currently being introduced by] Welch, Moss & Feehan Co., Haverhill."

Fig. 148. *Shoe Retailer*, September 15, 1923, p. 29. Advertisement by Tober-Saifer Shoe Co., St. Louis, for in-stock shoes. "No. 8017—Pat[ent] chrome, 2 button cutout strap pump, 13/8 military, celluloid covered heel, turn sole. . . $4.50."

Fig. 149. *Shoe Retailer*, September 15, 1923, p. 29. Advertisement by Tober-Saifer Shoe Co., St. Louis, for in-stock shoes. "No. 816—Patent chrome, dull calf cut-out apron, turn sole, made over French last, 15/8 Spanish celluloid covered heel. . . . $5.25."

Fig. 150. *Shoe Retailer*, September 15, 1923, p. 50. "Combination of dull kid with patent colt trimming. French braid bound, three inch vamp, medium round toe with narrow strap and rivet button fastening. Full Louis covered heel and square turn edge. [Style currently being introduced by] Burrows Shoe Co., Rochester, N.Y."

Fig. 151. *Shoe Retailer*, September 15, 1923, p. 61. "Love knot one strap turn of chestnut ooze with brown kid trimming, medium French toe, three inch vamp and 16/8 Spanish heel. [Style currently being introduced by] Capital Shoemakers Inc., St. Louis."

Fig. 152. *Shoe Retailer*, September 15, 1923, p. 50. "All patent leather close edge turn with celluloid covered Louis heel, two-inch vamp, cut low near shank. [Style currently being introduced by] The Val Duttenhofer Sons' Co., Cincinnati."

Fig. 153. *Shoe Retailer*, September 15, 1923, p. 61. "Field mouse ooze one strap model with light brown kid trim. Medium vamp with 12/8 Cuban heel. [Style currently being introduced by] Hallahan & Sons, Philadelphia."

Fig. 154. *New York Styles, Charles Williams Stores* catalog #27, Spring/Summer, 1925, pp. 224–25. Shoe with black patent vamp, tan calf quarter, and braided instep strap, $2.98.

Fig. 155. *Shoe Retailer*, October 2, 1926, p. 48. "Styles Certified by Leading Retailers." This style is identified only as being recommended by "Frank More's Shop, San Francisco."

Fig. 156. *Ladies' Home Journal*, October 1928. "Brown and Navy Blue for Fall Shoes." "A modernized sandal-type slipper for street wear, combining black lizard with insets of black kid."

Fig. 157. *Shoe Retailer*, March 17, 1928, p. 53. "Walk-Over's new tie effect, the 'Vista' of special ooze vamp and quarter with tawny beige trout quarter collar. [Style currently being introduced by] George E. Keith Co., Campello, Brockton, Mass."

Fig. 158. *Sears Roebuck Catalog*, 1930, p. 226. Reprinted in Blum, *Everyday Fashions of the Thirties*, p. 17. Black patent or kid "center buckle one-strap . . . trimmed with black embossed lizard and 1¾-inch covered military heels on Boulevard last. . . . $4.00."

Fig. 159. Common type of eighteenth-century shoe buckle fastening with a chape. The finer ones were typically made of silver, often ornamented with paste stones. Buckles were also made of pewter, bronze, cut steel, japanned iron, plated or gilded metal, etc.

Fig. 160. Peabody Essex Museum, #128,039. Fold-down buckle on a bronze kid T-strap slipper with Louis heel and metallic ornamentation, ca. 1880–85. Barely legible label: Colon de Pons y Cᵃ. SO.Cᴰ en [—]."

Fig. 161. (a) *Sears Roebuck Catalog*, 1930, p. 226. Reprinted in Blum, *Everyday Fashions of the Thirties*, p. 17. Shoe buckle of hexagonal design from an illustrated shoe. (b) *Sears Roebuck Catalog*, 1930/31, p. 222. Reprinted in Blum, *Everyday Fashions of the Twenties*, p. 147. Shoe buckle with Art Deco design from an illustrated shoe. (c) *Sears Roebuck Catalog*, 1933, p. 208. Reprinted in Blum, *Everyday Fashions of the Thirties*, p. 52. Shoe buckle with Art Deco design from an illustrated shoe.

Fig. 162. Generic illustration of an open-tab latchet tie shoe.

Fig. 163. Generic illustration of an open-tab blucher shoe.

Fig. 164. Generic illustration of a closed-tab oxford shoe.

Fig. 165. Generic illustration of two types of slit-vamp shoe.

Fig. 166. Historic Northampton, #66.632. Figured-silk buckled shoe with oval toe, Louis heel, and square tongue, possibly from the 1765 wedding of Elizabeth Foye Munroe of Boston.

Fig. 167. Haverhill Historical Society, #9362. White, glazed wool buckled shoe with pointed toe, Italian heel, and pointed tongue, ca. 1775–90. Label: "Shoes made and sold by Nathaniel Fogg, Exeter."

Fig. 168. Rhode Island Historical Society, #6-30-54. Pink satin latchet tie shoe with pointed toe and low Italian heel, ca. 1790–1800.

Fig. 169. Peter Oakley collection. Cream serge open-tab shoe with oval toe, low stacked heel, and clasp fastening, ca. 1825. A ribbon rosette added to the vamp about 1870 is not shown in the illustration.

Fig. 170. Old Sturbridge Village, #12.14.112. Heavy leather welted brogan with square toe, low stacked heel, and pegged half sole, ca. 1840–60.

Fig. 171. Peabody Essex Museum, USMC #1111. Black patent leather latchet tie shoe with rounded square toe and low stacked heel, used as a sample by Lyman Blake when applying for a patent on the McKay sole-sewing machine in 1860.

Fig. 172. Peabody Essex Museum, USMC #1724. Latchet tie shoe with rounded square toe, low stacked heel, ca. 1870–80, identified in the USMC catalog as "Misses' Newports . . . uppers of grained kip with lining of blue twill. Well made shoes of the period."

Fig. 173. *Godey's Lady's Magazine*, May 1875. "Fig. 14.—High kid shoe for house or street wear."

Fig. 174. Peabody Essex Museum, USMC #2287. Black glazed kid latchet tie shoe with rounded square toe and knock-on heel, made by Goodrich and Porter of Haverhill, Mass., for exhibit at the Centennial Exposition in Philadelphia in 1876. This shoe has vamp cut-outs backed with purple silk, not shown in illustration. See color plate 7.

Fig. 175. *Hirth, Krause and Wilhelm* catalog, 1890. "Empress Tie Shoe, No. 38."

Fig. 176. *Montgomery Ward Catalog* No. 57, 1895, p. 511. Reprinted in facsimile by Dover Publications, 1969. "The Blucherette Oxford. The very latest novelty in footwear, made from the finest French dongola, with long diamond tip and turnsole . . . $1.75."

Fig. 177. *Shoe Retailer*, May 15, 1901, p. 45. "The Colonial," a new style introduced by Laird, Schober Co. of Philadelphia. "This is a sample of a style which has taken hold of the trade with more of a grip than any novelty shown of late. The slipper is both practical and handsome. It is in great demand among the dealers of fine shoes."

Fig. 178. *Sears Roebuck Catalog*, 1906, p. 1044. "Ladies' haired calf top blucher oxford. . . $2.50."

Fig. 179. *Sears Roebuck Catalog*, 1907, p. 841. "Newport Tie, $0.98. Made of a very fine selection of vici kid, over a comfortable, but good fitting last, quarters being lined with white kid, a specially comfortable, yet serviceable shoe throughout. Turned sole with a common sense heel. Just the kind for those who want an easy slipper. Sizes and half sizes, 3 to 8. Full widths only."

Fig. 180. *Shoe Retailer*, September 28, 1907, p. 50. Open-tab shoe with patent vamp made by Bemis and Wright of Lynn, Mass., for spring and summer 1908.

Fig. 181. Historic Northampton, #66.690. White kid latchet tie shoe with pointed toe and knock-on heel, worn by Rachel Moore Warren at her wedding in Somersworth, N.H., July 1, 1908.

Fig. 182. *Shoe Retailer*, September 17, 1921, p. 87. "Women's Advance Styles [for spring 1922]: Patent, three buckle blucher oxford, flexible McKay sewed sole, perforated straight tip, medium round toe last, low rubber heel. Shown by Harper & Kirschten Shoe Co., Chicago."

Fig. 183. *Sears Roebuck Catalog*, Fall/Winter, 1927. "Very latest . . . medium tan color, fancy embossed, leather three-eyelet tie, with lighter tan color tongue, pinked at vamp, and fancy perforations. 1¼-inch heel with rubber top lift. New Boulevard last, square toe. . . $3.89."

Fig. 184. *Ladies' Home Journal*, September 1928. Advertisement by the Selby Shoe Co., Portsmouth, Ohio. "For Street—Coralie. Mocha bisque kid, 3 eyelet tie, with suede underlay to match."

Fig. 185. *Sears Roebuck Catalog*, 1933, p. 255. Reprinted in Blum, *Everyday Fashions of the Thirties*, p. 53. "Snakeskin . . . three-eyelet tie you'll see everywhere this year—morning, afternoon, and even evenings! Graceful two-inch continental heels, snakeskin covered. . . $2.98."

Fig. 186. Generic illustration of first type of slit-vamp shoe.

Fig. 187. Generic illustration of second type of slit-vamp shoe.

Fig. 188. Peabody Essex Museum, #104,997. Pale-blue kid slit-vamp shoe with oval toe, low stacked heel, and pale-blue ribbons, ca. 1825. Label: "Joseph Morton's Fashionable Variety Shoe Store, No. 39 Marlboro Street, Boston."

Fig. 189. Peabody Essex Museum, USMC #1541. Brownish-black kid oxford with square toe, made by Edward Swain Davis of Lynn, Mass., and exhibited with other examples of his work at the Exposition of the Mass. Charitable Mechanics Association of New England in 1839. See also figs. 211, 374, and 455.

Fig. 190. Peabody Essex Museum, USMC #593. Black leather (probably calf) slit-vamp shoe with square toe and pegged sole, ca. 1835–50.

Fig. 191. Connecticut Historical Society, #1956-5-5. Slit-vamp square-toed shoe of purplish-beige serge figured in a honeycomb pattern and foxed with tan morocco, worn by Mary Anna Warner Pierpont at her wedding in Waterbury, Conn., on April 20, 1846.

Fig. 192. Old Sturbridge Village, #12.14.61. Black leather (possibly calf) slit-vamp shoe with rounded square toe and twelve pairs of lace holes, ca. 1850–65.

Fig. 193. Ferrar-Mansur House, Costume #138. Black grained leather slit-vamp shoe with rounded square toe and low stacked heel, ca. 1855–70. Sole stamped "Sole Leather Counters."

Fig. 194. Museum of Fine Arts, Boston, #44.530. Black kid oxford with rounded square toe, high Louis heel, red leather lining, and embroidery on vamp and quarter, ca. 1875. Sole stamped "Limoges."

Fig. 195. Connecticut Historical Society, #1971-15-1. White kid oxford with rounded square toe and thick Louis heel, made by William J. Kinsella in a style already old-fashioned for his daughter Christine to wear at her wedding in 1894.

Fig. 196. *Harper's Bazar*, May 25, 1889, p. 384. Reprinted in Blum, *Victorian Fashions from Harper's Bazar, 1867–1898*. Part of a group identified as "walking and traveling shoes."

Fig. 197. Peabody Essex Museum, USMC #2470. Oxford shoe with oxblood calfskin vamp and patent leather tip and counter, oval toe, Louis heel, and turned sole, made by Selz-Schwab for the World's Columbian Exposition in Chicago in 1893.

Fig. 198. *Sears Roebuck Catalog*, 1897. "Ladies' fine chocolate Vici Kid oxford, made over the new coin last, with long perforated tip toe. This shoe is McKay sewed, very flexible, is suitable for dress or every day wear . . . $1.50."

Fig. 199. *Sears Roebuck Catalog*, 1902. "Ladies' patent leather oxford, $1.45, made from good patent leather stock, medium wide sole, with extension edges, and full perforated vamp, tip and heel foxing."

Fig. 200. *Shoe Retailer*, July 2, 1902, p. 55. Advertisement by D. Armstrong and Co., Rochester, N.Y., for "Louis Heel Shoes."

Fig. 201. *Sears Roebuck Catalog*, 1906, p. 1044. Black vici kid oxford with patent tip and chocolate-colored quarter. "A most unique pattern . . . $1.05."

Fig. 202. *Dorothy Dodd Catalog*, 1908, p. 30. "Number 1682 is a dress oxford of patent finished kidskin. Light, flexible turn sole; high louis heel."

Fig. 203. *B. Altman Catalog*, No. 103, Spring/Summer, 1911, pp. 106–7. "2370 Women's black kid oxfords, patent leather tip . . . $3.50."

Fig. 204. *Ladies' Home Journal*, May 15, 1915. Advertisement for Red Cross Shoes, made by the Krohn-Fechheimer Co. of Cincinnati, Ohio. "Model No. 395. The 'Avenue.' A charming oxford with fawn cloth quarter."

Fig. 205. *Bellas Hess Catalog*, Spring 1918, p. 242. "A neat, well-fitting oxford tie with vamp of glossy black patent leather, and quarters of dull black kid . . . light weight soles and leather Louis Cuban heels. . . . just what you need for a dressy street shoe."

Fig. 206. *Sears Roebuck Catalog*, 1920, p. 204. "Dark brown leather brogue oxford—fancy perforations—military heel—sewed sole. $4.95."

Fig. 207. *Ladies' Home Journal*, September 1924. Advertisement for Foot Saver shoes made by the Julian and Kokenge Co., Cincinnati, Ohio. "From eleven to three for shopping, walking for health, or while at active business, she should wear the Foot Saver next beneath."

Fig. 208. *Shoe Retailer*, December 4, 1926, p. 49. Advertisement. "Natural bridge arch black kid wh. qr. bal oxford, 13/8 leather heel, rubber tap, Goodyear welt, 986-X Comb. Last. . . . Priced at $3.35."

Fig. 209. *Ladies' Home Journal,* September 1927, p. 124. Advertisement for Arch Rest shoes, made by Drew of Portsmouth, Ohio. Style name: "Astor."

Fig. 210. *The Ladies' Home Journal,* July 1929. Style name: "Lucretia."

Fig. 211. Peabody Essex Museum, USMC #1539. Side-lacing square-toed shoe with upper of plaid wool and vamp of brown morocco, made by Edward Swain Davis of Lynn, Mass., and exhibited with other examples of his work at the Exposition of the Mass. Charitable Mechanics Association of New England in 1839. See also figs. 189, 374, and 455.

Fig. 212. Lynn Museum, #1217. Black kid side-lacing shoe with pointed toe, stacked heel, patent tip and front stay, and white kid lining, made by the George E. Barnard Co. of Lynn, Mass, 1890–95, probably for the World's Columbian Exposition in Chicago in 1892–93.

Fig. 213. *Sears Roebuck Catalog,* 1908. "Fine patent colt oxford with dull mat kid top. It has an artistic side lace of fine Barathea silk and is easy to fit to the foot. . . $1.64."

Fig. 214. Peabody Essex Museum, USMC #2237. Black kid button shoe with rounded square toe, stacked heel, and turned sole, made by Goodrich and Porter of Haverhill and exhibited at the Philadelphia Centennial Exposition in 1876.

Fig. 215. *Jordan Marsh & Co. Almanac,* 1883 (illustrates styles of late 1882). "Ladies French kid button slipper, hand-sewed turn. Price, $3.50, Fr. kid. Am. kid, $3.00, $2.50 and $2.00."

Fig. 216. *Hirth, Krause and Wilhelm Catalog,* 1890. "Empress Button Shoe, No. 32."

Fig. 217. *Shoe Retailer,* April 3, 1901, p. 32. Advertisement by the Batchelder and Lincoln Co., Boston, for ladies' oxfords. "Stock No. 5155—Patent vamp, southern button, New York imitation tip, turn. 'Ruby,' Price $1.50."

Fig. 218. *Shoe Retailer,* September 16, 1903, p. 57. "Slipper Styles: Four Recent Low-cut Fancies: 'The Flora' patent calf openwork. Wm. Lane."

Fig. 219. *Shoe Retailer,* September 28, 1904, p. 102. Advertisement by the J. J. Lattemann Shoe Mfg. Co. of New York, for the Lattemann "Corset Shoe which is unique, in that it has a patent ankle-stiffening device which may be added to or totally removed, as is most needed."

Fig. 220. *McCall's Magazine,* June 1904, p. 744. Advertisement by The Radcliffe Shoe Co. of Boston, illustrating a "chrome patent four button oxford, a dressy Summer shoe. . . $2.50."

Fig. 221. *Shoe Retailer,* September 28, 1907, p. 53. "Patent colt, 2-button, plain toe, kid top oxford, Spanish heel, 'Pinta'

last. Sampled [style currently being introduced] by F. J. Currier & Co., Lynn, Mass."

Fig. 222. *Shoe Retailer,* September 25, 1909, p. 45. "Spring and Summer, 1910: Gypsy five button oxford of 'Boston gray' calf, scalloped button fly, 14-8 Cuban heel. Shown by Harney Bros., Lynn."

Fig. 223. *Ladies' Home Journal,* April 1912. Advertisement for Red Cross Shoes. Model No. 247, not described.

Fig. 224. *Shoe Retailer,* September 18, 1915, p. 36. Advertisement by Hazen B. Goodrich & Co., Haverhill, Mass., for spring 1916 shoes. Style name: "Mazie."

Fig. 225. *Ladies' Home Journal,* September 1927. Advertisement by The Irving Drew Co. of Portsmouth, Ohio. Three-button shoe with instep cutouts. Style name: "Della." Not described.

Fig. 226. Elizabeth S. Brown collection, Buddington #4.75.5. White kid slipper with rounded toe, knock-on heel, and elastic strap with bow, worn by Mary Wheeler Buddington at her wedding, ca.1883.

Fig. 227. Peabody Essex Museum, USMC #1797. Black grained leather shoe with rounded square toe, low stacked heel, and vamp slit for elastic insertion, ca. 1865–75. Old USMC card dates this shoe to 1858 without explanation.

Fig. 228. Peabody Essex Museum, USMC #2231. Black kid shoe with rounded square toe, low stacked heel, cutout vamp with blue silk underlay, white machine embroidery, and two gussets of elastic goring on the instep. Made by Goodrich and Porter and shown at the Philadelphia Centennial Exposition in 1876.

Fig. 229. Valentine Museum, #65.150.1. Black kid shoe with rounded square toe, low stacked heel, white machine embroidery, and band of elastic connecting the quarters under the tab, ca. 1875.

Fig. 230. *Godey's Lady's Book,* April 1881. "Fig. 29.—Shoe with elastic at the sides and open straps across the instep; it is made of French kid stitched."

Fig. 231. *Montgomery Ward Catalog* No. 57, 1895, p. 511. "Ladies' Prince Albert: the stock is a fine Vici kid, light sole, flexible, medium opera heel, fancy patent leather trimmed up the front . . . for a neat summer shoe it has no equal. . . $1.60."

Fig. 232. *Sears Roebuck Catalog,* 1897. "Ladies Elastic Front Slippers. . . . This is one of the leading novelties in low shoes, out this season. Made from a good selection of Vici Kid, chocolate color, hand turn flexible sole and elastic front, which conforms to the shape of the foot whether high or low instep. The shoe is made over the new Dime Toe Last, with tip, kid lined . . . $1.50."

Fig. 233. *Shoe Retailer,* April 3, 1901, p. 12. Advertisement by The Rich Shoe Company, Milwaukee, for Julia Marlowe footwear. Only description of this shoe says, "None genuine unless bearing this stamp on every sole: Rich's Julia Marlowe Lace Oxford, Pat. Oct. 23rd 1900."

Fig. 234. *Shoe Retailer*, September 16, 1903, p. 135. "New Styles Designed for House and Evening Wear: Fancy goring applied to oxfords and combined with beading, produces some handsome effects, as shown by the two illustrations herewith. They were designed by Samuel H. Hayden of Haverhill."

Fig. 235. *The Shoe Retailer*, September 28, 1904, p. 81. "Spring and Summer 1905: Women's sixteen threads gore ouskin, lined in duck and leathers. A repetition of 'Ye Olden Days;' Made by G. A. & E. A. Mansfield, Lynn."

Fig. 236. *Sears Roebuck Catalog*, 1907, p. 839. "Star Nullifier, $1.15. Made of a nice medium weight vici kid, patent tip and with a rubber heel. This makes it a sort of a combination shoe, for either an indoor slipper or an outdoor shoe."

Fig. 237. *Shoe Retailer*, September 15, 1923, p. 64. "Side gore turn model of black ooze with patent leather collar and trim. Cut-out front, 3 1/4 inch vamp and covered Cuban heel. [Style currently being introduced by] P. Sullivan & Co., Cincinnati."

Fig. 238. *Charles Williams Stores Catalog*, Spring/Summer, 1925, p. 217. "The 'Swan' . . . modeled of lustrous patent leather with smartly cut-out elastic gored instep strap. Closely trimmed leather sole and stylish covered military heel. This identical pattern also comes in tan calf leather with rubber capped military heel. . . $2.98."

Fig. 239. *Sears Roebuck Catalog*, Fall/Winter, 1927. "Latest sport shawl pump . . . in tan calfskin with shawl tip and quarter in brown Scotch design leather. New round boulevard last, 1-inch heel and genuine Goodyear welt soles. Elastic front goring under bow insures perfect fit. . . . $4.95."

Fig. 240. *Sears Roebuck Catalog*, Fall/Winter 1934, p. 285. "House slippers. Black kid with patent leather overlay up the front. Wear them to do your housework."

Fig. 241. Peabody Essex Museum, USMC #1981. Front-lacing boot of pebbled calf with patent tip, rounded square toe, low stacked heel, and McKay-sewn sole, ca. 1865–70. Label: "Extra Quality, Manufactured Expressly for Geo. W. Cutting & Son, Weston, Mass, by John Fletcher & Sons, Acton, Mass."

Fig. 242. Peabody Essex Museum, USMC #2917. Buttoned boot of red glazed kid with high toe, high stacked heel, and "Sorosis" label, made by A. E. Little of Lynn, Mass., ca. 1914–15. See plate 10.

Fig. 243. Peabody Essex Museum, USMC #2260. Gored boot of black serge with stacked heel made by Goodrich and Porter of Haverhill, Mass., and exhibited at the Centennial Exposition in Philadelphia in 1876.

Fig. 244. Historic Northampton, #66.696. Side-lacing boot of black serge with black kid tip and square toe, ca. 1840–50.

Fig. 245. Colonial Dames, #1952.50. Front-lacing boot of green kid with pointed toe and low Italian heel, 1795–1805. See fig. 36.

Fig. 246. Peabody Essex Museum, USMC #880. Front-lacing boot of black calf(?) with oval toe, low stacked heel, welted sole, and rosette and steel buckle on vamp, ca. 1805–15. See fig. 56.

Fig. 247. Metropolitan Museum of Art, Costume Institute, #11.60.202. Front-lacing boot of purplish-brown kid with oval toe, spring heel, purple silk binding, and dark maroon fringe, ca. 1815–25.

Fig. 248. Valentine Museum, #43.23.1. Front-lacing boot of green kid, with oval toe, stacked heel, welted sole, green silk bow, and red and green fringe, ca. 1825–30. See plate 4.

Fig. 249. Los Angeles County Museum of Art, #37.15.7. Front-lacing boots of white kid with gypsy (top to toe) seam and knock-on heel, ca. 1860–65.

Fig. 250. Lynn Museum, #3146. Front-lacing boots of black serge with patent toe-cap, lace stay and binding, metal eyelets, McKay-sewn sole, and small stacked heel, ca. 1865. Labels: "Patent July 6[?] 1864. Warranted The C.O.D. Man." "Pat. Jan 26, 1864 & June 13, '65." "Bancroft & Purinton. Warranted. Lynn, Mass." See fig. 64.

Fig. 251. SPNEA, #1940.1012. Front-lacing boot of black serge with rounded square toe, low stacked heel, McKay-stitched sole, rosette with steel buckle on vamp and green leather facing at top, ca. 1865–75.

Fig. 252. Peabody Essex Museum, USMC #2294. Front-lacing boot of black kid with fancy vamp/quarter seam, white ornamental stitching, McKay-sewn sole, and high stacked heel. Made by Goodrich and Porter of Haverhill, Mass., and exhibited in the Philadelphia Exposition in 1876.

Fig. 253. Peabody Essex Museum, USMC #1733. Front-lacing boot of black calf, with round toe, stacked heel, and standard screw sole, ca. 1885. Stamped on sole: "Registered Trademark—Standard [picture of screw] Fastened."

Fig. 254. *Sears Roebuck Catalog*, 1897, p. 191. "Fine Needle Toe Lace. No. 3545. Ladies' [black] Paris Kid Lace . . . with long drawn out needle toe, hand turn flexible sole and long, narrow patent leather tip. This shoe has medium heel, fancy patent leather lace stays and the new heel foxing, making a shoe which will be very popular the coming season . . . $2.98."

Fig. 255. *Shoe Retailer*, July 2, 1902, p. 55. Advertisement by D. Armstrong and Co., Rochester, N.Y., includes this front-lacing boot with black patent slipper foxing and high Louis heel.

Fig. 256. *Sears Roebuck Catalog*, 1907, p. 835. "'Chicago Belle,' $1.89. This is the very latest design in a ladies' shoe.

The vamp is made of guaranteed patent coltskin cut in such a manner as to give the high instep effect, while the soles are solid oak and quite flexible. The shoe carries the very latest style military heel and is very desirable for dress wear."

Fig. 257. *Ladies' Home Journal*, April 1908. Advertisement by the Krohn-Fechheimer Co., Cincinnati, Ohio, for Red Cross Shoes. "A dress boot for summer wear. No. 91 Red Cross Blucher Patent Colt, $4.00."

Fig. 258. *Shoe Retailer*, September 20, 1913, p. 5. Advertisement by the Boardman Shoe Co., Boston, Mass. "Drusilla—in stock. No. 441. Gun metal blucher, Goodyear welt, $2.20."

Fig. 259. *Ladies' Home Journal*, October and November 1915. Advertisement by the Krohn-Fechheimer Co., Cincinnati, Ohio, for Red Cross Shoes. "No. 409. The 'Hampton' Lace Boot. Fashioned of patent colt with black cloth top."

Fig. 260. *Ladies' Home Journal*, November 1919. Advertisement by Utz and Dunn Co., of Rochester, N.Y., for "Ease-All" shoes.

Fig. 261. *La Belle Assemblée*, September 1828. "Second Walking Dress . . . Lapis-coloured boots of kid buttoned on one side, with mother-of-pearl buttons, are worn with this dress."

Fig. 262. *Every Lady Her Own Shoemaker*, Diagram 2. See fig. 512 for a similar boot.

Fig. 263. *Godey's Lady's Book*, June 1860. Advertisement by Oakford's, a Philadelphia hat and shoe retailer, for "Oakford's Fashions for Spring," Fig. 5, "English walking boot."

Fig. 264. SPNEA #1935.1. Ten-button boot of black satin embroidered on the vamp with white silk and silver thread, with oval toe and Louis heel, ca. 1877–80. Top facing of red sateen stamped in gold "Grande Assortimente di Calzature d'Ogni Genere. Erasmo Maurelli. Fornitore di S. M. La Regina d'Italia. Successore di Sno. Antinucci. Rome, Via due Macelli 101. Florence, Borgo Ognissanti 2. On parle francais. English Spoken."

Fig. 265. Peabody Essex Museum, USMC #2418. Black kid buttoned boot with oval toe, stacked heel, and McKay-sewn sole, ca. 1885–92. Circular gummed paper royalty stamp on bottom of heel states "Standard Boot & Shoe Lasting Company. License Stamp 3927. Pat. Aug. 11, '85. Reiss. Sep. 1, '85. Lasted Without Tacks."

Fig. 266. *Sears Roebuck Catalog*, 1897, p. 191. "Sears' Special Goodyear Welt Button. A $5.00 Shoe for $3.00. No. 3566. . . . made from the best of vici kid, with a fine satin finish, long, drawn out needle toe, patent leather tips, foxed heel. Goodyear welt bottoms, which are cut from the best of oak tan sole leather, and will wear like iron. This particular style of toe is very popular, and it gives the foot a very stylish appearance. We can thoroughly recommend this shoe to those of our patrons who wish something up-to-date, good fitting, and suitable for general wear."

Fig. 267. *Shoe Retailer*, September 14, 1904, p. 14. Advertisement for the Lindner Shoe Co., Carlisle, Pa. "Our newest styles for Spring and Summer, 1905."

Fig. 268. *Shoe Retailer*, September 20, 1913, p. 38. Advertisement for the Riley Shoe Mfg. Co., Columbus, Ohio. "No. 3571. McKay Welt—in Stock. Patent ¾ vamp, button, dull straight top, trotter last, 1¾-inch military heel, 7½ iron McKay welt sole. . . . $2.10."

Fig. 269. *Shoe Retailer*, September 18, 1915, p. 30. "Women's Styles for Spring & Summer 1916 . . . Gypsy Gaite. All kid gypsy gaiter button boot, white silk fitted, diamond tip with small perforations, 16/8 Louis leather heel, light welt, 7 ½-inch top. Shown by the Julian & Kokenge Co., Cincinnati, O."

Fig. 270. *Shoe Retailer*, September 22, 1917, p. 53. "Women's Spring & Summer Styles—1918. Women's eight-inch button boot, brown Russia calf vamp, fawn buck top, imitation wing tip. Shown by Krohn-Fechheimer Co., Cincinnati, O."

Fig. 271. Left: *La Belle Assemblée*, September 1829. "French Fashions. Walking Dress. . . . Half boots of the same colour as the dress [light willow-green]." Right: *La Belle Assemblée*, November 1828. "Walking Dress. . . . Half-boots of light-grey corded silk, with tips of kid."

Fig. 272. SPNEA, #1936.611. Tan cotton (possibly jean) side-lacing boot bound with tan silk and trimmed with fringe around the top and a tassel on the instep, 1828–30. The tan rand between sole and upper is rarely found after the 1770s. The thin covered heel slip is not common after 1820.

Fig. 273. Peabody Essex Museum, USMC #1878. Side-lacing boot of off-white wool with a small black woven square, foxed at the narrow square toe with black kid, and bound with black, ca. 1830–35.

Fig. 274. SPNEA, #1930.187. Side-lacing boot of bluish-gray silk foxed at the rounded square toe with black patent, ca. 1850–55. Worked eyelets and upper stitching of orange silk.

Fig. 275. Natural History Museum of Los Angeles County, #A3580-193. Side-lacing boots of faded purple silk moiré, foxed at the rounded square toe with black patent, ca. 1850. Circular stamp on soles reads, "22. Jeanneau Hervé & Cie. Paris. Élèves de Renault." From a Spanish family settled in Los Angeles before it became an American territory.

Fig. 276. Historic Northampton, #66.701. Side-lacing boot of bright red kid with rounded square toe and stacked heel, ca. 1860.

Fig. 277. Connecticut Historical Society, #X1996.38.0. White satin side-lacing boot with rounded square toe and low Louis heel, ca. 1865–70. Label: "Mssr Lapaque-Hoffmann F FAVRE Succr Boul^d des Capucines 27."

Fig. 278. Peabody Essex Museum, USMC #2252. Black satin side-lacing boot with black kid vamp and foxing, rounded square toe, and stacked heel. Made by Goodrich and Porter of Haverhill, Mass., and exhibited at the Philadelphia Exposition in 1876.

Fig. 279. *Hirth, Krause & Wilhelm Catalog*, 1890. "Ladies' Side Lace, No. 9. Circle Seam, or Seam from Top to Toe."

Fig. 280. *Ladies' Home Journal*, September 1915. Advertisement for Bellas Hess and Co. of New York. Shown with suit #1L61.

Fig. 281. Lynn Museum, #4184. Glossy black kid boot with elastic side gores of shirred goods, ca. 1850–60.

Fig. 282. Lynn Museum, #3147. Black serge boot with elastic side gores of fabric having the elastic threads woven in, ca. 1865–75. See fig. 64.

Fig. 283. SPNEA, #1924.332. Bronze leather side-gore boot with rounded square toe and the kind of goring in which the elastic threads are woven in, ca. 1850–60.

Fig. 284. Peabody Essex Museum, USMC #2010. Black serge boot with elastic side gores with elastic threads woven in, black patent toe cap, thick McKay-sewn sole, and stacked heel, ca. 1865–75. USMC card says, "Period 1865. Made for C. W. Cutting & Sons, Boston, Mass. by Fletcher & Sons, Acton, Mass. At time of purchase sold at retail for $3.50 per pair. Part of the stock of C. W. Cutting Co. of Weston, Mass. Purchased in 1935."

Fig. 285. Peabody Essex Museum, USMC #2016. Black serge side-gore boot with scalloped toe cap of black patent, stacked heel, and imitation buckle front, 1865–75. Bears on heel a rectangular paper stamp stating, "McKay Sew Mach Co License Stamp Pat^d Aug 14 1860." Handwritten stamp #50123.

Fig. 286. Peabody Essex Museum, USMC #2233. Black kid side-gore boot with rounded square toe, stacked heel, decorative white machine stitching imitating a buttoned front, and a fancy stitched patent tip. Made by Goodrich and Porter and exhibited at the Centennial Exposition in Philadelphia, 1876. Circular Exposition stamps on sole.

Fig. 287. SPNEA, #B3146. White satin-weave linen side-gore shoe with covered knock-on heel and turned sole, ca. 1865–75. The goring was woven so that when in a relaxed state, the white warps obscured the black rubber elastic wefts (which themselves alternated with two pairs of cream-colored wefts).

Fig. 288. Peabody Essex Museum, USMC #1838. Black pebble-grain leather side-gore boot with black patent toe cap, pegged sole, and low stacked heel, ca. 1865–75. Said to be part of the stock of Jonathan W. Maine of Scotland, Conn., and to date from 1872.

Fig. 289. *Montgomery Ward Catalog* No. 57, 1895, p. 512. "The Elite. 52146. This is a new departure in the line of stylish footwear. The stock in this shoe is of a very fine selection of Dongola. French tannage, very soft and durable. This being the first season for this very stylish Congress, we look for a large sale on same. The accompanying cut represents this very accurately. It has a very neat patent leather stay up the front and a light turn sole with thin edge, and a medium heel, which makes a very comfortable and stylish dress shoe. . . $2.75."

Fig. 290. *Sears Roebuck Catalog*, 1902. "Ladies' Serge Congress, $0.85. This shoe is made from a good quality of serge, leather soles and counters, common sense last, and is not only a very cool and comfortable shoe, but will give excellent service."

Fig. 291. *Sears Roebuck Catalog*, 1907, p. 835. "The Elite, $1.85. Ladies' up to date Congress shoe, made from finest chrome vici kid, over the late style coin toe last, with fancy pattern leather tip and front stay. The sole is cut from flint stone oak sole leather, is very flexible, and will outwear any sole tanned. It fits like a glove, has no buttons or laces to annoy you, can be put on or taken off in an instant, is suitable for house or street wear, and is 50 per cent cheaper than any similar shoe of the same quality."

Fig. 292. *Ladies' Home Journal*, January 1908.

Fig. 293. *Shoe Retailer*, September 18, 1915, p. 33. "Named the 'Nancy Hanks,' all black kid gypsy Congress, patent front stay, welt sole, 2-inch leather Louis heel, welt. Shown by [style currently being introduced by] the Miller Shoe Mfg. Co., Cincinnati, O."

Fig. 294. *Charles Williams Stores Catalog*, Spring/Summer 1925, p. 229. "A Common Sense Juliet. Every woman should have a pair of these easy-fitting Juliets while working around the house, or for comfort during her leisure hours. Made of pliable black kid-finish leather over a comfortable wide toe last, elastic side gore, good leather soles, cushion rubber heels, smoothly finished inside. . . . $1.89."

Fig. 295. *Harper's Bazar*, March 4, 1876, p. 149. "Fig. f: this black kid boot has a high heel covered with leather. The sides are furnished with elastic. An ornamental piece of kid is stitched on the toe of the foot. The top buttoned on the boot is of kid lined with purple satin, and consists of two parts, which are closed with buttons. . . . A rosette of black silk ribbon and lace trims the middle of the top."

Fig. 296. *Sears Roebuck Catalog*, 1897. "Rich's Patent 'Julia Marlowe' Lace Boot . . . Pat. Aug 11—'96. . . . No. 3607. . . . Made from finest selection of Vici Kid, coin toe with patent leather tips, patent leather lace stay, fancy vamp and heel foxing . . . it yields to every action of the foot. It conforms in vital points to the shape of the wearer's foot instead of pressing the foot into the shape of the shoe."

Fig. 297. *Sears Roebuck Catalog*, 1902. "Latest style elastic instep lace, $2.38 . . . with elastic goring fitted to the instep in such a manner as to produce a perfectly elastic foot fitting boot. . . . This boot will conform to the shape of the foot whether the instep be high or low. Made from the very finest selection of Vici kid stock over our handsome Cincinnati last with plain stitched tip toe. The style of heel foxing is the very latest and we fit the shoe with a medium concave heel."

Fig. 298. *Sears Roebuck Catalog,* 1907, p. 839. "New gore lace, $2.19. A shoe that has jumped into popularity from the start . . a real health shoe and a true friend to the foot. The improved elastic goring allows the muscles of the foot free action as the goring (while footfitting) does not bind as tight as a lace shoe. Patent colt stock with dull mat calf top, strong combination, pull strap, perforated tip, military heel."

Fig. 299. Historic Northampton, #66.782. Black velvet boot with rounded square toe, Louis heel, and eight eyeleted tabs over an open front, ca. 1875–85.

Fig. 300. Connecticut Historical Society, #1978-45-29. White kid boot with rounded square toe, knock-on heel, open front and ankle-high back, fastening with gold silk laces through six pairs of eyelets. Made by Laird Schober of Philadelphia, ca. 1875–80.

Fig. 301. Peabody Essex Museum, #131,886. Bronze kid ankle-high boot with oval toe, knock-on heel, and four straps buttoning over an open front, ca. 1877–83.

Fig. 302. *Godey's Lady's Book,* December 1877. "Fig. 16.— Black satin boot for the house, laced upon the side, and fastened up the front with straps to show the fancy stocking underneath."

Fig. 303. *Shoe Retailer,* 1901. "This handsome, 'eight-strap sandal,' in black velvet and gilt, is one of the latest products of the N.D. Dodge & Bliss Co., of Newburyport, Mass. It is a shoe which the coming season will bring into vogue."

Fig. 304. *Sears Roebuck Catalog,* 1906, p. 1040. "The Stage Favorite, $2.13. . . . Vamp cut of best Corona patent colt, genuine hand turned sole, medium French heel, and handsomely beaded cross straps. Top made of best box kid, producing a novelty for house, party, or dancing, at a price within the reach of all."

Fig. 305. *Bellas Hess Catalog,* Fall 1914, p. 248. "High-Class Novelties in Ladies' Shoes. New Gaby Tango Boot for Dancing or Street Wear. . . . An extremely smart novelty which the up-to-date dresser will be sure to admire." Vamp of patent leather with steel buckle. Quarter of heavy black and white brocaded silk cloth. Turn sole, high spool leather heel.

Fig. 306. *Shoe Retailer,* September 17, 1921, p. 76. "Women's Advance Styles [available for sale by early in 1922]. A new four buckle slipper, called the 'Swiss,' all patent leather, red silk fitted vamp, quarter foxing and straps, three bar vamp perforation with red kid underlay and red stitched vamp, medium round toe, short vamp, turn sole. Shown by B. Adler, New York."

Fig. 307. *Sears Roebuck Catalog,* 1928–29, p. 275. Reprinted in Blum, *Everyday Fashions of the Twenties,* p. 129. "'Grecian Beauty' Boot . . . gleaming patent leather, cleverly topped by

reptile embossed calfskin. 1¾-inch covered heel. Marcelle last."

Fig. 308. *Ladies' Home Journal,* February 1915. "High Russian boots" in an article on "Spring's First New Dresses."

Fig. 309. *Sears Roebuck Catalog,* 1922, p. 235. Reprinted in Blum, *Everyday Fashions of the Twenties,* p. 56. "The Russian Boot . . . $4.95."

Fig. 310. Four major types of heel construction, generic pictures.

Fig. 311. Six major styles of heels with American fashion names, generic pictures.

Fig. 312. Peabody Essex Museum, #128,306. Slipper with pointed toe, Italian heel, white satin quarter, and embroidered blue satin vamp, worn by Maria Greene Sumner, ca. 1785–95. Label: "Women's Shoes & Slippers of all Sorts made and sold By James Newell, Middle Street, Boston."

Fig. 313. Valentine Museum, #61.97. Slipper of white kid stamped with a small black figure, with pointed toe and low Italian heel, ca. 1790–1805.

Fig. 314. Peabody Essex Museum, USMC #2164. White kid sandal with round toe, very low Italian heel, and eyeleted tabs for lacing with a silk ribbon, ca. 1805–10. See fig. 35.

Fig. 315. Lynn Museum, #2978. See credit for fig. 130.

Fig. 316. Historic Northampton, #1979.30.83. Pale-blue kid slipper with oval toe, short Louis heel (without the wedge typical of this period), and cutout vamp back with embroidered satin, worn by Helena Burrows Breese at her wedding on December 29, 1801. Label: "Reuben Bunn, Ladies Shoe Maker, No. 60, William Street, Formerly No. 39, Smith Street, Between Wall Street and Maiden-Lane."

Fig. 317. Bedford Historical Society, #C-24. Slippers of white silk with a foxing of white kid worn by Prudence Dean at her wedding in 1797.

Fig. 318. Connecticut Historical Society, #X1996.38.0. See credit for fig. 277.

Fig. 319. Museum of Fine Arts, Boston, #44.530. See credit for fig. 194.

Fig. 320. Connecticut Historical Society, #1971-15-1. See credit for fig. 195.

Fig. 321. *Jordan Marsh Almanac,* 1883 (illustrates styles of late 1882), Boot and Shoe Department. "Ladies' alligator Edson tie, Louis XV heel, hand-sewed turn, price $6.00."

Fig. 322. *Shoe Retailer,* September 21, 1904, p. 25. "New Fall Styles—Purple kid 'Francis' slipper, white kid insertion, Louis heel; made by Griffin-White Shoe Co., New York City."

Fig. 323. *Shoe Retailer,* September 18, 1915, p. 34. Advertisement by the Moore-Shafer Shoe Mfg. Co. for a button boot, "No. R962—Black corkscrew cloth top, patent vamp and foxing, medium welt sole, Spanish heel. . . . $2.60."

Fig. 324. *Shoe Retailer,* September 20, 1919, p. 87. "Women's

Spring and Summer Styles [for 1920]:" "New pattern in a patent opera pump with high throat giving tongue effect, heavy edge turn sole, full Louis celluloid covered wood heel. The Carfagno Shoe Co., Rochester."

Fig. 325. *Shoe Retailer*, October 2, 1926, p. 49. "Styles Certified by Leading Retailers." Oxford-type shoe with high spike heel recommended by Levy Bros. Dry Goods Co. of Houston.

Fig. 326. Connecticut Historical Society, #210. Pink satin slipper with round toe, spring heel, and silver embroidery on the vamp, ca. 1805–15.

Fig. 327. Danvers Historical Society, #60.7.1. White kid slipper with oval toe and no heel, worn by Tabitha Dana Leach at her wedding in 1812. For labels, see fig. 3.

Fig. 328. Old Sturbridge Village, #12.14.61. See credit for fig. 192.

Fig. 329. Black silk quilt-woven shoe foxed with morocco, with square toe, spring heel, furlike edging, and two pairs of ribbon ties, ca. 1845–55. Owned privately. See fig. 25.

Fig. 330. *Montgomery Ward Catalog*, No. 57, 1895, p. 509. "Ladies' Spring Heel [buttoned boot]. . . This shoe is made from fine glazed dongola kid and a shoe that will meet the desired wants of a great many. In the past the largest size attainable in this style was No. 2. In the last year we have had hundreds of orders, which we are unable to fill. Now we can offer you a shoe we can recommend, and we trust will be appreciated by those of our customers that could not obtain them heretofore. . . $2.15."

Fig. 331. SPNEA, #1936.203. Gold ribbed silk buttoned boot with rounded square toe, knock-on heel covered with white satin, and a rosette on the vamp, worn by Mary Richmond Buffington at her wedding in 1866.

Fig. 332. Danvers Historical Society, #DH2360. White kid slipper with bow on vamp and knock-on heel, said to date 1872.

Fig. 333. Peabody Essex Museum, USMC #2242. White satin side-lacing boot with rounded square toe, high knock-on heel, and hand-done embroidery down the front, made by the Bradley-Goodrich Co. for the Philadelphia Centennial Exposition in 1876.

Fig. 334. Morristown Historical Society, #83.13. White kid slipper with knock-on heel and rosette worn at a wedding on October 21, 1891.

Fig. 335. *John Wanamaker Catalog* No. 50, Spring/Summer, 1901, p. 153. Illustration of opera heel.

Fig. 336. Morristown Historical Society. White satin one-strap shoe with high knock-on heel and tulle rosette, worn at a wedding in 1911.

Fig. 337. *Shoe Retailer*, September 15, 1923, p. 51. "Autumn brown suede two button strap pump with cut-out strap,

without tip and covered military heel. The Kenworth Shoe Co., Cincinnati."

Fig. 338. *Sears Roebuck Catalog*, Fall/Winter, 1927–28. "Lorraine . . . $3.45 . . . patent leather covered wood heel, 1¾ inches high."

Fig. 339. *Ladies' Home Journal*, July 1929. One strap with contrast foxing, style name "Eva."

Fig. 340. Peabody Essex Museum, USMC #880. See credit for fig. 246.

Fig. 341. Peabody Essex Museum, USMC #1721. White figured silk slipper with oval toe, stacked heel, and a portrait of General Lafayette printed on vamp. Worn by Eliza Jane Kelley in 1824 at a ball honoring Lafayette. Label: "Warranted Boots & Shoes Sold Wholesale and Retail by [—] Greenough, [—] Middle Street [——, Mass?]."

Fig. 342. Topsfield Historical Society, #T-069. Slit-vamp tie shoe with square toe, low stack heel, tan morocco vamp, and brown serge quarters, ca. 1835–45.

Fig. 343. SPNEA, #1942.806. Blue serge side-lacing boot with turned soles and low stacked heels, marked 1852, and probably associated with a wedding. A piece of the blue plaid silk dress they were presumably worn with is preserved with the boots.

Fig. 344. Connecticut Historical Society, #1958-42-7. White kid slippers with ridiculously small stacked heels probably added after they were made, worn by Mary Elizabeth Carter Brinley at her wedding in 1871.

Fig. 345. Peabody Essex Museum, USMC #2294. See credit for fig. 252.

Fig. 346. Peabody Essex Museum, USMC #2418. See credit for fig. 265.

Fig. 347. Museum of Fine Arts, Boston, #43.2514. Tan colonial slipper with oval toe, stacked heel, and ornamental metal buckle, worn by Sarah Lord Day McCormick, ca.1904–5.

Fig. 348. Dorothy Dodd Catalog, Autumn/Winter, 1908, p. 26. "This kid boot is made with light flexible turn sole, on a high arched last . . . $3.50."

Fig. 349. Dorothy Dodd Catalog, Autumn/Winter, 1908, p. 27. "Patent kid boot. Made with light, flexible sole, medium heel and toe. . . . $3.00."

Fig. 350. SPNEA, #1990.51. Button boot with black patent vamp and foxing, brown cloth top, and stacked leather heel, ca. 1914–16. Label: Thayer McNeil Co., Boston.

Fig. 351. *Shoe Retailer*, September 22, 1917, p. 31. Advertisement for front-lacing boots by Hallahan and Sons, Inc., Philadelphia. "Style 88. Finest Black Glace Kid, Liberty height (nine-inch) laced boot, leather Louis heel, plain toe, Brighton (825) last, light welted sole. Price $5.75."

Fig. 352. *Shoe Retailer*, September 22, 1917, p. 53. "Women's

Spring & Summer Styles—1918: Eight-inch Russia calf lace boot, small perforations on tip, quarter and vamp, 10/8 heel. Shown by The Manss-Owens Co., Cincinnati, O."

Fig. 353. *Shoe Retailer*, December 4, 1926, p. 49. Advertisement by the Craddock-Terry Co., of Lynchburg, Va. Three strapped shoes and one oxford, all with welted soles, show the same "leather heel, rubber tap."

Fig. 354. Haverhill Historical Society, #9362. See credit for fig. 167.

Fig. 355. Bedford Historical Society, #C-24. See credit for fig. 317.

Fig. 356. Historic Northampton, #66.635. Dark bluish-green morocco latchet tie shoe with pointed toe and very low Italian heel worn by Anna Stoddard Williams at her wedding on April 28, 1799.

Fig. 357. Tioga County Historical Society, #80.19.3. Slipper of gold silk with tiny woven dot, with pointed toe, spring heel, and black silk binding, ca. 1800–1805. Worn by Sarah Swan, born 1777, married 1795.

Fig. 358. Peter Oakley collection. Heavy black leather slippers with pointed toe and very low stacked heel, ca. 1800–1810.

Fig. 359. Peabody Essex Museum, USMC #2164. See credit for fig. 314.

Fig. 360. Museum of Fine Arts, Boston, #51.346. Sandal-type shoe of nankeen foxed with red morocco and bound with red silk, with oval toe, low Italian heel, red silk ribbons, ca. 1805–10.

Fig. 361. Lynn Museum, #2978. See credit for fig. 130.

Fig. 362. Peabody Essex Museum, USMC #880. See credit for fig. 246.

Fig. 363. Historic Northampton, #1976.137.1 White kid slipper with oval toe, spring heel, and vamp cutouts backed with embroidered satin, worn by Sarah Poole Brewer at her wedding in 1810. Label almost identical to that in fig. 4.

Fig. 364. Danvers Historical Society, #60.7.1. See credit for fig. 327. For labels, see fig. 3.

Fig. 365. Haverhill Historical Society, #2821. See credit for fig. 104.

Fig. 366. Peabody Essex Museum, #135,384. White kid slipper with oval toe, spring heel, and a vamp that has been slit and laced, marked "1816." Label: "S. Driver, 3d & Co. Fashionable Boot and Shoe Store, No. 7 Old Paved Street, Salem, Rips mended gratis."

Fig. 367. Rhode Island Historical Society, #1983.14.8. Tan and brown striped silk slipper with pointed toe and spring heel said to have been worn by Nan Osborne of S. Danvers, Mass., at her wedding in 1820.

Fig. 368. Peabody Essex Museum, USMC #1721. See credit for fig. 341.

Fig. 369. Peabody Essex Museum, #104,997. See credit for fig. 188.

Fig. 370. SPNEA, #1936.611. See credit for fig. 272.

Fig. 371. Connecticut Historical Society, #1972-63-2. See credit for fig. 106.

Fig. 372. Danvers Historical Society, #37.10.6. Off-white twilled wool slippers with square toe, no heel, and pleated silk ribbon at throatline, worn by Polly Gould Weston of Middleton, Mass., at her wedding in 1831.

Fig. 373. Connecticut Historical Society, #1960-24-5. White kid slipper with square toe and no heel worn by Eliza Heyer Polhumus at her wedding in 1835.

Fig. 374. Peabody Essex Museum, USMC #1538. Side-lacing shoe of fancy black serge foxed with black kid, with a narrow square toe, made by Edward Swain Davis of Lynn, Mass., and exhibited with other examples of his work at the Exposition of the Mass. Charitable Mechanics Association of New England in 1839. See also figs. 189, 211, and 455.

Fig. 375. Topsfield Historical Society, #T-069. See credit for fig. 342.

Fig. 376. Connecticut Historical Society, #1956-5-5. See credit for fig. 191.

Fig. 377. Peabody Essex Museum, USMC #593. See credit for fig. 190.

Fig. 378. Rhode Island Historical Society, #1985.22.19. White satin side-lacing boots with rounded square toe and no heel worn by Abigail Angenetta Blake at her wedding in 1852.

Fig. 379. Peabody Essex Museum, USMC #1959. Black calf slit-vamp shoe with rounded square toe and pegged sole, ca. 1850–60. See fig. 62.

Fig. 380. SPNEA, #1942.806. See credit for fig. 343.

Fig. 381. Peabody Essex Museum, USMC #1838. See credit for fig. 288.

Fig. 382. Peabody Essex Museum, USMC #2005. Black serge front-lacing boot with scalloped patent toe cap and low stacked heel. Bears 1860 license stamp for McKay Sewing Machine, 1860–70.

Fig. 383. Peabody Essex Museum, USMC #1851. Black serge elastic-sided boot with rounded square toe, stacked heel, and sole ornamented at the waist, 1865–75.

Fig. 384. Los Angeles County Museum of Art, #37.15.7. See credit for fig. 249.

Fig. 385. Connecticut Historical Society, #x1996.38.0. See credit for fig. 277.

Fig. 386. Peabody Essex Museum, USMC #1714. Black grained kip single-latchet tie ("Newport") with rounded square toe, low stacked heel, and pegged sole, 1870–80.

Fig. 387. Haverhill Historical Society, #10.099. White kid slipper with rounded square toe, knock-on heel, square tongue, pinked leather rosette, and silver buckle, worn by Sara S. H. Cheney at her wedding January 16, 1873.

Fig. 388. Peabody Essex Museum, USMC #2249. White kid side-lacing boot with knock-on heel made by Goodrich and Porter of Haverhill for the Philadelphia Centennial Exposition in 1876.

Fig. 389. Peabody Essex Museum, USMC #2252. See credit for fig. 278.

Fig. 390. Peabody Essex Museum, USMC #2251. Bronze kid side-lacing boot with duckbill toe, stacked heel, and ornamented sole, made by Goodrich and Porter of Haverhill for the Philadelphia Centennial Exposition in 1876.

Fig. 391. Peabody Essex Museum, USMC #1342. Pink kid buttoned boot with rounded square toe and knock-on heel, purchased at Rogers and Co., Boston for $15 in 1877.

Fig. 392. SPNEA, #1920.61. Black satin one-strap shoe with rounded toe, Louis heel, and embroidered vamp, ca. 1877–80. Label: "Perchellet, 26 Rue Louis le Grand, du coin de la rue du 4 Septembre. L. Perchellet, Breveté S.G.D.G. Fab^t des Chaussure à Ressorts pour Hommes et pour dames, Paris."

Fig. 393. Connecticut Historical Society, #1961-64-45. White satin buttoned shoe with rounded toe and Louis heel, ca. 1877–85.

Fig. 394. Vermont Historical Society, #54.35.5. White kid slipper with rounded toe, knock-on heel, and layered bow, worn at a wedding in 1881.

Fig. 395. Peabody Essex Museum, USMC #1733. See credit for fig. 253.

Fig. 396. Peabody Essex Museum, USMC #2418. See credit for fig. 265.

Fig. 397. SPNEA, #1943.637. Black kid cross-strap shoe with rhinestone buttons, oval toe and Louis heel, ca. 1885–90. Marked "Jolly, Paris."

Fig. 398. Morristown Historical Society, #56.293. Black kid buttoned boot with oval toe and stacked heel worn by Emma Massey Cheney at her wedding on August 21, 1890.

Fig. 399. Peabody Essex Museum, USMC #2457. Brown calf front-laced boot with oval toe, low stacked heel, and vamp and trimming of black patent leather, made by Selz-Schwab of Chicago for the World's Columbian Exposition in Chicago in 1893.

Fig. 400. Peabody Essex Museum, USMC #2351. See credit for fig. 135.

Fig. 401. Peabody Essex Museum, USMC #2312. Dark-brown kid oxford shoe with long pointed toe and stacked heel made by Rice and Hutchins of Marlboro, Mass., in 1898.

Fig. 402. *Shoe Retailer*, May 22, 1901, p. 28. Patent calf and black velvet tie shoe with high Louis heel made by B. Cohen and Sons of New York.

Fig. 403. Museum of Fine Arts, Boston, #42.2514. See credit for fig. 347.

Fig. 404. Museum of Fine Arts, Boston, #53.1067. Tan suede one-eyelet tie shoe with pointed toe, knock-on heel, pointed tongue, and broad silk laces, dated by donor 1908. Label: "Jones, Peterson & Newhall, 48 & 50 Temple Pl, Boston."

Fig. 405. Morristown Historical Society. See credit for fig. 336.

Fig. 406. Peabody Essex Museum, USMC #2130. Buttoned boot with black enamel foxing, black serge top, rounded toe, and stacked heel, ca. 1911–14. Made by A. E. Little and Co., Lynn, Mass. Label: "Sorosis."

Fig. 407. *Ladies' Home Journal*, November 1915. Advertisement for Cat's Paw rubber heels.

Fig. 408. Peabody Essex Museum, USMC #1491. High front-lacing boot with calf vamp, gray suede top, rounded toe, and high Louis heel, the first shoe made by the Cornell Shoe Co., Brooklyn, in 1916.

Fig. 409. *Shoe Retailer*, September 18, 1915, p. 37. Advertisement for the G and R Shoe Company, Lynn, Mass., showing six different toe styles.

Fig. 410. *Ladies' Home Journal*, August, 1918. Advertisement for Neolin Soles.

Fig. 411. Peabody Essex Museum, USMC #2344. Black kid and patent cross-strap shoe made on a French-style short-vamp last with very round toe and high knock-on heel by Rice and Hutchins of Marlboro, Mass., in 1922.

Fig. 412. Vermont Historical Society, #70.14.15. White kid one-strap shoe with pointed toe, high Louis heel, and ribbon tie, associated with a wedding of 1923.

Fig. 413. Peabody Essex Museum, USMC #2417. Black kid and calf buttoned shoe with oval toe and knock-on heel made by Dr. Kahler of Boston in 1923.

Fig. 414. SPNEA, #1932.2301. Open-tab tie shoe of calf and imitation snakeskin with oval toe and knock-on heel, worn by Mrs. E. F. Larrabee in spring 1931. Label: "Made for Hanan & Son Retail Stores, Boston."

Fig. 415. Peabody Essex Museum, USMC #2293. Tan kid cross-strap shoe with rounded toe and high covered wood heel, said to have been made in 1928.

Fig. 416. *Shoe Retailer*, February 18, 1928, p. 64. Advertisement by the Essex Rubber Co. of Trenton, N.J., for Plytex soles and heels.

Fig. 417. *Sears Roebuck Catalog*, 1933, p. 208. Reprinted in Blum, *Everyday Fashions of the Thirties*, p. 52. Two-tone sports shoe with rubber sole and one-inch heel with rubber top lift, $1.59.

Fig. 418. Diagram of a recede toe in a turn shoe.

Fig. 419. Diagram of a recede toe in a McKay shoe.

Fig. 420. Diagram of a blunt toe with toe box.

Fig. 421. Danvers Historical Society, #60.7.1. See credit for fig. 327. For labels, see fig. 3.

Fig. 422. Philadelphia Museum of Art, #28.38.12. Brown serge slit-vamp shoe with oval toe, domed waist, and one-inch stacked heel, ca. 1825.

Fig. 423. Historic Northampton, #66.644. See credit for fig. 107.

Fig. 424. Old Sturbridge Village, #12.14.61. See credit for fig. 192.

Fig. 425. Peabody Essex Museum, USMC #1714. See credit for fig. 386.

Fig. 426. Colonial Dames, #1949.60. Blue-and-green plaid wool buttoned boot with black patent foxing, rounded square toe, and Louis heel, ca. 1872–76. See plate 8.

Fig. 427. SPNEA, #1920.61. See credit for fig. 392.

Fig. 428. Peabody Essex Museum, USMC #2292. Black serge side-lacing boot with black kid foxing, stacked heel, and square domed toe, made by Goodrich and Porter for the Philadelphia Centennial Exposition in 1876.

Fig. 429. *Ladies' Home Journal*, January, 1892. Advertisement by H. Fargo and Co. of Chicago for "Fargo's $2.50 Ladies' Boot."

Fig. 430. *Sears Roebuck Catalog*, 1897. "Ladies' Oxford Vici Kid Lace . . . No. 3534 . . . dark wine (ox blood) color, long drawn out needle toe and tip . . . $2.35."

Fig. 431. Peabody Essex Museum, USMC #2367. Front-lacing boot with brown kid top and black kid vamp, flat forepart, and shallow domed toe, ca. 1900.

Fig. 432. *Shoe Retailer*, September 28, 1907, p. 47. "Lynn Styles in Women's Footwear For Spring and Summer, 1908 . . . Narrow toe, 'Prince Chap' oxford. Shown by Levirs & Sargent, Lynn, Mass."

Fig. 433. *Shoe Retailer*, September 16, 1911, p. 3. Advertisement by the Rich Shoe Company, Milwaukee, Wisc., for Julia Marlowe footwear, "Spring 1912 Beauties."

Fig. 434. *Shoe Retailer*, September 20, 1919, p. 81. "Women's Spring & Summer [1920] Styles: Havana brown kid two strap pump, four inch vamp, plain toe, covered Louis wood heel, light welt sole, close trimmed edge. The O'Donnell Shoe Mfg. Co., St. Paul, Minn."

Fig. 435. *Shoe Retailer*, December 18, 1926, p. 37. Advertisement by Murphy & Saval Co., Chicago, for "Tom Boy" welt type McKays. . . . $8.50 and $10.00." Style name, "Giggles."

Fig. 436. Diagram of soles, straights.

Fig. 437. Diagram of soles, minimal right/left differentiation.

Fig. 438. Diagram of soles, strong right/left differentiation (swing).

Fig. 439. Historic Northampton, #1985.29.4. Slipper made of early-eighteenth-century floral silk with pointed toe and spring heel, worn by Elizabeth Martin of Woodstock, Conn., ca. 1800–1805.

Fig. 440. Historic Northampton, #1979.30.83. See credit for fig. 316.

Fig. 441. Rhode Island Historical Society, #1928.8.1. Black satin slipper with pointed toe, spring heel, and vamp cutouts

backed with gray silk, worn by Frances Mary Eldredge Lyman of Brooklyn, Conn., at her wedding on June 26, 1811.

Fig. 442. Historic Northampton, #1976.137.1. See credit for fig. 363.

Fig. 443. Museum of Fine Arts, Boston, #51.346. See credit for fig. 360.

Fig. 444. Peabody Essex Museum, #112,941. Pink figured-silk slipper with round toe, thin covered heel, and gold sequin embroidery on the vamp. Label: "Duchamp, Cordonnier, rue l'Hôpital St. André, no. 8 à Bordeaux."

Fig. 445. Vermont Historical Society, #1986.10 (Old Constitution House #75-55-62). Yellow kid slipper printed with black, with oval toe, spring heel, and a rosette of paillettes and silver bouillon, ca. 1810.

Fig. 446. Colonial Dames, Boston, #1952.532. Yellow kid slipper with fringe and buckle ornament, ca. 1810. See plate 2. For label, see fig. 4.

Fig. 447. Danvers Historical Society, #60.7.1. See credit for fig. 327. For labels, see fig. 3.

Fig. 448. Danvers Historical Society, #37.10.6. See credit for fig. 372.

Fig. 449. Peabody Essex Museum, USMC #1721. See credit for fig. 341.

Fig. 450. Old Sturbridge Village, #26.25.78. Slipper made of blue and white ticking worked in cross-stitch on the white stripes, with oval toe, spring heel pegged on, and a blue ribbon bow on the vamp, ca. 1815.

Fig. 451. Connecticut Historical Society, #1981-15-10. White kid shoe with oval toe and two bows on the vamp, ca. 1815–25.

Fig. 452. Rhode Island Historical Society, #1980.86.16. Tan serge slipper with oval toe, low stacked heel, and small rosette at the throat worn by Mary Wilbur Hazard of Hopkinton, R.I., at her wedding on October 2, 1828. Label: "G & R Johnson, Norwich, CT, Boot & Shoe Manufacturer, Rips Sewed Gratis."

Fig. 453. Colonial Dames, #71E. Beige serge slipper with oval toe and stiffly pleated rosette at the throat, ca. 1825–30. See plate 3.

Fig. 454. Rhode Island Historical Society, #1983.14.4. Bronze slippers with square toe and small bow at throat, ca. 1835–45.

Fig. 455. Peabody Essex Museum, USMC #1537. Black kid slipper with square toe and small flat bow held in place with a gold buckle, made by Edward Swain Davis of Lynn, Mass., and exhibited with other examples of his work at the Exposition of the Massachussetts Charitable Mechanics Association of New England in 1839. See also figs. 189, 211, and 374.

Fig. 456. Peabody Essex Museum, #103,126. White satin

slipper with rounded square toe, no heel, and tiny bow, ca. 1850. Esté label of type illustrated in fig. 5c.

Fig. 457. Connecticut Historical Society, #1956-5-5. See credit for fig. 191.

Fig. 458. Historic Northampton, #66.656. See credit for fig. 108.

Fig. 459. Peabody Essex Museum, #120,574. White satin slipper with rounded square toe, no heel, and large bow added at throat, ca. 1850–55. Esté label of type illustrated in fig. 5c.

Fig. 460. Black kid shoe with thin black satin rosette backed with black lace and topped with a pleated length of black velvet ribbon edged with white, ca. 1855–65. Label: Viault-Esté. Owned privately.

Fig. 461. *Godey's Lady's Book*, December 1861. "Shoe Rosette."

Fig. 462. Peabody Essex Museum, #127,013. White twilled cotton slipper with rounded square toe and pompon-style rosette, ca. 1860–70.

Fig. 463. Connecticut Historical Society, #1960-57-2E. Black kid slipper with rounded square toe, low stacked heel, and large velvet bow, ca. 1865–75.

Fig. 464. Historic Northampton, #66.660. Bronze kid slipper with rosette of brown silk ribbon pleated into leaflike vandykes, ca. 1865–70. Worn by Jane Damon Smith.

Fig. 465. Historic Northampton, #66.669. White kid slipper with rounded square toe, knock-on heel, and leather bow edged with braid, worn by Amelia Clark at her high school graduation in 1871.

Fig. 466. Peabody Essex Museum, #126,721. White natural silk slipper with binding and embroidery of purple silk, 1855–65.

Fig. 467. Historic Northampton, #66.658. Bronze kid with rounded square toe, no heel, and vamp cutouts backed with light blue silk, ca. 1855–65.

Fig. 468. Historic Northampton, #66.659. Bronze kid with rounded square toe, no heel, and vamp cutouts backed with rose silk, ca. 1865–70. Label: "Jolly 125."

Fig. 469. Peabody Essex Museum, USMC #2235. Black kid one-strap shoe with rounded square toe, stacked heel, and a cutout vamp with purple silk underlay and cut-steel buckle, made by Goodrich and Porter for the 1876 Philadelphia Centennial Exposition.

Fig. 470. Peabody Essex Museum, USMC #2297. Black patent shoe with rounded square toe, knock-on heel, and cutout vamp with gold kid underlay made by Bradley, Goodrich of Haverhill for the 1876 Philadelphia Centennial Exposition.

Fig. 471. Historic Northampton #66.673. Bronze kid slipper with rounded toe, knock-on heel, and cutout vamp lined with rough-textured brown wool, ca. 1880.

Fig. 472. SPNEA, #1932.2695. Black patent side-gore shoe with pointed toe, Louis heel, and trellislike cutouts on the vamp, edged with black beads, ca. 1890.

Fig. 473. Valentine Museum, #65.150.1. See credit for fig. 229.

Fig. 474. Museum of Fine Arts, Boston, #44.530. See credit for fig. 194.

Fig. 475. SPNEA, #1920.61. See credit for fig. 392.

Fig. 476. *Godey's Lady's Magazine*, May 1881. "Fig. 25.— Slipper for evening wear, made of white satin embroidered with gold thread." Also illustrated in *Harper's Bazar*, January 22, 1881, p. 52, as "lady's ball slipper with Spanish embroidery."

Fig. 477. *Harper's Bazar*, January 21, 1882, p. 36. "Embroidered kid slipper."

Fig. 478. *Harper's Bazar*, May 25, 1889, p. 384. Illustrated in a group of "walking and traveling shoes."

Fig. 479. Historic Northampton, #66.671. White kid slipper with rounded square toe, knock-on heel, large white silk rosette, and mother-of-pearl buckle, worn by Laura Agnes Shaw Hudson of Plainfield, Mass., at her wedding on September 8, 1871. Label: "A Moll [?] The Great Leading Fashionable Shoe Emporium, 1125 & 1187 Broadway & 28th St. [New York]." See fig. 39.

Fig. 480. Haverhill Historical Society, #10.099. See credit for fig. 387.

Fig. 481. Valentine Museum, #65.150.2. Black kid slipper with rounded square toe, stacked heel, scalloped tongue, and leather bow, 1871–76. Patent date on sole, August 16, 1870.

Fig. 482. Historic Northampton #66.672. White satin slipper with oval toe, knock-on heel, and tiered bow, worn by Fannie Burr Look at her wedding on October 20, 1880. See fig. 39.

Fig. 483. Vermont Historical Society, #54.35.5. See credit for fig. 394.

Fig. 484. Connecticut Historical Society, #1974-114-2. See credit for fig. 110.

Fig. 485. Danvers Historical Society, #DH-2358. White kid slippers with oval toe, knock-on heel, satin bow, and pleating at throat, said to date 1887.

Fig. 486. Colonial Dames, #x2000.4. Black kid slipper with rounded toe, low stacked heel, steel-beaded vamp, and steel-beaded black satin bow and pleating at the throat, ca. 1880–90.

Fig. 487. Peabody Essex Museum, #103,495. Off-white satin slippers with oval toe, Louis heel, beaded vamp, and narrow bow, ca. 1890.

Fig. 488. Historic Northampton, #66.683. Black satin slippers with pointed toe, Louis heel, tiered bow, and beaded vamp, ca. 1895. Label: "Thayer, McNeil & Hodgkins, 47 Temple Place, London."

Fig. 489. Historic Northampton, #66.675. White kid slipper with narrow oval toe, low knock-on heel, and tailored bow, worn by Annie Porter at her wedding in 1891. See fig. 42.

Fig. 490. Haverhill Historical Society, #6595. White kid slipper with oval toe, low stacked heel, and beaded bow on the strap, said to have been worn in 1895.

Fig. 491. Historic Northampton, #1978.15.1. Tan kid one-strap shoe with pointed toe, high knock-on heel, and grosgrain ribbon bow, ca. 1910.

Fig. 492. *Shoe Retailer*, September 16, 1911, 58. Advertisement by the Julian & Kokenge Co., Cincinnati, for their pumps and Colonials.

Fig. 493. Historic Northampton, #66.499. White satin slipper with pointed toe, Louis heel, and tulle rosette, worn by Mrs. Charles Hills at her wedding in 1909.

Fig. 494. Peabody Essex Museum, #134,694. Blue velvet "Tango" slipper with narrow oval toe, jeweled Louis heel, and long blue satin ribbons to tie around the ankle, ca. 1914.

Fig. 495. *Shoe Retailer*, March 17, 1928, p. 50. "A decidedly chic pump effect in this black patent step-in of Lape & Adler Co., Columbus, Ohio, with beaded buckle and concealed goring."

Fig. 496. *Shoe Retailer*, January 21, 1928, p. 79. Advertisement by Abe Manheimer and Co., Inc., St. Louis, "No.10199—Leather, Per doz. pair . . . $9.00."

Fig. 497. *Shoe Retailer*, January 21, 1928, p. 79. Advertisement by Abe Manheimer and Co., Inc., St. Louis. "No. 10217, Satin or grosgrain ribbon with rhinestone ornament. Per dozen pair . . . $9.00."

Fig. 498. *Shoe Retailer*, March 17, 1928, p. 57. "Printed linen one strap pattern, black patent trimming and heel by The Riley Shoe Mfg. Co., of Columbus, Ohio."

Fig. 499. Peabody Essex Museum, USMC #2207. Black enamel kid shoe with narrow oval toe, knock-on heel, and two straps, one beneath a flaring three-part tongue and another beneath a velvet bow, made by Goodrich and Porter of Haverhill for the World's Columbian Exposition in Chicago in 1893.

Fig. 500. *Sears Roebuck Catalog*, 1902. "The Goodyear Welt Colonial Dame, $1.95."

Fig. 501. *Shoe Retailer*, September 28, 1907, p. 8. Advertisement by the Lindner Shoe Co. of Carlisle, Pa. No description.

Fig. 502. Museum of Fine Arts, Boston, #53.1067. See credit for fig. 404.

Fig. 503. *Shoe Retailer*, September 16, 1911, p. 84. Advertisement by the P. J. Harney Shoe Co., Lynn, Mass., for Colonials for spring 1912.

Fig. 504. *Shoe Retailer*, September 20, 1913, p. 32. "Patent colt colonial pump, high arch and narrow recede toe, close trimmed edge, 2-inch wood kidney enamel heel, cut steel buckle,

welt. Shown by [style currently being introduced by] Irving Drew Co., Portsmouth, O."

Fig. 505. *Shoe Retailer*, September 18, 1915, p. 36. Advertisement by Hazen B. Goodrich and Co., Haverhill, Mass., for their spring 1916 line. Style name, "Plaza."

Fig. 506. *Shoe Retailer*, September 20, 1919, p. 87. "Women's Spring & Summer [1920] Styles: One eyelet colonial pump, black glazed kid, quarter over, worn with buckle or ribbon tie, 3 3/4-inch vamp, narrow toe, light welt, leather Louis heel. John Ebberts Shoe Co., Buffalo, N. Y."

Fig. 507. *Shoe Retailer*, December 18, 1926, p. 37. Advertisement by Murphy and Saval Co., Chicago, for "'Tom Boy' Welt Type McKays: 'Bow Wow.'"

Fig. 508. *Savage's Catalog*, 1927/28, p. 53. Reprinted in Blum, *Everyday Fashions of the Twenties*, p. 106.

Fig. 509. Peabody & Essex Museum, USMC #880. See credit for fig. 246.

Fig. 510. Valentine Museum, #43.23.1. See credit for fig. 248.

Fig. 511. *Petit Courrier des Dames*, June 1831, #813.

Fig. 512. SPNEA, #1936.203. See credit for fig. 331.

Fig. 513. SPNEA, #1940.1012. See credit for fig. 251.

Fig. 514. *Godey's Lady's Book*, February 1869, fig. 19. "Walking boot of light-colored cloth, ornamented with gray fur and the heads of the animal."

Fig. 515. *Godey's Lady's Book*, August, 1872, fig. 8. "Promenade boot to button. Glove kid tops, patent leather fronts, and trimmed with patent leather, stitched with white silk."

Fig. 516. Haverhill Historical Society, #4.2.a-b (in Centennial Showcase). Black serge side-lacing boot with rounded square toe, knock-on heel, and decorative white machine stitching up the center front seam, 1876.

Fig. 517. Peabody Essex Museum, USMC #2242. See credit for fig. 333.

Fig. 518. *Harper's Bazar*, July 15, 1882, p. 437, fig. g.

Fig. 519. Peabody Essex Museum, USMC #2457. See credit for fig. 399.

Fig. 520. *Montgomery Ward Catalog*, 1895. "The Juliet. 52148 . . . very fine French dongola kid, with hand turned soles, fancy patent leather stay up the front. . . . $2.50."

Fig. 521. *Sears Roebuck Catalog*, 1897. "No. 3906. Ladies' Beaver Congress, felt lined throughout, with leather sole and heel; also leather side patches. . . . $1.00."

Fig. 522. *Sears Roebuck Catalog*, 1897, p. 193. "Ladies' calf Polish, made from the best all calf stock, half double soles and hand pegged. This is a strictly western custom made shoe, and there is nothing better for heavy wear at any price. . . . $1.70."

Fig. 523. *Sears Roebuck Catalog*, 1900, p. 488. "Ladies' Changeable Silk Vesting Top Shoes, tan or black. . . . kid back stay and a kid lace stay, both of which come just high enough to protect the vesting top from coming in contact with the skirts. The silk vesting cloth top is the very best French made, being a gold brown with black figures which produces altogether the daintiest combination we have seen. . . $1.95.”

Fig. 524. *Shoe Retailer*, April 3, 1901, p. 27. Advertisement by Hoag and Walden Makers, Lynn, Mass., for “Ladies’ Swell Shoes . . . Modern Shapes . . . Extreme Edges.”

Fig. 525. *Shoe Retailer*, September 28, 1907, p. 8. Advertisement by The Lindner Shoe Co., Carlisle, Pa.

Fig. 526. *Shoe Retailer*, September 18, 1915, p. 28. “For the white season [Spring and Summer 1916], genuine white buck bal., perforated ball strap, tip, vamp and lace stay, light-weight white rubber sole with reinforced toe piece. Shown by Slater & Morrill, Inc., So. Braintree, Mass.”

Fig. 527. *Shoe Retailer*, September 18, 1915, p. 30. “New black and white combination. A 14-button, black kid gypsy cut boot, white calf tip and front stay combined, white calf covered two-inch Louis wood heel with black top lift. Light welt sole. Shown by the Murray Shoe Co., Lynn [for spring/summer 1916].”

Fig. 528. *Sears Roebuck Catalog*, Fall/Winter, 1927. Winter boot “made of black genuine kid leather, fleece lined. Roomy round toe. 1-inch heel with rubber top lift.”

Index of Illustrated and Cited Shoes

Alphabetically by Museum

(W) = associated with a wedding

(E) = associated with an exhibition or trade show

Date	Description	Catalog No.	Illustration/Page No.
Albany Institute of History and Art, 125 Washington Ave., Albany, NY 12210-2296			
1850–1860	Rubber overshoes, man's		p. 155
1856	Side-lacing boot, red wool, riding	1941.45	plate 16, p. 133
Barre Historical Society, Aldrich Public Library, Barre, VT 05641			
1880–90	Button shoe, purple brocade top	——	p. 193
Bedford Historical Society, 15 The Great Road, Bedford, MA 01730			
1797 (W)	Slipper, white silk & kid	C-24	Figs. 317, 355, pp. 216, 223
Brown, Elizabeth S., Belle Mead, NJ 08502			
1883 (W)	Slipper, white kid, elastic strap	Buddington, 4.75.5	Fig. 226
Colonial Dames (National Society of the Colonial Dames in the Commonwealth of Massachusetts), 55 Beacon St., Boston, MA 02108			
1790–1800	Tie shoe, blue satin, Hon Sing label	1948.50	Plate 2, p. 11, 184
1795–1805	Boot, front-lace, green kid	1952.50	Figs. 36, 245, pp. 74, 198
1795–1805	Slipper, purple kid stamped in tan	1952.7	Plate 2, p. 239
1805–1810	Slipper, red satin	1952.533	Plate 2
1805–15	Slipper, yellow kid, fringe & buckle	1952.532	Plate 2, Figs. 4, 446, p. 11
1815–25	Tie shoe, tan kid, blue binding	1952.105	Plate 3, p. 244
1815–25	Slipper, green figured silk	1952.101	Plate 3
1815–25	Slipper, pale pink kid, tassel	1952.102	Plate 3
1825–30	Slipper, tan serge, rosette	71E	Plate 3, Fig. 453
1865–67	Side-lacing boot, green silk	1960.169	Plate 8
1865–70	Button boot, bronze kid, tassel	1956.115	Plate 8, p. 258
1872–76	Button boot, blue-green plaid silk	1949.60	Plate 8, Fig. 426
1878–80	Slipper, tan silk, large rosette	1949.45	Plate 9
1880–1920	Bathing boot, black knit	1957.81	p. 138
1885–90	Slipper, black kid, beaded rosette	x2000.4	Fig. 486
1885–90	Button boot, rust-brown silk	1955.1	Plate 8

Date	Description	Catalog No.	Illustration/Page No.
Colonial Dames (*cont.*)			
1885–90	Tie shoe, bronze kid, beaded	1961.23	Plate 9
1890 (W)	Slipper, pink satin, embroidered	1961.32	Plate 9
1890–95	Slipper, chartreuse silk	1938.97-8	Plate 9
1893–1900	Tie shoe, tan kid, perforated	1952.189	Plate 11
1900–1905	Colonial, tan kid, French label	1956.143	Plate 11
1900–1905	Four-strap shoe, cream suede	1989.22	Plate 11
1915	Slipper, red satin, throat ornament	1965.188D	Plate 12
1915–16	Button shoe, gray suede, cutout, beads	1956.134	Plate 11
1917–21	Slipper, silver fabric	1947.1	Plate 12
1921–24	Cross-strap, black and gold brocade	1982.39	Plate 12
1923–26	Slipper, black satin, jeweled heel	x2000.1	Plate 12
1924–30	T-strap, white canvas, black patent	1956.138	Plate 11
1933	T-strap, purple, gold, cutouts	1981.85	Plate 12
Connecticut Historical Society, 1 Elizabeth St., Hartford, CT 06105			
1795–1805	Slipper, white kid, pointed toe	1960-57-2A	Fig. 102
1798 (W)	Slipper, white satin	1958-2-1-6	Fig. 121, p. 216
1805–15	Slipper, pink satin, silver embroidery	210	Fig. 326
1810 (W)	Slipper, blue kid, loops for ribbons	1983-80-1	pp. 223, 357
1810–30	Gaiters, nankeen, leather strap	1963-8-6	p. 161
1815–25	Slipper, white kid, two bows	1981-15-10	Fig. 451
1830 (W)	Slipper, white satin, square toe	1972-63-2	Figs. 106, 371
1835 (W)	Slipper, white kid, square toe	1960-24-5	Fig. 373, p. 225
1845–60	Rubbers, imitate oxford shoe pattern	1963-33-1&2	Fig. 85a, p. 155
1846 (W)	Tie shoe, tan kid, patterned serge	1956-5-5	Figs. 191, 376, 457, p. 188
1862 (W)	Slipper, white satin, large bow	1974-24-2	p. 225
1865–70	Side-lacing boot, white satin	x1996.38.0	Figs. 277, 318, 385
1865–75	Slipper, black kid, velvet bow	1960-57-2E	Fig. 463
1865–75	Rubber-coated over-boot with buckle	1960-37-14G	Fig. 85b, p. 156
1871 (W)	Slipper, white kid, rosette, tiny heel	1958-42-7	Fig. 344
1875–80	Open-front boot, white kid, gold laces	1978-45-29	Fig. 300
1877–85	Button shoe, white satin, bow	1961-64-45	Fig. 393
1885 (W)	Slipper, white kid, tiered rosette	1974-114-2	Figs. 110, 484
1891 (W)	Cross-strap white suede, beaded	1942	Fig. 133
1894 (W)	Tie shoe, white kid, Louis heel	1971-15-1	Figs. 195, 320, p. 189
1895–1930	Bathing shoes, cross-strap, black	1959-72-20	Fig. 72j, p. 138
1896–1900	Bicycling boots	1983-45-1	p. 139
Danvers Historical Society, 7 Page St., PO Box 381, Danvers, MA 01923			
1812 (W)	Slippers, white kid Perkins/Vose labels	60.7.1	Figs. 3, 327, 364, 421, 447, pp. 11, 218, 223
1831 (W)	Slippers, white serge, pleated edge	37.10.6	Figs. 372, 448
1869 (W)	Slippers, white kid, rosette, elastic	45.5.3	Fig. 109
1872 (W)	Slippers, white kid, rosette	DH-2360	Fig. 332
1887 (W)	Slippers, white kid, pleated satin bow	DH-2358	Fig. 485
1920–25	Bathing boots, green satin	91.34.319	p. 325
Ferrar-Mansur House, Weston Historical Society, Weston, VT 05161			
1855–70	Slit-vamp shoe, grained leather	Costume #138	Fig. 193

Date	Description	Catalog No.	Illustration/Page No.

Haverhill Historical Society, 240 Water Street, Haverhill, MA 01830

Date	Description	Catalog No.	Illustration/Page No.
1770–90	Buckled shoe, white wool	9362	Figs. 167, 354
1815 (W)	Slipper, white kid, pleated edging	2821	Fig. 104, 365, p. 175
1862 (W)	Slipper, white kid, oval rosette	9534	p. 225
1866 (W)	Slipper, white velvet, pompon	5429	p. 242
1873 (W)	Slipper, white kid, rosette, silver buckle	10.099	Figs. 387, 480
1876 (E)	Side-lacing boot, black embroidered serge	4.2.a-b	Fig. 516
1895 (W)	One-strap with beaded bow, white kid	6595	Fig. 490

Historic Northampton (Northampton Historical Society), 46 Bridge St., Northampton, MA 01060

Date	Description	Catalog No.	Illustration/Page No.
1760–70	Buckle shoe and clog	66.632	Plate 1, Fig. 166
1770–90	Buckle shoe, glazed black wool	66.633	Plate 1
1799 (W)	Tie shoe, dark blue-green kid	66.635	Plate 1, Fig. 356, p. 222
1800–1805	Slipper, floral silk, rosette	1985.29.4	Fig. 439
1801 (W)	Slipper, blue kid, cutout vamp	1979.30.83	Figs. 316, 440, p. 240
1810 (W)	Slipper, white kid, cutout vamp	1976.137.1	Figs. 363, 442, p. 240
1830–50	Moccasins, brown suede, embroidered	66.795	Plate 13, p. 99
1830–50	Moccasin, brown suede, buckle strap	66.796	p. 99
1835–50	Side-lacing boot, black serge and kid	66.696	Fig. 244
1835–50	Side-lacing boot, brown serge and kid	66.695	Plate 6
1837	Slipper, white silk, small bow	66.644	Figs. 107, 423
1845–55	Slipper, black kid, gilt-stamped vamp	66.656	Fig. 108, 458
1845–55	Slipper, white kid, Mrs. Hurrell label	66.646	Fig. 9, p. 16
1850–55	Side-lacing boot, tan top, patent fox	66.698	Plate 6
1850–60	Leggings, black knitted wool	01.426	p. 163
1850–70	Slipper, pink-yellow knitted silk	66.799	Plate 13, p. 97
1850–75	Leggings, green and gray knit wool	01.425	p. 163
1855–65	Slipper, bronze kid, fancy blue inlay	66.658	Fig. 467
1855–1870	Slipper, pink-scarlet knitted wools	66.798	Plate 13
1860–65	Side-lacing boot, red kid, heel	66.701	Plate 6, Fig. 276, p. 258
1863 (W)	Side-lacing boot, rosettes, butterflies	1979.39.86	Fig. 46, pp. 91–92, 259
1865–70	Slipper, bronze kid, fancy red inlay	66.659	Plate 13, Fig. 468
1865–70	Slipper, bronze kid, brown rosette	66.660	Fig. 464
1868 (W)	Slipper, white satin, rosette	66.662	Figs. 6, 39, pp. 93, 225
1869–74	Slipper, white kid, leather rosette	66.670	Figs. 54, 122
1871	Slipper, white kid, leather bow	66.669	Fig. 465
1871 (W)	Slipper, white kid, satin bow	66.671	Figs. 39, 479
1875–85	Open-front boot, black velvet, laces	66.782	Fig. 299
1880 (W)	Slipper, white satin, bow	66.672	Figs. 39, 482
1880–85	Slipper, bronze, brown wool inlay	66.673	Fig. 471
1885–90	Three-strap, black kid, beaded	66.677	Fig. 132
1891 (W)	Slipper, white kid, silk bow	66.675	Figs. 42, 489
1895–1900	Slipper, black satin, beads, rosette	66.683	Fig. 488
1899 (W)	One-strap, white kid, beaded bow	1978.82.18	Fig. 42
1907–9	Latchet tie, white kid, silk ribbon	66.685	Fig. 42
1908 (W)	Latchet tie, white kid	66.690	Fig. 181
1909 (W)	Slipper, white satin, tulle rosette	66.499	Fig. 493
ca. 1910	One-strap, tan kid, bow, high heel	1978.15.1	Fig. 491

Date	Description	Catalog No.	Illustration/Page No.
Historic Northampton (*cont.*)			
1914–16	Slipper, bronze kid, beaded vamp	66.692	Fig. 116
1917–19	Boots, white canvas, very high	1976.121.2	Plate 15, p. 125
1920–30	Boots, brown canvas, ankle-high	1984.33.22	Plate 15
1920–30	Bathing boots, red satin, rubber sole	1976.121.1	Plate 15, p. 138

The Kansas City Museum Association, 30 West Pershing., Kansas City, MO 64108-2422

1895–1915	Gymnasium shoes, black leather	76.121.5	Fig. 75
1920–30	Bathing shoes, black and white canvas	67.43	p. 138

Los Angeles County Museum of Art (LACMA), Department of Costume and Textiles, 5905 Wilshire Blvd., Los Angeles, CA 90036

1860–65	Front-lacing boot, white kid	37.15.7	Figs. 249, 381
ca. 1876	Boots, solid leg, fine stitching	TR9025	p. 20

The Lynn Museum (Lynn Historical Society), 125 Green St., Lynn, MA 01902

1804	Patten, pointed toe, iron ring	118, 119	Fig. 78
1805–10	One-strap, black kid, wedge heel	2978	Figs. 130, 315, 361, p. 178
1806 (W)	Slipper, white kid stamped in black	2973	Fig. 59, p. 110
1810–30	Tie shoe, thick covered cork sole	1423	Fig. 86, pp. 156–57
1838	Side-lacing boot, tan silk, morocco	1088	Fig. 60, p. 204
1850–60	Gored boot, black kid, shirred goods	4184	Fig. 281
1850–70	Tie shoe, heavy leather, pegged sole	3207	p. 114
1865–70	Front-lacing boot, black serge	3146	Figs. 64, 250
1865–75	Gored boot, black serge, woven elastic	3147	Figs. 64, 282
1869 (W)	Slipper, white kid, heel added later	5554	Fig. 45, p. 91
1877–85	Slit-vamp tie, black kid, rosette	1735	Fig. 66
1882–87	Oxford tie shoe, black kid	4179	Fig. 66
1893 (E?)	Cross-strap, bronze kid	4177	Fig. 55
1893 (E?)	Side-lacing shoe, patent front stay	1217	Fig. 55, 212, p. 192
1893 (E?)	Oxford tie, light-blue serge, patent	4175	Fig. 55
1900–1910	Oxford tie, wooden sole	6377	Fig. 80, p. 147
1920–30	Tennis shoes, brown canvas	6842	Fig. 76

Metropolitan Museum of Art, Costume Institute, Fifth Ave. at 82d St., New York, NY 10028

1804–10	Sandal shoes, pink kid	60.22.23	Fig. 128
1815–25	Front-lacing boots, red-brown kid, fringe	11.60.202	Fig. 247

Morristown Historical Society, Noyes House, Morristown, VT 05661

1890 (W)	Button boots, brown kid	56.293	Fig. 398
1891 (W)	Slipper, white kid, leather rosette	83.13	Fig. 334
1911 (W)	One-strap, white satin, chiffon rosette		Fig. 336, 405

Museum of Fine Arts, Boston, Department of Costume and Textiles, 465 Huntington Ave., Boston, MA 02115

1805–10	Sandal, red kid, nankeen, red ribbons	51.346	Figs. 360, 443, p. 240
1805–15	Slipper, silvered kid	49.1021	p. 239
1810–20	Slipper, purple silk, leather overshoe	43.1737	Fig. 81a, p. 148
1817	Front-lacing boot, green silk, fringe	1988.1160	p. 74
1875–80	Oxford tie, black kid, embroidered	44.530	Figs. 194, 319, 474, p. 189
1904–5	Colonial pump, tan kid, oval buckle	43.2514	Figs. 347, 403
1908	Tie shoe, tan suede, wide silk laces	53.1067	Figs. 404, 502

Natural History Museum of Los Angeles County, 900 Exposition Blvd., Los Angeles, CA 90007

1820–45	Slipper, white satin, stamped sole	A.3580-1322	Fig. 18
1820–45	Slipper, dark blue satin, stamped sole	A.3580-197	Fig. 18

Date	Description	Catalog No.	Illustration/Page No.
Peabody Essex Museum (*cont.*)			
1835–50	Slit-vamp, tan morocco, fancy rosette	133,695	Plate 5
1835–50	Slipper, brightly printed cotton	125,959	Plate 14
1839 (E)	Oxford tie, black kid, E. S. Davis	USMC 1541	Fig. 189
1839 (E)	Slipper, black kid, bow, E. S. Davis	USMC 1537	Fig. 455
1839 (E)	Side-lacing shoe, black serge, E. S. Davis	USMC 1538	Fig. 374
1839 (E)	Side-lacing shoe, tan serge, E. S. Davis	USMC 1539	Fig. 211
1844 (W)	Button shoe, white quilted silk	122,803	Fig. 49, p. 99
1845–50	Slipper, white satin, Esté label	136,315	Plate 5
1847 (W)	Slit-vamp, tan kid	122,427	Plate 5
1847–55	Slipper, white satin, Esté label	103,126b.1-2	Fig. 456
1850–55	Slipper, white satin, Esté label	120,814	Fig. 459
1850–60	Slit-vamp tie, black calf, pegged sole	USMC 1959	Figs. 62, 379, p. 114
1850–60	Slit-vamp tie, black kid, welted sole	USMC 584	Fig. 62
1853–60	Slipper, white, Esté & Rogers labels	123,335	pp. 12–13
1855–65	Slipper, white silk, purple embroidery	126,721	Fig. 466
1855–65	Slipper, bronze kid, fancy cutouts	123,789	Fig. 54
1858 (W)	Slipper, white satin in satin box	127,626	p. 37
1860	Latchet tie, black, Lyman Blake Patent	USMC 1111	Fig. 171, pp. 184–85
1860–70	Slipper, Berlin-work purple ground	122,969	Plate 14
1860–70	Slipper, white cotton twill, pompon	127,013	Fig. 462
1860–70	Front-lacing boot, black serge, McKay	USMC 2005	Fig. 382, p. 18
1860–75	Side-gore boot, black serge, patent tip	USMC 2010	Fig. 284
1865–70	Front-lacing boot, pebble calf, black tip	USMC 1981	Fig. 241
1865–75	Side-gore boot, imitation buckle flap	USMC 2016	Fig. 285, pp. 18, 207–8, 258
1865–75	Side-gore boot, grained leather, pegged	USMC 1838	Figs. 288, 381
1865–75	Side-gore boot, black serge	USMC 1851	Fig. 383
1865–75	Instep-gore shoe, black leather	USMC 1797	Fig. 227, p. 196
1865–75	Slit-vamp tie, black calf, pegged sole	USMC 1807	Fig. 62
1870–80	Latchet tie, grained kip Newports	USMC 1724	Fig. 172, pp. 121, 185
1870–80	Latchet tie, grained kip, pegged sole	USMC 1714	Figs. 386, 425, pp. 121, 185
1876 (E)	Gored shoe, black kid, blue inlay	USMC 2231	Fig. 228, 195
1876 (E)	Side-gore boot, imitation buttons	USMC 2233	Fig. 286
1876 (E)	One-strap, black kid, purple inlay	USMC 2235	Fig. 469
1876 (E)	Button shoe, black kid	USMC 2237	Fig. 214
1876 (E)	Side-lacing boot, embroidered white satin	USMC 2242	Figs. 333, 517
1876 (E)	Side-lacing boot, white kid	USMC 2249	Fig. 388
1876 (E)	Side-lacing boot, bronze kid	USMC 2251	Fig. 390
1876 (E)	Side-lacing, black satin, kid foxing	USMC 2252	Figs. 278, 389
1876 (E)	Side-gore boot, black serge	USMC 2260	Fig. 243
1876 (E)	Tie shoe, black kid, purple inlay	USMC 2287	Plate 7, Fig. 174
1876 (E)	Side-lacing boot, black serge, black kid	USMC 2292	Fig. 428
1876 (E)	Front-lacing boot, black kid, white thread	USMC 2294	Figs. 252, 345
1876 (E)	Slipper, gilded kid, purple inlay	USMC 2296	Plate 7
1876 (E)	Slipper, black patent, gold kid inlay	USMC 2297	Fig. 470
1877	Button boots, pink kid	USMC 1342	Fig. 391

Date	Description	Catalog No.	Illustration/Page No.
Peabody Essex Museum (*cont.*)			
1877–83	Open-front boot, black kid, four straps	131,886	Fig. 301
1877–85	One-strap, bronze kid, beaded	132,447.2	Plate 7
1880–85	T-strap, bronze, fancy beading	128,039	Fig. 160, p. 182
1880–90	One-strap, black kid, buckles	121,705	Plate 7
1880–90	Front-lacing boot, black calf, screw sole	USMC 1733	Figs. 253, 395
1880–1930	Bathing slipper with ankle tapes	131,162.2	p. 138
1885–90	Button boot, black kid, 1885 Patent	USMC 2418	Figs. 265, 346, 396
ca. 1890	Slipper, white satin, beaded vamp	127,398	Fig. 111
ca. 1890	Slipper, gray satin, beaded vamp	103,495	Fig. 487
1890–95	Button boot, black felt, scarlet lining	137,676	p. 260
1890–1919	Instep gore shoe, black canvas	137,689	p. 196
1892–95	House slippers, red kid, tassel	134,743	Plate 14
1893 (E)	One-strap, fancy tongue, black kid, bow	USMC 2207	Fig. 499
1893 (E)	Front-lacing boot, brown, black kid	USMC 2457	Figs. 399, 519
1893 (E)	Oxford tie, oxblood and patent	USMC 2470	Fig. 197
1893–96	Front-lacing boot, vesting top, tan kid	USMC G387	Plate 10
1896	T-strap, light green silk	USMC 2351	Figs. 135, 400, p. 179
1898	Oxford tie, dark brown kid	USMC 2312	Fig. 401
ca. 1898	Slipper, black kid, pointed toe	USMC 690	Fig. 112
1898–1902	Front-lacing boot, fancy black vamp	USMC 2367	Fig. 431
1911–13	Button boot, tan calf, high toe	USMC 2566	Plate 10
1911–14	Button boot, black serge, enamel vamp	USMC 2130	Fig. 406
1912	Slipper, navy-blue felt	USMC 2512	Plate 14
1912	Slipper, tan plaid felt, fuzzy collar	USMC 2504	Plate 14
1914–15	Slipper, blue velvet, jeweled heel	134,694	Fig. 494, pp. 95, 177
1914–15	Button boot, red kid, Sorosis label	USMC 2917	Plate 10, Fig. 242
1916	Front-lacing boot, gray suede, calf vamp	USMC 1491	Fig. 408
1919	Front-lacing boot, plush top, tan vamp	USMC 1522	Plate 10
1920–30	Riding boot, ankle lacing	135,574	Fig. 70k, p. 135
1922	Slipper, black kid, jeweled heel, buckle	USMC #2285	Fig. 118
1922	Double cross-strap, black patent	USMC 2344	Fig. 411
1923	Button shoe, black calf, serge top	USMC 2417	Fig. 413
1928	Cross-strap, tan kid, cutouts, high heel	USMC 2393	Fig. 415
1850–1930	English clog shoe	USMC 596	Fig. 79

Philadelphia Museum of Art, Department of Costume and Textiles, Benjamin Franklin Pkwy., Box 7646, Philadelphia, PA 19101-7646

Date	Description	Catalog No.	Illustration/Page No.
1825–30	Slit-vamp, tan serge, stacked heel	28.28.12	Fig. 422

Rhode Island Historical Society, 52 Power St., Providence, RI 02906

Date	Description	Catalog No.	Illustration/Page No.
1790–1800	Latchet tie, pink satin	6-30-54	Fig. 168, p. 184
1811 (W)	Slipper, black satin, cutouts	1928.8.1	Fig. 441, p. 222
1820 (W)	Slippers, tan striped silk	1983.14.8	Fig. 367
1828 (W)	Slipper, tan serge, stacked heel	1980.86.16	Fig. 452
1835–45	Slipper, bronze kid, brown silk bow	1983.14.4	Fig. 454
1852 (W)	Side-lacing boots, white satin	1985.22.19	Fig. 378

Society for the Preservation of New England Antiquities (SPNEA), 141 Cambridge St., Boston, MA 02114

Date	Description	Catalog No.	Illustration/Page No.
1795–1805	Slipper, white kid, pointed toe	1936.823	p. 351
1805–15	Over-boot, red morocco, flannel lined	1937.1079	p. 150

Date	Description	Catalog No.	Illustration/Page No.
Society for the Preservation of New England Antiquities (*cont.*)			
1815–30	Slipper, brown satin, fancy sole	1966.42	p. 30
1828–30	Side-lacing boots, tan cotton, fringe	1936.611	Figs. 272, 370, p. 204
1850–55	Side-lacing boot, blue-gray silk, foxed	1930.187	Fig. 274
1850–60	Side-gore boot, black kid	1924.332	Fig. 283
1852 (W)	Side-lacing boot, blue serge, stack heel	1942.806	Figs. 343, 380
1855–60	Button boot, gray serge, black foxing	1930.255	pp. 76, 203
1855–75	Overshoe, red and white knit wool	1923.102	p. 152
1865–75	Front-lacing boot, black serge, buckle	1940.1012	Figs. 251, 513
1865–75	Side-gore boot, white sateen	B3146	Fig. 287, p. 93
1866 (W)	Button boot, gold silk, white rosette	1936.203	Figs. 331, 512, p. 202
1877–80	Button boot, black satin, embroidered	1935.1	Fig. 264
1877–80	One-strap, black satin, embroidered	1920.61	Figs. 392, 427, 475, p. 20
1885–90	Cross-strap, black kid, paste buttons	1943.637	Fig. 397
1890	Mule, mustard-yellow kid, Turkish toe	1933.1142	p. 354
1890	Mule, gray satin, beaded	1933.1141	p. 354
ca. 1890	Rubber with attached sock	1933.1236	p. 160
ca. 1890	Rubber with attached sock	1946.339	p. 160
ca. 1890	Rubber with attached sock	1953.515	p. 160
ca. 1890	Side-gore shoe, bronze kid, cutouts	1932.2695	Fig. 472
ca. 1916	Buttoned boot, tan cloth, patent foxing	1990.51	Fig. 350
1931	Tie shoe, imitation snakeskin	1932.2301	Fig. 414
Tioga County Historical Society, PO Box 724, Wellsboro, PA 16901			
1800–1805	Slipper, gold silk, black binding	80.19.3	Fig. 357
Topsfield Historical Society, Howlett St., Topsfield, MA 01983			
1835–45	Tie shoes, tan morocco and serge, heel	T-069	Figs. 342, 375
United Shoe Machinery Company (USMC) shoe collection. *See* Peabody Essex Museum			
Valentine Museum, 1015 East Clay St., Richmond, VA 23219			
1790–1800	Slipper, white silk vamp, kid quarters	60.160.2	p. 240
1790–1805	Slipper, black stamped on white kid	61.97	Fig. 313
1825–30	Front-lacing boot, green kid, fringed	42.23.1	Plate 4, Figs. 248, 510, p. 199
1871–76	Slipper, black kid, kid bow & tongue	65.150.2	Fig. 481
ca. 1875	Gored shoe, black kid, white stitching	65.150.1	Fig. 229, 473, p. 195
Vermont Historical Society, 109 State St., Montpelier, VT 05602			
1805–15	Slipper, yellow kid stamped in black	1986.10. (OCHS 74-55-62)	Fig. 445
1881 (W)	Slipper, white satin, tiered bow	54.35.5	Figs. 394, 483
1884 (W)	Buttoned boot, white kid	71.11.2	p. 93
1923 (W)	One-strap, white kid, ribbon tie	70.14.15	Fig. 412
Private Collections			
1845–55	Tie shoes, quilted black silk, foxed		Fig. 25, 329
1855–65	Slipper, black patent, rosette		Fig. 460

Index

Women's Shoes in America, 1795–1930
was designed by Christine Brooks;
composed in 10.5/14.5 Plantin Light Old Style
with display type in Wembley Light
on a Macintosh G4 using PageMaker 6.5;
printed by sheet-fed offset lithography
on 128 gsm Japanese White A gloss enamel stock,
Smyth sewn and bound over binder's boards in Brillianta cloth,
and wrapped with dust jackets printed in three colors
by King's Time Printing Press, Ltd., Hong Kong;
and published by
The Kent State University Press
Kent, Ohio 44242